# Veterinary Science and Disease Management

# Veterinary Science and Disease Management

Edited by Shawn Kiser

SYRAWOOD
PUBLISHING HOUSE
New York

Published by Syrawood Publishing House,
750 Third Avenue, 9th Floor,
New York, NY 10017, USA
www.syrawoodpublishinghouse.com

**Veterinary Science and Disease Management**
Edited by Shawn Kiser

International Standard Book Number: 978-1-68286-439-5 (Hardback)

**Cataloging-in-publication Data**

Veterinary science and disease management / edited by Shawn Kiser.
        p. cm.
Includes bibliographical references and index.
ISBN 978-1-68286-439-5
1. Veterinary medicine. 2. Animals--Diseases. 3. Animals--Diseases--Control. 4. Livestock--Diseases. I. Kiser, Shawn.
SF745 .V48 2017
636.089--dc23

Printed in the United States of America.

# TABLE OF CONTENTS

**Permissions**

**List of Contributors**

**Index**

# PREFACE

The branch of medicine dealing with the causes, investigation and treatment of diseases and injuries of animals is referred to as veterinary science. The aim of this book is to present researches that have transformed this discipline and aided its advancement. It provides a comprehensive study of various disease managing skills that are of vital importance to the field of veterinary science and to those who are practicing it. The text is an essential resource for understanding the varied aspects of animal health and disease, genetics and biotechnology. Different approaches, evaluations, methodologies and advanced studies on veterinary science have been included in this book. It will serve as a resource guide for veterinary doctors, scientists, practitioners and students involved in this field.

The information contained in this book is the result of intensive hard work done by researchers in this field. All due efforts have been made to make this book serve as a complete guiding source for students and researchers. The topics in this book have been comprehensively explained to help readers understand the growing trends in the field.

I would like to thank the entire group of writers who made sincere efforts in this book and my family who supported me in my efforts of working on this book. I take this opportunity to thank all those who have been a guiding force throughout my life.

**Editor**

# Vaccine Safety and Efficacy Evaluation of a Recombinant Bovine Respiratory Syncytial Virus (BRSV) with Deletion of the SH Gene and Subunit Vaccines Based On Recombinant Human RSV Proteins: N-nanorings, P and M2-1, in Calves with Maternal Antibodies

Krister Blodörn[1], Sara Hägglund[1]*, Jenna Fix[2], Catherine Dubuquoy[2], Boby Makabi-Panzu[3], Michelle Thom[3], Per Karlsson[4], Jean-Louis Roque[5], Erika Karlstam[6], John Pringle[1], Jean-François Eléouët[2], Sabine Riffault[2], Geraldine Taylor[3], Jean François Valarcher[1,4]

1 Swedish University of Agricultural Sciences, Host Pathogen Interaction Group, Department of Clinical Sciences, Uppsala, Sweden, 2 INRA, Unité de Virologie et Immunologie Moléculaires, Jouy-en-Josas, France, 3 The Pirbright Institute, Pirbright, Surrey, United Kingdom, 4 National Veterinary Institute, Department of Virology, Immunology, and Parasitology, Uppsala, Sweden, 5 Clinique Veterinaire des Mazets, Riom es Montagnes, France, 6 National Veterinary Institute, Department of Pathology and Wildlife Diseases, Uppsala, Sweden

## Abstract

The development of safe and effective vaccines against both bovine and human respiratory syncytial viruses (BRSV, HRSV) to be used in the presence of RSV-specific maternally-derived antibodies (MDA) remains a high priority in human and veterinary medicine. Herein, we present safety and efficacy results from a virulent BRSV challenge of calves with MDA, which were immunized with one of three vaccine candidates that allow serological differentiation of infected from vaccinated animals (DIVA): an SH gene-deleted recombinant BRSV (ΔSHrBRSV), and two subunit (SU) formulations based on HRSV-P, -M2-1, and -N recombinant proteins displaying BRSV-F and -G epitopes, adjuvanted by either oil emulsion (Montanide ISA71$^{VG}$, SUMont) or immunostimulating complex matrices (AbISCO-300, SUAbis). Whereas all control animals developed severe respiratory disease and shed high levels of virus following BRSV challenge, ΔSHrBRSV-immunized calves demonstrated almost complete clinical and virological protection five weeks after a single intranasal vaccination. Although mucosal vaccination with ΔSHrBRSV failed to induce a detectable immunological response, there was a rapid and strong anamnestic mucosal BRSV-specific IgA, virus neutralizing antibody and local T cell response following challenge with virulent BRSV. Calves immunized twice intramuscularly, three weeks apart with SUMont were also well protected two weeks after boost. The protection was not as pronounced as that in ΔSHrBRSV-immunized animals, but superior to those immunized twice subcutaneously three weeks apart with SUAbis. Antibody responses induced by the subunit vaccines were non-neutralizing and not directed against BRSV F or G proteins. When formulated as SUMont but not as SUAbis, the HRSV N, P and M2-1 proteins induced strong systemic cross-protective cell-mediated immune responses detectable already after priming. ΔSHrBRSV and SUMont are two promising DIVA-compatible vaccines, apparently inducing protection by different immune responses that were influenced by vaccine-composition, immunization route and regimen.

Editor: John S. Tregoning, Imperial College London, United Kingdom

Funding: This work was funded by the Swedish Research Council (Formas, Sweden), the Biotechnology and Biological Sciences Research Council (BBSRC, UK), and L'Agence Nationale de la Recherche (ANR, France), through EMIDA ERA NET (Grant no FP#87). The funders had no role in study design, data collection and analysis, decision to publish, or preparation of the manuscript. (http://www.formas.se/; http://www.bbsrc.ac.uk/; http://www.agence-nationale-recherche.fr/; http://emida-era.net/).

Competing Interests: The authors have read the journal's policy and have the following conflicts: Jean-Franc̦ois Ele´oue¨t and Sabine Riffault (co-inventors) hold two patents on N-rings usage for RSV vaccination (WO/2006/117456) and N-rings as immunogenic carrier for heterologous antigens (WO/2007/119011).

* E-mail: sara.hagglund@slu.se

## Introduction

Bovine respiratory syncytial virus (BRSV), a pneumovirus in the family *Paramyxoviridae*, is a major cause of respiratory disease in young calves [1]. By causing high morbidity and mortality, this virus impacts dramatically on animal welfare and productivity, resulting in significant economic losses to farmers, and is even a public health-concern through the risk of antibiotic-resistance developing from the massive use of antibiotics to treat secondary bacterial infections [2].

Clinical signs of respiratory disease are modulated by the presence of BRSV-specific immunity and since BRSV seroprevalence is high in adult cattle [3], disease is mainly observed in young calves, even in the presence of low to moderate levels of

BRSV-specific maternal antibodies (MDA) [4]. Although high levels of MDA protect against disease, even low levels impact negatively on the development of humoral immune responses induced by BRSV vaccination or infection in calves [5]. This, and the inherent immaturity of the immune system of young animals, is a hurdle that needs to be overcome in developing a protective vaccine for this target group [6].

Similar to BRSV in cattle, human (H)RSV, is a major cause of acute lower respiratory infection in humans, which in turn is a leading cause of child morbidity and mortality worldwide [7]. Although host-specific, BRSV and HRSV are genetically and antigenically closely related, and have a similar pathogenesis and clinical expression upon infection of calves and young children, respectively [1]. The similarity of these viruses makes research into either field complementary, and is utilized in vaccine development.

The RSV genomes consist of a single stranded, negative-sense RNA containing ten genes encoding eleven proteins [1]. Among these proteins, the fusion protein F (F) and the glycoprotein G (G) induce protective humoral responses [8,9], in the form of virus-neutralizing systemic antibodies [10], and mucosal IgA [11]. Mucosal IgA can be induced in the respiratory tract by parenteral immunization [12], but mucosal immunization is more likely to prime mucosal immunity in the presence of MDA [13]. Furthermore, the F, N, M2 [14] and P (G. Taylor, unpublished observations) proteins are recognized by bovine CD8+ T cells, known to be important for clearance of BRSV and clinical recovery [15].

Knowledge of these protein-specific immunogenic characteristics is essential to develop effective vaccines to control RSV. Although extensive research has been performed to develop RSV vaccines, no vaccine is yet commercially available for humans [16], largely due to the potential for vaccine-induced exacerbation of HRSV disease by inactivated vaccines, first reported by Kim et al. in 1969 [17]. Conversely, several BRSV vaccines have been commercially available since the 1970's. The early modified live BRSV vaccines were attenuated by serial cell culture passage, and were exclusively for parenteral use until 2007 when one became licensed for intranasal (i.n.) use due to its greater efficacy in calves with MDA [18]. However, intranasal administration of a modified live vaccine carries the risk of spread and reversion to virulence, and the use of modified live vaccine has been associated with exacerbated clinical BRSV disease when administered in presence of a natural BRSV infection [19].

For this reason, and to achieve greater protective durability, as well as cost-efficiency and practicality of vaccine handling, adjuvanted inactivated vaccines have also been developed and commercialized. Although these inactivated BRSV vaccines have been used very extensively, there is evidence of exacerbated BRSV disease upon natural infection of vaccinated calves, similar to that in man, which has also been experimentally reproduced [20,21]. Despite the concurrent development of adjuvants that can induce balanced immune responses, which may avoid disease exacerbation and increase efficacy, none of these commercially available, classic inactivated BRSV vaccines have proven to be completely effective against severe experimental challenge when administrated to young calves in the presence of BRSV-specific MDA [22].

To improve both BRSV and HRSV vaccine efficacy and safety, genetic engineering has been used to produce DNA vaccines, vectored vaccines and attenuated candidate strains with mutations and/or deletions in one of six viral genes (NS1, NS2, SH, G, F and M2-1) [1,23]. One of the most promising HRSV vaccine candidates is an attenuated strain containing a combination of three temperature sensitive (*ts*) phenotypical point-mutations, in addition to deletion of the SH gene, which have shown sufficient attenuation and indications of protection in clinical trials in infants [23]. Its bovine counterpart, a recombinant BRSV with a deletion of the SH gene, is attenuated in calves and has been shown to be safe and to induce good protection in colostrum-restricted calves [24]. However, the use of genetically modified viruses is not always acceptable, even if the modification is made by deletion, which drastically reduces the risk of reversion to wild-type. Therefore, new inactivated vaccines are also required, such as subunit vaccines containing RSV-specific proteins and epitopes [12,25]. Both these vaccine approaches have the added advantage that by omitting virus genes or proteins, vaccinated animals can be serologically distinguished among infected (DIVA). Thus, vaccination does not interfere with seroepidemiological surveillance. Furthermore, due to the natural and gradual genetic changes in circulating BRSV, the DIVA characteristic is essential to track vaccine safety and efficacy in the field at a population level.

In the current study, we have evaluated and compared the safety, immunogenicity and protective potential of an attenuated recombinant BRSV lacking the SH gene (ΔSHrBRSV) using i.n. administration, and a subunit vaccine (SU) composed of recombinant RSV proteins. The SU, which consisted of HRSV-M2-1 and -P proteins, and nanorings with 10 or 11 protomers of HRSV-N protein displaying BRSV-F and -G epitopes, was evaluated following formulation with two different adjuvants, and was administered either intramuscularly (i.m.) or subcutaneously (s.c.). Protection afforded by immunization was determined in a virulent BRSV challenge, five weeks after first vaccination.

## Materials and Methods

### Ethics Statement

The experiment was carried out in compliance with the E.U. Directive 86/609, and approved by the Ethical Committee of the district court of Uppsala, Sweden (Ref. no. C330/11).

### Cells and Viruses

Bovine turbinate (BT) cells, fetal calf kidney (CK) cells and Vero cells were propagated at low passages, as previously described [12,26]. All cells were free from bovine viral diarrhea virus (BVDV) and mycoplasmas.

Deleted SH recombinant BRSV (ΔSHrBRSV) was derived from full-length cDNA of BRSV strain A51908 [27], variant Atue51908 (GenBank accession no. AF092942), as previously described [28]. Stocks of ΔSHrBRSV were prepared in Vero cell monolayers and verified to be free of BVDV, as previously described [29].

Virulent BRSV used for the experimental challenge was prepared using bronchoalveolar lavage (BAL) from a gnotobiotic calf, six days after inoculation with the Snook strain of BRSV [30], which had previously been passaged twice in gnotobiotic calves [29]. The BAL was free from BVDV, mycoplasmas, and bacteria as assessed by inoculation of tissue culture or mycoplasmal or bacterial media (data not shown).

Virus titers were determined by plaque assay on fetal calf kidney (CK) cells or Vero cell monolayers in 35-mm-diameter petri dishes as described previously [26].

### Subunit Vaccine Production and Formulation

**Construction, expression and purification of recombinant RSV proteins.** The plasmids pGEX-M2-1, pGEX-P and pGEX-PCT (coding for residues 161–241 of the phosphoprotein (PCT)) derived from the pGEX-4T3 expression vector (Pharmacia), and pET-N derived from pET28a(+) vector

(Novagen) plasmids which contain sequences from the HRSV Long strain have been described previously [31–33]. *E.* coli BL21(DE3) (Novagen) cells were transformed with pGEX- or pET-derived plasmids for expression of recombinant proteins (Table 1), as previously described [31–34]. The co-expression and co-purification of pET-N and pGEX-PCT to produce N nanorings ($N^{SRS}$) composed of 10 or 11 protomers, has been previously described [32,35]. For insertion of the F and G epitopes of BRSV strain 9402022 [36] into N to create epitope-decorated nanorings (eN; Table 1), complementary oligonucleotides coding for either: i) an F mimotope (HWSISKPQ) [37], ii) F residues 255–278 (SELLSLINDMPITNDQKKLMSSNV) [38], iii) F residues 422–438 (CTASNKNRGIIKTFSNG) [38], or iv) G residues 174–187 (STCEGNLACLSLCQ) [39], were annealed and inserted at *Age*I-*Xho*I sites (for fusion at the C-terminus of N) or *Nde*I-*Bam*HI sites (for fusion at the N-terminus of N) in the pET-N-GFP [34] and pET-N plasmids, respectively. Expression and purification of eN was performed as described for $N^{SRS}$. All constructs were verified by sequencing. Proteins were quantified by absorption at 280 nm, except for eN proteins, which contain RNA and were quantified by the Bradford method.

**Subunit vaccine formulation.** Each dose of subunit BRSV vaccine contained 25 µg of each of the recombinant proteins (Table 1) in PBS, which were either: for the subunit Montanide vaccine (SUMont), mixed and emulsified with 1.4 ml of Montanide ISA71$^{VG}$ (SEPPIC, France) in a 3:7 (aqueous:oil) ratio, and a final volume of 2 ml; or for the subunit AbISCO vaccine (SUAbis), mixed with 144 µl (390 µg) AbISCO-300 (Novavax, Sweden), and diluted in PBS to a final volume of 2 ml. Each dose of placebo vaccine consisted of 390 µg AbISCO-300 diluted in PBS to a final volume of 2 ml.

## Calves and Experimental Design

Twenty-three conventionally-reared bull calves of Swedish Holstein and Swedish red and white breed were obtained from the certified BVDV-free Swedish Livestock Research Centre (Lövsta, Sweden). Natural infections of BRSV in the herd were ruled out by continuous seromonitoring of 5 seronegative animals for BRSV-specific $IgG_1$ antibodies, for 2 months prior to the experiment. Twenty healthy calves were allocated into 4 groups of 5 calves based on their age and titers of BRSV-specific MDA (Table 2). In addition, 3 BRSV-seronegative calves were selected

to act as sentinels to study the potential transmission of ΔSHrBRSV. After arrival at the animal facility, during the week of acclimatization, all the calves were treated with procaine benzyl penicillin (20 mg/kg/day intramuscularly) for five days. Each calf was vaccinated for the first time 34 days before the day of experimental BRSV challenge (PID 0), with either: (a) $5 \times 10^6$ pfu of ΔSHrBRSV vaccine i.n. in a volume of 6 ml DMEM; (b) 2 ml of the SUMont vaccine i.m.; (c) 2 ml of the SUAbis vaccine s.c.; or (d) 2 ml placebo s.c. (Fig. 1). Approval to use a genetically modified microorganism within the context of this experiment was obtained from the Swedish Work Environment Authority (registration number 202100-1868 v8a1). Three weeks later, group b, c and d were boosted with the same formulation and route as in the first immunization (Fig. 1). Clinical signs including post-vaccination swellings at injection sites in the calves immunized with SU or adjuvant alone, classified as mild ($<5 \times 5$ cm), moderate ($<10 \times 10$ cm), marked ($<15 \times 15$ cm) or severe ($>15 \times 15$ cm), were monitored. The calves immunized with ΔSHrBRSV, along with the 3 in-contact sentinel calves, were kept in an isolated unit in the animal facility until three weeks after first vaccination, while the other groups were kept in separate rooms in another unit. The two units had separate ventilation and staff, and showers were required to exit each unit. To avoid direct contamination of sentinels with inoculum virus, sentinel calves were housed in a separate room until one day after vaccination, when 2 out of 3 were transferred to the room (20 m²) housing the ΔSHrBRSV-vaccinated calves, while 2 out of 5 ΔSHrBRSV-vaccinated calves were transferred to the room (20 m²) of the remaining sentinel calf. Co-housing lasted for six days, then the sentinel calves were again isolated from the ΔSHrBRSV-vaccinated calves, to avoid potential reinfection of the ΔSHrBRSV-vaccinated calves. The sentinel calves were clinically, immunologically and virologically monitored for two additional weeks (Fig. 1). Three weeks after inoculation with ΔSHrBRSV, calves were moved to a separate room in the same unit as the other calves in the animal facility. One calf vaccinated once with SUAbis (calf c5) 3 weeks previously, was euthanized for welfare concerns caused by a traumatic leg injury. Five weeks after the initial vaccination, calves were challenged by aerosolization [12] of $10^4$ pfu BRSV strain Snook in 4 ml BAL, diluted up to 5 ml in DMEM. Throughout the experiment, each calf was examined clinically on a daily basis and scored as previously described [12].

**Table 1.** RSV proteins and epitopes used in subunit vaccine formulation.

| Protein product[a] | Description | Sequence origin |
|---|---|---|
| M2-1 | Full length M2-1 protein[c] | HRSV[b] |
| P | Full length P protein[d] | HRSV[b] |
| eN-F$_{255–278}$ | Residues 255–278 of F at N terminus of N in eN[f] (AA: SELLSLINDMPITNDQKKLMSSNV) | BRSV[e] |
| eN-F$_{422–438}$ | F residues 422–438 at C terminus of N in eN[f] (AA: CTASNKNRGIIKTFSNG) | BRSV[e] |
| eN-F$_{mimo}$ | Residues mimicking epitope on F[g] at C terminus of N in eN[f] (AA: HWSISKPQ) | Combinatorial peptide |
| eN-G$_{174–187}$ | G residues 174–187 at N terminus of N in eN[f] (AA: STCEGNLACLSLCQ) | BRSV[e] |

[a]Protein product included in subunit vaccine formulations, as abbreviated in the current paper.
[b]HRSV Long strain (GenBank accession no. AY911262) was used to construct recombinant protein.
[c]Full length HRSV M2-1 protein (Long strain).
[d]Full length HRSV P protein (Long strain).
[e]BRSV strain 9402022 (Larsen et al. 1998) was used to construct recombinant protein.
[f]Selected residues were recombinantly attached to the N or C terminus of HRSV N protein (Long strain) and co-expresses with a fragment of HRSV P protein (Long strain, AA residues 161–241) to form N-nanorings with attached epitopes (eN) on each of 10 or 11 protomers.
[g]Antigenic site II (AA residues 422–438) on F, as described by Chargelegue et al. (1998).

**Table 2.** Vaccine effect on virus load, clinical disease and lung pathology after BRSV challenge.

| Immunization[a] | Calf | Age (weeks)[b] | MDA ($\log_{10}$ titer$^{-1}$)[c] | BRSV RT-PCR ($\log_{10}$ TCID$_{50}$ eq.)[d] Accum. NS | BAL | Virus isolated from BAL (passage)[e] | Accumulated clinical score[f] | Extent of macroscopic lesions (%)[g] |
|---|---|---|---|---|---|---|---|---|
| ΔSHrBRSV once i.n. | a1 | 9 | 2.0 | 0.0 | 2.1 | – | 0 | 4 |
| | a2 | 8 | 2.2 | 0.0 | 2.2 | – | 3 | 10 |
| | a3 | 7 | 2.0 | 1.0 | 3.0 | – | 8 | 4 |
| | a4 | 6 | 3.0 | 0.0 | 1.4 | – | 1 | 1 |
| | a5 | 4 | 2.2 | 1.8 | 1.9 | | 7 | 1 |
| SUMont twice i.m. | b1 | 10 | 1.9 | 0.0 | 3.0 | – | 10 | 4 |
| | b2 | 8 | 1.9 | 1.1 | 3.5 | – | 43 | 25 |
| | b3 | 6 | 2.9 | 2.3 | 4.4 | +P3 | 9 | 13 |
| | b4 | 3 | 3.3 | 1.0 | 3.9 | – | 17 | 1 |
| | b5 | 3 | 2.1 | 0.0 | 1.0 | – | 13 | 1 |
| SUAbis twice s.c. | c1 | 9 | 2.2 | 2.8 | 4.5 | +P3 | 48 | 22 |
| | c2 | 8 | 1.9 | 1.6 | 4.3 | +P3 | 28 | 18 |
| | c3 | 8 | 2.4 | 2.7 | 4.3 | +P3 | 12 | 11 |
| | c4 | 6 | 2.0 | 1.4 | 3.8 | – | 37 | 32 |
| | c5 | 2 | 2.3 | † | † | † | † | † |
| Control twice s.c. | d1 | 11 | 1.9 | 3.0 | 4.2 | +P1 | 70 | 64 |
| | d2 | 8 | 2.6 | 2.0 | 5.0 | +P1 | 27 | 36 |
| | d3 | 6 | 2.1 | 3.0 | 5.8 | +P1 | 106 | 38 |
| | d4 | 4 | 2.9 | 2.9 | 4.5 | +P2 | 78 | 45 |
| | d5 | 2 | 2.3 | 2.6 | 5.3 | +P1 | 86 | 57 |

[a]Conventional colostrum-fed calves were immunized with either ΔSHrBRSV, SUMont, SUAbis or adjuvant alone, as indicated in the table. All animals were immunized on post-infection day (PID) −34, and all animals except those immunized with ΔSHrBRSV were immunized again on PID −14, and all were challenged with BRSV on PID 0, as indicated in Figure 1.

[b]Age at first vaccination (weeks).

[c]Serum titer of BRSV-specific maternal antibodies (MDA) before first vaccination (PID −36) as determined ELISA.

[d]Accumulated viral-shed in nasal secretions and virus RNA detected in 1 ml of bronchoalveolar lavage (BAL) collected as indicated in figure 1. Samples were analyzed using BRSV-F real-time PCR after total RNA extraction. The unit TCID$_{50}$ equivalent is determined by including standard dilution series of virus with a known TCID$_{50}$ in the real-time PCR analysis.

[e]Virus isolated from post-mortem BAL cell samples, after inoculation of bovine turbinate epithelium cells in 25 cm$^2$ flasks in three consecutive passages. In any of the three passages, cell cultures with evident cytopathic effects within seven days of culture were determined to be positive for BRSV in passage one (+P1), two (+P2) or three (+P3). Samples that were negative after three passages are noted as negative (−).

[f]Accumulated clinical score, calculated as the area under the curve of daily clinical scores, in turn determined by clinical examination.

[g]Extent of lung lesions were determined post mortem and are presented as a percentage of lesioned lung tissue per calf.

†Calf c5 was euthanized before challenge due to traumatic injury.

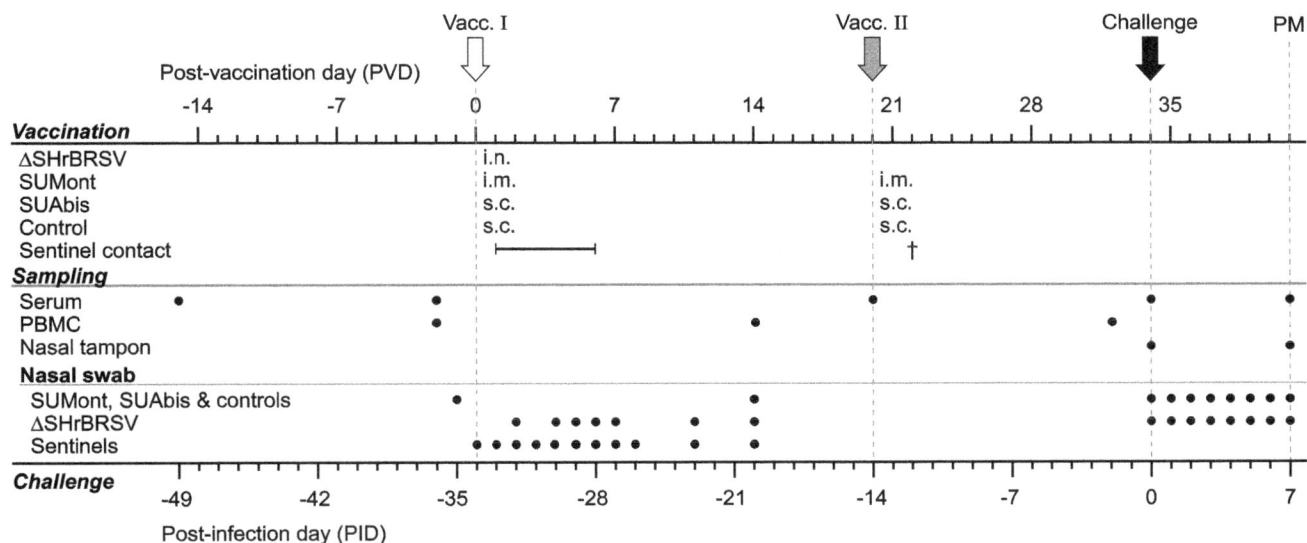

**Figure 1. Experiment timeline, vaccination and sampling.** Twenty calves with moderate titers of BRSV-specific serum antibodies (MDA) were allocated into 4 groups and vaccinated as indicated in the figure; all were vaccinated on post-vaccination day (PVD) 0 (Vacc. I, white arrow) with either (a) $5 \times 10^6$ pfu of ΔSHrBRSV intranasally (i.n.); (b) BRSV and HRSV recombinant protein subunits (SU) adjuvanted by Montanide (SUMont) intramuscularly (i.m.), (c) SU adjuvanted by AbISCO-300 (SUAbis) subcutaneously (s.c.), or (d) adjuvant alone s.c. (Controls). On PVD 20, all animals except those immunized with ΔSHrBRSV, were boosted with the same formulation and route as for Vacc. I (Vacc. II, gray arrow). Three BRSV-seronegative calves were housed in contact with ΔSHrBRSV-infected animals to determine transmission of the vaccine virus (Sentinel calves), and monitored until euthanized (†) on PVD 22. On PVD 20, one calf in group c was euthanized due to traumatic injury. On post-infection day (PID) 0, all calves were challenged i.n. with $10^4$ pfu virulent BRSV (black arrow), and clinically scored daily until PID 7. Throughout the experiment, samples were collected, as indicated in the figure, to analyze antibodies in serum and nasal secretions, *ex-vivo* response of peripheral blood mononuclear cells (PBMC) to restimulation with BRSV, and virus shedding in nasal secretions (Nasal swab). At post-mortem examination (PM), lung lesions were recorded and tissue samples collected, as well as bronchoalveolar lavage (BAL) samples for antibody, BRSV RT-PCR and virus isolation.

## Sampling

Heparinized and unmodified venous blood samples were collected from all calves as indicated in Figure 1. Peripheral blood mononuclear cells (PBMC) and serum were extracted from heparinized and unmodified blood, respectively. PBMCs were used directly in lymphocyte proliferation assays, whereas serum was stored at $-20°C$.

Nasal secretions were collected as indicated in Figure 1, and stored at $-70°C$, as previously described [12] using sterile cotton-tipped swabs (NS) and tampons (NT). On PID 7, the calves were euthanized by an overdose of general anesthesia (5 mg/kg ketamine and 15 mg/kg pentobarbital sodium) followed by exsanguination.

Lungs were excised and lesions photographed, palpated and recorded on a standardized chart; after scanning and digitalization, the proportion of consolidated lung parenchyma was calculated as a percentage of the total lung area (Adobe Illustrator CS5, version 15.1 for Mac). BAL samples were collected post-mortem from the left lung of all challenged calves, as previously described [10]. After aliquoting, BAL cells corresponding to 10 ml of BAL fluid were pelleted by centrifugation ($200 \times g$, 10 min), counted manually in a Bürker chamber, and resuspended in 350 μl RLT buffer (Qiagen) or 1 ml DMEM containing 20% fetal calf serum and stored at $-70°C$, along with the recovered supernatant, for further analysis. Samples of lung tissue were collected post-mortem, preferentially from consolidated areas, of each of the lobes in the right lung (cranial part of cranial lobe, caudal part of cranial lobe, caudal lobe and accessory lobe), fixed in 10% buffered formalin, embedded in paraffin and sectioned.

## Detection of BRSV

**Detection of BRSV RNA.** BRSV RNA coding for the F protein present in nasal secretions or in BAL cells corresponding to 10 ml of BAL, was quantified by RT-PCR as previously described [12]. The unit $TCID_{50}$ equivalent ($TCID_{50}$ eq.) was used since the standard curve in this assay was based on a BRSV infected cell lysate with a known titer ($10^{5.8}$ $TCID_{50}$).

**Isolation of BRSV from BAL cells.** Isolation of BRSV present in BAL cell samples was attempted by inoculating 95% confluent BT cells in 25 cm$^2$ tissue culture flasks, as described previously [12]. Inoculated cells were examined daily for seven consecutive days for cytopathic effects. Supernatants from samples not showing cytopathic effects were passed a further two times in new 25 cm$^2$ flasks.

## Humoral Responses

**ELISA for detection of BRSV- and protein-specific IgG and IgA.** BRSV-specific $IgG_1$ antibody titers were determined using a commercially available kit (SVANOVIR BRSV-Ab ELISA, Boehringer Ingelheim Svanova, Sweden) in accordance with the manufacturer's instructions. HRSV-F, -N, -P and -M2-1 IgG antibodies were analyzed as described previously for $N^{SRS}$ [25], using ELISAs based on the relevant purified protein described herein for N, P and M2-1, and previously for F [40]. BRSV-specific IgA antibodies were detected by capture ELISA, as previously described by Uttenthal et al. 2000 [41] and modified as earlier reported [12]. RSV-N-specific IgA antibodies were detected using $N^{SRS}$-coated microtiter plates as previously described [34], with the following alterations: blocking after coating was achieved by 1h incubation with 2% BSA in PBS; mouse anti-bovine IgA (Serotec, MCA2438) was used to detect

IgA in samples; and rat anti-mouse $IgG_{2a}$ conjugated to HRP (Serotec, MCA1588P) was used to elucidate anti-IgA. BRSV-G specific IgG antibodies were determined by ELISA as previously described [15] using a lysate of chick embryo fibroblasts (CEF) infected with recombinant fowlpox virus (rFPV) expressing the G protein of the Snook strain of BRSV, produced as described previously for rFPV expressing other BRSV proteins [14]. A lysate of CEF infected with wild-type FPV was used as a control. Sera were serially diluted and end-point titers calculated from corrected optical density (COD), as previously described [12]. Nasal secretions were not titrated, but instead diluted :20 and the level of BRSV-specific IgA expressed as percentage of a positive control sample.

**Virus neutralizing antibody assay.** Neutralizing antibodies to BRSV in heat-inactivated serum were determined by a plaque reduction assay on fetal calf kidney cells as described previously [42].

## Cellular Responses

**BRSV-specific lymphocyte proliferation assay.** Peripheral blood mononuclear cells (PBMC) were isolated from heparinized blood of all animals, as described previously [10]. Additionally, tracheobronchial lymph nodes (LN) of ΔSHrBRSV-immunized and control calves, collected on PID 7, were mechanically disrupted and lymphocytes were isolated by centrifugation over Ficoll Paque Plus (GE Healthcare) during 8 minutes at $800 \times g$. PBMC and lymph node cells were restimulated with heat-inactivated ($56°C$ for 30 min) BRSV-infected (no. 9402022, Denmark [43]) or uninfected BT cell lysate. After 7 days of incubation, Alamar Blue (Invitrogen, Sweden) was added and, following an additional 8 (PBMC) or 24 (LN cells) hours of incubation, optical absorbance (OD) was measured at 570 nm and 595 nm (Multiskan EX 355, Thermo Fisher Scientific, USA) and adjusted according to the manufacturer's instruction. Corrected OD (COD) was calculated by subtracting $OD_{595nm}$ from $OD_{570nm}$, and then $OD_{control}$ from $OD_{BRSV}$. After determination of proliferative response to restimulation and following centrifugation at $200 \times g$, supernatants were recovered and stored at $-80°C$ for cytokine analysis.

**Flow cytometric analysis of BRSV-specific IFNγ-producing lymphocytes.** Tracheobronchial LN cells were restimulated as above, in duplicates of $5 \times 10^6$ cells/calf for 18 hours. Brefeldin A (Sigma) was added for the last 15 hours at 10 μg/ml. Cells were stained for viability (*LIVE/DEAD* Fixable *Near-IR* Dead Cell Stain, Life Technologies) and for expression of surface markers, CD4 and CD8 (MCA1653F:FITC (CD4), MCA837A647: AlexaFlour 647 (CD8), AbD Serotec). Cells were then fixed for 10 min with 4% (w/v) paraformaldehyde in PBS, and cell membranes were permeabilized (FACS permeabilization solution 2, BD Biosciences) prior to intracellular staining for IFNγ (MCA1783PE: RPE (IFNγ), AbD Serotec). Cells were assayed using a flow cytometer (FACSVerse, BD Biosciences) and data were analyzed using FACSuite software. Non-aggregating, live cells (3300–20000, mean 17500) were gated based on light-scattering properties and fluorescence at 783/56 nm. Gates for CD8, CD4 and IFNγ were set based on Fluorescence Minus One controls.

**ELISA for detection of bovine IL-4 and IFNγ.** Bovine interleukin-4 (IL-4) and interferon gamma (IFNγ) were detected in supernatant from restimulated lymphocytes using commercially available kits (Bovine IL-4 ELISA, MCA5892KZZ, and Bovine IFNγ ELISA, MCA5638KZZ, Bio-Rad), in accordance with the manufacturer's instructions. Concentrations were derived by

including dilution series of supplied standard samples of recombinant protein, and expressed as ng/ml.

## Histology

Histological sections of lung tissue were stained with hematoxylin and eosin (HE) or carbol chromotrope (CC) histochemical stain to demonstrate eosinophils, and were evaluated in a blinded manner. Cell subpopulation characteristics and any inflammation in each section was morphologically described and scored as either normal (0), mild (1), moderate (2) or severe (3), as previously described [12]. Individual severity of histopathology in consolidated areas was calculated as the mean score of all sections (described above) per calf.

## Data Analysis

**Statistical analysis.** Statistically significant differences between groups, with regard to each set of collected and aggregate data, was determined using either one-way ANOVA followed by Student's *t*-test, or Kruskal–Wallis analysis followed by Wilcoxon test (JMP 10 for Mac, SAS Institute Inc.), if not otherwise specified. Significance was assumed when $p \leq 0.05$ (*), $p \leq 0.01$ (**), $p \leq 0.005$ (***) or $p \leq 0.001$ (****).

**Accumulated clinical score and viral shedding.** Accumulated clinical score (ACS) and accumulated viral shedding (AVS) from PID 0 to PID 7 was calculated as the area under curves using the trapezoidal rule.

**Ranking.** The ACS and AVS represent the sum of individual clinical disease and viral load, respectively, regardless of the time they occurred during the challenge experiment. Likewise, the proportion of consolidated lung tissue post-mortem represents accumulated lung injury. Based on these criteria, three ranks were constructed and all calves were ranked (1–19) to indicate the individual level of disease and viral replication following challenge. The highest rank (19) was assigned to the most affected calf, and in decreasing order to the least affected, with a high clinical rank indicating a high accumulated clinical score (ACS); a high lung lesion rank indicating a high percent of macroscopic lung lesions post-mortem; a high viral-shed rank indicating a high accumulated viral-shed (AVS). Statistical differences between groups were calculated using individual rank sum, defined as the sum of these three ranks for each calf. In addition, group rank sums were calculated for each of the three ranks and corrected for number of calves per group (n), since one of the calves (d5) in the SUAbis-vaccinated group was excluded, by division by n followed by multiplication by 5, and a total rank sum calculated.

## Results

### Post Vaccination Monitoring

**Intranasally administered ΔSHrBRSV appeared to be clinically safe and did not transmit to sentinels.** Following i.n. vaccination with ΔSHrBRSV, only very slight upper respiratory signs (e.g. slight nasal discharge and infrequent coughing) were irregularly observed in all animals, in the week following vaccination. Marginal amounts of viral RNA were detected in nasal secretions of only one of these calves (calf a2; ≤ 0.36 $TCID_{50}$ eq. unit; 5–7 days post-vaccination). In the 3 seronegative sentinel calves housed with the ΔSHrBRSV calves, clinical signs of respiratory disease were not observed, and virus was not detected in nasal secretions by RT-PCR (data not shown). Furthermore, an increase in BRSV-specific serum $IgG_1$ was not detected in sentinel animals, three weeks after first contact with ΔSHrBRSV-vaccinated calves (data not shown). The absence of clinical signs, viral shedding and seroconversion indicated that transmission of ΔSHrBRSV to the sentinels had not occurred.

**Vaccination by parenteral route with SUMont, SUAbis and AbISCO-300 alone generated transient local and general adverse reactions.** Following the first vaccination with SUMont, all the calves were slightly depressed and developed elevated rectal temperatures (mean max ± SD 40.8±0.29°C) for 2–3 days post-vaccination, but no or only mild diffuse swelling was seen at the injection sites. The SUMont-vaccinated animal's reaction to the second vaccination was similar (mean max ± SD rectal temperature 40.0±0.11°C), except for moderate to marked swelling at injection sites.

Calves immunized with SUAbis had elevated rectal temperatures following the first vaccination (mean max ± SD 40.3±0.19°C), with mild to moderate swellings at injection sites, which waned within 2–3 days. Following the vaccination boost, no or mild to moderate swellings were seen, but calves did not develop significantly elevated rectal temperatures. The general and local clinical signs observed in calves immunized with AbISCO-300 alone were similar to those described for SUAbis, except for one control calf (calf d5) which demonstrated elevated rectal temperatures following both first and second vaccination (peaked at 39.5°C and 40.1°C, respectively).

## ΔSHrBRSV and SUMont Induced Strong and Good Clinical Protection, Respectively, Against Virulent BRSV Challenge

Despite moderate titers of MDA at the time of challenge, control calves developed marked to severe clinical signs as previously observed in this model [12] (Blodorn et al, in preparation). The clinical scores of the control calves presented in figure 2A reflect the progression from mild respiratory signs appearing on PID 3, to severe upper and lower respiratory disease on PID 7. Severe signs included a severely depressed general state and fever (max 40.2–41.2°C mean max 40.8°C); markedly reduced or absent appetite; coughing; nasal discharge; moderate to severe abdominal dyspnea; wheezing lung sounds on auscultation and increased respiratory rate (mean max 81.6 SD±4.6 breaths/min). One control (calf d3), reached the end-point at the time of euthanization on PID7. The mean accumulated clinical score from PID 0 to PID 7 (ACS) of the control group was 73.2 (SD±29.1; Fig. 2B).

In contrast to the controls, all vaccinated animals exhibited varying degrees of clinical protection (Fig. 2A–B). Clearly, the most clinically protected were animals immunized once i.n. with ΔSHrBRSV, with a mean ACS of 3.7 (SD±3.6), which was significantly lower than that of control calves (p≤0.001) or animals immunized twice with SUAbis (p≤0.05), and also tended to be lower than those immunized twice with SUMont (p = 0.06; Fig. 2B). Throughout the challenge, none of the ΔSHrBRSV-vaccinated calves had a reduced appetite or depressed general state. Apart from one calf (a1), which showed no clinical signs, and one calf (a5), which exhibited mild dyspnea and slight wheezing lung sounds on PID 7, calves immunized with ΔSHrBRSV showed very mild signs of respiratory disease. These mild signs were recorded on the last two days of the challenge (PID 6 and PID 7), and included slight serous nasal discharge, coughing on provocation, and slightly enhanced lung sounds. From PID 0 to 7, only one of the ΔSHrBRSV immunized calves had a peak rectal temperature exceeding 39.5°C (calf a2, 39.6°C on PID 7), and none had more than slightly elevated respiratory rate (mean max 49.6 SD±3.6 breaths/min).

Compared to controls, significant clinical protection was also observed in calves immunized with either of the subunit vaccines

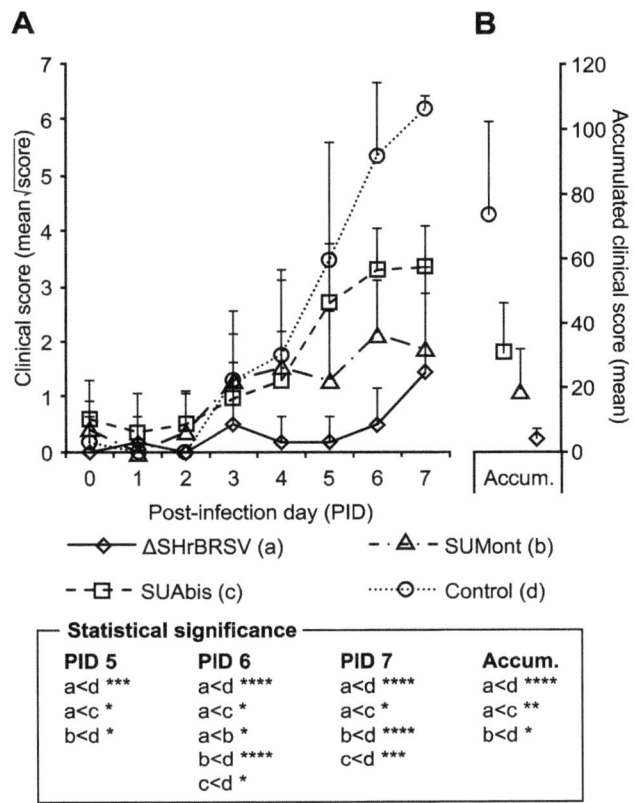

**Figure 2. Vaccination protects against clinical signs of BRSV disease.** Four groups of 5 calves were vaccinated as described in Fig. 1 and challenged with BRSV, 5 weeks after vaccination, on post-infection day (PID) 0. Following challenge, calves were examined daily until euthanization on PID 7, and the severity of clinical signs of diseases were scored as previously described [12]. (A) presents the mean square root of clinical scores per day (to approximate normal distribution for statistical analysis), and (B) the accumulated clinical score from PID 0 to PID 7, with standard deviations indicated by upward deflecting lines. Statistically significant differences are indicated by asterisks p≤0.05 (*); p≤0.01 (**); p≤0.005 (***); p≤0.001 (****); p≤0.0001 (*****).

(Fig. 2A–B). In calves immunized with SUMont, respiratory signs were first observed on PID3, and peaked at moderate levels on PID6, when the group mean clinical score was significantly higher than that of ΔSHrBRSV (p≤0.05; Fig. 2A). These mild and moderate clinical signs included serous nasal discharge, spontaneous coughing, slight to moderate dyspnea, slight wheezing lung sounds and elevated respiratory rate (mean max 54.4 SD±8.3 breaths/min). From PID 0 to PID 7, only 2/5 calves immunized with SUMont demonstrated rectal temperatures above 39.5°C (calf b2, 39.9°C on PID 4; calf b4, 39.7°C on PID 2). Compared to that of controls, the level of clinical disease observed in the SUMont calves was significantly lower on PID 5 (p≤0.05), PID 6 (p≤0.001) and PID 7 (p≤0.001), yielding a highly significantly lower ACS (mean ± SD 18.0±14.0, p≤0.005) (Fig. 2 and Table 2A–B).

Although the calves immunized with SUAbis were afforded clinical protection compared to controls on PID 6 (p≤0.05) and 7 (p≤0.005), they were less protected than calves vaccinated with SUMont (p = 0.26), and significantly less protected than calves vaccinated with ΔSHrBRSV (p≤0.05), in terms of ACS (mean ± SD 31.0±15.0; Fig. 2A–B). The severity of clinical signs observed in calves immunized with SUAbis was intermediate to those observed in calves vaccinated with SUMont and control animals (Fig. 2A–B), with a mean peak respiratory rate of 61.0 breaths/min (SD±6.8 breaths/min), and with 3/4 calves having peak rectal temperatures over 39.5°C after challenge (calf c1, 40.2°C on PID 6; calf c2, 39.7°C on PID 3; calf c4, 39.7°C on PID 7).

In summary, whereas a single i.n. administration of ΔSHrBRSV in calves with moderate to high titers of BRSV-specific MDA induced almost complete clinical protection against virulent challenge, two parenteral administrations of SUMont induced a good level of clinical protection, while SUAbis afforded some clinical protection, compared to controls (Table 2, Fig. 2A–B).

## ΔSHrBRSV and SUMont Afforded Almost Complete and Good Protection, Respectively, Against Pathologic Changes in the Lungs

The pathological observations were well in agreement with the clinical data. Whereas a high percentage of gross pneumonic consolidation was observed in controls at necropsy, 7 days after challenge, significantly less macroscopic lesions were observed in the lungs of all vaccinated calves ($p \leq 0.05$; Fig. 3A). Among the vaccinated animals, the ΔSHrBRSV-vaccinated calves had less lesions, compared to the SUMont-vaccinated calves, but the difference was not statistically significant ($p = 0.66$). Furthermore, while calves immunized with either ΔSHrBRSV or SUMont had less lesions compared to those immunized with SUAbis (Fig. 3A), this was only statistically significant for ΔSHrBRSV ($p \leq 0.05$). Overall, the majority of lesions were in the cranial parts of the lungs, but the extent of consolidated tissue varied from small and scattered lesions in the animals immunized with ΔSHrBRSV, to massive areas of consolidation involving almost half the lungs in the controls (Fig. 3B). Apart from areas of consolidation, two calves (d3 and d4) in the control group also exhibited moderate lung pleural emphysema.

Tissue from consolidated areas of the lungs from all calves were histologically examined, and proliferative and exudative bronchiolitis with accompanying alveolar collapse and peribronchiolar infiltration by mononuclear cells was observed, as previously described for BRSV-infection in calves [44]. These lesions were severe in control animals, with decreasing intensity in SUAbis-, SUMont- and ΔSHrBRSV-immunized animals, in that order.

Lesions were most pronounced in sections from the cranial lobes, whereas the caudal and accessory lobes were less severely affected. Histological lesions were most marked in controls (score 2.8–3.0, mean 2.9), followed by animals immunized with SUAbis (score 2.0–3.0, mean 2.5), followed by animals immunized with SUMont (score 0.6–2.5, mean 1.6), and least severe in animals immunized with ΔSHrBRSV (score 0.8–2.3, mean 1.3) (Fig. 3A). Panels C (I–IV) in figure 3 show representative histological images from each of the vaccinated and unvaccinated groups of animals. Whereas panel C (I) shows lung parenchyma from a ΔSHrBRSV-immunized calf (a2), with minimal thickening of the alveolar walls, panel C (II) shows lung parenchyma with mild pathological changes from a SUMont-immunized calf (b3), with slight thickening of the alveolar walls, but where alveolar spaces are still clear. On the other hand, calves immunized with SUAbis (panel C (III), calf c2) demonstrated moderate pathological changes in the lung parenchyma, with moderate thickening of the alveolar walls, and mononuclear inflammatory cells and a few neutrophils in the alveolar spaces. In the unvaccinated control animals (panel C (IV), calf d1) severe pathological changes were evident in the lung parenchyma, with severe thickening of alveolar walls, and scattered type II-cells lining the alveoli. Furthermore, in these animals, alveolar spaces were filled with numerous mono-

nuclear inflammatory cells, some neutrophils and occasional syncytial cells. For all calves, inflammatory cell infiltration consisted of mononuclear cells and neutrophils, with very few eosinophils.

BAL cells count showed that control animals had significantly more cells in BAL ($p \leq 0.01$; mean±SD $11.0 \pm 3.7$ cells × $10^5$/ml), compared to animals immunized with ΔSHrBRSV (mean±SD $5.2 \pm 3.5$ cells × $10^5$/ml), SUMont (mean±SD $3.1 \pm 1.8$ cells × $10^5$/ml) and SUAbis (mean±SD $3.2 \pm 1.9$ cells × $10^5$/ml).

In summary, among vaccinated calves, ΔSHrBRSV-immunized calves were best protected based on lung pathology after challenge, followed by calves immunized with SUMont, and the least protected SUAbis-immunized calves. There was no evidence of exacerbated pulmonary pathology in any of the vaccinated calves.

## Vaccine-induced Virological Protection Consistent with Clinical and Pathological Protection

The extent of BRSV infection in the controls was demonstrated by high levels of BRSV RNA detected in nasal secretions of all control calves from PID 3 to PID 7, with a peak on PID 5 (mean ± SD $2.2 \pm 0.36$ $\log_{10}$ $TCID_{50}$ eq. unit; Fig. 4A). In the lower respiratory tract, high levels of viral RNA were detected in BAL cells from control calves, collected on PID7 (mean ± SD $5.0 \pm 0.62$ $\log_{10}$ $TCID_{50}$ eq. unit; Fig. 4B). Accordingly, live BRSV was isolated from the lower respiratory tract of the controls, after inoculation of BAL cells on cell cultures, followed by one or two passages (Table 2). The accumulated virus shed (AVS) in nasal secretions of the control calves was $11.0 \pm 2.2$ $\log_{10}$ $TCID_{50}$ eq. unit.

In contrast to the control calves, calves immunized with ΔSHrBRSV were very well protected against BRSV replication following challenge, since only low quantities of BRSV RNA were detected in nasal secretions (max mean ± SD $0.1 \pm 1.1$ $\log_{10}$ $TCID_{50}$ eq. unit; Fig. 4A, Table 2), and only in 2/5 calves (calves a3 and a5, Table 2) for 2 and 3 days respectively. Furthermore, the mean AVS in the upper respiratory tract for the group of calves immunized with ΔSHrBRSV (mean ± SD $1.4 \pm 2.2$ $\log_{10}$ $TCID_{50}$ eq. unit) was highly significantly reduced compared to controls ($p \leq 0.0001$), and the mean AVS of controls were $10^9$ times higher. In addition, only low quantities of BRSV RNA could be detected in the BAL collected on PID 7 (mean ± SD $2.1 \pm 0.6$ $\log_{10}$ $TCID_{50}$ eq. unit, Fig. 4) and virus could not be isolated in cell culture, even after three passages (Table 2).

Virologically, calves immunized with SUMont were also well protected, since BRSV RNA was only detectable in NS for 2–4 days (mean 3.4 days), amounting to a significantly lower AVS (mean ± SD $3.6 \pm 2.6$ $\log_{10}$ $TCID_{50}$ eq. unit; $p \leq 0.001$) compared to controls, which had a $10^7$ times higher AVS. Moreover, the BRSV RNA in BAL of SUMont animals was significantly reduced ($p \leq 0.001$), compared to controls (Fig. 4B), and virus was isolated only from one SUMont calf (calf b3, 3rd passage; Table 2). However, compared to ΔSHrBRSV animals, the mean AVS of the SUMont-vaccinated animals was $10^2$ times greater, although this was not significant due to individual variation ($p = 0.2$).

Finally, calves immunized with SUAbis showed some degree of virological protection compared to controls, but less than that in vaccinated calves from other groups, since BRSV RNA could be detected in NS for 4–5 days (mean 4.5 days), with an AVS (mean ± SD $7.9 \pm 3.4$ $\log_{10}$ $TCID_{50}$ eq. unit) which was less than one-thousandth ($1/10^3$) that of controls, but $10^6$ times higher than the ΔSHrBRSV calves ($p \leq 0.005$), and $10^4$ times higher than the SUMont calves ($p \leq 0.05$, Fig. 4A). The virological protection of the lower airways of the SUAbis calves was similarly intermediary,

Vaccine Safety and Efficacy Evaluation of a Recombinant Bovine Respiratory Syncytial Virus (BRSV) with Deletion...

9

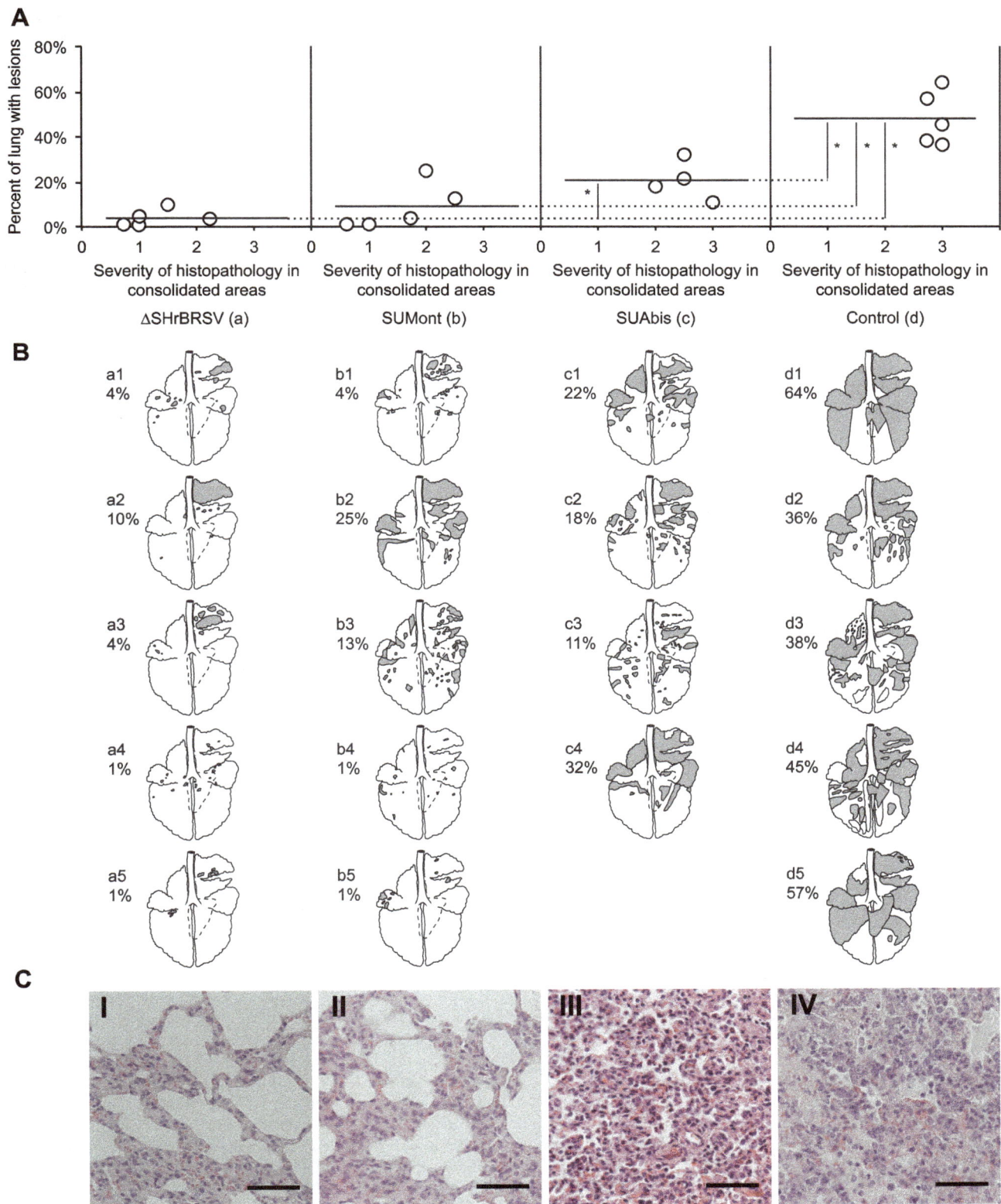

**Figure 3. Vaccination reduces the extent of lung lesions following BRSV challenge.** Four groups of 5 calves were vaccinated as described in Fig. 1 and challenged with BRSV, 5 weeks after vaccination. Two weeks before challenge, one calf (c5) was euthanized due to traumatic injury. Lungs were removed after exsanguination, lesions were recorded on a lung chart after visual examination and palpation, and the proportion of lung showing pneumonic consolidation was calculated. Formalin-fixed tissue samples from each lobe in the right lung were analyzed for the severity of histopathological changes and scored as either normal (0), mild (1), moderate (2) or severe (3). (A) shows the extent of macroscopic lesions on the y-axes, and the microscopic severity of inflammation (mean score of four sections per calf) on the x-axes. Statistically significant difference is indicated

by asterisks (p≤0.05). (B) shows the percent of pneumonic consolidation in each animal (also depicted as filled areas in lung-charts), and emphysema (outlined areas in calves d3 and d4). Panels C (I–IV) show representative histological images from each of the four groups of calves. Bar indicate 100 μm. Panels C (I) (ΔSHrBRSV), C (II) (SUMont), C (III) (SUAbis) and C (IV) (Control) show lung parenchyma with minimal, mild, moderate and severe pathological changes, respectively.

as less BRSV RNA was detected by RT-PCR in BAL samples from these calves, compared to the control calves, but more than in BAL from the other vaccinated groups (Fig. 4B). Furthermore, whereas infectious virus was isolated from the BAL cells of all control calves in passage one or two, virus could only be isolated from BAL cells from 3 out of 4 calves vaccinated with SUAbis, and only in passage three (Table 2).

In summary, the vaccine-induced virological protection was in accordance with the clinical and pathological protection observed. Calves immunized with i.n. ΔSHrBRSV, followed by calves immunized with i.m. SUMont, were better protected virologically in the upper and lower respiratory tracts against challenge with virulent BRSV, compared to animals immunized with SUAbis or adjuvant alone (Fig. 4A–B).

## Ranking

The three ranks: clinical rank, viral-shed rank and lung lesion rank; reflected the significant differences detected between groups in clinical signs, extent of lung lesions, and virus shed. Thus, the relative order of group rank sums was consistent across clinical, virological and pathological ranking, yielding consistent group total rank sums (Fig. 5): i) the ΔSHrBRSV-immunized animals were significantly protected compared to SUMont-immunized animals (p≤0.05), to SUAbis-immunized animals (p≤0.001) and to control animals (p≤0.001), ii) SUMont-vaccinated animals were significantly more protected than the SUAbis-vaccinated animals (p≤0.05) and controls (p≤0.001), and iii) SUAbis-immunized animals in turn, were significantly protected compared to controls (p≤0.05).

## Immunology

**Systemic humoral immune responses.** Serum IgG antibodies against total BRSV; F, N, P, M2-1 of HRSV and G of BRSV were measured by ELISA. All calves except the sentinels had moderate to high, and statistically homogenous, titers of maternal BRSV-specific serum $IgG_1$ antibodies at the time of first vaccination (Fig. 6A, Table 2). In the three weeks following first vaccination, BRSV-specific serum antibodies either continued to decline or remained unchanged (Fig. 6A). However, in the two weeks following the second vaccination, a slight increase in BRSV-specific serum antibody titers were observed in calves immunized with either SUMont or SUAbis, and these reached their highest levels one week after challenge, at the termination of the experiment. Following the second vaccination, the mean titer of BRSV-specific serum antibody titers in calves immunized with SUMont was consistently higher than that of calves immunized with SUAbis (Fig. 6A), but the difference was not statistically significant.

In the animals immunized once i.n. with ΔSHrBRSV, BRSV-specific $IgG_1$ serum antibodies continued to decline after vaccination until one week after challenge, when they had rapidly increased (Fig. 6A).

The inhibitory effect of MDA on priming did not affect antibody responses to all BRSV proteins equally (Fig. 6A–G). Indeed, despite the apparent continued decrease of total BRSV-specific serum $IgG_1$ (Fig. 6A), titers of IgG antibodies in serum directed against the N, P and M2-1 proteins in the SU, were already increasing after the first vaccination (Fig. 6D–F). In contrast, titers of F- and G-specific serum antibodies in SU-vaccinated animals were not significantly different compared to controls (Fig. 6B–C).

In calves immunized with ΔSHrBRSV, an increase in serum IgG antibodies against N, P, M2-1, G or F was not detected before challenge. However, one week after challenge, antibody titers specific to the F and G proteins were significantly higher in these animals, compared to animals in all other groups (p≤0.05; Fig. 6B–C). The ΔSHrBRSV animals also demonstrated a relative increase in antibody titers specific to N, P and M2-1 following challenge, compared to controls (p≤0.01, p = 0.45 and p≤0.05, respectively),

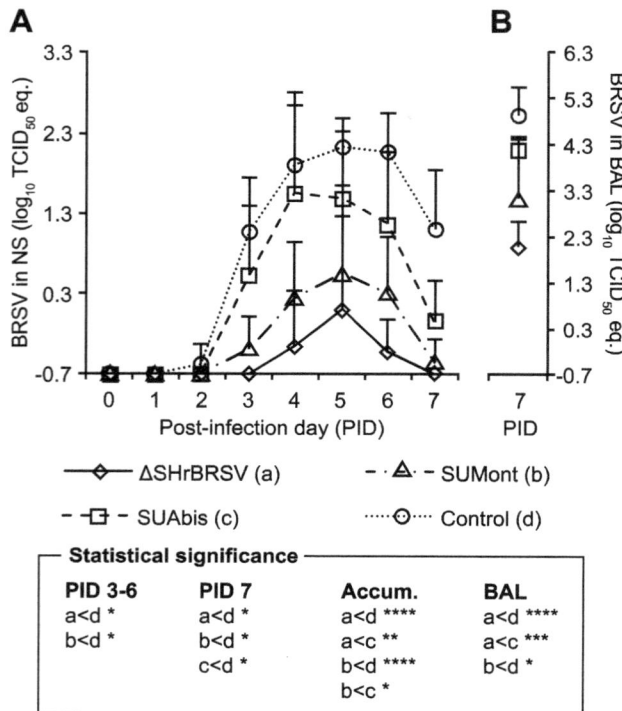

**Figure 4. Vaccination reduces virus load in upper and lower airways following virulent BRSV challenge.** Four groups of 5 calves were vaccinated as described in Fig. 1 and challenged with BRSV, 5 weeks after vaccination, on post-infection day (PID) 0. Two weeks before challenge, one calf (c5) was euthanized due to traumatic injury. The figure presents mean viral load in nasal swabs collected from PID 0 to PID 7 in panel A and post-mortem bronchoalveolar lavage (BAL) in panel B, as determined by BRSV F-gene RT-PCR after total RNA extraction, and is expressed as $TCID_{50}$ equivalent, calculated from standard dilution series of virus with a known $TCID_{50}$. The area under mean curves in panel A represents the accumulated detected virus shed (AVS): calves immunized with either ΔSHrBRSV or SUMont had significantly lower AVS (1.4±2.2 $eqTCID_{50}$, p≤0.005 and 3.6±2.6 $eqTCID_{50}$, p≤0.05 respectively), compared to calves immunized with either SUAbis (7.9±3.4 $eqTCID_{50}$) or adjuvant alone (11.0±2.2 $eqTCID_{50}$). Statistically significant difference with Student's t-test are indicated by asterisks and the corresponding groups; p≤0.05 (*); p≤ 0.01 (**); p≤0.005 (***); p≤0.001 (****).

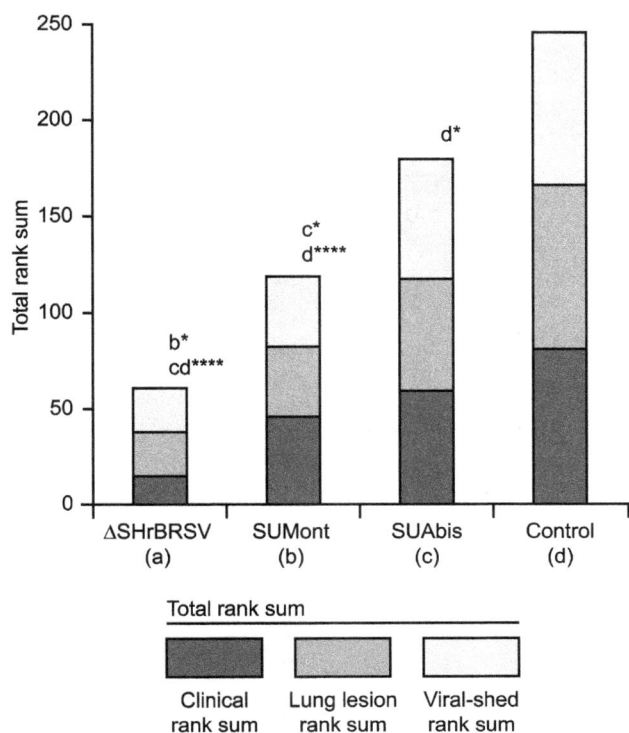

**Figure 5. Vaccination reduces clinical signs, lung pathology and viral replication, following virulent BRSV challenge.** Four groups of 5 calves were vaccinated as described in Fig. 1 and challenged with BRSV, 5 weeks after vaccination. Two weeks before challenge, one calf (c5) was euthanized due to traumatic injury. Calves were ranked (1–19) in each of three post-challenge parameters, with a high clinical rank indicating a high accumulated clinical score (Fig. 2); a high lung lesion rank indicating a high percent of macroscopic lung lesions post-mortem (Fig. 3); and a high viral-shed rank indicating a high accumulated viral-shed following challenge (Fig. 4). The figure shows the group sum of each of these ranks. To correct for the unequal number of calves per group (n), each rank sum was divided by n, and multiplied by 5. The stacked bars per group represent the sum of rank sums (total rank sum). Statistically significant differences in individual rank sums are indicated by asterisks and the corresponding group; p≤ 0.05 (*); p≤0.001 (****).

but the antibody responses were less than those seen in animals vaccinated with SU (Fig. 6D–F).

BRSV neutralizing antibodies were also quantified in sera. Before challenge, no significant increase in neutralizing antibodies was detected in sera from any of the vaccinated calves (Fig. 6G). However, following challenge, ΔSHrBRSV-vaccinated calves demonstrated a significant increase in neutralizing antibodies (p≤0.001), and had significantly higher titers on PID 7, compared to all other animals (p≤0.001; Fig. 6D).

**Local humoral immune responses.** Before challenge, on PID 0, BRSV-specific IgA was detected in nasal secretions only from animals immunized with SUMont (Fig. 7A). However, 7 days after BRSV challenge, BRSV-specific IgA was detected in nasal secretions from all vaccinated calves, although, the increase was statistically significant only in those calves that had been vaccinated i.n. with ΔSHrBRSV (Fig. 7A, p<0.01, PID *0 vs. 7*).

Similar to findings in the upper respiratory tract, all vaccinated animals demonstrated significantly higher levels of BRSV-specific

IgA in BAL after challenge, compared to controls (ΔSHrBRSV and SUMont p≤0.001; SUAbis p≤0.01; Fig. 7B).

In agreement with the HRSV N-specific serum IgG responses after challenge, animals immunized with either SUMont or ΔSHrBRSV had significantly higher titers of IgA antibodies against HRSV-N in BAL, compared to controls (p≤0.001 and, p≤0.05 respectively; Fig. 7C). Furthermore, titers of HRSV-N specific IgA in BAL from the SUMont calves were also significantly higher than titers in animals in both the ΔSHrBRSV and the SUAbis groups (p≤0.05; Fig. 7C). In contrast to IgA, BRSV specific IgG$_1$ antibodies were not detected in BAL or nasal secretions.

**BRSV-specific cell mediated immune responses.** BRSV-specific T lymphocyte proliferative responses in PBMCs measured 2 weeks after first and second vaccination, were statistically significant only in animals immunized with SUMont, both after first (p≤0.001) and second vaccination (p≤0.05), compared to all other groups (Fig. 8A). Whereas IL-4 was only detected at very low concentrations (<0.05 ng/ml) in supernatant from restimulated PBMCs from all animals 2 weeks after boost, PBMCs from SUMont-immunized animals produced significant higher levels of IFNγ, compared to those from animals in all other groups (Fig. 8B; p≤0.05; 2 weeks after first vaccination not analysed). Although not detected in PBMCs from ΔSHrBRSV-immunized animals, BRSV-specific proliferative responses were detected in cells from tracheobronchial lymph nodes of these calves, collected 1 week after challenge, and were greater than in cells from controls (Table 3, p≤0.05). These responses were of similar magnitude as those seen in PBMCs from SUMont-immunized animals before challenge (Fig. 8A and Table 3). Lymph nodes from SUMont and SUAbis groups were not analysed, since these could not be prepared following necropsy due to logistical limitations. There was, moreover, a statistically significant increase in proportion of IFNγ-producing CD4$^+$ lymphocytes after restimulation of the lymph node cells with BRSV-infected compared to uninfected cell lysate, in ΔSHrBRSV-vaccinated calves (p = 0.02) but not controls (p = 0.14), using paired Student's *t*-test (Table 3). Despite using inactivated BRSV for restimulation, the proportion of IFNγ-producing CD8$^+$ lymphocytes also increased following BRSV-infected compared to uninfected cell lysate stimuli, in ΔSHrBRSV-vaccinated calves (p = 0.06) but not controls (p = 0.4). When IFNγ and IL-4 production was measured in supernatants from BRSV-restimulated LN cells by ELISA, there was no significant difference in IL-4 production, whereas LN cells from ΔSHrBRSV-immunized animals produced significantly more IFNγ, compared to those from controls (p = 0.03; Table 3).

## Discussion

In the present study, two very promising DIVA-compatible BRSV vaccine candidates were identified, when evaluated in young calves with BRSV-specific MDA in a BRSV challenge with severe clinical expression, compared to many published evaluation studies for commercial vaccines [22]. Based on efficacy in reducing clinical signs of disease, consolidated lung lesions and viral load, the vaccine candidates consistently exhibited three distinct levels of protection. ΔSHrBRSV, a live attenuated SH gene-deleted recombinant BRSV, induced almost total clinical protection, and a high level of virological protection, five weeks after a single i.n. immunization. In the same experiment, calves immunized twice i.m. with SUMont, a HRSV subunit vaccine with epitopes from BRSV adjuvanted by Montanide ISA71$^{VG}$, were also well protected, when challenged with virulent BRSV two weeks after the second vaccination. Although high, the protection observed in

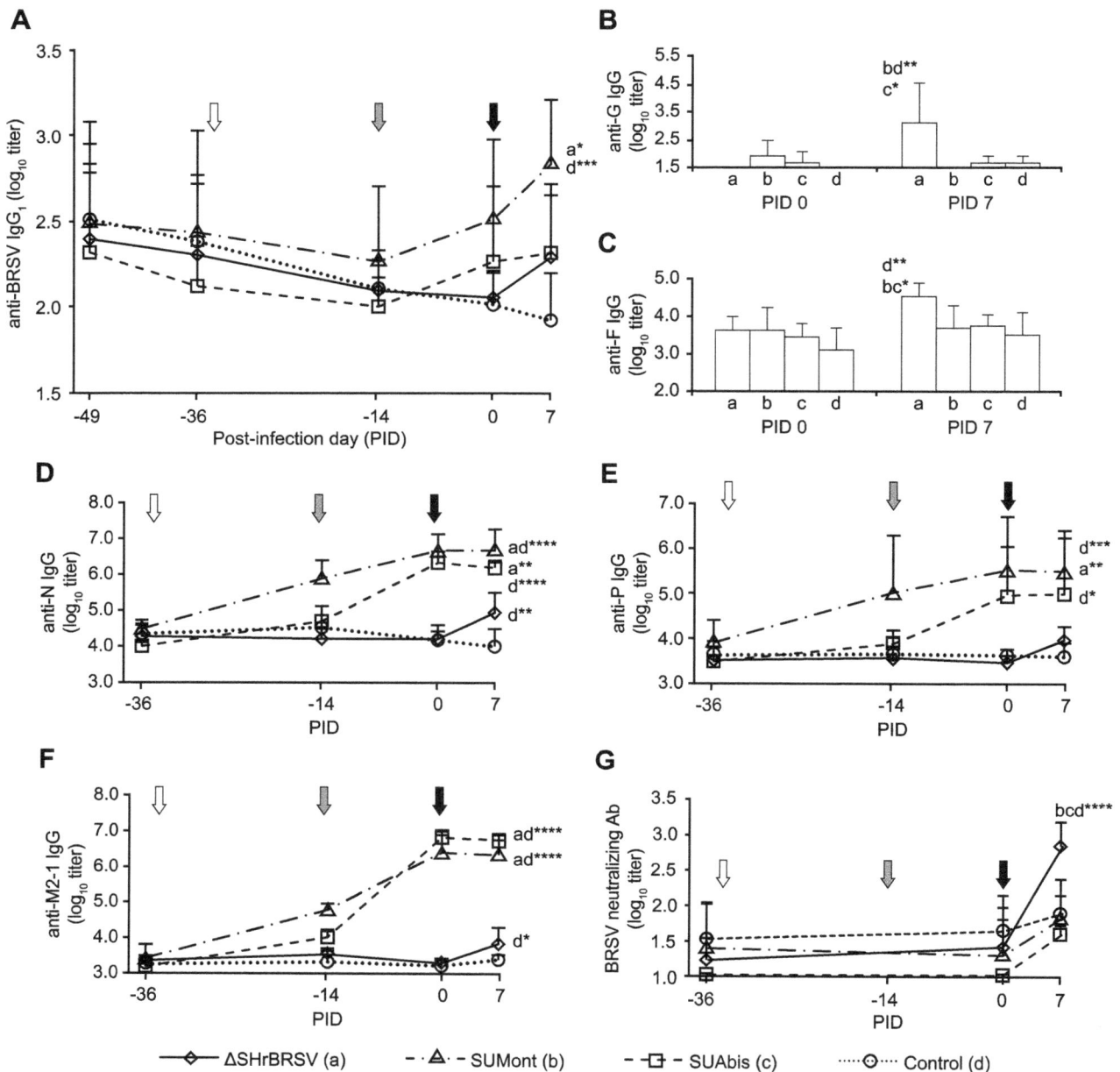

**Figure 6. RSV-specific serum antibodies in calves before and after immunization and subsequent challenge with virulent BRSV.** Four groups of 5 calves were vaccinated as described in Fig. 1 (white and grey arrows) and challenged with BRSV, 5 weeks after vaccination (black arrow) on post-infection day (PID) 0. Two weeks before challenge, one calf (C5) was euthanized due to traumatic injury. Panels show group mean $\log_{10}$ serum titers of: (A) BRSV-specific IgG$_1$ (by ELISA); (B) IgG directed against BRSV G on PID 0 and PID 7 (by ELISA); (C) IgG directed against HRSV F on PID 0 and PID 7 (by ELISA); (D) IgG directed against HRSV N (by ELISA); (E) IgG directed against HRSV P (by ELISA); and (F) IgG directed against HRSV M2-1 (by ELISA) (G) BRSV-neutralizing antibodies (by plaque reduction assay). Note that the scale of the y-axis is not uniform between panels. Statistically significant difference on PID 7 is indicated by asterisks and the corresponding group; $p \leq 0.05$ (*); $p \leq 0.01$ (**); $p \leq 0.005$ (***); $p \leq 0.001$ (****).

SUMont immunized animals was not as great as that observed in ΔSHrBRSV immunized animals. In contrast, the same subunits adjuvanted by AbISCO-300 and administered s.c., twice at an interval of three weeks, afforded statistically significant, but limited protection two weeks after the second vaccination.

The strong protection induced by ΔSHrBRSV confirmed previous results obtained in 1 to 4 week-old, BRSV-seronegative calves, vaccinated i.n. and intratracheally with ΔSHrBRSV and challenged with virulent BRSV, 6 months after vaccination [24].

This vaccine virus appears to be attenuated compared to wild type rBRSV by replicating less well in the lower respiratory tract and inducing little or no pathological lesions in 2 to 3 week-old gnotobiotic calves [24]. In the present study, only low levels of virus RNA were detected in nasal swabs from only one out of five conventional calves after vaccination, and furthermore, sentinel calves did not become infected after 6 days of contact with ΔSHrBRSV vaccinated calves. This contrasts with the higher levels of virus shedding detected in the upper respiratory tract in

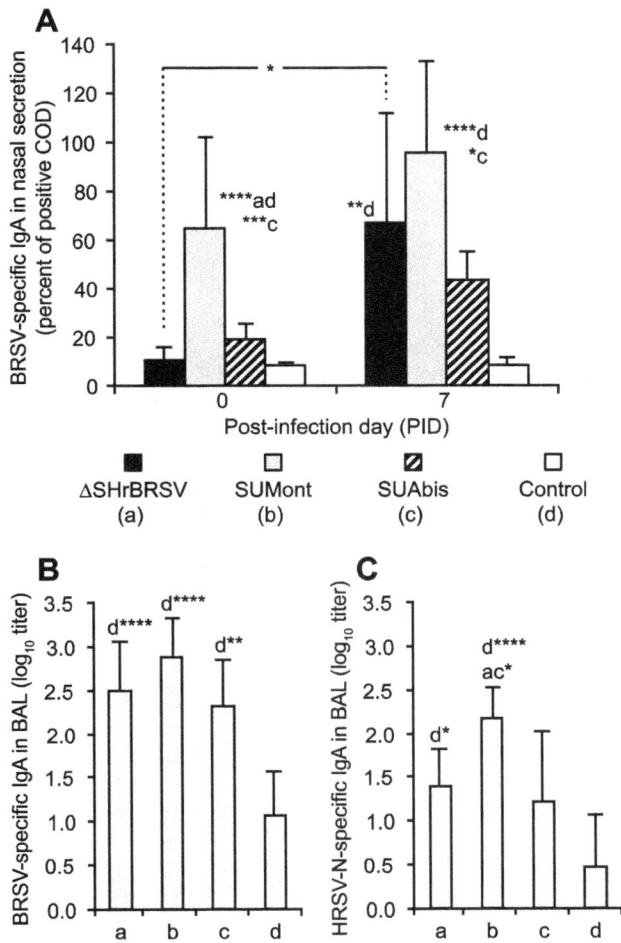

**Figure 7. Mucosal IgA antibodies in the upper and lower airways, before and after BRSV challenge.** Four groups of 5 calves were vaccinated as described in Fig. 1 and challenged with BRSV, 5 weeks after vaccination. Two weeks before challenge, one calf (c5) was euthanized due to traumatic injury. BRSV-specific IgA antibodies were analyzed by ELISA. (A) shows group mean levels of BRSV-specific IgA in nasal secretions on post-infection day (PID) 0 and 7, whereas (B) and (C) show group mean titers of total BRSV- and HRSV-N-specific IgA in bronchoalveolar lavage (BAL) on PID 7, respectively. BAL samples were titrated, whereas antibody levels in nasal secretions were semi-quantitatively determined and expressed as a percentage of a positive control sample, due to lack of sample material. Standard deviations are indicated by upward deflecting lines. Statistically significant differences between PID 0 and PID 7 in panel A are indicated by a horizontal line, whereas in all panels significant differences between groups for the same time-point are indicated by asterisks and the corresponding group letter; $p \leq 0.05$ (*); $p \leq 0.01$ (**); $p \leq 0.005$ (***); $p \leq 0.001$ (****).

gnotobiotic calves seen in previous studies [24] and might partly be explained by the presence of BRSV-specific MDA, which inhibited virus replication. Altogether, this suggests that the very mild clinical signs observed following i.n. immunization with ΔSHrBRSV were unlikely caused by viral replication, but were probably due to other factors. Even if further studies need to be performed to confirm the good innocuity of ΔSHrBRSV, these observations and the nature of the gene-deletion approach, which makes ΔSHrBRSV more refractory to wild-type reversion compared to live vaccines attenuated by point mutations [23], suggests that the use of ΔSHrBRSV in young calves is safe. The

**Table 3.** BRSV-specific lymphocyte responses from tracheobronchial lymph nodes of ΔSHrBRSV vaccinated calves.

| Calf group[a] | FACS[b] | | | | | | Lymphocyte proliferation (COD)[c] | | ELISA[d] | |
| | CD4+IFNg+ (%) | | CD8+IFNg+ (%) | | | | | | | |
| | BRSV stim. | Control stim. | BRSV stim. | Control stim. | | | | | IFNγ (ng/ml) | IL-4 (ng/ml) |
|---|---|---|---|---|---|---|---|---|---|---|
| ΔSHrBRSV | 0.27 (±0.13)* | 0.16 (±0.07)* | 0.09 (±0.04) | 0.06 (±0.02) | | | 0.14 (±0.12)* | | 1.10 (±1.08)* | 0.24 (±0.28) |
| Control | 0.22 (±0.10) | 0.19 (±0.13) | 0.05 (±0.03) | 0.05 (±0.02) | | | 0.02 (±0.03)* | | 0.20 (±0.10)* | 0.32 (±0.27) |

[a]Four groups of 5 calves were vaccinated as described in Fig. 1 and challenged with BRSV, 5 weeks after vaccination, on post-infection day (PID) 0. Lymphocytes were isolated on PID 7 from tracheobronchial lymph nodes of calves vaccinated with ΔSHrBRSV and controls, and stimulated ex-vivo with either BRSV-infected or uninfected cell lysate (heat-inactivated).
[b]After 18 hours of incubation, production of IFNγ by CD4+ and CD8+ lymphocytes were assayed using a flow cytometer (FACSVerse, BD Biosciences) and data were analyzed using FACSuite software (BD Biosciences). Results are expressed as % of CD4+ or CD8+ cells producing IFNγ.
[c]After 7 days of incubation, proliferative responses were determined by corrected optical density (COD) of Alamar Blue (Invitrogen, Sweden). Results are expressed as the mean corrected OD (COD, $OD_{BRSV} - OD_{cell\ lysate}$).
[d]After 9 days of incubation, IFNγ and IL-4 were analysed in supernatants of BRSV-restimulated cells by ELISA (BioRad).
*Statistically significant difference between groups is indicated by asterisks; $p \leq 0.05$ (*). Standard deviations are presented within parenthesis.

**A**

**B**

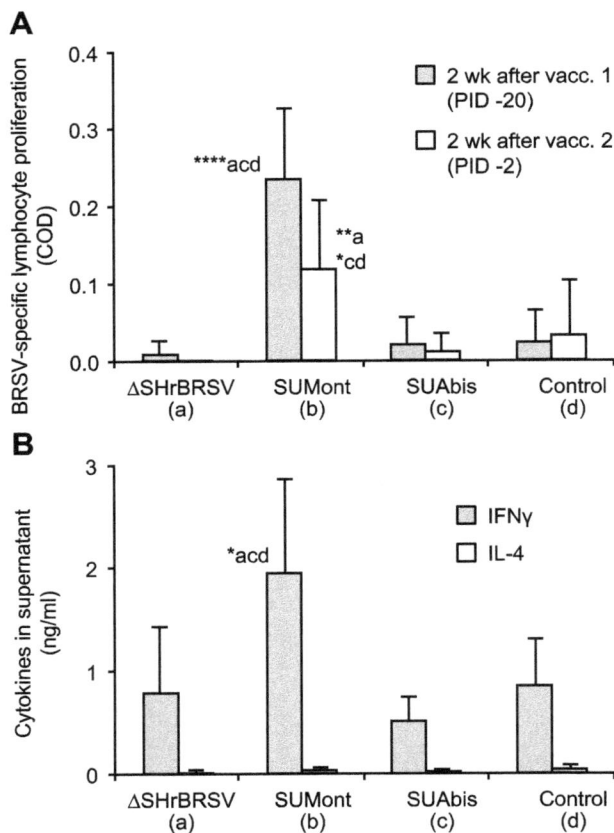

**Figure 8. BRSV-specific lymphocyte proliferative response in vaccinated calves.** Four groups of 5 calves were vaccinated as described in Fig. 1 and challenged with BRSV, 5 weeks after vaccination, on post-infection day (PID) 0. Two weeks before challenge, one calf (c5) was euthanized due to traumatic injury. Peripheral blood mononuclear cells (PBMC) were purified from blood two weeks after first and second vaccination, as indicated in Fig. 1, and stimulated ex-vivo with either BRSV-infected or uninfected cell lysate. (A) Corrected optical density (COD) of Alamar Blue (Invitrogen, Sweden), indicating proliferative response after seven days of incubation. (B) IFNγ and IL-4 in supernatant from PBMC restimulated with BRSV-infected cell lysate, expressed as group means (ng/ml). Standard deviations are indicated by upward deflecting lines. Statistically significant differences are indicated by asterisks and the corresponding group; $p \leq 0.05$ (*); $p \leq 0.01$ (**); $p \leq 0.001$ (****).

safety of this vaccine, like the adjuvanted SU vaccines, was further confirmed by the absence of exacerbated histopathological lesions or an influx of eosinophils in the lungs, following BRSV challenge of the vaccinated calves, which have been observed with some inactivated vaccines both in the field and experimentally [20,21].

Surprisingly, BRSV-specific immune responses could not be demonstrated in animals immunized with ΔSHrBRSV, until after challenge with virulent BRSV. Following challenge, the strong protection induced by ΔSHrBRSV was in part associated with rapid and strong anamnestic, local and systemic humoral immune responses. In agreement with previous studies, these were characterized by BRSV-specific IgA in respiratory secretions and BRSV-neutralizing serum antibodies directed against the F and G proteins [5,10,12,13,18]. Although undetectable in PBMC before challenge, the BRSV-specific T cell responses detected in tracheobronchial lymph nodes after challenge similarly indicated anamnestic cellular responses, which may have contributed to

protection. These responses were dominated by IFNγ rather than IL-4 production, partly by CD4+ and possibly by CD8+ lymphocytes, which are important for BRSV clearance [15].

Whereas ΔSHrBRSV-induced protection seems to have been largely mediated by BRSV-neutralizing systemic antibodies, BRSV-specific local IgA and T cell responses directed against native viral proteins, protection observed in SUMont-vaccinated animals were mediated mainly by T-cell cross-reactions against the internal proteins N, P and M2-1 of HRSV. Unfortunately, we were not able to assess the local T cell immunity in SUMont-vaccinated animals, however, Riffault et al. [25] demonstrated $N^{SRS}$-specific IFNγ production of tracheobronchial lymph node cells in calves vaccinated with $N^{SRS}$ and Montanide ISA71$^{VG}$, compared to unvaccinated controls, 20 days after BRSV challenge. In further agreement with that study, serum antibodies were also induced against these proteins but were not neutralizing, and it is likely that induced mucosal IgA antibodies had similar characteristics. In relation to $N^{SRS}$ evaluated in seronegative calves, protection appears to have been strongly enhanced by the inclusion of additional internal HRSV proteins P and M2-1, with known CD8+ epitopes [14] (G. Taylor, unpublished observations). SUAbis, containing the same subunits but adjuvanted by AbISCO-300, induced immune responses of a similar type but of lower magnitude.

The route of immunization, the presence of BRSV-specific MDA, the composition of the vaccine, and/or the type of adjuvant in the SU vaccines may contribute to the differences in vaccine-induced protection observed in this study. One reason for the superior protection provided by the intranasal administration of a live virus vaccine may be due to the homing-mechanisms of antigen-specific memory lymphocytes that migrate from lymphoid tissue to mucosal effector sites including the site of infection [45]. Immune responses induced by mucosal vaccination are, moreover, considered to be less inhibited by antigen-specific MDA than those induced by parenteral vaccination [5,13]. One i.n. BRSV vaccine is commercially available for use in young calves with MDA in the field and seems effective in this target animal group, but it is not DIVA compatible. Despite the limited virus replication following i.n. vaccination with ΔSHrBRSV, and the absence of a detectable BRSV-specific immune response before challenge in this study, BRSV-specific MDA did not appear to inhibit priming of protective immunity induced by ΔSHrBRSV.

The superior protection induced by ΔSHrBRSV may be explained by the expression of full-length glycoproteins with the native conformation, even if they were expressed in low quantities due to limited viral replication. In addition, the virus replication and presence of viral pathogen-associated molecular patterns would be expected to activate the innate immune system and to present antigens on major histocompatibility complex class I, which will initiate a CTL response.

The antigenic epitopes used in the SU vaccines in the present study, were carefully selected epitopes from the F and G proteins, which were grafted onto N nanorings. Specifically, $F_{422-438}$ corresponds to a linear epitope on the fusion protein, antigenic site IV, which is the target of MAb19 [38] and 101F [46], and is also recognized by a protective, BRSV-neutralizing bovine mAb [47] (P Whyte & G Taylor, unpublished observations). MAb19 also binds with high affinity to $F_{mimo}$, a combinatorial peptide mimicking the same epitope, and which was reported to induce neutralizing antibodies [37]. $F_{255-278}$ corresponds to antigenic site II on F, which is the target of Palivizumab and Motavizumab, and is recognized by a protective BRSV-neutralizing mAb [38,47]. $G_{174-187}$ corresponds to a dominant protective epitope on the attachment protein, which induces partially protective, but non-neutralizing, antibodies in calves [48]. These epitopes have not been shown to be T-cell epitopes in cattle [49], but their contribution to cellular immunity is possible and needs to be further elucidated. All purified nanorings with grafted epitopes were recognized by the respective epitope-specific monoclonal antibody, as determined by ELISA (data not shown). However, antibodies detected by ELISA in animals immunized with SUMont were directed against HRSV N, P and M2-1 but not against F and G. The lack of antibodies directed against the F and G proteins in calves immunized with SU might be explained by problems of conformation or accessibility, or by the relatively low quantity of these epitopes in the SU preparations, compared to the quantity of full-length HRSV-N, -P and -M2-1. Indeed, a recent study demonstrated enhanced immunogenicity, when the influenza epitope (M2e) attached to N-nanorings were repeated [50].

Increases of N-, P- and M2-1-specific IgG in the SU-vaccinated animals were detected after vaccination but were not evident by measuring total BRSV-specific serum $IgG_1$ antibodies. This might be explained by a masking effect of declining MDA specific to other proteins (*e.g.* BRSV F [8]) after first vaccination, or differences in test sensitivity, possibly due to differences in the amount of these proteins in ELISAs based on BRSV-infected lysate and recombinant proteins, respectively. The contribution of N-, P- and M2-1-specific antibodies to SU-induced protection should be marginal, since these are all internal virus proteins. Taken together, these findings suggest that the F and G epitopes played a very limited role in the protection observed in SU-vaccinated calves and that cross-protective T-cell responses are induced by HRSV-N in calves, as previously described [25] and likely also by P and M2-1. Indeed, N, P and M2-1 are highly conserved, with 93%, 81% and 80% amino acid homology between BRSV and HRSV, respectively [51–53], which strengthens the possibility that all of them could have contributed to the observed cross-protection. This level of cross protection has not been observed in previous investigations with live RSV in different animal species. Immunization with BRSV provided cotton rats with limited protection against HRSV challenge [54] and recombinant BRSV with glycoproteins F and G from HRSV was overly attenuated in chimpanzees, with marginal viral replication, humoral response and protective efficacy [55]. Likewise, HRSV replicates poorly in calves and induces only mild lung lesions after intranasal and intratracheal administration [56] (Valarcher & Taylor, unpublished observations). Therefore the lack of viral replication due to the species barrier, which might explain a poor protective immune response, can be bypassed by direct administration of conserved recombinant viral proteins combined with a powerful adjuvant, as demonstrated by SUMont in the present study.

The SUMont-immunized animals were the only calves that demonstrated a systemic BRSV-specific proliferative T-cell response after first and second vaccination, with production of IFNγ. The F, N, P and M2 proteins are the major antigens recognized by CD8+ T cells [14] (Taylor unpublished observations) and N, P and M2-1 were present in high quantities in the SU vaccines. Recall responses in PBMCs stimulated with either BRSV lysate or $N^{SRS}$ have been observed in calves immunized with N or $N^{SRS}$ alone [10,25]. In the present study, however, only BRSV lysate restimulation of PBMCs was performed, so the contribution of the individual proteins to T-cell priming was not determined. Nonetheless, our data suggest that the T-cell responses plays a very important role in the protection against RSV and that SUMont could be a good base for the development of a vaccine against BRSV as well as HRSV. Further improvement of the protective efficacy could be likely obtained by including the pre-fusion F-

protein of BRSV or HRSV [57] instead of decorating N with epitopes from F and G.

Not only the proteins included in SU but also the adjuvant played an important role in the efficacy of these vaccines. The adjuvant effects of water-in-oil emulsion vaccines, such as SUMont, are not fully understood, but include the induction of inflammation and recruitment of cells to the site of immunization, as well as a depot effect [58]. In this work, IFNγ was detected in the supernatant from BRSV-stimulated PBMC collected from animals vaccinated with SUMont after boost, but only minimal amounts of IL-4, suggesting a T helper cell type 1 (Th 1) orientation of the immune response. Although not confirmed herein, Iscomatrices such as AbISCO-300, is similarly known to induce Th1 responses and prime CTL by antigen cross-presentation on dendritic cells and B-cells [59,60] and activate dendritic cells through recruitment of IFNγ-producing NK cells to draining lymph nodes [61]. The limited protection induced by SUAbis in the present study, contrasts with the high protective efficacy of s.c. administered classic BRSV-ISCOMs, containing similar adjuvant quantities [12,62], but additionally the F, G, SH and M proteins [63].

The difference in protection between SUMont and SUAbis may be explained by the use of two different route of immunization. However, to our knowledge, the subcutaneous route of immunization has not previously shown to be disadvantageous in cattle.

Combining different types of vaccines, adjuvants and routes of administration, in a heterologous prime-boost, may be a way to improve the efficacy as well as the duration of protection induced by vaccination. Although not evaluated herein, the duration of protection might be limited after a single mucosal administration [64], and theoretically, a homologous mucosal boost of ΔSHrBRSV might be ineffective, due to vaccine neutralization by secretory IgA antibodies. Boosting intramuscularly with ΔSHrBRSV or SUMont could thus prolong and potentiate protective immunity, by activating several arms of the immune system.

Finally, one characteristic of this combined or separate vaccine approach is to enable DIVA, by measuring antibodies against a protein that is absent in the vaccine. The concept was introduced as a way to implement disease eradication programs in veterinary medicine, to limit the spread of a disease, while not being serologically blinded by vaccination [65]. However, the DIVA-aspect can also be used at a population level in the field to serologically monitor the virological protection induced by vaccination, in cattle as well as in man, since vaccine efficacy and duration of protection may change over time due to genetic evolution of field strains [66]. The envisaged DIVA-target in the present study is the SH protein, which has been excluded from both vaccines: by genetic manipulation in ΔSHrBRSV, and by rational design in the subunit vaccines. As serum antibodies against SH are induced by natural BRSV infection [63], detection of these antibodies will presumably enable the differentiation of infected animals from those vaccinated with either vaccine in the present study. In calves, the detection of $IgG_2$ antibodies would increase the specificity, since this isotype is not present in high quantities in MDA [13].

In conclusion, our data suggest that several types of immune response, influenced by vaccine composition and vaccination regimen, may provide protection against BRSV in calves with MDA. A single intranasal administration of ΔSHrBRSV was sufficient to safely induce anamnestic neutralizing systemic and mucosal IgA responses as well as local T cell immune responses affording almost complete protection against BRSV challenge, 5 weeks later. In contrast, SUMont induced good protection in absence of neutralizing antibodies, possibly through strong cross-reactive T-cell responses against the recombinant HRSV proteins N, P and M2-1. We believe that the combination of both vaccines (live and inactivated) in a heterologous prime-boost regimen might afford sterilizing long lasting protection against BRSV and this hypothesis is under evaluation.

## Acknowledgments

We thank the technical staff at SVA for maintaining the challenged animals, Annika Rikberg and Karin Selin-Wretling, SLU, for helping with logistics and the preparation of histological samples, Prof. L. E. Larsen, DTU, Denmark for generously sharing the BRSV isolate no. 9402022, Prof. J.S. McLellan, Geisel School of Medicine at Dartmouth, USA for kindly providing the HRSV-F-ELISA antigen, Juliette Ben Arous, SEPPIC, Vaccines & Injectables Business Unit, for providing us with Montanide ISA71 VG and the material to prepare an emulsion with our antigens, Dr. Dolores Gavier-Widen, SVA, for organizing histological work and for photomicrographs, as well as Dr. Mikael Andersson Franko, SLU, for his feedback on statistical analysis.

## Author Contributions

Conceived and designed the experiments: KB SH JP JFE SR GT JFV. Performed the experiments: KB SH JF CD BMP MT PK JLR EK JP JFE SR GT JFV. Analyzed the data: KB SH JF CD BMP MT EK JP JFE SR GT JFV. Contributed reagents/materials/analysis tools: KB SH JFE SR GT JFV. Wrote the paper: KB SH JF CD BMP MT PK JLR EK JP JFE SR GT JFV.

## References

1. Valarcher J-F, Taylor G (2007) Bovine respiratory syncytial virus infection. Vet Res 38: 153–180. doi:10.1051/vetres:2006053.

2. Seiffert SN, Hilty M, Perreten V, Endimiani A (2013) Extended-spectrum cephalosporin-resistant gram-negative organisms in livestock: An emerging problem for human health? Drug Resist Updat. doi:10.1016/j.drup.2012.12.001.

3. Fulton RW (2009) Bovine respiratory disease research (1983–2009). Anim Health Res Rev 10: 131–139. doi:10.1017/S146625230999012X.

4. Kimman TG, Zimmer GM, Westenbrink F, Mars J, van Leeuwen E (1988) Epidemiological study of bovine respiratory syncytial virus infections in calves: influence of maternal antibodies on the outcome of disease. Vet Rec 123: 104–109.

5. Kimman TG, Westenbrink F, Straver PJ (1989) Priming for local and systemic antibody memory responses to bovine respiratory syncytial virus: effect of amount of virus, virus replication, route of administration and maternal antibodies. Vet Immunol Immunopathol 22: 145–160.

6. Chase CCL, Hurley DJ, Reber AJ (2008) Neonatal immune development in the calf and its impact on vaccine response. Vet Clin North Am Food Anim Pract 24: 87–104. doi:10.1016/j.cvfa.2007.11.001.

7. Nair H, Nokes DJ, Gessner BD, Dherani M, Madhi SA, et al. (2010) Global burden of acute lower respiratory infections due to respiratory syncytial virus in young children: a systematic review and meta-analysis. Lancet 375: 1545–1555. doi:10.1016/S0140-6736(10)60206-1.

8. Westenbrink F, Kimman TG, Brinkhof JM (1989) Analysis of the antibody response to bovine respiratory syncytial virus proteins in calves. J Gen Virol 70 (Pt 3): 591–601.

9. Walsh EE, Hall CB, Briselli M, Brandriss MW, Schlesinger JJ (1987) Immunization with glycoprotein subunits of respiratory syncytial virus to protect cotton rats against viral infection. J Infect Dis 155: 1198–1204.

10. Taylor G, Thomas LH, Furze JM, Cook RS, Wyld SG, et al. (1997) Recombinant vaccinia viruses expressing the F, G or N, but not the M2, protein of bovine respiratory syncytial virus (BRSV) induce resistance to BRSV challenge in the calf and protect against the development of pneumonic lesions. J Gen Virol 78 (Pt 12): 3195–3206.

11. Taylor G, Bruce C, Barbet AF, Wyld SG, Thomas LH (2005) DNA vaccination against respiratory syncytial virus in young calves. Vaccine 23: 1242–1250. doi:10.1016/j.vaccine.2004.09.005.

12. Hägglund S, Hu K, Vargmar K, Poré L, Olofson A-S, et al. (2011) Bovine respiratory syncytial virus ISCOMs-Immunity, protection and safety in young conventional calves. Vaccine 29: 8719–8730. doi:10.1016/j.vaccine.2011.07.146.

13. Kimman TG, Westenbrink F, Schreuder BE, Straver PJ (1987) Local and systemic antibody response to bovine respiratory syncytial virus infection and reinfection in calves with and without maternal antibodies. J Clin Microbiol 25: 1097–1106.

14. Gaddum RM, Cook RS, Furze JM, Ellis SA, Taylor G (2003) Recognition of bovine respiratory syncytial virus proteins by bovine CD8+ T lymphocytes. Immunology 108: 220–229.

15. Taylor G, Thomas LH, Wyld SG, Furze J, Sopp P, et al. (1995) Role of T-lymphocyte subsets in recovery from respiratory syncytial virus infection in calves. J Virol 69: 6658–6664.

16. Rudraraju R, Jones BG, Sealy R, Surman SL, Hurwitz JL (2013) Respiratory syncytial virus: current progress in vaccine development. Viruses 5: 577–594. doi:10.3390/v5020577.

17. Kim HW, Canchola JG, Brandt CD, Pyles G, Chanock RM, et al. (1969) Respiratory syncytial virus disease in infants despite prior administration of antigenic inactivated vaccine. Am J Epidemiol 89: 422–434.

18. Ellis J, Gow S, West K, Waldner C, Rhodes C, et al. (2007) Response of calves to challenge exposure with virulent bovine respiratory syncytial virus following intranasal administration of vaccines formulated for parenteral administration. J Am Vet Med Assoc 230: 233–243. doi:10.2460/javma.230.2.233.

19. Kimman TG, Sol J, Westenbrink F, Straver PJ (1989) A severe outbreak of respiratory tract disease associated with bovine respiratory syncytial virus probably enhanced by vaccination with modified live vaccine. Vet Q 11: 250–253. doi:10.1080/01652176.1989.9694231.

20. Schreiber P, Matheise JP, Dessy F, Heimann M, Letesson JJ, et al. (2000) High mortality rate associated with bovine respiratory syncytial virus (BRSV) infection in Belgian white blue calves previously vaccinated with an inactivated BRSV vaccine. J Vet Med B Infect Dis Vet Public Health 47: 535–550.

21. Antonis AFG, Schrijver RS, Daus F, Steverink PJGM, Stockhofe N, et al. (2003) Vaccine-induced immunopathology during bovine respiratory syncytial virus infection: exploring the parameters of pathogenesis. J Virol 77: 12067–12073.

22. Meyer G, Deplanche M, Schelcher F (2008) Human and bovine respiratory syncytial virus vaccine research and development. Comp Immunol Microbiol Infect Dis 31: 191–225. doi:10.1016/j.cimid.2007.07.008.

23. Karron RA, Wright PF, Belshe RB, Thumar B, Casey R, et al. (2005) Identification of a recombinant live attenuated respiratory syncytial virus vaccine candidate that is highly attenuated in infants. J Infect Dis 191: 1093–1104. doi:10.1086/427813.

24. Taylor G, Wyld S, Valarcher J-F, Guzman E, Thom M, et al. (2014) Recombinant bovine respiratory syncytial virus with deletion of the SH gene induces increased apoptosis and pro-inflammatory cytokines in vitro, and is attenuated and induces protective immunity in calves. J Gen Virol. doi:10.1099/vir.0.064931-0.

25. Riffault S, Meyer G, Deplanche M, Dubuquoy C, Durand G, et al. (2010) A new subunit vaccine based on nucleoprotein nanoparticles confers partial clinical and virological protection in calves against bovine respiratory syncytial virus. Vaccine 28: 3722–3734. doi:10.1016/j.vaccine.2010.03.008.

26. Stott EJ, Thomas LH, Collins AP, Crouch S, Jebbett J, et al. (1980) A survey of virus infections of the respiratory tract of cattle and their association with disease. J Hyg (Lond) 85: 257–270.

27. Mohanty SB, Ingling AL, Lillie MG (1975) Experimentally induced respiratory syncytial viral infection in calves. Am J Vet Res 36: 417–419.

28. Karger A, Schmidt U, Buchholz UJ (2001) Recombinant bovine respiratory syncytial virus with deletions of the G or SH genes: G and F proteins bind heparin. J Gen Virol 82: 631–640.

29. Valarcher J-F, Furze J, Wyld S, Cook R, Conzelmann K-K, et al. (2003) Role of alpha/beta interferons in the attenuation and immunogenicity of recombinant bovine respiratory syncytial viruses lacking NS proteins. J Virol 77: 8426–8439.

30. Thomas LH, Gourlay RN, Stott EJ, Howard CJ, Bridger JC (1982) A search for new microorganisms in calf pneumonia by the inoculation of gnotobiotic calves. Res Vet Sci 33: 170–182.

31. Tran T-L, Castagné N, Dubosclard V, Noinville S, Koch E, et al. (2009) The respiratory syncytial virus M2-1 protein forms tetramers and interacts with RNA and P in a competitive manner. J Virol 83: 6363–6374. doi:10.1128/JVI.00335-09.

32. Tran T-L, Castagné N, Bhella D, Varela PF, Bernard J, et al. (2007) The nine C-terminal amino acids of the respiratory syncytial virus protein P are necessary and sufficient for binding to ribonucleoprotein complexes in which six ribonucleotides are contacted per N protein protomer. J Gen Virol 88: 196–206. doi:10.1099/vir.0.82282-0.

33. Castagné N, Barbier A, Bernard J, Rezaei H, Huet J-C, et al. (2004) Biochemical characterization of the respiratory syncytial virus P-P and P-N protein complexes and localization of the P protein oligomerization domain. J Gen Virol 85: 1643–1653.

34. Roux X, Dubuquoy C, Durand G, Tran-Tolla T-L, Castagné N, et al. (2008) Sub-nucleocapsid nanoparticles: a nasal vaccine against respiratory syncytial virus. PLoS ONE 3: e1766. doi:10.1371/journal.pone.0001766.

35. Tawar RG, Duquerroy S, Vonrhein C, Varela PF, Damier-Piolle L, et al. (2009) Crystal structure of a nucleocapsid-like nucleoprotein-RNA complex of respiratory syncytial virus. Science 326: 1279–1283. doi:10.1126/science.1177634.

36. Larsen LE, Uttenthal A, Arctander P, Tjørnehøj K, Viuff B, et al. (1998) Serological and genetic characterisation of bovine respiratory syncytial virus (BRSV) indicates that Danish isolates belong to the intermediate subgroup: no evidence of a selective effect on the variability of G protein nucleotide sequence by prior cell culture adaption and passages in cell culture or calves. Vet Microbiol 62: 265–279.

37. Chargelegue D, Obeid OE, Hsu SC, Shaw MD, Denbury AN, et al. (1998) A peptide mimic of a protective epitope of respiratory syncytial virus selected from a combinatorial library induces virus-neutralizing antibodies and reduces viral load in vivo. J Virol 72: 2040–2046.

38. Arbiza J, Taylor G, López JA, Furze J, Wyld S, et al. (1992) Characterization of two antigenic sites recognized by neutralizing monoclonal antibodies directed against the fusion glycoprotein of human respiratory syncytial virus. J Gen Virol 73 (Pt 9): 2225–2234.

39. Furze JM, Roberts SR, Wertz GW, Taylor G (1997) Antigenically distinct G glycoproteins of BRSV strains share a high degree of genetic homogeneity. Virology 231: 48–58. doi:10.1006/viro.1997.8490.

40. McLellan JS, Yang Y, Graham BS, Kwong PD (2011) Structure of respiratory syncytial virus fusion glycoprotein in the postfusion conformation reveals preservation of neutralizing epitopes. J Virol 85: 7788–7796. doi:10.1128/JVI.00555-11.

41. Uttenthal A, Larsen LE, Philipsen JS, Tjørnehøj K, Viuff B, et al. (2000) Antibody dynamics in BRSV-infected Danish dairy herds as determined by isotype-specific immunoglobulins. Vet Microbiol 76: 329–341.

42. Kennedy HE, Jones BV, Tucker EM, Ford NJ, Clarke SW, et al. (1988) Production and characterization of bovine monoclonal antibodies to respiratory syncytial virus. J Gen Virol 69 (Pt 12): 3023–3032.

43. Viuff B, Uttenthal A, Tegtmeier C, Alexandersen S (1996) Sites of replication of bovine respiratory syncytial virus in naturally infected calves as determined by in situ hybridization. Vet Pathol 33: 383–390.

44. Bryson D (1993) Necropsy findings associated with BRSV pneumonia. Vet Med 88: 894–899.

45. Belyakov IM, Ahlers JD (2009) What role does the route of immunization play in the generation of protective immunity against mucosal pathogens? J Immunol 183: 6883–6892. doi:10.4049/jimmunol.0901466.

46. Wu S-J, Schmidt A, Beil EJ, Day ND, Branigan PJ, et al. (2007) Characterization of the epitope for anti-human respiratory syncytial virus F protein monoclonal antibody 101F using synthetic peptides and genetic approaches. J Gen Virol 88: 2719–2723. doi:10.1099/vir.0.82753-0.

47. Thomas LH, Cook RS, Wyld SG, Furze JM, Taylor G (1998) Passive protection of gnotobiotic calves using monoclonal antibodies directed at different epitopes on the fusion protein of bovine respiratory syncytial virus. J Infect Dis 177: 874–880.

48. Bastien N, Taylor G, Thomas LH, Wyld SG, Simard C, et al. (1997) Immunization with a peptide derived from the G glycoprotein of bovine respiratory syncytial virus (BRSV) reduces the incidence of BRSV-associated pneumonia in the natural host. Vaccine 15: 1385–1390.

49. Fogg MH, Parsons KR, Thomas LH, Taylor G (2001) Identification of CD4+ T cell epitopes on the fusion (F) and attachment (G) proteins of bovine respiratory syncytial virus (BRSV). Vaccine 19: 3226–3240.

50. Hervé P-L, Raliou M, Bourdieu C, Dubuquoy C, Petit-Camurdan A, et al. (2014) A novel subnucleocapsid nanoplatform for mucosal vaccination against influenza virus that targets the ectodomain of matrix protein 2. J Virol 88: 325–338. doi:10.1128/JVI.01141-13.

51. Samal SK, Zamora M, McPhillips TH, Mohanty SB (1991) Molecular cloning and sequence analysis of bovine respiratory syncytial virus mRNA encoding the major nucleocapsid protein. Virology 180: 453–456.

52. Mallipeddi SK, Samal SK (1992) Sequence comparison between the phosphoprotein mRNAs of human and bovine respiratory syncytial viruses identifies a divergent domain in the predicted protein. J Gen Virol 73 (Pt 9): 2441–2444.

53. Zamora M, Samal SK (1992) Sequence analysis of M2 mRNA of bovine respiratory syncytial virus obtained from an F-M2 dicistronic mRNA suggests structural homology with that of human respiratory syncytial virus. J Gen Virol 73 (Pt 3): 737–741.

54. Piazza FM, Johnson SA, Darnell ME, Porter DD, Hemming VG, et al. (1993) Bovine respiratory syncytial virus protects cotton rats against human respiratory syncytial virus infection. J Virol 67: 1503–1510.

55. Buchholz UJ, Granzow H, Schuldt K, Whitehead SS, Murphy BR, et al. (2000) Chimeric bovine respiratory syncytial virus with glycoprotein gene substitutions from human respiratory syncytial virus (HRSV): effects on host range and evaluation as a live-attenuated HRSV vaccine. J Virol 74: 1187–1199.

56. Thomas LH, Stott EJ, Collins AP, Crouch S, Jebbett J (1984) Infection of gnotobiotic calves with a bovine and human isolate of respiratory syncytial virus. Modification of the response by dexamethasone. Arch Virol 79: 67–77.

57. McLellan JS, Chen M, Joyce MG, Sastry M, Stewart-Jones GBE, et al. (2013) Structure-based design of a fusion glycoprotein vaccine for respiratory syncytial virus. Science 342: 592–598. doi:10.1126/science.1243283.

58. Aucouturier J, Dupuis L, Ganne V (2001) Adjuvants designed for veterinary and human vaccines. Vaccine 19: 2666–2672.

59. Duewell P, Kisser U, Heckelsmiller K, Hoves S, Stoitzner P, et al. (2011) ISCOMATRIX Adjuvant Combines Immune Activation with Antigen Delivery to Dendritic Cells In Vivo Leading to Effective Cross-Priming of CD8+ T Cells. J Immunol. Available: http://www.ncbi.nlm.nih.gov/pubmed/21613613. Accessed 30 May 2011.

60. Robson NC, Donachie AM, Mowat AM (2008) Simultaneous presentation and cross-presentation of immune-stimulating complex-associated cognate antigen by antigen-specific B cells. Eur J Immunol 38: 1238–1246. doi:10.1002/eji.200737758.

61. Schnurr M, Orban M, Robson NC, Shin A, Braley H, et al. (2009) ISCOMATRIX adjuvant induces efficient cross-presentation of tumor antigen by dendritic cells via rapid cytosolic antigen delivery and processing via tripeptidyl peptidase II. J Immunol 182: 1253–1259.

62. Hägglund S, Hu K-F, Larsen LE, Hakhverdyan M, Valarcher J-F, et al. (2004) Bovine respiratory syncytial virus ISCOMs–protection in the presence of maternal antibodies. Vaccine 23: 646–655. doi:10.1016/j.vaccine.2004.07.006.

63. Hägglund S, Hu K, Blodörn K, Makabi-Panzu B, Gaillard A-L, et al. (2014) Characterization of an experimental vaccine for bovine respiratory syncytial virus. Clin Vaccine Immunol: CVI.00162-14. doi:10.1128/CVI.00162-14.

64. Ellis JA, Gow SP, Mahan S, Leyh R (2013) Duration of immunity to experimental infection with bovine respiratory syncytial virus following intranasal vaccination of young passively immune calves. J Am Vet Med Assoc 243: 1602–1608. doi:10.2460/javma.243.11.1602.

65. Paton DJ, de Clercq K, Greiner M, Dekker A, Brocchi E, et al. (2006) Application of non-structural protein antibody tests in substantiating freedom from foot-and-mouth disease virus infection after emergency vaccination of cattle. Vaccine 24: 6503–6512. doi:10.1016/j.vaccine.2006.06.032.

66. Valarcher JF, Schelcher F, Bourhy H (2000) Evolution of bovine respiratory syncytial virus. J Virol 74: 10714–10728.

# 2

# Demographic Processes Drive Increases in Wildlife Disease following Population Reduction

**Jamie C. Prentice**[1,2,3], **Glenn Marion**[2]*, **Piran C. L. White**[3], **Ross S. Davidson**[1], **Michael R. Hutchings**[1]

**1** Disease Systems Team, SRUC, Edinburgh, United Kingdom, **2** Biomathematics and Statistics Scotland, Edinburgh, United Kingdom, **3** Environment Department, University of York, York, United Kingdom

## Abstract

Population reduction is often used as a control strategy when managing infectious diseases in wildlife populations in order to reduce host density below a critical threshold. However, population reduction can disrupt existing social and demographic structures leading to changes in observed host behaviour that may result in enhanced disease transmission. Such effects have been observed in several disease systems, notably badgers and bovine tuberculosis. Here we characterise the fundamental properties of disease systems for which such effects undermine the disease control benefits of population reduction. By quantifying the size of response to population reduction in terms of enhanced transmission within a generic non-spatial model, the properties of disease systems in which such effects reduce or even reverse the disease control benefits of population reduction are identified. If population reduction is not sufficiently severe, then enhanced transmission can lead to the counter intuitive perturbation effect, whereby disease levels increase or persist where they would otherwise die out. Perturbation effects are largest for systems with low levels of disease, e.g. low levels of endemicity or emerging disease. Analysis of a stochastic spatial meta-population model of demography and disease dynamics leads to qualitatively similar conclusions. Moreover, enhanced transmission itself is found to arise as an emergent property of density dependent dispersal in such systems. This spatial analysis also shows that, below some threshold, population reduction can rapidly increase the area affected by disease, potentially expanding risks to sympatric species. Our results suggest that the impact of population reduction on social and demographic structures is likely to undermine disease control in many systems, and in severe cases leads to the perturbation effect. Social and demographic mechanisms that enhance transmission following population reduction should therefore be routinely considered when designing control programmes.

**Editor:** Maciej F. Boni, University of Oxford, Viet Nam

**Funding:** SRUC and Biomathematics and Statistics Scotland (BioSS) receive funding from the Scottish Government. This work was also supported by the EU (project number 212414). The funders had no role in study design, data collection and analysis, decision to publish, or preparation of the manuscript.

**Competing Interests:** The authors have declared that no competing interests exist.

* E-mail: glenn@bioss.ac.uk

## Introduction

The relevance of ecology to understanding the dynamics and persistence of infectious disease has long been recognised [1], and ecological factors are critical to wildlife disease systems. Control of disease in wildlife is of considerable importance for managing risks to humans [2,3] and livestock [4,5], as well as for the conservation of wildlife species themselves [3,6–8]. Population reduction is a commonly employed strategy used to control disease in wildlife [9,10] with the aim of reducing the number of infected animals and the overall size of key populations, leading to a reduction in rates of transmission, disease prevalence and risks to other populations. Application of this strategy is supported by theoretical evidence of a threshold for disease persistence below which disease does not spread quickly enough to persist, and eventually dies out [9,11,12]. However, there is growing evidence that population reduction may be less effective than standard analyses predict, and in some cases be counter-productive (see below). Such unexpected increases in disease prevalence following population reduction have been termed the "perturbation effect" [13]. The theoretical basis and empirical evidence for disease thresholds in wildlife has

been reviewed [14], concluding that important elements of wildlife ecology are neglected by current theories.

It is known that the social and spatial structure of host populations has significant implications for disease persistence and prevalence [15,16]. Population reduction disrupts existing social structures and this may lead to increased numbers of contacts [17] and/or a greater proportion of agonistic encounters within or between groups [18,19]. Similarly, a change in susceptibility of individual hosts may also occur as a consequence of population reduction due to stress [20]. Both effects will enhance disease transmission and are likely to be widespread and reduce or even reverse the efficacy of population reduction measures.

For example, management of rabies in foxes (*Vulpes vulpes*) has shown that vaccination is more suitable than culling, as the latter can destabilise social structure and lead to enhanced transmission rates [10,21]. Studies of the management of classical swine fever (CSF) in wild boar (*Sus scrofa*) recommend that hunting should cease following detection of the disease [22], in order to discourage dispersal of infected individuals, and reduce risks to neighbouring groups [10]. The U.K. Randomised Badger Control Trial (RBCT) [23] showed that reactive culling of badgers (*Meles meles* in response to a confirmed bovine tuberculosis (*Mycobacterium bovis*, bTB) herd breakdown in cattle, was associated with a 27% increase in the incidence of confirmed breakdowns, relative to survey-only trials [24]. Repeated reactive culling was also associated with increased bTB prevalence in badgers [25].

In this paper we study the potential for behavioural and demographic aspects of the ecology of wildlife species to reduce or reverse the efficacy of population reduction as a means of disease control. Our results are based on the analytical and numerical treatment of generic models of demography and disease dynamics in wildlife populations. In a non-spatial context we analyse the potential that individual and collective behavioural responses to population reduction have on disease control. We use this framework to explore the demographic and epidemiological characteristics of wildlife disease systems that make them susceptible to such effects. We then demonstrate that such impacts arise as an emergent property of spatial models of wildlife disease systems with density dependent dispersal. Finally we discuss the significance of these results for disease control in wildlife.

## Methods

### A non-spatial deterministic model of demography and disease dynamics

We examine a generic single pathogen wildlife disease system with a fluctuating host population. The number of susceptible and infected individuals in the population at time $t$ are $S(t)$ and $I(t)$ respectively, and the total population size is given by $N(t) = S(t) + I(t)$. We assume density dependent (logistic) growth, with intrinsic reproduction rate $r$ (the maximum rate that individuals can reproduce in optimal circumstances), limited by a carrying capacity $c$ (the population size for which the density limited per-capita birth rate reaches zero — note this is not necessarily the same as the population equilibrium [26,27], since mortality, including that induced by disease and population reduction, will prevent the population from attaining this maximum). Natural mortality (from causes unrelated to disease or explicit population reduction measures) occurs at constant per-capita rate $d$, while disease induced mortality occurs at constant per-capita rate $e$. The rate of infection is a combination of susceptibility and contact rates between susceptible and infective individuals and here we consider density dependent infection (i.e. disease transmission depends on the density of infectives, $I$) with horizontal transmission rate $\beta$.

We model population reduction as a constant per-capita death rate $p$ which applies to all individuals regardless of disease status. As noted earlier such measures can alter host behaviour and hence contact rates. We therefore model the horizontal disease transmission rate as $\beta + kp$. Here $k > 0$ represents any mechanism or combination of mechanisms that lead to increased contact rates or susceptibility in a host population subjected to population reduction at rate $p$. Note that this formulation represents a simplification in that the effect is linear in $p$, there is no lag as $p$ changes and the effect is constant for the duration of the population reduction event.

In Appendix S1 (see Supporting Information, File S1), we show how to formulate a simple non-spatial deterministic model that encapsulates the above assumptions. We also simplify this representation, removing the variables $c$ and $r$ by respectively scaling the variables $S$, $I$ and $N$ by $1/c$ to obtain values between 0 (empty) and 1 (at carrying capacity) and rescaling time by $r$ (see Appendix S1.2, Eqn. S1 in File S1). Analysis can then focus on the effects of population characteristics (parameters $d$ and $e$), disease dynamics ($\beta$), population reduction ($p$), enhanced transmission ($k$) and the interactions between them. However, results for specific values of $c$ and $r$ can still be obtained by appropriate back scaling.

The rescaled deterministic ordinary differential equations (ODEs) that combine the demography and disease dynamics described above with population reduction and a corresponding enhanced transmission resulting from explicit behavioural and implicit ecological (system) responses are given by:

$$\dot{S} = N(1 - N) - (d + p)S - (\beta + kp)SI \tag{1}$$

$$\dot{I} = -(d + e + p)I + (\beta + kp)SI$$

Three fixed points of this system of equations are derived in the Supporting Information: population extinction, where $\{S, I\} = \{0, 0\}$; the disease free equilibrium, where $\{S, I\} = \{1 - d - p, 0\}$; and the endemic equilibrium $\{S, I\} = \{S^*(p), I^*(p)\}$, where both the population and the disease persist (note that it is possible for $I^*(p)$ to be negative, in which case $I(t) \to 0$, since there cannot be a negative number of individuals). The stability properties of these equilibria are discussed in Appendix S1.4 in File S1. Note that we write the endemic equilibrium as a function of the reduction rate $p$, even though it also depends on other parameters, because we are particularly interested in the effect of population reduction.

### A spatial stochastic model of demography and disease dynamics

In the stochastic spatial model we consider a set of sites where, at time $t$, the integer number of susceptibles and infectives in site $i$ are $S_i(t)$ and $I_i(t)$ respectively. Since we are dealing with numbers of individuals these are not rescaled as above. The demography and disease dynamics of each sub-population are governed by the same processes as for the non-spatial model, with the addition of dispersal and disease transmission within and between groups.

Dispersal is the movement of individuals between social groups, for the purposes of obtaining more resources such as food or reproductive opportunities (including inbreeding avoidance). In the model dispersal from any given site occurs at constant per-capita rate $m$, into any of its nearest neighbouring sites. However, since this process may be mediated by the population levels in the destination site [28–30] this is modified by a function $f(N_j)$, where $N_j$ is the population at neighbouring site $j$. We consider a step function

$$f(N_j) = \begin{cases} 1 & \text{if } N_j < \alpha N_{DF}^* \\ 0 & \text{if } N_j \geq \alpha N_{DF}^* \end{cases} \tag{2}$$

where $N_{DF}^* = c(1 - d/r)$ is the population size in the disease free equilibrium, and $\alpha$ is the fraction of the disease free equilibrium at which the neighbouring site becomes accessible. Dispersal rates may also be affected by conditions in the source area, e.g. due to overpopulation, social exclusion, or lack of resources, lack of mating opportunities in small populations; however, we do not consider these effects here.

Disease transmission rates within and between groups are denoted $\beta_w$ and $\beta_b$ respectively. The horizontal disease transmission rate in site $i$ is therefore given by

$$H_i = \beta_w S_i I_i + \beta_b S_i \sum_j I_j$$

where the sum is over neighbouring sites of $i$. The total infection rate is given by $H = \sum_i H_i$ and the effective disease transmission rate is defined as

$$\beta_{\text{eff}} = \frac{H}{(\sum_i S_i)(\sum_i I_i)}$$

The spatial model is implemented as a discrete state-space Markov process, to account for demographic stochasticity, with events and associated rates shown in Table 1, and simulated using the Gillespie algorithm [31]. In the spatial model population reduction is parametrised by the probability that a site is targeted $p_1$ and the rate of removal of individuals within targeted sites $p_2$.

## Measuring the perturbation effect

We define the magnitude of the perturbation effect at time $t$ after the application of population reduction at rate $p$ to be

$$\Pi(t;p) = I(t;p) - I(t;0) \qquad (3)$$

A population that is in equilibrium $I^*(0)$ prior to the application of population reduction at rate $p$, will reach a new equilibrium $I^*(p)$. We define the persistent perturbation effect

$$\Pi_{\text{eqm}} = \max\{I^*(p),0\} - \max\{I^*(0),0\} \qquad (4)$$

Note that $I^*(p)$ may be negative, in which case the equilibrium is no longer stable and cannot be reached, and so $I(t) \to 0$, hence the restrictions (see Appendix S1.4 in File S1 for more details). In the results, we study both the persistent $\Pi_{\text{eqm}}$ and transient $\Pi(t;p)$ perturbation effects. In the spatial case we also examine the proportion of sites containing infectives, $P_I(t;p)$, as the basis for measuring the perturbation effect

$$\Pi_{\text{sites}}(t;p) = P_I(t;p) - P_I(t;0) \qquad (5)$$

## Results

### Explicit enhancement of disease transmission induced by population reduction

We first consider the perturbation effect in the deterministic non-spatial model. Several features of the perturbation effect caused by increased horizontal disease transmission in response to population reduction are demonstrated in Fig. 1. For different levels of transmission enhancement $k$, a range of outcomes are possible when a population in the endemic equilibrium $I^*(0)$

(disease endemic before intervention starts), is subjected to sustained population reduction at rate $p$ (see Fig. 1A). The long term equilibrium $I^*(p)$ increases with $k$ (i.e. the effectiveness of population reduction reduces) and when $k$ is greater than some critical value $k_p$, $\Pi_{\text{eqm}} > 0$. However, another behaviour is also apparent: when $k$ approaches a lower threshold $k_t$, there is a temporary increase in $I(t)$, which results in $\Pi(t;p) > 0$ for a short period, despite no perturbation effect in the long term ($\Pi_{\text{eqm}} < 0$). We call these two increases the persistent and the transient perturbation effect, and examine their properties in the following sections. Both persistent and transient perturbation effects are also possible in the case of emerging disease (when starting from close to the disease free equilibrium) (see Fig. 1B).

Behaviour in the long-term equilibrium can be seen by plotting the endemic equilibrium $I^*(p)$ versus population reduction rate $p$, for several values of the horizontal transmission rate $\beta$. Three important points are evident (see Fig. 1C). First, persistent population reduction at a sufficiently intense rate does reduce the level of disease, leading to $I^*(p) < I^*(0)$. Second, the maximum size of the persistent perturbation effect reduces as the horizontal transmission rate increases, with no perturbation effect present in the deterministic model for $\beta$ sufficiently high. Finally, increased horizontal transmission induced by population reduction can allow the disease to persist, where it would otherwise fade out in the absence of culling.

## Persistent perturbation effect with no disease induced mortality

We now explore the properties of the persistent perturbation effect $\Pi_{\text{eqm}}$ in more detail. For clarity we focus on the algebraically simpler case where there is no disease induced mortality, $e = 0$, and technical details of the analysis are given in Appendix S1.5 (in File S1). Subsequently we apply numerical analysis to Eqn. 1 with disease induced mortality $e > 0$.

Case 1: Disease persists without population reduction, $I^*(0) > 0$
In this case there is a perturbation effect if

$$\Pi_1 = \Pi_{\text{eqm}} = -p - \frac{d+p}{\beta+kp} + \frac{d}{\beta} > 0$$

**Minimum disease enhancement required to produce perturbation effect.** Note that when $k = 0$, we obtain $\Pi_1 = -p(1 + 1/\beta)$, which is always negative, showing that culling reduces disease when there is no mechanism enhancing disease transmission. Rearranging gives a threshold value of $k$, above which a perturbation effect is possible

**Table 1.** Default event rates for the stochastic *SI* model.

| Event | Rate | $\delta S_i$ | $\delta I_i$ | $\delta S_j$ | $\delta I_j$ |
|---|---|---|---|---|---|
| Birth of $S_i$ | $rN_i(1 - N_i/c)\delta t$ | +1 | 0 | 0 | 0 |
| Death of $S_i$ | $dS_i\delta t$ | −1 | 0 | 0 | 0 |
| Death of $I_i$ | $(d+e)I_i\delta t$ | 0 | −1 | 0 | 0 |
| Infection of $S_i$ | $H_i\delta t$ | −1 | +1 | 0 | 0 |
| Dispersal of $S_i$ to site $j$ | $mzS_if(N_j)\delta t$ | −1 | 0 | +1 | 0 |
| Dispersal of $I_i$ to site $j$ | $mzI_if(N_j)\delta t$ | 0 | −1 | 0 | +1 |

Event rates and corresponding effects in the spatial stochastic model. $H_i$ and $f(N_j)$ are defined in the methods.

**Table 2.** List of parameters used in the deterministic and stochastic *SI* models.

| Parameter | Symbol | Non-spatial | Spatial |
|---|---|---|---|
| Intrinsic reproduction rate | $r$ | 1 | 1 |
| Carrying capacity | $c$ | 1 | 20 |
| Natural mortality rate | $d$ | 0.2 | 0.01 |
| Disease induced mortality rate | $e$ | 0.1 | 0.1 |
| Horizontal transmission rate | $\beta$ | 0.4 | — |
| background | $\beta_e$ | — | 0 |
| within group | $\beta_w$ | — | 0.5 |
| between groups | $\beta_b$ | — | 0 |
| Dispersal rate | $m$ | — | 0.1 |
| threshold value | $\alpha$ | — | 0.7 |
| Population reduction rate | $p$ | 0.1 | — |
| coverage | $p_1$ | — | 0.2 |
| removal within sites | $p_2$ | — | 0.5 |
| Disease enhancement | $k$ | 5 | — |

A summary of the parameters and their symbols used in the non-spatial and spatial models are described here. Values shown indicate both the parameters and their default values used in the spatial and non-spatial models.

$$k > k_1 = \frac{\beta(1+\beta)}{d - p\beta}$$

There is a lower bound on this threshold, such that $k_1 > \beta(1+\beta)/d > (1+\beta) > 1$ (since the disease is able to persist, which requires that $\beta > d/(1-d) > d$, hence $\beta/d > 1$).

**High disease prevalence precludes a perturbation effect.** As $\beta \to \infty$, $\Pi_1 \to -p$, showing that for sufficiently high $\beta$, the perturbation effect cannot occur in the deterministic model. In fact in this case there is an upper bound, $\beta_u$, on the value of $\beta$ for which $\Pi_1 > 0$,

$$\beta < \beta_u = \frac{1}{2}\sqrt{(1+pk)^2 + 4dk} - \frac{1}{2}(1+pk)$$

and $\Pi_1 > 0$ only when $\beta < \beta_u$ (see Fig. 2A for high $\beta$). Similarly, as $d \to 0$, $\Pi_1 \to -p(1+1/(\beta+kp)) < 0$, showing that the perturbation effect is possible only for higher mortality rates. There is a corresponding lower bound on $d$ for which $\Pi_1 > 0$, at

$$d > d_l = \beta(1+\beta+kp)/k$$

(see Fig. 2B, for low $d$). For low $d < d_l$, infectives are removed from the population slowly, and for high $\beta > \beta_u$, the disease spreads quickly; either situation leads to disease saturation, with insufficient susceptibles to allow for a perturbation effect.

**High rates of population reduction will reduce disease levels.** A simple observation is that a persistent perturbation effect is possible (for any model) only if the population size under persistent culling is greater than the equilibrium number of infected individuals without population reduction i.e. $N^*(p) > I^*(0)$ which implies that there is an upper bound on the culling rate, $p = d/\beta$, above which population reduction will reduce disease (see Appendix S1.5 in File S1). This is also evident in $k_1$ (the lower bound for $k$) which diverges as $p \to d/\beta$ from below implying that, in order to see a perturbation effect, population reduction must produce ever greater enhanced transmission $k$ as $p$

approaches this critical level. Furthermore (see Appendix S1.5 in File S1), we show that the range of $p$ that permits the perturbation effect also depends on $k$ and is given by

$$0 < p < \frac{d}{\beta} - \frac{1+\beta}{k}$$

This is illustrated in Fig. 1C, where the range of $p$ for which $I^*(0) < I^*(p)$ decreases with $\beta$, and that for sufficiently large $p$, $I^*(p) < 0$ for all $\beta$.

Case 2: Disease does not persist without population reduction, $I^*(0) > 0$

**Population reduction can allow disease to persist where it would naturally fade out.** In this case there is a persistent perturbation effect if the disease is only able to persist under continued population reduction for a given $p$ and $k$, i.e. when

$$\Pi_2 = \Pi_{eqm} = 1 - d - p - \frac{d+p}{\beta+kp} > 0$$

The conditions for which the disease is only able to persist under population reduction are detailed in Appendix S1.4 in File S1. The minimum $k$ in order to make the endemic equilibrium $I^*(p) > 0$ following population reduction is

$$k > k_2 = \frac{d+p-\beta(1-d-p)}{p(1-d-p)}$$

and therefore sufficiently large $k$ can lead to a perturbation effect under these conditions. For example, given $d = 0.2, p = 0$, $I^*(0) < 0$ for $\beta < 0.25$; however, given $d = 0.2, \beta = 0.2$, (thus unable to persist for $p = 0$), when population reduction is applied at rate $p = 0.1$, then $I^*(p = 0.1) > 0$ for $k > k_2 = 2.286$, therefore the disease can persist as long as population reduction is sustained, leading to a perturbation effect (see Fig. 1C, for $\beta = 0.2$).

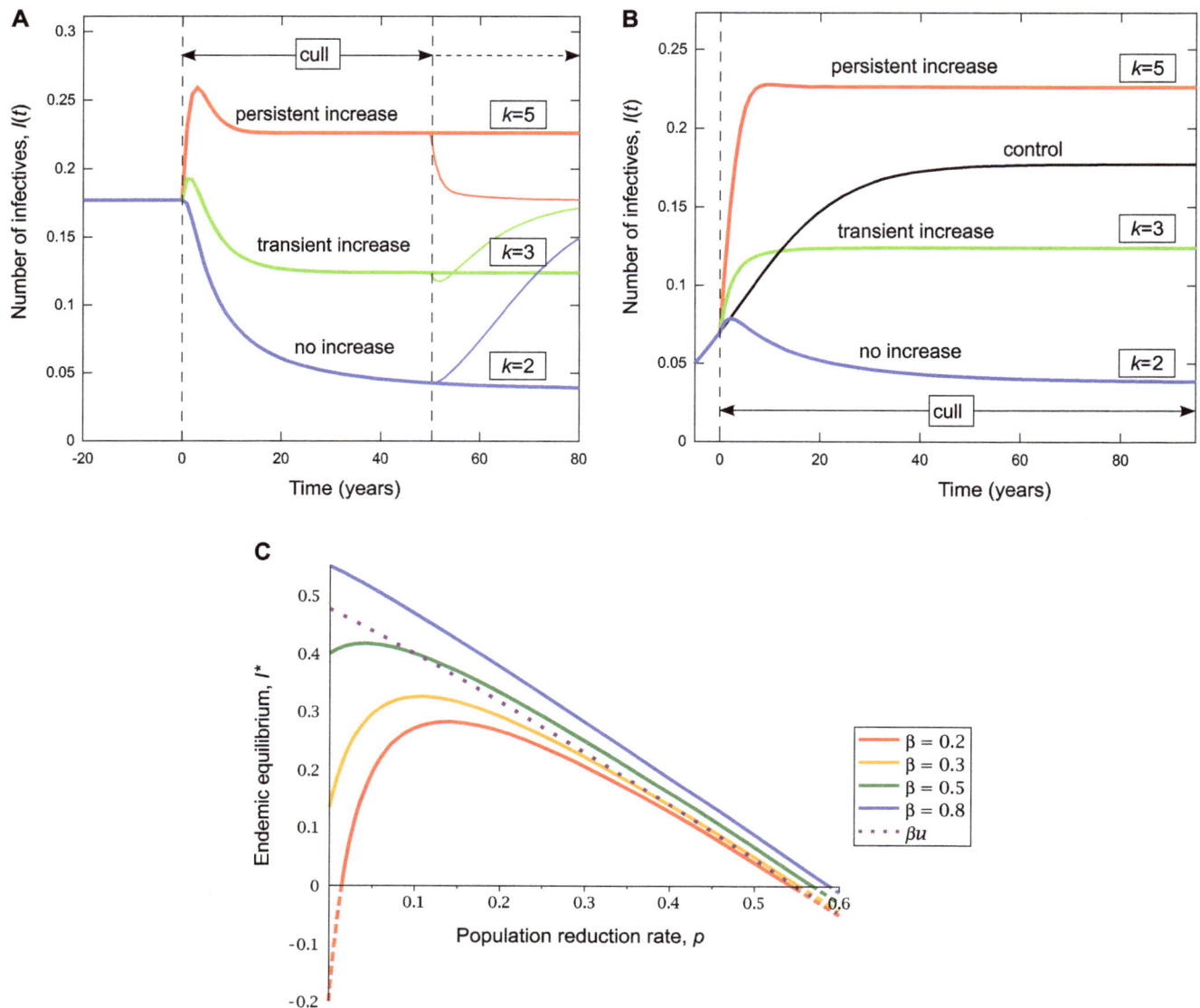

**Figure 1. Deterministic simulation of $I(t)$, and algebraic solution of $I^*(p)$.** The results of ongoing population reduction are shown for various levels of disease enhancement $k$ in (A) endemic disease, (B) emergent disease (starting near the disease free equilibrium, $I(0) = 0.05$). (C) shows the endemic equilibrium for varying $\beta$. The lines cut the vertical axis at $I^*(0)$, and so the perturbation effect occurs whenever a line rises above this value. Note that for $\beta = 0.2$, the equilibrium is negative for small $p$ (which cannot be reached, since only a non-negative number of individuals is biologically possible), and so if any disease is introduced for $p = 0$, it moves to the disease free equilibrium $I^*_{DF} = 0$, and the perturbation effect does not occur until $p$ is sufficiently high. The dotted line shows $\beta_u$ (see text for details), marking the upper bound of $\beta$ for given $p$ for which the perturbation effect is possible, and crosses each line at the point where the increase no longer occurs for that value of $\beta$ ($\beta_u$ is also illustrated in Fig. 2A). Parameters are given in Table 2, except $p = 0.2$ in (A) and (B).

## Persistent perturbation effect with disease induced mortality

We now investigate the persistent perturbation effect in the more complex situation with disease induced mortality $e > 0$ by solving Eqn. 1 numerically to show how $\Pi_{eqm}$ varies with $e$ itself, and also with horizontal disease transmission $\beta$, background mortality $d$, and enhanced transmission $k$ resulting from population reduction.

Numerical analysis of the role of transmission rate $\beta$ is consistent with the analysis of the previous section (see Fig. 2A). Under case 1 (where $I^*(0) \geq 0$ and $\Pi = \Pi_1$), $\Pi$ decreases with $\beta$ and no perturbation is possible for $\beta > \beta_u$ because the disease has

saturated the population, whereas in case 2 (where $I^*(0) < 0$ and $\Pi = \Pi_2$), $\Pi$ increases with $\beta$, and there is a lower limit below which the disease becomes extinct despite enhanced disease transmission. This is in accordance with analysis of $\Pi_1$ and $\Pi_2$ (see Appendix S1.5 in File S1, and above).

The role of natural mortality $d$ is also consistent with the previous analysis (see Fig. 2B). In the region of case 1, there is a lower bound $d_l$, below which the perturbation effect is not possible due to disease saturation, and above which $\Pi$ increases with $d$. In the region of case 2, $\Pi$ decreases with $d$, and there is an upper limit on $d$, above which the disease becomes unable to persist despite

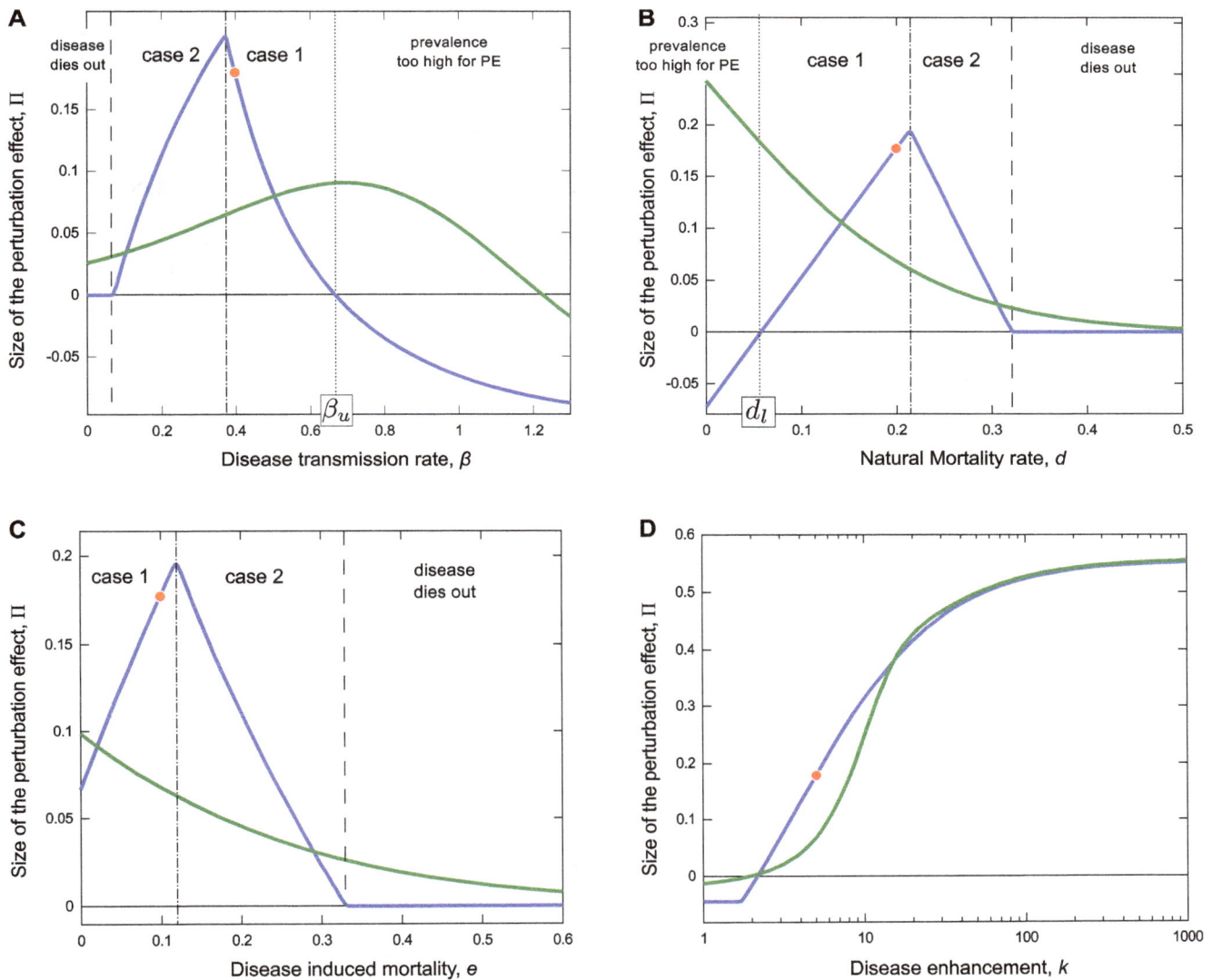

**Figure 2. Sensitivity analysis of the persistent and transient perturbation effects in the deterministic model.** Parameter values as in Table 2 and marked by a red dot when explicitly varied, the transient perturbation (green) is shown for $t = 5$, the persistent perturbation (blue) $\Pi_{eqm}$ is evaluated at $t = 1,000$. The transient perturbation: (A) has an optimum for intermediate $\beta$, decays with (B) natural and (C) disease induced mortality, and (D) increases with $k$. With the exception of (D), the behaviour of the persistent perturbation is more complex. In (A) to the left of $I^*(p) = 0$ (dashed vertical line) $\beta$ is low and there is no perturbation ($I^*(p) < 0$). To the right of $I^*(p) = I^*(0)$ (dotted vertical line corresponding to upper bound $\beta_u$, see text) the prevalence in the absence of culling is sufficiently high to prevent a perturbation. The central region between $I^*(p) = 0$ and $I^*(p) = I^*(0)$ is divided by a third vertical line $I^*(0) = 0$ (dot dashed), independent of $k$ and $p$, into regions corresponding to case 1 ($I^*(0) > 0$) where the disease persists the absence of population reduction, and case 2 ($I^*(0) < 0$) where it does not (see text for details). The maximum persistent perturbation occurs at this boundary. Under case 2, population reduction is sufficient to stabilise the endemic equilibrium. In (B) as natural mortality $d$ increases from zero (moving left to right) $I^*(0)$ *decreases*, and the pattern seen in (A) is reversed. Here the dotted vertical line $I^*(p) = I^*(0)$ denotes the lower bound $d_l$. (C) shows the impact of disease induced mortality $e$ is similar to that of natural mortality, but the chosen parameter values mean that prevalence is never too high to prevent a perturbation effect. Note: dotted and dashed lines are reversed when $k$ is too low for the perturbation effect to occur, leaving no room for cases 1 and 2. See Fig. 4 for analogous spatial model results.

enhanced transmission. The role of disease induced mortality $e$, is broadly similar to that of $d$ (see Fig. 2C).

The impact of the disease enhancement parameter $k$ on the perturbation effect is illustrated for case 1 in Fig. 2D. $\Pi$ increases with $k$, tending to an asymptote as $k \to \infty$, while there is no perturbation effect below the threshold $k_1$. The behaviour under case 2 (not shown) is broadly similar with a different lower bound $k_2$ and lower asymptote.

## Maximising the persistent perturbation effect

An important addendum to these results is related to the conditions that maximise the perturbation effect. For low mortality rates $d$ or $e$, or high transmission rate $\beta$, the disease is able to persist before and during population reduction, the prevalence is very high and there is little room for further increase. As mortality increases or transmission decreases, the size of the perturbation effect $\Pi_{eqm}$ increases until $\beta = (d + e)/(1 - d)$, where the endemic equilibrium becomes negative, and the disease becomes unable to persist for $p = 0$ (as in case 2). After this point, as mortality increases, or transmission decreases, $\Pi_{\text{eqm}}$ decreases, until mortality is too high, or transmission is too low to maintain the disease either before or during population reduction. This implies that the maximum perturbation effect occurs when $I^*(0) \approx 0$ and $I^*(p) > 0$. Therefore in practice, the persistent perturbation effect is most likely in a disease with very low prevalence. These results can be seen graphically in Fig. 2.

## Transient perturbation effect

The transient perturbation effect can be assessed by linearising the system and examining the rate of change of $\Pi(t; p)$ with respect to time, at time $t = 0$, which is positive (i.e. the disease increases faster under population reduction) only if $I \in (0, N - 1/k)$ (see Appendix S2.1 in File S1). To obtain an initial increase in disease levels there must be some infectives, but similar to the results in the persistent case, too many infectives will prevent a transient perturbation effect; as $k$ increases a transient perturbation effect is possible for ever larger numbers of infectives. The lower bound here is equivalent to $k > k_t = 1/S$ and since $S \in (0,1)$, this requires that $k_t > 1$; therefore, the transient perturbation effect does not occur in the absence of a change in behaviour. It is also possible to show that the transient perturbation effect increases fastest when $S = N/2 + 1/2k$ and $I = N/2 - 1/2k$ (i.e. roughly equal numbers of susceptibles and infectives) and that $\dot{\Pi}(0; p)$ increases with both $p$ and $k$ (see Appendix S2 in File S1 for details). Also, a temporary peak, where $I(t) > I^*(p)$ may occur, if the disease increases quickly before culling reduces the population size $N$; this can be observed in both endemic and emerging disease cases (see Fig. 1).

**Starting from the endemic equilibrium.** Consider the case where the disease is in the endemic equilibrium $\{S^*, I^*\}$ prior to disease intervention (as shown in Fig. 1A). We show in Appendix S2 (in File S1) that $k_t = \beta/(d + e)$ so that the minimum disease enhancement required for a transient perturbation effect is reduced when the infection rate $\beta$ is small and mortality rates $d$ and $e$ are large. In addition $k_t < k_p$ (where $k_p$ is the relevant $k_1$ or $k_2$) and the transient perturbation effect occurs for smaller $k$ than the persistent perturbation effect. Consequently, for small $k < k_t$, there is no perturbation effect. For larger $k \in (k_t, k_p)$, $I(t; p) > I(t; 0)$ for small $t$, i.e. the number of infectives is initially larger following disease intervention, however eventually $I(t) \to I^*(p)$ which is less than the initial level $I^*(0)$, and in this case the increase is temporary. However, for $k > k_p$, the number of infectives increases and remains higher than the control.

**Starting from near the disease free equilibrium.** The situation is somewhat different in the case of an emerging outbreak where $I(0) = \epsilon$ where $\epsilon > 0$ is small, and $S(0) = S_{\text{DF}}^* - \epsilon$, as shown in Fig. 1B ($S_{\text{DF}}^*$ is $S$ in the disease free equilibrium, see Appendix S1.3 in File S1). Here, $k_t = 1/(1 - d - \epsilon)$ (see Appendix S2.2 in File S1), and so the minimum disease enhancement required for a transient perturbation effect is reduced when the initial prevalence is low (although contrary to the persistent perturbation effect, when mortality rates are also low). Fig. 2 shows the impact of varying $d$, $e$, $\beta$ and $k$ on the transient perturbation effect for the case of an emerging outbreak where $I(0) = \epsilon$ where $\epsilon > 0$ is small, and $S(0) = S_{\text{DF}}^* - \epsilon$. These numerical results show that the transient perturbation effect monotonically decreases with both natural and disease induced mortality, whilst it monotonically increases with enhanced transmission $k$. The disease transmission rate $\beta$ affects the time disease takes to reach equilibrium, and therefore small $\beta$ can result in a slow initial increase (and small transient perturbation effect), while very large $\beta$ can saturate the population and prevent the transient perturbation effect from occurring at the time considered; the largest increase therefore occurs with an

intermediate value of $\beta$, although this will vary depending on the time at which the transient perturbation effect is assessed.

These results contrast with those for the persistent perturbation effect (also shown in Fig. 2), demonstrating that conditions required for the transient and persistent perturbation effect are not necessarily the same for both emerging and endemic disease.

## Implicit enhancement of disease transmission induced by population reduction

We now show how the intrinsic dynamics of a natural spatial formulation of disease transmission and demography may give rise to an increased effective horizontal transmission when population reduction is applied, leading to an implicit perturbation effect. The non-spatial results of the previous section suggest that perturbation is strongest when disease prevalence is relatively low and where population reduction is intermediate, and gives rise to a sufficiently large increase in the horizontal transmission rate.

We begin by demonstrating the importance of heterogeneity in the model, and show through analysis of the horizontal infection rate in a simple two-site model that in the spatial model such an enhancement of the transmission rate will be strongest in situations where infection levels are most heterogeneous between groups.

## Heterogeneity and the perturbation effect in the spatial model

Consider a simple two-site model, with density dependent dispersal between the two groups A and B. The global infection rate $H$ is

$$H = H_A + H_B = \beta_w(S_A I_A + S_B I_B) + \beta_b(S_A I_B + S_B I_A)$$

Assuming disease induced mortality rate $e = 0$, then $N_A = N_B = N$, and the number of infectives is $I_A + I_B = I$, thus $H$ can be simplified to

$$H = \text{constant} + 2(\beta_w - \beta_b)(I - I_A)I_A$$

revealing that when between-group infection rate $\beta_b$ is small, and $\beta_w > \beta_b$, $H$ is maximised when the infection is distributed evenly between sub-populations, and $I_A = I_B$. Conversely, $H$ is minimised when $I_A = 0$ or $I_A = I$ (i.e. all infectives are restricted to one of the groups).

In order to quantify enhanced transmission resulting from population reduction, consider the rate of change of the global infection rate $H$ (differentiated with respect to time) to obtain

$$\dot{H} = \beta_w(\dot{S}_A I_A + S_A \dot{I}_A + \dot{S}_B I_B + S_B \dot{I}_B)$$
$$+ \beta_b(\dot{S}_A I_B + S_A \dot{I}_B + \dot{S}_B I_A + S_B \dot{I}_A)$$

While $\dot{H}$ is affected by all processes, including birth, death, infection and dispersal, if we only examine the effect of dispersal on $\dot{H}$ by substituting only the relevant components ($\dot{S}_A = \ldots + m S_B f(N) - m S_A f(N)$ etc.) then we obtain

$$\dot{H}_{\text{dispersal}} = 2m(\beta_w - \beta_b)(I_A - I_B)^2 f(N)$$

Consequently, if $\beta_w > \beta_b$ and $I_A \neq I_B$, then the effect of dispersal is to increase $\dot{H}$. Moreover, this rate of increase in horizontal disease transmission is greatest for heterogeneously distributed disease (larger difference $I_A - I_B$), and for larger dispersal rate $m$. The presence of the density dependence function $f(N)$ shows that it is

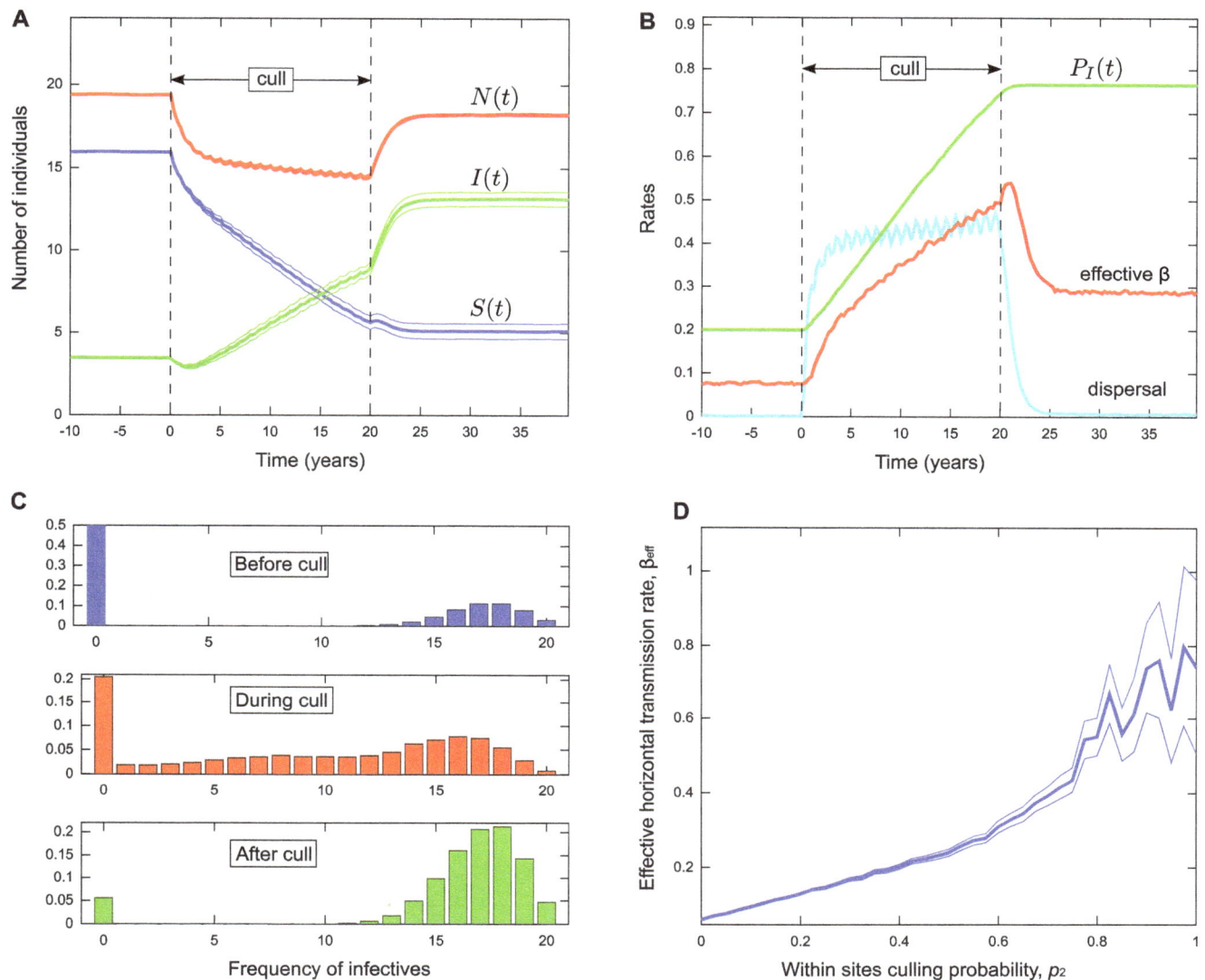

**Figure 3. Time trajectories and heterogeneity for emergent disease in the stochastic model.** (A) Population numbers, $S(t)$, $I(t)$, and $N(t)$. (B) Proportion of sub-populations containing infectives, $P_I(t)$, effective transmission rate $\beta$, and dispersal rate. (C) Distribution of $I$ across sites. (D) Effective transmission rate $\beta$ for disease transmission vs population reduction coverage $p_1$. Parameters are given in Table 2, and initial conditions are at the disease free equilibrium $\{S,I\} = \{20,0\}$, while in 20% of sites randomly chosen, a single individual is infected, resulting in $\{S,I\} = \{19,1\}$. Population reduction occurs annually from years 50–69, and in $p_1 = 20\%$ of sites (chosen randomly each year) the removal rate is set to $p_2 = 1.0$, without regard to disease status (equivalent to an overall culling rate of $p = 0.2$). An initial reduction in $I$ is rapidly replaced by an increase, which is due to the increased chance of invasion of naïve groups by infectives due to the density dependent dispersal. The CI for the effective transmission rate increases for large $p_1$ due to the increasing number of simulations where the disease becomes extinct.

greater for smaller $N$, which will follow as a consequence of population reduction. Note that the formula for $H$ shows that a large $\beta_b$ will lead to rapid spread between sites, quickly spreading to sub-populations, and reducing spatial heterogeneity in the distribution of disease.

## Initial conditions

Given the above discussion, when studying the spatial model we focus on cases where disease is distributed heterogeneously between groups and overall prevalence is low. This is most easily achieved when the system is close to the disease free equilibrium with: (i) disease maintained in each site by high within-site transmission rate $\beta_w$ and low mortality; (ii) low levels of disease transmission between sites; and (iii) relatively large and stable

populations at each site leading to low levels of dispersal between sites. Under this scenario, even in the absence of population reduction, the number of sites infected, and thus overall prevalence, tends to slowly increase (from close to the disease free equilibrium) as rare dispersal or transmission events spread disease. Fig. 3 (discussed in detail below) shows how transient perturbation effects occur in such a system. In contrast, we show in Appendix S3.2 (in File S1) that by making both disease and population less stable within sites it is possible to achieve a dynamic quasi-equilibrium (quasi- because the ultimate fate of all simulations of this model is total extinction) where the spread of disease to uninfected sites is balanced by spontaneous recovery of infected sites, e.g. through death of infectives and birth of susceptible individuals. When the system is in such an endemic

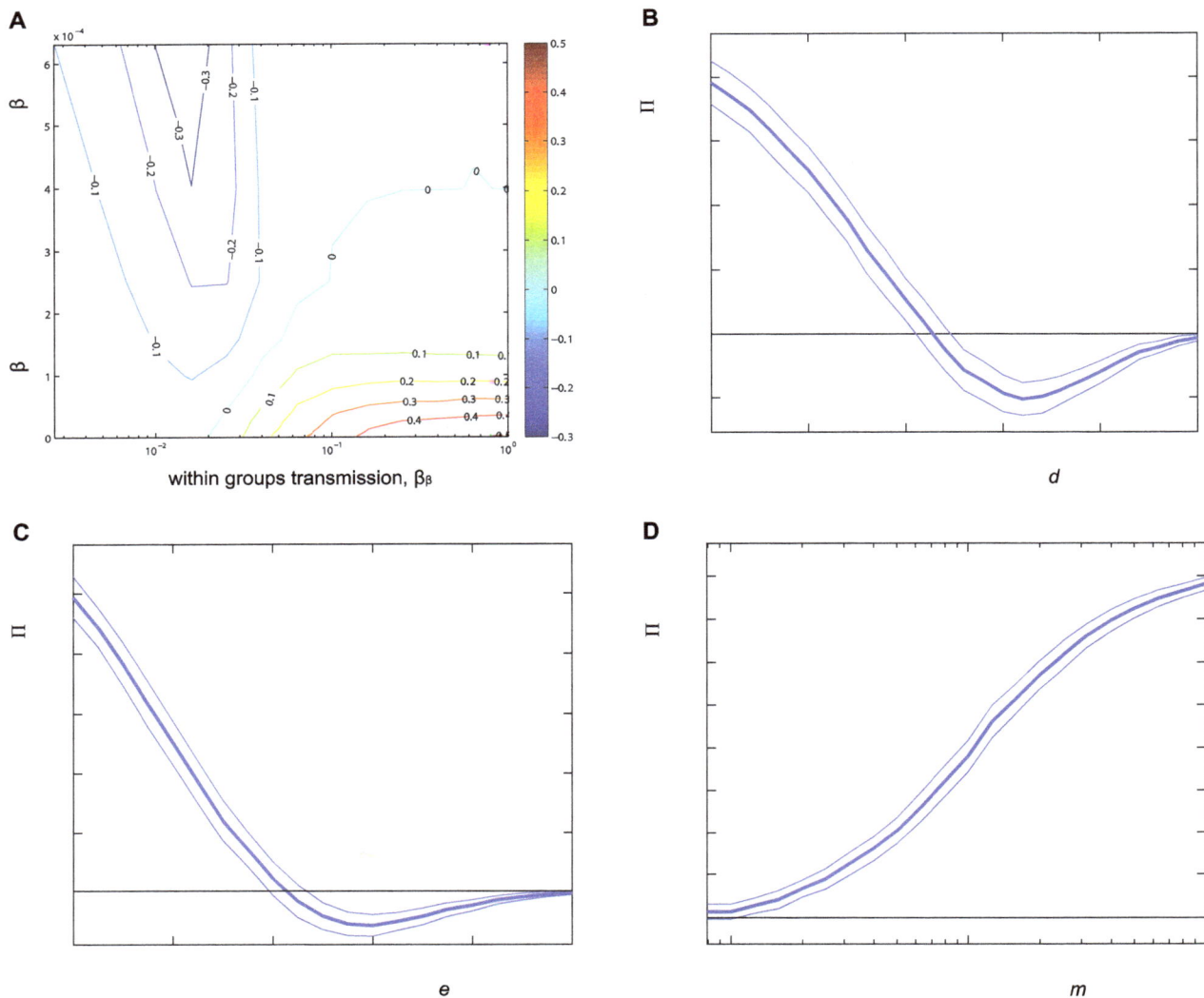

**Figure 4. Sensitivity analysis of $\Pi$ in the stochastic model.** The size of the perturbation effect, $\Pi_{\text{sites}}$, at time $t = 20$ starting near the disease free equilibrium for (A) Between and within-groups infection rates $\beta_b$ and $\beta_w$ (log scale). (B) Natural mortality rate $d$. (C) Disease induced mortality rate $e$. (D) Dispersal rate $m$ (log scale). Default parameters are given in Table 2, and one parameter is varied at a time. This is analogous to Fig. 2 for the non-spatial case. Initial conditions are such that 20% of sites are randomly chosen to start near the endemic equilibrium (with a minimum of 1 infective), while the remainder begin at the disease free equilibrium.

state population reduction leads to a persistent perturbation effect, as we saw in the non-spatial model (see Fig. S2 in File S1). However, this endemic state is very sensitive to the balance between site-level establishment and recovery of disease which makes it difficult to explore variation in the perturbation effect with respect to the value of key parameters. We therefore focus attention on the transient perturbation effect when starting close to the disease free state in the spatial model.

## Transient perturbation effect in the spatial model

The behaviour during population reduction in the spatial model is shown for the population values $S(t)$, $I(t)$, and $N(t)$ (see Fig. 3A), and the proportion of infected sites $P_I(t)$, dispersal rates and effective transmission rate $\beta_{\text{eff}}$ (see Fig. 3B). The distribution of infectives between sites is shown in Fig. 3C before, during, and after population reduction. Prior to population reduction, sites can

be classified as disease-free or infected. During population reduction, the typical level of disease within sites decreases, but the number of infected sites increases. When population reduction ceases, typical prevalence in infected sites returns to previous levels which, given that there are now more of them, leads to a rapid increase in global prevalence. Some light may be shed on the mechanisms behind such changes, as population reduction leads to a large increase in dispersal, followed by increasing rates of horizontal disease transmission, $H$ (see Fig. 3B). Population reduction disrupts the stable demographic structure (shown in Fig. 3C) leading to an increase in the dispersal rate and movement of infectives to previously disease free sites. This *vacuum effect* [5,26] emerges from the spatial model's density dependent dispersal and leads to increased transmission. The effective horizontal transmission rate parameter varies with population reduction effort $p_1$: for small $p_1$, there is an almost linear increase in $\beta_{\text{eff}}$ (see Fig. 3D), which agrees well with the explicit increase assumed to be $\beta_{\text{eff}} = \beta + kp$ in the non-spatial model. However, one key difference (as shown in Fig. 3B), is that the increase is not immediate, but grows linearly with time — an effect not accounted for by our earlier analysis.

We now explore the sensitivity of this perturbation effect with respect to key aspects of demography and disease dynamics. The results are broadly consistent with those obtained when starting close to the disease free equilibrium in the non-spatial model. Fig. 4 shows results for parameters analogous to those in Fig. 2, and that $\Pi$ decreases with mortality rates $d$ and $e$ and increases with dispersal rate $m$ (similar to $k$ in the non-spatial case). The role of disease transmission is more complex. The perturbation effect decreases with between-group infection rate $\beta_b$ which reduces the number of disease free sites, and increases with $\beta_w$, which increases disease persistence within sites. Thus for small $\beta_b$ and sufficient $\beta_w$, population reduction is able to spread disease to uninfected sites where it is able to persist. We also explore the impact of varying the threshold parameter $\alpha$ that determines how sensitive the rate of dispersal is to local reductions in the size of the population in the destination site (see Appendix S3.1 and Fig. S1 in File S1). Results show that a perturbation effect occurs for a wide range of values, although the largest effects are seen for $\alpha$ around 0.9 (we suspect the largest increase would be observed for $\alpha$ near $1 - p_2$). Perturbation effects were also found for alternative forms of the density dependent dispersal function $f(N_k)$ (results not shown).

## Discussion

In this paper we explored the impact on disease control of enhanced transmission resulting from individual or demographic responses to population reduction. Using a generic non-spatial and deterministic model of demography and disease dynamics we explored the potential for such effects to reduce and reverse the disease control benefits of population reduction. We found that there was a threshold of enhanced transmission above which a perturbation effect occurred, whereby the number of infected individuals increases during the period when population reduction is applied. However, sufficient population reduction (the level rising with mortality rates $d$ and $e$ and disease enhancement $k$, but decreasing with infection rate $\beta$) will always reduce numbers of infectives in the area it is applied. Disease systems with low levels of disease are more sensitive to the impacts of enhanced transmission. For systems with endemic disease, the potential for the perturbation effect increases with natural and disease induced mortality rates (due to reduced levels of endemic disease), with the opposite trend where disease is emerging, as higher mortality removes cases caused by enhanced transmission. With respect to the horizontal transmission rate, the perturbation effect in endemic disease is maximised for small to intermediate $\beta$ (at the point where the disease changes its ability to persist in the absence of population reduction). For emerging disease however, higher $\beta$ causes the disease to reach equilibrium sooner, but reduces the size of the perturbation effect, so the earlier the disease is measured, the higher the optimal $\beta$, but the weaker the perturbation. Enhanced transmission effects can also lead to disease being maintained by population reduction in systems where it would otherwise die out.

We also considered a spatially explicit model that represents demographic fluctuations and disease transmission within locally well mixed populations, and dispersal and disease transmission

between such groups. In this context we found that enhanced transmission emerged implicitly as a demographic response to population reduction when dispersal was density dependent. This enhancement would be increased if individuals explicitly changed their behaviour, e.g. by dispersing more or by increasing agonistic interactions and therefore disease contacts between groups (i.e. increasing $\beta_b$). However, the implicit dispersal mechanism alone was sufficient to give rise to a perturbation effect. We found that the system was susceptible to enhanced transmission in both the case of endemic and emerging diseases when infection was heterogeneously distributed among groups and when overall levels of disease were relatively low. For emerging disease we showed that the impact of mortality rates was qualitatively similar to the predictions of the non-spatial analysis. In the spatial model, dispersal rate played a similar role to the non-spatial enhancement parameter $k$, whereas the role of horizontal disease transmission is not directly comparable between the two cases. In the spatial context, higher within-group transmission increased the size of the perturbation effect, but even low rates of between-group transmission reduced it. Analysis of the effective contact rate in the spatial model reveals that enhanced transmission varied in time and this could be incorporated in future analysis of the non-spatial system. It is worth noting that the linear assumption $kp$ for disease enhancement is reasonable, at least early in disease intervention period, and for low removal rate $p$.

Many authors have noted problems related to disease control via population reduction in wildlife [10,21,22,24,32], including situations were disease risks are increased rather than reduced [13,25]. Individual behavioural [18–20] and demographic [33] responses to population reduction are thought to enhance disease transmission in wildlife. One system of particular relevance is TB in badgers, where the disease is spatially heterogeneous [34], transmission between groups is weak, and the host exhibits density dependent dispersal [29,30,35]. Thus TB in badgers is a disease system exhibiting many of the properties this paper shows are likely to lead to the perturbation effect, and we note that the RBCT [23] did indeed show that culling was associated with an increase in bTB prevalence in badgers [25]. Moreover, the results of this paper suggest that a wide range of wildlife disease systems are sensitive to such effects, and this is consistent with the marked inefficiencies of population reduction as a disease control strategy observed to date. However, the effects studied here are likely to be even more widespread than current empirical studies suggest as they undermine the efficacy of population reduction measures even in situations where they do not lead to a complete reversal of its effectiveness.

## Acknowledgments

We would like to thank three reviewers for their helpful comments which greatly improved the manuscript.

## Author Contributions

Conceived and designed the experiments: JCP GM RSD PCLW MRH. Performed the experiments: JCP GM RSD MRH. Analyzed the data: JCP GM RSD MRH. Wrote the paper: JCP GM RSD PCLW MRH.

# References

1. Anderson R (1991) Populations and infectious diseases: ecology or epidemiology? Journal of Animal Ecology 60: 1–50.
2. Jones KE, Patel NG, Levy MA, Storeygard A, Balk D, et al. (2008) Global trends in emerging infectious diseases. Nature 451: 990–994.
3. Daszak P, Cunningham AA, Hyatt AD (2000) Emerging infectious diseases of wildlife – threats to biodiversity and human health. Science 287: 443–449.
4. Frölich K, Thiede S, Kozikowski T, Jakob W (2002) Review of mutual transmission of important infectious diseases between livestock and wildlife in europe. Annals of the New York Academy of Sciences 969: 4–13.
5. Gortázar C, Ferroglio E, Höfle U, Frölich K, Vicente J (2007) Diseases shared between wildlife and livestock: a European perspective. European Journal of Wildlife Research 53: 241–256.
6. Cunningham AA (1996) Disease risks of wildlife translocations. Conservation Biology 10: 349–353.
7. Daszak P, Cunningham AA, Hyatt AD (2001) Anthropogenic environmental change and the emergence of infectious diseases in wildlife. Acta Tropica 78: 103–116.
8. Evensen DT (2008) Wildlife disease can put conservation at risk. Nature 452: 282.
9. Wobeser GA (1994) Investigation and management of disease in wild animals. New York: Plenum Press.
10. Artois M, Delahay R, Guberti V, Cheeseman C (2001) Control of infectious diseases of wildlife in Europe. The Veterinary Journal 162: 141–152.
11. Anderson RM, May RM (1979) Population biology of infectious diseases: Part I. Nature 280: 361–367.
12. Carter SP, Roy SS, Cowan DP, Massei G, Smith GC, et al. (2009) Options for the control of disease 2: targeting hosts. In: Delahay RJ, Smith GC, Hutchings MR, editors, Management of disease in wild mammals, Tokyo, Japan: Springer, chapter 7. pp. 121–146. doi:10.1007/978-4-431-77134-0-7
13. Carter SP, Delahay RJ, Smith GC, Macdonald DW, Riordan P, et al. (2007) Culling-induced social perturbation in Eurasian badgers *Meles meles* and the management of TB in cattle: an analysis of a critical problem in applied ecology. Proceedings of the Royal Society of London B 274: 2769–2777.
14. Lloyd-Smith JO, Cross PC, Briggs CJ, Daugherty M, Getz WM, et al. (2005b) Should we expect population thresholds for wildlife disease? Trends in Ecology and Evolution 20: 511–519.
15. Keeling M (1999) The effects of local spatial structure on epidemiological invasions. Proceedings of the Royal Society of London B 266: 859–867.
16. Davidson RS, Marion G, Hutchings MR (2008) Effects of host social hierarchy on disease persistence. Journal of Theoretical Biology 253: 424–433.
17. Tuyttens F, Delahay R, Macdonald D, Cheeseman C, Long B, et al. (2000a) Spatial perturbation caused by a badger (*Meles meles*) culling operation: implications for the function of territoriality and the control of bovine tuberculosis (*Mycobacterium bovis*). Journal of Animal Ecology 69: 815–828.
18. Swinton J, Tuyttens F, Macdonald D, Nokes D, Cheeseman C, et al. (1997) Comparison of fertility control and lethal control of bovine tuberculosis in badgers: the impact of perturbation induced transmission. Philosophical Transactions of the Royal Society of London B 352: 619–631.
19. Tuyttens F, Macdonald D (2000) Consequences of social perturbation for wildlife management and conservation. In: Gosling L, Sutherland W, editors, Behaviour and Conservation, Cambridge: Cambridge University Press. pp. 315–329.
20. Gallagher J, Clifton-Hadley R (2000) Tuberculosis in badgers; a review of the disease and its significance for other animals. Research in Veterinary Science 69: 203–217.
21. Macdonald D (1995) Wildlife rabies: the implications for Britain - unresolved questions for the control of wildlife rabies: social perturbation and interspecific interactions. In: Rabies in a Changing World, Cheltenham, UK: Proceedings of the British Small Animal Veterinary Association. pp. 33–48.
22. Guberti V, Rutili D, Ferrari G, Patta C, Oggiano A (1998) Estimate of the threshold abundance for the persistence of the classical swine fever in the wild population of Eastern Sardinia. In: Measures to control classical swine fever in European wild boar. pp. 54–61.
23. Independent Scientific Group (2007) Bovine TB: the scientific evidence. A science base for a sustainable strategy to control TB in cattle. Final report of the Independent Scientific Group on Cattle TB. Technical report, HMSO, London.
24. Donnelly C, Woodroffe R, Cox D, Bourne J, Gettinby G, et al. (2003) Impact of localized badger culling on tuberculosis incidence in British cattle. Nature 426: 834–837.
25. Vial F, Donnelly CA (2012) Localized reactive badger culling increases risk of bovine tuberculosis in nearby cattle herds. Biology Letters 8: 50–53.
26. Ginzburg LR (1992) Evolutionary consequences of basic growth equations. Trends in Ecology and Evolution 7: 133.
27. Hui C (2006) Carrying capacity, population equilibrium, and environment's maximal load. Ecological Modelling 192: 317–320.
28. Johst K, Brandl R (1997) The effect of dispersal on local population dynamics. Ecological Modelling 104: 87–101.
29. Bodin C, Benhamou S, Poulle ML (2006) What do European badgers (*Meles meles*) know about the spatial organisation of neighbouring groups? Behavioural Processes 72: 84–90.
30. Lintott R, Norma R, Hoyle A (2013) The impact of increased dispersal in response to disease control in patchy environments. Journal of Theoretical Biology 323: 57–68.
31. Keeling MJ, Rohani P (2007) Modelling Infectious Diseases in Humans and Animals. Princeton, NJ: Princeton University Press.
32. Woodroffe R, Donnelly CA, Cox D, Bourne FJ, Cheeseman C, et al. (2006a) Effects of culling on badger *Meles meles* spatial organization: implications for the control of bovine tuberculosis. Journal of Applied Ecology 43: 1–10.
33. Smith G, Cheeseman C, Wilkinson D, Clifton-Hadley R (2001b) A model of bovine tuberculosis in the badger *Meles meles*: the inclusion of cattle and use of a live test. Journal of Applied Ecology 38: 520–535.
34. Delahay R, Langton S, Smith G, Clifton-Hadley R, Cheeseman C (2000) The spatio-temporal distribution of *Mycobacterium bovis* (bovine tuberculosis) infection in a high-density badger population. Journal of Animal Ecology 69: 428–441.
35. Macdonald DW, Newman C, Buesching CD, Johnson PJ (2008) Male-biased movement in a highdensity population of the Eurasian badger (*Meles meles*). Journal of Mammalogy 89: 1077–1086.

# 3

# Long-Term Assessment of Wild Boar Harvesting and Cattle Removal for Bovine Tuberculosis Control in Free Ranging Populations

Gregorio Mentaberre[1]*, Beatriz Romero[2,3], Lucía de Juan[2,3], Nora Navarro-González[1], Roser Velarde[1], Ana Mateos[3], Ignasi Marco[1], Xavier Olivé-Boix[5], Lucas Domínguez[2,3], Santiago Lavín[1], Emmanuel Serrano[1,4]

1 Servei d'Ecopatologia de Fauna Salvatge (SEFaS), Departament de Medicina i Cirurgia Animal, Facultat de Veterinària, Universitat Autònoma de Barcelona, Bellaterra, Barcelona, Spain, 2 VISAVET Health Surveillance Centre. Universidad Complutense, Madrid, Spain, 3 Departamento de Sanidad Animal. Facultad de Veterinaria, Universidad Complutense, Madrid, Spain, 4 Estadística i Investigació Operativa, Departament de Matemàtica. Universitat de Lleida, Lleida, Spain, 5 Reserva Nacional de Caça dels Ports de Tortosa i Beseit, Roquetes, Tarragona, Spain

## Abstract

Wild boar is a recognized reservoir of bovine tuberculosis (TB) in the Mediterranean ecosystems, but information is scarce outside of hotspots in southern Spain. We describe the first high-prevalence focus of TB in a non-managed wild boar population in northern Spain and the result of eight years of TB management. Measures implemented for disease control included the control of the local wild boar population through culling and stamping out of a sympatric infected cattle herd. Post-mortem inspection for detection of tuberculosis-like lesions as well as cultures from selected head and cervical lymph nodes was done in 745 wild boar, 355 Iberian ibexes and five cattle between 2004 and 2012. The seasonal prevalence of TB reached 70% amongst adult wild boar and ten different spoligotypes and 13 MIRU-VNTR profiles were detected, although more than half of the isolates were included in the same clonal complex. Only 11% of infected boars had generalized lesions. None of the ibexes were affected, supporting their irrelevance in the epidemiology of TB. An infected cattle herd grazed the zone where 168 of the 197 infected boars were harvested. Cattle removal and wild boar culling together contributed to a decrease in TB prevalence. The need for holistic, sustained over time, intensive and adapted TB control strategies taking into account the multi-host nature of the disease is highlighted. The potential risk for tuberculosis emergence in wildlife scenarios where the risk is assumed to be low should be addressed.

**Editor:** Joao Inacio, National Institute for Agriculture and Veterinary Research, IP (INIAV, I.P.), Portugal

**Funding:** This work has been funded by the Ministry of Science and Innovation within the Programme of Interaction between wild animals and livestock (FAU2006-00011 and FAU2008-00021). The funders had no role in study design, data collection and analysis, decision to publish, or preparation of the manuscript. No additional external funding was received for this study.

**Competing Interests:** The authors have declared that no competing interests exist.

* E-mail: caprapyrenaica@gmail.com

## Introduction

### Epidemiology

The ever-growing impact of wildlife reservoirs in the epidemiology of bovine tuberculosis (TB) has become clear in the recent decades worldwide [1]. Hence, although the effectiveness of TB eradication programs in cattle has been considerable [2], success also depends on the absence or control of wildlife reservoirs [3–5]. Under natural conditions, the multi-host nature of this disease would render ineffective any control strategy that overlooks the ecology, susceptibility, behaviour and abundance of the whole host community [4–6]. As a result, understanding the role of each host species in the maintenance and transmission of the disease is essential to designing any measures for TB control [1,6].

In the last decade, a large number of species have been identified as spill-over, maintenance and/or reservoir hosts in the wild [1]. Wild boar (*Sus scrofa*) and, to a lesser extent, red deer (*Cervus elaphus*) are considered maintenance hosts of TB in the Iberian Peninsula and often suggested as reservoirs for livestock

[7–9]. The link between wild and domestic ungulates in the epidemiology of TB has been confirmed in southern Spain through genotype mapping [10,11]. This finding along with the persistence of high TB prevalence in wild boar populations isolated from livestock for decades and lesion pattern characteristics indicating infection and excretion routes have been key factors for recognizing its role as a true reservoir in the Mediterranean ecosystems [8]. This situation is especially concerning for EU animal health policies given the huge increase in wild boar populations [12]. The problem is magnified in southern Spain mainly by the existence of estates where extensive livestock coexist with managed wild ungulate populations with up to 90 individuals/km$^2$ aimed at commercial hunting [12,13]. In contrast to this, game management of wildlife is anecdotal in the northern part of the country and generally in Europe [7,9,14].

### Management

In line with compulsory tests and slaughter campaigns implemented in livestock, enormous efforts are underway for TB control in wildlife [6,15–18]. Different strategies have been adopted for this purpose, with culling of the reservoir the most common in the case of game, feral or pest species. In some cases, wildlife culling may be socially unacceptable [19], not sufficiently effective [16] or even counter-productive [20] in such a way that additional or alternative measures for TB control are necessary [15,21]. However, since game ungulates are common TB reservoirs in the wild, this strategy may be a suitable option that can be applied as major indiscriminate depopulation exercises or more restricted culling protocols aimed at reducing reservoir density below the theoretical persistence threshold [15,22] or using "capture-test-and-slaughter" protocols where only positive animals are culled [23] in order to appease social and economic concerns [19]. Regarding wild boar, little and contradictory information on the effectiveness of intensive culling for TB control has been recently published. Under similar field (fencing and high densities of ungulates) and treatment conditions, Boadella and cols. succeeded in decreasing TB prevalence by 21–48% after reducing wild boar abundance to half [17], while Garcia-Jimenez and cols. failed to do so [18].

Herein we report the output of eight years of TB monitoring in wild boar, cattle and Iberian ibex (*Capra pyrenaica hispanica*) in a different scenario to that previously described for the Mediterranean ecosystems. Specifically, this is the first high prevalence focus of tuberculosis in wildlife in northern Spain, occurring in a free-ranging (non-fenced), non-intensively managed wild boar population sharing habitat with cattle and ibexes in a national game reserve. In addition, this area lacks other known wild reservoirs of TB in the Iberian Peninsula, red deer (*Cervus elaphus*) and fallow deer (*Dama dama*). This focus of tuberculosis was first detected in 2004 in hunter-harvested wild boar thanks to active disease surveillance in wildlife. We also show the outcome of the combination of two different disease management strategies consisting of intensive culling of wild boar populations and removal of a sympatric infected cattle herd. This is the first attempt to address control of TB in a wild boar population through eradication of sympatric infected cattle (most probably, the original source of infection for wild boar in our study area) in the Mediterranean context. Our main objectives were: (i) to characterize the epidemiology of TB amongst sympatric wild boar, cattle and Iberian ibexes through both the study of macroscopic lesion patterns in wild boar and the genotyping of *Mycobacterium tuberculosis* complex isolates obtained; (ii) to describe spatial and temporal TB patterns in this scenario; (iii) to evaluate whether the implemented disease management strategies succeeded in the control of TB; (iv) and to explore the effects of the intensive culling on the wild boar population structure to better understand the effect of this measure on TB evolution.

## Materials and Methods

### Ethics statement

No approval was needed from any Ethics committee since the animals used in the present study were not sacrificed for research purposes. The harvested wild boar and ibexes included in the present study have been legally hunted (shot) or box-trapped in their own habitat by authorized gamekeepers and hunters within the framework of an annual hunting plan approved by the Departament d'Agricultura, Ramaderia, Pesca, Alimentació i Medi Natural - Generalitat de Catalunya (DARPAMN -the Regional authority in charge of livestock and wildlife management-). Box-trapping and euthanasia of wild boar was promoted and approved by the DARPAMN as an exceptional measure for the control of bovine tuberculosis in the affected area. The bovine tuberculosis positive cows were slaughtered (shock and bleed) in an authorised abattoir according to the guidelines of the Council Directive 64/432/EEC and subsequent modifications on animal health problems affecting intra-Community trade in bovine animals and swine. Hence, no animals were harvested in order to perform this study, but we took advantage of the harvested animals for this aim. Standard protocols of anaesthesia and euthanasia were used to minimize stress and suffering of the box-trapped wild boar and carried out by veterinarians.

### Study area

This focus of tuberculosis is located in the National Game Reserve "Ports de Tortosa i Beseit" (NGRPTB) in north-eastern Spain (40°48′ 28″N, 0 19′ 17″ E) and within the Iberian bio-region 5, as described in [24]. It is a limestone mountain massif of about 28,000 ha that shows a high level of orographic complexity, which results in a rugged and abrupt terrain formed by numerous canyons, ravines and steep slopes. About 28% of the surface is above 1000 m.a.s.l., with the highest peak being Mont Caro (1442 m) and the lower heights around 300 m.a.s.l. The mean annual temperature in the reserve is 13.7°C (min = 1.6°C in December – February, max = 30°C in July – August), while the mean annual accumulated rainfall is 697 mm (min = 536 in 2009, max = 889 in 2011) [25]. The vegetal stratum is characterized by a typical Mediterranean forest dominated by *Quercus ilex* and *Pinus halepensis* with dense scrublands of *Quercus coccifera*, *Pistacea lentiscus* and *Chamaerops humilis*, among others. Patches of non-irrigated crops are also common in the study area, mainly those with olive trees (*Olea europaea*), European carobs (*Ceratonia siliqua*) and almond trees (*Prunus amygdalus*). The average density of Iberian ibexes is 11.1 individuals/km$^2$ (Personal communication; Distance sampling® estimate by the NGRPTB managers) and of wild boar is 3 individuals/km$^2$ (estimate based on hunting bags for the whole NGRPTB), the only wild ungulates that share grazing areas with cattle (cross-breed of Spanish fighting bull) year-round. The farming conditions of cattle in the study area are free-ranging (extensive farming) with supplemental feeding in the dry season (summer).

Ravines and other natural barriers may play an important role driving transmission of infectious diseases [26]. Hence, based on the local orography and the preliminary observations on the TB distribution, we defined three different zones within the study area (Figure 1): TBA (defined as "tuberculosis area"), an area of 2,150 ha where the first cases of TB in wild boar were detected and the disease management has been carried out; OA ("outlying areas") covers 6,380 ha of the surrounding areas that could be potentially affected by the spread of TB from TBA; and DA ("distant areas to TBA"; 8,810 ha.), consisting of two different zones [DA1 and DA2; 3,920 and 4,890 ha., respectively], where TB-positive wild boar have also been detected and TB surveillance has been maintained during the whole study period. No disease management actions have been carried out in either OA or DA.

### Study period

Tuberculosis-like lesions (TBLL) were first detected in the TBA in December 2004, while performing field necropsies of hunter-harvested wild boar, and were later confirmed by culture and isolation of *Mycobacterium bovis*. Since then, wild boar have been harvested by hunting and box-trapping captures year-round, with a peak harvest time in autumn-winter (September – March), coinciding with the regular game season. For this reason, we divided the TB study period (2004–2012) into eight harvesting periods covering July to June of the following year (from 2004–05 to 2011–12). These periods were conceived to include the regular

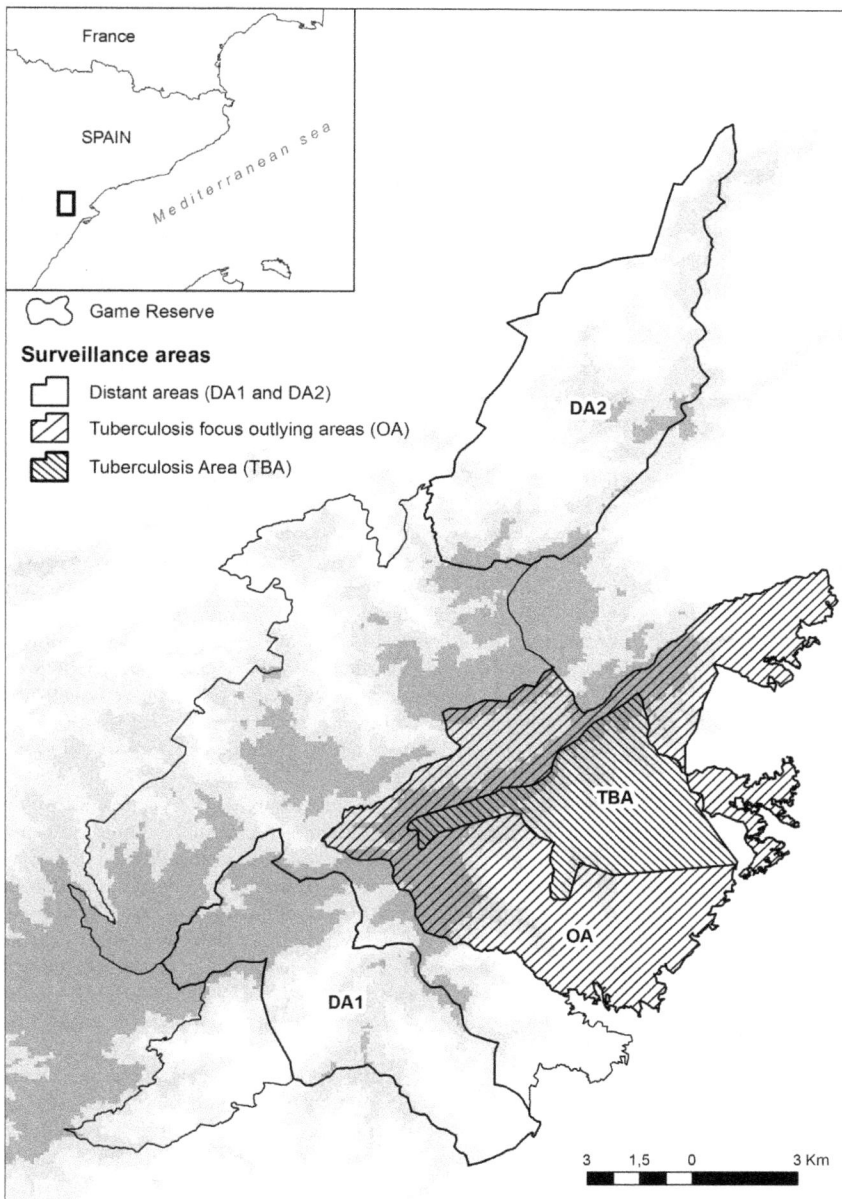

**Figure 1. Study area.** The study area is located in the National Game Reserve "Ports de Tortosa i Beseit", Catalonia region, north-eastern Spain. Three different areas were defined according to preliminary apparent TB distribution: the main tuberculosis area (TBA), outlying areas to TBA (OA) and two distant areas (DA1 and DA2) to TBA.

game seasons in the middle of every harvesting period. To analyse the accumulated effect of culling, data regarding hunting pressure and wild boar abundance was used from 2001 onward. Thus, the first harvesting period (2001-2002) corresponds to number 1, and so on.

## Animal inspection and sampling

During the study period, 745 wild boar (436 in TBA, 209 in OA and 100 in DA), 355 Iberian ibexes (throughout NGRPTB) and five cows (from the TB affected bullfighting herd in TBA and with a positive result for the tuberculin skin test) were inspected for TBLL. Wild boar were either hunter-harvested during the regular game seasons (in the whole NGRPTB; n = 591) or box-trapped

and later euthanatized year-round (only in TBA and in harvesting periods number 6 to 11; n = 154). Complete post-mortem examination and, thus, determination of the distribution of the lesions was possible in 115 (39 box-trapped and 76 hunter-harvested) tuberculous wild boar. In agreement with the authorities responsible for the management of game in the NGRPTB, their game rangers were trained to identify the normal aspect of organs and responsible for collecting apparently abnormal organs and all the mandibular and retropharyngeal lymph nodes of Iberian ibexes hunter-harvested during the regular game season for this species (two annual periods in spring -March to June- and autumn -September to December-, respectively). Finally, the five cows were inspected and sampled in the slaughterhouse facilities following the established official channels. Once inspected for

TBLL, selected samples were either refrigerated in a cold box (4°C) and immediately dispatched to the laboratory for detection of Mycobacteria within the first 48–72 hours (wild boar and cows) or stored at −20°C until processing (ibex).

Sex and age of the animals was recorded. Wild boar were aged by tooth replacement and by dental attrition [27] but ultimately assigned to four age classes for minimizing determination errors: piglets (0–6 months; n = 115), juveniles (6–12 months; n = 152), yearlings (13–24 months; n = 95) and adults (over 24 months; n = 383). The age of ibexes was determined in years by counting horn segments [28].

## Bacteriology

Selected samples (mostly head and cervical lymph nodes and including TBLL if present) from every animal were subjected to bacteriological culture regardless of TBLL presence or not. Samples from each animal were pooled, homogenized with sterile distilled water and decontaminated with 0.35% hexadecylpyridinium chloride for 30 minutes [29], centrifuged at 1300 g for 30 min and cultured onto Coletsos and 0.2% (w/v) pyruvate-enriched Löwenstein-Jensen media (Biomedics, Madrid, Spain) at 37°C. Isolates were heat-treated and identified by PCR amplification of Mycobacterium genus-specific 16 S rRNA fragment and the MPB70 sequence for the *M. tuberculosis* complex (MTBC) isolates [30].

## Fingerprinting

The DVR-spacer oligonucleotide typing (DVR-spoligotyping) method was later performed as previously described [31] to identify the mycobacterium species of the MTBC and to characterize the isolates. In addition, data of spoligotypes detected in cattle grazing in our study area were obtained from the Spanish Database of Animal Mycobacteriosis (mycoDB) [32] and the authorities in charge of the compulsory test and slaughter campaigns. Mycobacterial Interspersed Repetitive Units - Variable Number Tandem Repeats (MIRU-VNTR) typing was also performed using nine VNTR markers (ETR-A, ETR-B, ETR-D, ETR-E, MIRU26, QUB11a, QUB11b, QUB26 and QUB3232) [33].

For further analysis, TB infection status was based on both gross tubercle-like lesions (TBLL) and/or microbiological culture, in order to alleviate disease underestimation [34].

## Increase of wild boar harvesting

Once bovine tuberculosis was detected (in 2004), it was decided to increase wild boar harvesting in the affected area with the aim of disease control. Specifically, the strategy was based on the authorization of additional hunting battues and the implementation of a box-trapping system in the TBA. This consists of six box-traps permanently baited with acorns and activated monthly. Box-trapped boars were anaesthetized with a combination of xylazine (3 mg/kg IM; Xilagesic®, Calier Laboratories), zolazepam and tiletamine (3 mg/kg IM each; Zoletil®, Virbac Laboratories) delivered by blowpipe and then euthanized with T-61 euthanasia solution (0.1 mL/kg IV; T-61®, Intervet Laboratories).

## Cattle removal

Bovine tuberculosis is subjected to compulsory tests and slaughter campaigns in cattle (EC No 64/432 and the Spanish transposition R.D. 2611/1996) with the higher infection rates occurring in beef and bullfighting cattle, mainly in south-central Spain [35]. Due to repeated TB positive cases amongst tested cattle (bullfighting) in the TBA area, compulsory removal and slaughter ("stamping out") of the entire herd population was officially decreed by May 2008 and, after a 13-month period, a new TB-free herd was reintroduced into the TBA.

## Statistical analysis

Different statistical analyses were performed depending on the objectives of the study. To assess the spatial pattern of TB in the game reserve, the differences in TB prevalence among TBA, OA and DA zones were analysed by a Fisher's exact test [36]. To assess the effects of disease management on TB control, we first checked whether the yearly increases in harvesting pressure, including both hunting and box-trapping sessions, resulted in an increase in harvested boars. This was checked by a linear regression between the number of harvesting sessions and the number of wild boar harvested. After that, we fitted a set of generalized additive models (GAM) [37] that explored the effects of the disease management strategies on TB control. In this case, TB infection status (the categorical dependent variable with two modalities: 1 if TBLL were present or a positive culture obtained, and 0 otherwise) was analyzed taking into account as dependent variables the harvesting season, the number of harvested wild boar, age of animals (only juveniles, yearling and adults were retained for this analysis due to the chronic character of bovine tuberculosis and because few TB infected piglets were captured during the study period), cattle removal (a categorical variable with two modalities: pre-cattle removal and post-cattle removal) and their two-way interactions. The variable harvesting season was included in all models given that we aimed to explore temporal trends in TB infection rate.

Since the effects of harvesting pressure on TB occurrence would not be immediate, we considered several harvesting pressure-related variables by accounting for the accumulated number of wild boar harvested in one, two, and three harvesting seasons previous to the current one. It was impossible to consider beyond the three previous seasons because these data were not available for harvesting season 4. Nevertheless, owing to the correlation between these variables (e.g., $R^2 = 87\%$, t = 6.3, p>0.001 for the correlation between the accumulated number of wild boar harvested three and two seasons before the current one), only two explanatory harvesting pressure-related variables were retained for the analysis: the number of wild boars harvested in the previous harvesting season (Harv1) and the accumulated number of wild boar harvested in the three previous seasons (Harv3). Following the same rationale, no model simultaneously included harvesting season and the Harv3 as explanatory variables due to high correlation ($R^2 = 79\%$, t = 4.83, p>0.001). Finally, we explored whether the observed TB trends in TBA differed from those in OA and DA by a model (GAM) including the interaction between harvesting season and zone (TBA, OA and DA).

Finally, we explored the potential mechanisms through which increased wild boar harvesting influenced population structure and hence TB dynamics. For this purpose, we fitted a set of linear models (LM) to explore whether total wild boar abundance or the percentage of juveniles were influenced by Harv1 or Harv3. Closed scrublands on steep slopes predominate in our region, which hinders census through direct observation of animals as well as application of indirect methods based on faecal droppings for abundance estimates [12]. For this reason, the number of sighted wild boar (including those hunted) divided by the number of participating hunters in the hunting journey was considered a proxy for wild boar abundance (see [38] for a revision on census methods for wild boar).

In all cases, we followed a model selection procedure based on the information-theoretic approach and the Akaike's Information

Criterion [39]. Subsequently, we estimated the Akaike weight ($wi_i$), defined as the relative probability that a given model is the best model among those being compared. Once the best model was selected we confirmed the general assumptions of GAM and LM following the previously published recommendations [37,40]. Statistical analyses were performed using "mgcv" package version 1.7-12 [37] of the statistical software R version 3.0.2 [41].

## Results

### Prevalence of TB and genotype mapping

Twenty-four percent of wild boars showed TBLL (179/745). Sixteen percent had a positive culture of *Mycobacterium* sp. (121/745) and, based on both TBLL and/or a MTBC positive culture, the overall prevalence of TB in the NGRPTB was 24.7% (21.6–27.9 at 95% CI; n = 184). Distribution of isolates into mycobacterium species and spoligotypes is presented in Table 1. Tuberculous infection by members of the MTBC was confirmed in 103 wild boars (97 *M. bovis* y 6 *M. caprae* isolates). The remaining eighteen isolates corresponded to species of the genus *Mycobacterium* other than MTBC. Moreover, eighteen wild boars without TBLL displayed positive mycobacteria cultures (four to *M. bovis*, one to *M. caprae* and 13 to non-tuberculous mycobacteria), and no mycobacteria were recovered from 76 wild boars with TBLL. Two wild boars detected in DA with miliary TBLL in the lung parenchyma were ultimately diagnosed as pulmonary botryomycosis due to infection with *Staphylococcus aureus*. None of the ibexes harvested had TBLL or a positive *Mycobacterium* sp. culture.

Ten different spoligotypes have been identified from the 103 MTBC-infected wild boar and the most frequent profiles were SB0121 (n = 36) and SB1195 (n = 31), detected in the reserve from 2004 to 2012. The remaining eight spoligotypes were sporadically isolated in wild boar (n = 36). In the five isolates from cattle, four spoligotyes were identified (SB0121, SB1095, SB1192 and SB1685) and three of them (SB0121, SB1095, and SB1192) were also shared with wild boar. Five of the spoligotypes detected in TBA (SB0121, SB0294, SB0415, SB1095 and SB1192) have also been isolated from wild boar harvested in OA, whereas only the *Mycobacterium caprae* (SB0415) has been detected in DA. Ninety-nine out of 103 MTBC isolates (no DNA was available for four isolates) were also characterized by MIRU-VNTR typing with 9 loci, and 13 MIRU-VNTR types were obtained when ETR-A,

ETR-B, QUB11a and QUB322 loci were analysed, with the most frequent being MIRU-VNTR (MV) type MV0006 (n = 59)(see Table S1). In general, the five remaining VNTR markers (QU11b, MIRU4, MIRU31, MIRU26 and QUB26) did not provide additional information and the isolates were clustered using only the four most polymorphic loci (see Table S2).

Attending to age classes, the prevalence of TB was 58.6% amongst adults, 32.2% in juveniles and yearlings and 6.3% in piglets. The occurrence of TBLL in different anatomical regions (localized versus more extended or generalized) are presented in Table 2. Most tuberculous wild boar had lesions in the head lymph nodes (109/115, 95%), while only 14/115 and 6/115 had lesions only in intrathoracic (mediastinic or bronchial) or mesenteric lymph nodes, respectively.

### Spatial pattern of TB in the game reserve

85.3% of the TB positive boars (168/197) were harvested in TBA, which accounts for an overall prevalence of 38.5% in this zone (33.9–43.2 95% CI, 168/436 examined wild boar) and results between 4 and 6.42 times higher than in OA or DA, respectively (Fisher test = 85.62, d.f. = 2, p-value <0.001, Figure 2).

### Effects of disease management on TB control

Harvesting pressure nearly tripled (e.g., increased 2.6 times); in fact, only 3.7 beats per game season occurred previous to TB detection (period 2001–2004), whereas 9.6 harvesting actions per game season (including both hunting and box-trapping) occurred after TB detection in wild boar. In general, the increase in the number of harvesting sessions resulted in a higher number of harvested boars during the whole study period ($\beta = 4.3$, SE = 0.22, t-value = 19.36, p<0.001, $R^2 = 36.9\%$, Figures 3a and 3b). But the number of harvested boars in every harvesting period was also positively correlated to their abundance in the corresponding period ($\beta = 218.14$, SE = 9.26, t-value = 23.55, p<0.001, $R^2 = 60.7\%$, Figures 3c and 3d). Hence, the peak in the number of harvested wild boar in the game season 3 would be more related to the high abundance in this season whereas the peak observed in harvesting seasons 7 and 8 would be more related to harvesting effort.

On the other hand, the prevalence of TB infection displayed a temporary pattern in TBA (Figure 4). According to our model

**Table 1.** Distribution of 121 isolates into mycobacterium species and spoligotypes in eight harvesting seasons.

| Harvesting season | Mycobacterium bovis | | | | | | | | | Mycobacterium caprae | Non-MTBC mycobacteria |
|---|---|---|---|---|---|---|---|---|---|---|---|
| *4 | | | SB0121 (2) | | | | SB1095 (2) | SB1192 (1) | | | |
| *5 | SB0119 (1) | SB0120 (1) | **SB0121** (7) | | | | SB1095 (1) | SB1192 (2) | SB1336 (6) | SB0415 (1) | NA (2) |
| *6 | | | SB0121 (4) | | | SB0295 (2) | SB1095 (4) | SB1192 (1) | SB1336 (4) | | NA (3) |
| *7 | | | **SB0121** (15) | | | SB0295 (2) | **SB1095** (5) | **SB1192** (1) | | SB0415 (3) | NA (6) |
| 8 | | | SB0121 (2) | SB0140 (1) | SB0294 (1) | SB0295 (1) | SB1095 (7) | | | SB0415 (1) | NA (2) |
| 9 | | | SB0121 (1) | | SB0294 (3) | | SB1095 (1) | | | SB0415 (1) | |
| 10 | | | SB0121 (2) | | SB0294 (1) | | SB1095 (3) | | | | NA (1) |
| 11 | | | SB0121 (3) | SB0140 (1) | | | SB1095 (8) | SB1192 (2) | | | NA (4) |
| TOTAL | 1 | 1 | 36 | 2 | 5 | 5 | 31 | 6 | 10 | 6 | 18 |

*Mycobacterium tuberculosis* complex spoligotypes and number of isolates (in brackets) in 121 harvested wild boars in eight harvesting seasons starting in the period 2004-05 (4th) and ending in 2011–12 (11th). Asterisks indicate those harvesting seasons in which TB-infected cattle were present in TBA. In bold, TB spoligotypes also isolated from cattle in the respective season.

**Table 2.** Occurrence of tuberculosis-like lesions in different anatomical regions of wild boar.

| TB LESION DISTRIBUTION PATTERNS (n = 115) | |
|---|---|
| **One anatomical region** | 89%(102) |
| **Head only** | 83.5%(96) |
| **Thorax only** | 4.3%(5) |
| **Abdomen only** | 0.8%(1) |
| **Two or more anatomical region** | 11%(13) |
| **Head an thorax** | 7%(8) |
| **Head and abdomen** | 3.5%(4) |
| **Thorax and abdomen** | 0 |
| **Head, thorax and abdomen** | 0.9%(1) |
| **Submandibular lymph nodes** | 92%(106) |
| **Retropharyngeal lymph nodes** | 16.5%(19) |
| **Bronquial or mediastinic lymph nodes** | 12%(14) |
| **Lungs parenchyma** | 1.7%(2) |
| **Mesenteric lymph nodes** | 5%(6) |
| **Abdominal viscera** | 0 |

Percentage of wild boars showing localized of generalized specific TBLL in different anatomical regions amongst 115 individuals in which complete post-mortem examination was performed.

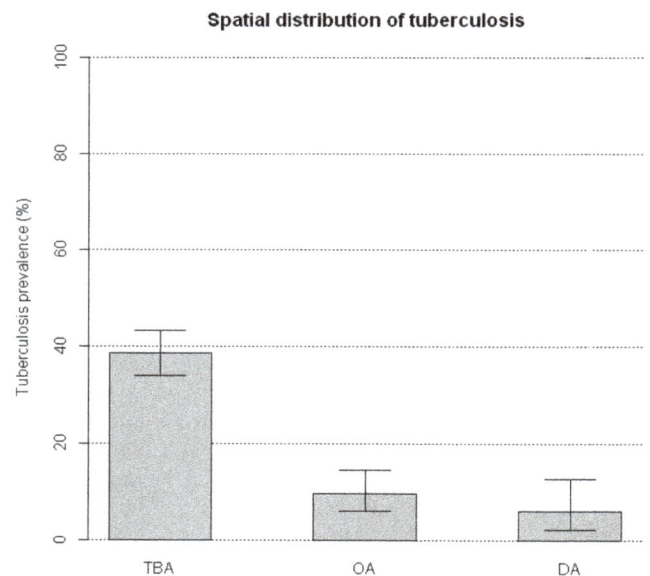

**Figure 2. Spatial pattern of tuberculosis in the National Game Reserve "Ports de Tortosa i Beseit".** Prevalence of tuberculosis in wild boars harvested in the National Game Reserve "Ports de Tortosa i Beseit" in three defined areas: the main tuberculosis area (TBA), outlying areas to TBA (OA) and distant areas to TBA (DA1 and DA2 were pooled). Confidence interval at 95% is represented.

selection procedure, the cattle removal, the accumulated number of wild boar harvested in the last three harvesting seasons (Harv3) and the age of wild boar were the main factors for explaining the probability of TB in the wild boar ($W_i$ Harv3 * Cattle removal + Age = 1; that explained 15% of the observed variability in the probability of TB infection; Table 3). The second competing model, which included Harv3 and age, was at 31.23 units from the best model, and thus a candidate with little support for explaining the observed patterns [39]. On the other hand, both juveniles and adults followed the same temporal pattern (the model including the interaction with age was at 32.13 units from the best model), but as expected, the probability of TB infection for the young animals was half that for the adults ($\beta$ Yearlings = −1.0023, SE = 0.2231, Z = −4.492, p-value <0.001). Concerning the effect of TB management, neither cattle removal nor wild boar harvesting were able to shape temporal TB dynamics independently (models including the single effects of these management strategies were more than 54 units from the best model).

In general (all age classes included), the TB prevalence before cattle removal was 49% (42–56 at 95% CI; n = 221) and decreased to 28% (22–34 CI 95%; n = 215) after cattle removal, with an odds ratio of 2.46. Such odds ratio increases to 3.3 when considering only individuals aged over 1 year (69% TB prevalence before vs 40% after cattle removal). However, only the interaction of the two measures resulted in the decrease in the probability of TB infection. Furthermore, intensive wild boar harvesting was more effective in reducing TB infection rates before (deviance explained = 16 %) than after cattle removal (deviance explained = 9%), perhaps because the TB prevalence was 1.9 times lower after cattle removal (e.g., for an accumulated number of wild boar harvested of 500, the probability of TB infection was 1.2 times greater before cattle removal; Figure 5). Finally, TB dynamics differed between TBA, where the management actions were carried out, and OA or DA, as shown by the significant interaction between harvesting

season and the study area (Chi-square = 12.38, p-value 0 0.005, 28.5% deviance explained).

## Effects of intensive harvesting on the wild boar population structure

The intense harvesting of wild boar in TBA had an effect on that wild boar population. The age structure of the TBA wild boar population varied over the study period due to an increment of young (juveniles + yearlings) animals and a decrease of adult boars (Figure 6). This was not reflected in OA or DA. Actually, this trend could be a consequence of TB management because of the relationship between the harvesting pressure in the previous seasons and the increment of young boars harvested in the TBA ($\beta$ Harv1 = 0.05, SE = 0.02, Z = 2, p-value <0.05, $R^2$ = 35.2%). On the other hand, the increment of harvesting pressure did not influence wild boar population abundance ($\beta$ Harv1 = −0.0003, SE = 0.0003, Z = −0.9, p-value = 0.4).

## Discussion

Whereas southern Spain is a hotspot of tuberculosis in wildlife, reports of the disease are scarce in the northern part of the country, where conditions of wildlife are more similar to those in the rest of Europe (no fencing, no artificial feeding and lower densities). This study provides evidence that high TB prevalence is also possible in free-ranging and non-intensively managed (i.e., not overcrowded, non-fenced and without supplemental feeding) wild boar populations living in the absence of deer (fallow deer and red deer). In fact, deer are present in most of the tuberculosis scenarios in which wild boar is implicated [13,42], including large natural protected areas (e.g., Doñana National Park (DNP)) [43]. Instead, the Iberian ibex, a wild caprinae, is present in the scenario considered here. Previous studies have suggested that this wild caprinae does not play a significant role in the epidemiology of TB [44], and the presented results increase the previous sample size

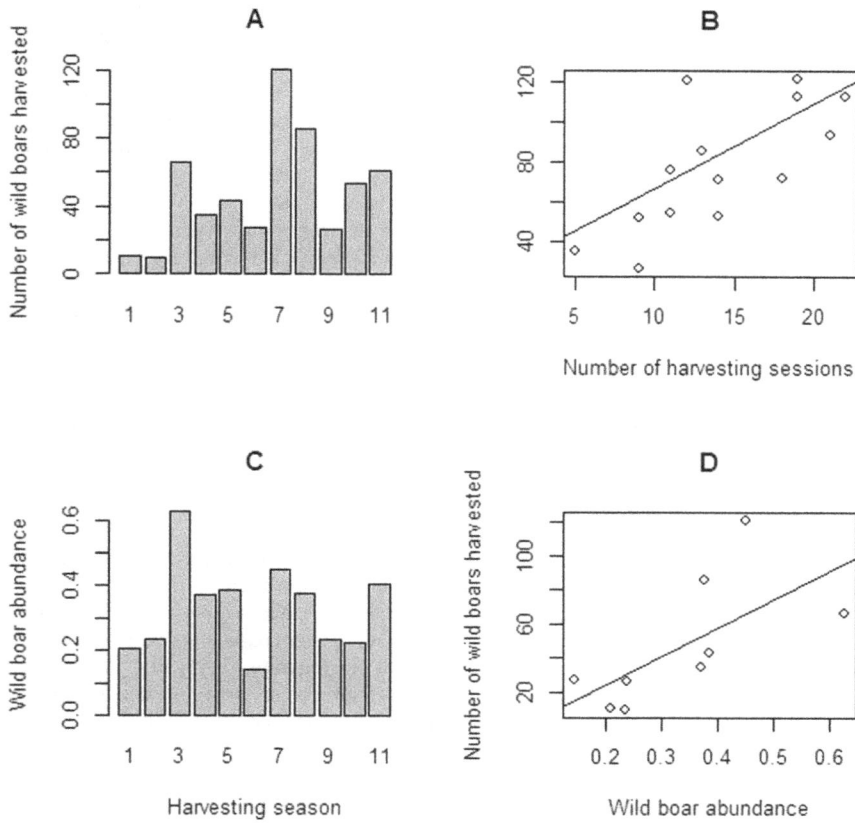

**Figure 3. Relationship amongst hunting pressure, wild boar abundance and the number of wild boar harvested.** Number of harvested wild boars (a) and abundance (b) per game season; Graphical representation of positive correlation between the number of harvesting sessions (c) and abundance (d) and the number of harvested wild boars.

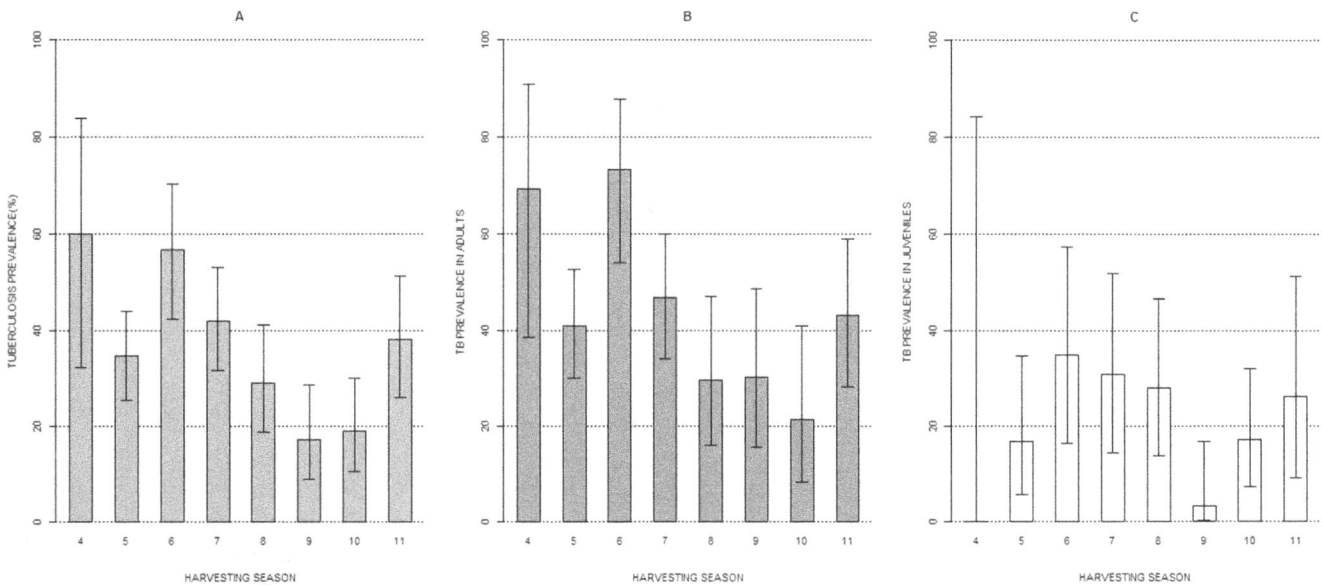

**Figure 4. Temporal evolution of tuberculosis prevalence in wild boar.** Overall prevalence of tuberculosis (a), prevalence in adults (b) and in juveniles (c) per harvesting seasons in TBA from 2004 to 2011. Cattle removal occurred in May 2008 (this is by the end of harvesting season 7).

**Table 3.** Models considered for explaining the probability of tuberculosis infection in the wild boar.

| Biological models | K | AIC | $\Delta_i$ | $w_i$ |
|---|---|---|---|---|
| **Harv3 * Cattle removal + Age** | 8 | 590.09 | 0.00 | 1 |
| Harv3 + Age | 5 | 621.32 | 31.23 | 0 |
| Harv3 * Age + Cattle removal * Age | 8 | 622.22 | 32.13 | 0 |
| Harv3 + Age + Cattle removal | 6 | 622.94 | 32.85 | 0 |
| Harv3 * Age | 6 | 636.89 | 46.80 | 0 |
| Game season + Age + Cattle removal * Harv1 | 8 | 641.6 | 51.51 | 0 |
| Game season + Age | 5 | 642.7 | 52.61 | 0 |
| Game season + Age + Cattle removal + Harv1 | 7 | 643.07 | 52.98 | 0 |
| Game season + Age + Harv1 | 6 | 643.17 | 53.08 | 0 |
| Game season * Harv1 + Age | 6 | 644.03 | 53.94 | 0 |
| Game season + Age + Cattle removal | 6 | 644.54 | 54.45 | 0 |
| Game season + Age * Harv1 | 7 | 644.85 | 54.76 | 0 |
| Game season + Age * Cattle removal | 7 | 645.59 | 55.50 | 0 |
| Game season + Cattle removal * Age + Harv1* Age | 9 | 646.16 | 56.07 | 0 |
| Mo | 1 | 774.22 | 184.13 | 0 |

Model selection based on generalized additive modelling for exploring the temporal variation in the probability of tuberculosis infection determined in 267 adult, 97 juvenile and 70 yearling wild boars harvested in the main tuberculosis area and outlying areas (TBA and OA) in the National Game Reserve "Ports de Tortosa i Beseït". Harv1 means the total number of wild boars harvested in the previous harvesting season, whereas Harv3 is the total number of wild boars harvested during the three seasons before the current one. K = effective number of parameters in the additive modelling, AIC = Akaike Information Criterion, $\Delta_i$ = difference of AIC with respect to the best model, $w_i$ = Akaike weight, Mo = null model only with the constant term. In bold the best model for explaining the observed TB probability of infection.

reinforcing this idea. The TB prevalence (TBLL and/or culture positive) found in our study area is amongst the highest described in wildlife, reaching values around 70% in adults in some harvesting seasons (see Fig. 5). Similar values have been observed in overcrowded and intensively managed wild boar populations in the central Iberian Peninsula [9], and higher, up to 92% in free-ranging wild boars from DNP [43] and 100% in feral pigs from New Zealand [6]. The post-mortem examination is an easy-to-perform and inexpensive first option for the presumptive diagnosis of TB in game species. However, prevalence of TB in our study may have been slightly underestimated since histopathology was not routinely performed and a low percentage of infected wild boar with microscopic lesions and a false-negative bacteriological culture result could have gone unnoticed. Actually, a negative culture status is not a guarantee that a wild boar is not infected [34], as reinforced in our study by animals with TBLL and a negative culture (76/179) or vice versa, positive culture without TBLL (18/566). Overestimation of TB prevalence based on TBLL has been suggested due to infection by other pathogens [9]. The *Staphylococcus aureus* causing pulmonary botryomycosis was detected in DA, far from TBA, whereas infection by MTBC was confirmed in a significant percentage (90/157) of the wild boar with TBLL in TBA, and thus overestimation is improbable.

Generalized lesions in wild boar from the NGRPTB were rare (11%) as compared to populations from south central Spain, where values around 60% have been repeatedly observed and attributed to the early infection of young animals favoured by unnaturally high densities and spatial aggregation [9,45]. In fact, disease progression is likely to be more severe in immature individuals because of reduced immunocompetence [45,46]. The importance of the route of infection on the TB lesion pattern is still unclear. De Lisle, for example, associated the localized lesions in the head lymph nodes of feral pigs from New Zealand to infection through scavenging of tuberculous carrion [46], whereas Martin-Hernando and cols. attributed both localized and generalized patterns to either respiratory (air-borne infection by frequent direct oronasal contact behaviour between wild boar) or digestive (food and water) infection routes [45]. Based in the literature and our own data, we could hypothesize that lesion distribution may be positively correlated to exposure, as it would increase the probability of a wild boar getting infected in early life and by several routes. But

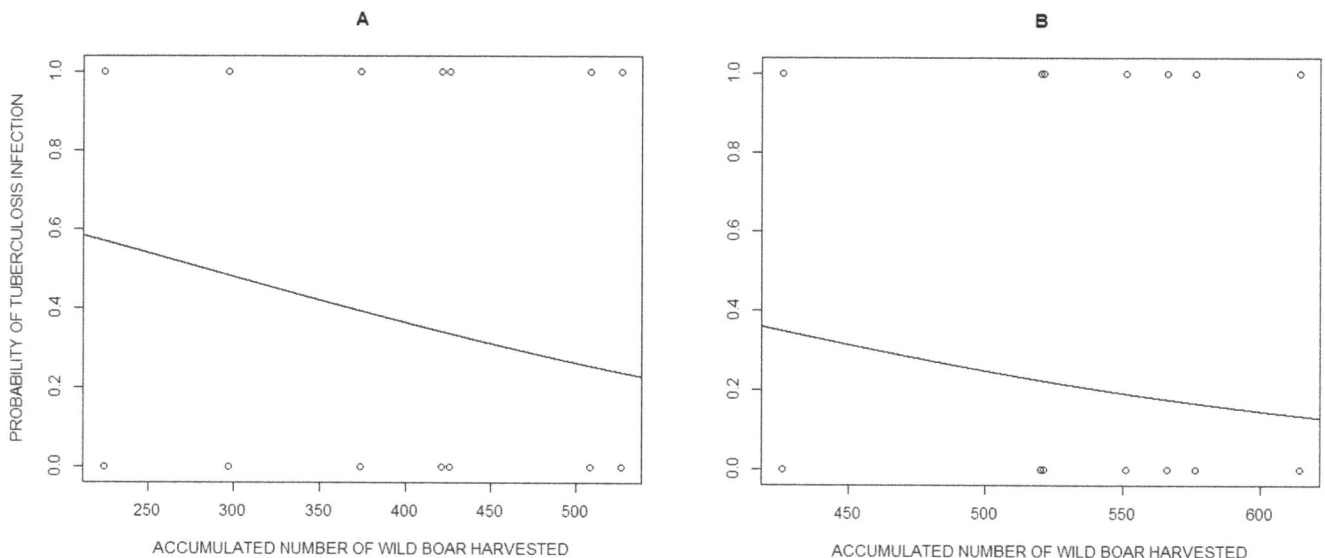

**Figure 5. Effect of wild boar harvesting on the probability of tuberculosis infection.** Effect of wild boar harvesting before (a) and after (b) cattle removal on the probability of TB infection in wild boars harvested in the main tuberculosis area (TBA) in the National Game Reserve "Ports de Tortosa i Beseït", Catalonia, north-eastern Spain.

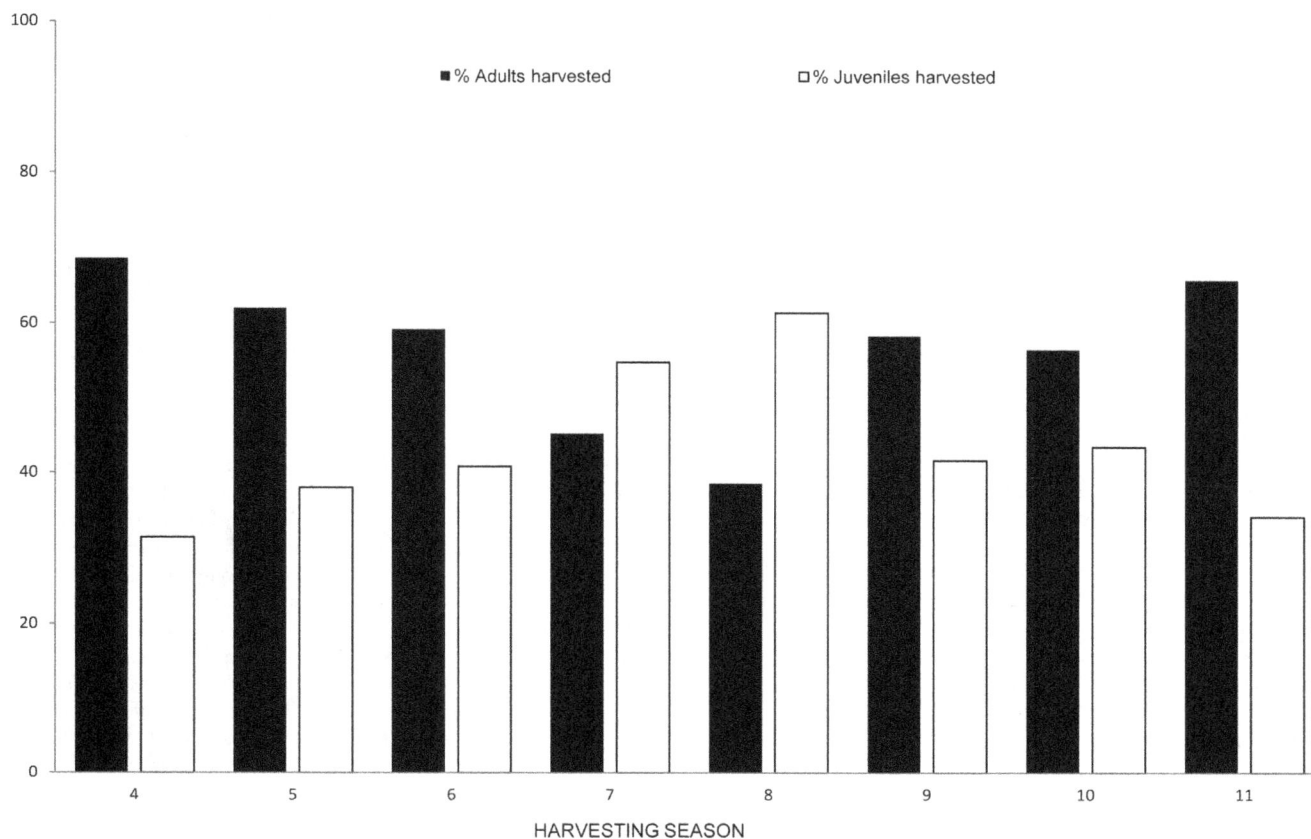

**Figure 6. Temporal evolution of wild boar population age structure.** Percentage of adult (a) and young (juveniles and yearlings) b) wild boars harvested in TBA per harvesting season.

other factors may also determine lesion pattern. Garcia-Jimenez and cols., for example, described a higher load of mycobacteria in lesions caused by *M. caprae* (scarce in our study), which could result in higher excretion rates and, subsequently, exposure for other individuals in the population [47]. Additionally, genetic factors have been related to the ability of both wild boar to limit infection (host resistance) and *Mycobacterium bovis* to circumvent host immune responses and establish infection (pathogen mechanisms of virulence) [48]. Furthermore, climate and food availability would also be key factors driving disease severity. In fact, the problem of tuberculosis in wild boar seems to be concentrated in south-west Spain [9], where long dry summers [49] and the homogeneous habitat and high densities of ungulates [24] often result in food and water shortages for nearly half the year. Our study is located in the northern third of the Iberian bio-region 5 [24], corresponding to coastal areas where seasonal food shortages are not likely to lessen the ability of wild boar to cope with TB infection. The landscape composition may also play a role, as the heterogeneous habitat of our study area could revert to greater availability and variety of food and water resources, thus minimising shortage periods and improving micronutrient intake. Altogether, these factors may determine fitness, immunocompetence and even coinfection-related variations in susceptibility to infections by regulation of the pathogen community and pathogen load of animals [50,51]. However, all of these arguments are to date speculative, and hence further research is necessary to explain the lack of generalized lesions in our study area.

To our knowledge this study reveals a local MTBC spoligotype diversity never before described in the scientific literature [10,52,53]. The strains shared with sympatric livestock point to cattle as the original source of infection for wild boar in the TBA. This diversity of spoligotypes may suggest repeated introductions of infected cattle in TBA in the past, which favoured the spread of new spoligotypes to the wild boar population. On the other hand, the genotyping analysis grouped several spoligotypes within the same MIRU-VNTR type. The MV0006 type (n = 59) included the majority of the isolates with the spoligotypes SB0121, SB1095, and SB1685 (only found in cattle), and the loss of spacers within the DR locus could also suggest the evolution and fitness of the new strains in this area, as previously described in other regions [52]. The fitness of the SB0121 and SB1095 strains in wild boar became clear when TB increased at seasons 10 and 11, and these profiles were maintained in the area whereas other genotypes disappeared. The SB0121 is the most prevalent spoligotype in the Iberian Peninsula in cattle, goats and wildlife [53,54] and also the most frequent profile in our study area. By contrast, the second predominant spoligotype in our study area, SB1095, may be biased toward northern Spain [54]. On the other hand, the appearance of only one spoligotype of *M. caprae*, SB0415, and in distant areas probably indicates that past infections remain from infected flocks of domestic goats, very common a few decades ago. Currently, the presence of caprine livestock in the NGRPTB is anecdotic.

The marked spatial pattern of TB in the present study is, at least, unexpected given the absence of physical barriers in the study area other than orography. This concentration of tuberculosis reinforces the hypothesis of cattle as a source of infection for wild boar in TBA. The intensive culling of badgers has been observed to produce unexpected effects such as TB dispersal or increased prevalence both in cattle and badger populations in the UK [16] due to increased movements of surviving individuals [55]. In our study, the spatial concentration of wild boar TB in our study was maintained throughout the study period despite culling. This is probably due to their preference to staying in TBA, where water springs and food (fruit trees and farming by-products) are available year-round. Moreover, wild boar leaving the TBA can be hunted in OA or more distant areas since wild boar is hunter-harvested everywhere in the surrounding areas.

As mentioned, the efficacy of the culling method for disease management in wildlife is subject to some controversy [16,19], also in the specific case of the European wild boar [17,18]. In our study, a temporary reduction of TB prevalence in wild boar as a result of both increasing harvesting and removing cattle was achieved between harvesting seasons 7 and 10. For comparison, the prevalence of TB in feral swine decreased from 20% in 1980 to 3.2% in 1983 in the Hawaiian island of Molokai, after an infected cattle herd was removed and intense hunting pressure reduced feral swine density [56]. Our model selection supported the same temporally decreasing pattern in TB occurrence for both juveniles and adults, which could be due to the reduction of force of infection in juveniles, to the incorporation of young TB-free animals and the reduction of infected adults, respectively. However, it was impossible to disentangle the effects of wild boar culling and cattle eradication on TB reduction. Nonetheless, the role of cattle as a source of TB infection appears clear as the prevalence in wild boar fell to half after livestock removal. On the other hand, intensive culling did not result in a reduction of wild boar abundance, maybe due to the dispersion of young animals from neighbouring areas or to increased turnover derived from compensatory reproduction observed in intensively-hunted wild boar populations [57,58]. Hence, the use of culling as a measure for reducing density of infected animals and consequently opportunities for disease transmission did not seem to work in our study system. Thus, the rejuvenation of wild boar populations and the reduction of force of infection would be the most plausible mechanism for explaining the reduction observed in TB prevalence. This highlights the need for integrated holistic control strategies.

It is important to highlight that the wild boar harvesting was more effective before cattle removal, indicating that intensive culling is an effective first intervention measure, especially in areas with high TB prevalence [17]. It is also interesting to observe that the disease still remains in our wild boar population several years after eradication in cattle. This fact lends clear support to the role of wild boar as a true reservoir of TB in the Mediterranean context [8], even at low densities if other risk factors take place. Apart from that, the re-introduced herd in TBA remains negative based on the periodical skin tests performed to date, probably due to the improvement of farming practices. Despite the efforts made, TB increased in wild boar at the end of the study period (e.g., harvesting period 11 or 2011-2012), which would confirm the lack of effectiveness of intensive harvesting for TB control when prevalence is low. This could be attributed to the collateral increase of juveniles and to the decrease in the harvesting efforts during the last years after peaking in periods 7 and 8. This supports that disease control measures must be continued over time and intensively enough to achieve the required efficacy and to counteract the temporary nature of beneficial effects. Intensive culling has achieved TB eradication in the wild only through

massive and sustained programs [59]. This is crucial if we bear in mind that we are dealing with an abundant species such as wild boar that locally reaches pest levels and whose ecological elasticity and behaviour allows them to cope with high harvesting rates [57,58]. In fact, some authors propose more selective harvesting strategies to improve efficacy for achieving population reduction [57]. For example, Bieber and Ruf propose that reducing juvenile survival will have the largest effect on population growth rate under good environmental conditions, whereas strong hunting pressure on adult females will lead to the most effective population control in years with poor conditions [60]. Box-trapping was quite selective for young animals in our study (70% of box-trapped wild boar in our study were below 2 years old), hence this could be a good methodological option for the first assumption.

## Concluding remarks

Active disease surveillance in wildlife makes clear its value and discloses the first high prevalence focus of tuberculosis described in wildlife in the northern half of the Iberian Peninsula. Until now, this focus went unnoticed despite affecting a high percentage of the local wild boar population. Moreover, although TB in wildlife was not assumed to be a cause of concern in these latitudes, the conditions necessary for the onset of this focus have occurred within a protected area where risk factors such as fencing, feeding, overcrowding and/or varied host communities are lacking. Hence, the potential risk for tuberculosis emergence in wildlife populations under certain conditions should not be neglected in the future. Both our evidence and that found in the literature point to exposure as a key factor to understanding lesion patterns of affected individuals. Nevertheless, a better understanding of this question as well as of other factors determining susceptibility and virulence could derive implications for management aimed at reducing generalized patterns and, consequently, curbing infected individuals and exposure of healthy susceptible ones. Factors determining the movements of wild boar may also be of interest to TB management in unfenced areas.

Active disease surveillance in wildlife makes clear its value and discloses the first high prevalence focus of tuberculosis described in wildlife in the northern half of the Iberian Peninsula. Until 2004, this focus went unnoticed despite affecting a high percentage of the local wild boar population. A TB in wildlife was not anticipated to be of concern in these latitudes since the assumed conditions necessary for the onset of the disease such as fencing, feeding, overcrowding and/or varied host communities were lacking. Hence, the potential risk for tuberculosis emergence in wildlife populations under more natural conditions should not be neglected in the future. Both, our evidence and documented cases in the literature point towards early and intense exposure as a key factor to understand lesion patterns of affected individuals. Nevertheless, a better understanding of this question as well as of other factors that drive susceptibility and virulence, it will help to design management practices to reduce generalized patterns and, consequently, reduce exposure of healthy susceptible ones. Factors determining the movements of wild boar may also be of interest to TB management in unfenced areas.

Some evidence suggests that poor farming practices may have occurred in this area in the past. This should be noted especially by the managers of natural areas where interaction between livestock and wildlife may occur, in order to apply preventive measures. Once again, but for the first time in TB, we have shown that it is possible to address the control of a multi-host pathogen in a wild host population via the management of the domestic counterpart [61]. However, the need for holistic control strategies is highlighted, as reduction but not eradication was achieved with the applied measures. Culling is probably the least expensive measure that can be applied, which makes it valuable in the current scenario of economic shortages in the EU (affecting countries in the Mediterranean basin more severely, where this problem [TB in wild boar populations] occurs). Our "culling" experience in TB-infected wild boar adds to the recent ones [17,18] with clarifying intermediate results. As observed by Boadella and cols., culling seems to be an effective first intervention measure to be applied in high prevalence foci, whereas efficacy tends to decrease as prevalence does [17]. However, estimating the threshold required for a significant reduction under natural conditions can be difficult. Hence, to achieve either eradication or a significant decrease of prevalence, culling must be continued over time and intensively enough to achieve the required efficacy and to counteract the temporary nature of beneficial effects. Alternatively, the applicability of more selective harvesting strategies to improve efficacy for achieving population reduction are another area to explore.

## Supporting Information

**Table S1  MIRU-VNTR results and analysis of the *M. bovis* and *M. caprae* isolated from wild boar.** [a] MIRU-VNTR loci with corresponding alias. [b] MIRU-VNTR types obtained with the four-loci approach including ETR-A, ETR-B, QUB11a and QUB3232. Table is arranged according to the MVtype in ascending order. [c] Eight out of 99 isolates are not included in the table due to failure in one or more loci or multiple bands in some loci. Grey indicates the MIRU-VNTR profile of the five cattle isolates. The bovine isolate with the SB1685 profile (not included in the table because was only present in cattle) showed the most frequent MV0006 type and the SB0121 spoligotype.

**Table S2  Genotyping analysis of the *M. bovis* and *M. caprae* isolated from wild boar.** Genotyping analysis (combination of spoligotypes and MIRU-VNTR types) of the *M. bovis* and *M. caprae* isolated from wild boar. [a] Eight out of 99 isolates genotyped by MIRU-VNTR are not included in the table due to failure in one or more loci or multiple bands in some loci. [b] MIRU-VNTR types obtained with the four-loci approach including ETR-A, ETR-B, QUB11a and QUB3232. Grey indicates the season and genotype of the cattle isolates. The bovine isolate with the SB1685 profile belongs to season 7 but is not included in the table since no wild boar were detected with this spoligotype.

## Acknowledgments

We express our gratitude to the Departament d'Agricultura, Ramaderia, Pesca, Alimentació i Medi Natural of the Generalitat de Catalunya (DARPAMN) for promoting active disease surveillance in wildlife. We are also very grateful to the staff of the National Game Reserve and Natural Park "Els Ports de Tortosa i Beseit" for their involvement, especially Jordi Romeva, Rafael Balada and Josep Maria Forcadell, to the forest rangers (Cos d'Agents Rurals -CAR-) from Terres de l'Ebre and to the wild boar hunters from the NGRPTB, especially to those from Roquetes and Mas de Barberans. The map of the study area was kindly provided by José M. López-Martín, from the Àrea d'Activitats Cinegètiques de la Direcció General del Medi Natural i Biodiversitat (DARPAMN).

## Author Contributions

Conceived and designed the experiments: GM SL LD AM ES. Performed the experiments: GM BR XO LJ ES NN RV IM. Analyzed the data: GM ES BR. Contributed reagents/materials/analysis tools: SL LD AM. Wrote the paper: GM BR ES. Revised critically, improved and approved the final manuscript: GM BR LJ NN RV AM IM XO LD SL ES.

## References

1. Corner LA (2006) The role of wild animal populations in the epidemiology of tuberculosis in domestic animals: How to assess the risk. Vet Microbiol 112: 303–312.
2. de la Rua-Domenech R, Goodchild AT, Vordermeier HM, Hewinson RG, Christiansen KH, et al. (2006) Ante mortem diagnosis of tuberculosis in cattle: A review of the tuberculin tests, gamma-interferon assay and other ancillary diagnostic techniques. Res Vet Sci 81: 190–210.
3. Nishi JS, Shury T, Elkin BT (2006) Wildlife reservoirs for bovine tuberculosis (*Mycobacterium bovis*) in canada: Strategies for management and research. Vet Microbiol 112: 325–338.
4. Renwick AR, White PC, Bengis RG (2007) Bovine tuberculosis in Southern African wildlife: A multi-species host-pathogen system. Epidemiol Infect 135: 529–540.
5. Delahay RJ, Smith GC, Barlow AM, Walker N, Harris A, et al. (2007) Bovine tuberculosis infection in wild mammals in the south-west region of England: A survey of prevalence and a semi-quantitative assessment of the relative risks to cattle. Vet J 173: 287–301.
6. Ryan TJ, Livingstone PG, Ramsey DS, de Lisle GW, Nugent G, et al. (2006) Advances in understanding disease epidemiology and implications for control and eradication of tuberculosis in livestock: The experience from New Zealand. Vet Microbiol 112: 211–219.
7. Gortázar C, Delahay RJ, McDonald RA, Boadella M, Wilson GJ, et al. (2012) The status of tuberculosis in European wild mammals. Mamm Rev 42: 193–206.
8. Naranjo V, Gortazar C, Vicente J, de la Fuente J (2008) Evidence of the role of European wild boar as a reservoir of *Mycobacterium tuberculosis* complex. Vet Microbiol 127: 1–9.
9. Vicente J, Hofle U, Garrido JM, Fernandez-De-Mera IG, Juste R, et al. (2006) Wild boar and red deer display high prevalences of tuberculosis-like lesions in Spain. Vet Res 37: 107–119.
10. Gortazar C, Vicente J, Samper S, Garrido JM, Fernandez-De-Mera IG, et al. (2005) Molecular characterization of *Mycobacterium tuberculosis* complex isolates from wild ungulates in south-central Spain. Vet Res 36: 43–52.
11. Parra A, Fernandez-Llario P, Tato A, Larrasa J, Garcia A, et al. (2003) Epidemiology of *Mycobacterium bovis* infections of pigs and wild boars using a molecular approach. Vet Microbiol 97: 123–133.
12. Acevedo P, Vicente J, Hofle U, Cassinello J, Ruiz-Fons F, et al. (2007) Estimation of European wild boar relative abundance and aggregation: A novel method in epidemiological risk assessment. Epidemiol Infect 135: 519–527.

13. Vicente J, Hofle U, Garrido JM, Fernandez-de-Mera IG, Acevedo P, et al. (2007) Risk factors associated with the prevalence of tuberculosis-like lesions in fenced wild boar and red deer in south central Spain. Vet Res 38: 451–464.
14. Boadella M, Acevedo P, Vicente J, Mentaberre G, Balseiro A, et al. (2011) Spatio-temporal trends of Iberian wild boar contact with *Mycobacterium tuberculosis* complex detected by ELISA. Ecohealth.
15. O'Brien DJ, Schmitt SM, Rudolph BA, Nugent G (2011) Recent advances in the management of bovine tuberculosis in free-ranging wildlife. Vet Microbiol 151: 23–33.
16. Jenkins HE, Woodroffe R, Donnelly CA (2010) The duration of the effects of repeated widespread badger culling on cattle tuberculosis following the cessation of culling. PLoS One 5: e9090.
17. Boadella M, Vicente J, Ruiz-Fons F, de la Fuente J, Gortazar C (2012) Effects of culling Eurasian wild boar on the prevalence of *Mycobacterium bovis* and Aujeszky's disease virus. Prev Vet Med.
18. Garcia-Jimenez WL, Fernandez-Llario P, Benitez-Medina JM, Cerrato R, Cuesta J, et al. (2013) Reducing Eurasian wild boar (*Sus scrofa*) population density as a measure for bovine tuberculosis control: Effects in wild boar and a sympatric fallow deer (*Dama dama*) population in central Spain. Prev Vet Med.
19. Dandy N, Ballantyne S, Moseley D, Gill R, Quine C, et al. (2012) Exploring beliefs behind support for and opposition to wildlife management methods: A qualitative study. Eur J Wildl Res 58: 695–706.
20. Donnelly CA, Woodroffe R, Cox DR, Bourne FJ, Cheeseman CL, et al. (2006) Positive and negative effects of widespread badger culling on tuberculosis in cattle. Nature 439: 843–846.
21. Buddle BM, Skinner MA, Chambers MA (2000) Immunological approaches to the control of tuberculosis in wildlife reservoirs. Vet Immunol Immunopathol 74: 1–16.
22. Cowled BD, Garner MG, Negus K, Ward MP (2012) Controlling disease outbreaks in wildlife using limited culling: Modelling classical swine fever incursions in wild pigs in Australia. Vet Res 43: 3-9716-43-3.
23. Keet DF, Kriek NP, Bengis RG, Grobler DG, Michel A (2000) The rise and fall of tuberculosis in a free-ranging chacma baboon troop in the Kruger national park. Onderstepoort J Vet Res 67: 115–122.
24. Munoz PM, Boadella M, Arnal M, de Miguel MJ, Revilla M, et al. (2010) Spatial distribution and risk factors of brucellosis in Iberian wild ungulates. BMC Infect Dis 10: 46.

25. Servei Meteorologic de Catalunya website. Available: http://www.meteocat.cat. Accessed 2012 Dec 11.

26. Blanchong JA, Samuel MD, Scribner KT, Weckworth BV, Langenberg JA, et al. (2008) Landscape genetics and the spatial distribution of chronic wasting disease. Biol Lett 4: 130–133.

27. Boitani L, Mattei L (1992) Aging wild boar (Sus scrofa) by tooth eruption. In: Spitz F, Janeau G, González G, Aulagnier S, editors. Ongules/Ungulates 91. Toulouse: SFEPM-IRGM. pp. 419–421.

28. Fandos P (1995) Factors affecting horn growth in male Spanish ibex (Capra pyrenaica). Mammalia 59: 229–236.

29. Corner LA, Trajstman AC (1988) An evaluation of 1-hexadecylpyridinium chloride as a decontaminant in the primary isolation of Mycobacterium bovis from bovine lesions. Vet Microbiol 18: 127–134.

30. Wilton S, Cousins D (1992) Detection and identification of multiple mycobacterial pathogens by DNA amplification in a single tube. PCR Methods Appl 1: 269–273.

31. Kamerbeek J, Schouls L, Kolk A, van Agterveld M, van Soolingen D, et al. (1997) Simultaneous detection and strain differentiation of Mycobacterium tuberculosis for diagnosis and epidemiology. J Clin Microbiol 35: 907–914.

32. Rodriguez-Campos S, Gonzalez S, de Juan L, Romero B, Bezos J, et al. (2012) A database for animal tuberculosis (mycoDB.es) within the context of the Spanish national programme for eradication of bovine tuberculosis. Infect Genet Evol 12: 877–882.

33. Rodriguez-Campos S, Aranaz A, de Juan L, Saez-Llorente JL, Romero B, et al. (2011) Limitations of spoligotyping and variable-number tandem-repeat typing for molecular tracing of Mycobacterium bovis in a high-diversity setting. J Clin Microbiol 49: 3361–3364.

34. Santos N, Geraldes M, Afonso A, Almeida V, Correia-Neves M (2010) Diagnosis of tuberculosis in the wild boar (Sus scrofa): A comparison of methods applicable to hunter-harvested animals. PLoS One 5: 10.1371/journal.pone.0012663.

35. Allepuz A, Casal J, Napp S, Saez M, Alba A, et al. (2011) Analysis of the spatial variation of bovine tuberculosis disease risk in Spain (2006–2009). Prev Vet Med 100: 44–52.

36. Zar JH (2009) Biostatistical analysis. New Jersey: Prentice Hall.

37. Wood S (2006) Generalized additive models: An introduction with R. Boca Raton, USA: CEC Statistic.

38. Acevedo P, Vicente J, Alzaga V, Gortázar C (2009) Wild boar abundance and hunting effectiveness in atlantic Spain: Environmental constraints. Galemys 21(2): 13–19.

39. Burnham KP, Anderson DR (2002) Model selection and multimodel inference: A practical information-theoretic approach. New York, USA: Springer-Verlag.

40. Zuur AF, Ieno EN, Walker NJ, Saveliev AA, Smith GM (2009) Mixed effects models and extension in ecology with R. New York, USA: Springer. 530 p.

41. R Development Core Team 3.0.2. A language and environment for statistical computing. R foundation for statistical computing, Vienna, Austria. http://www.R-project.org. Accessed 2012 Dec 11.

42. Parra A, Garcia A, Inglis NF, Tato A, Alonso JM, et al. (2006) An epidemiological evaluation of Mycobacterium bovis infections in wild game animals of the Spanish Mediterranean ecosystem. Res Vet Sci 80: 140–146.

43. Gortazar C, Torres MJ, Vicente J, Acevedo P, Reglero M, et al. (2008) Bovine tuberculosis in Doñana biosphere reserve: The role of wild ungulates as disease reservoirs in the last Iberian lynx strongholds. PLoS One 3: e2776.

44. Mentaberre G, Serrano E, Velarde R, Marco I, Lavin S, et al. (2010) Absence of TB in Iberian ibex (Capra pyrenaica) in a high-risk area. Vet Rec 166: 700.

45. Martin-Hernando MP, Hofle U, Vicente J, Ruiz-Fons F, Vidal D, et al (2007) Lesions associated with Mycobacterium tuberculosis complex infection in the European wild boar. Tuberculosis (Edinb) 87: 360–367.

46. de Lisle GW (1994) Mycobacterial infections in pigs. Surveillance 21: 23–25.

47. Garcia-Jimenez WL, Benitez-Medina JM, Fernandez-Llario P, Abecia JA, Garcia-Sanchez A, et al. (2013) Comparative pathology of the natural infections by Mycobacterium bovis and by Mycobacterium caprae in wild boar (Sus scrofa). Transbound Emerg Dis 60: 102–109.

48. Galindo RC, Ayoubi P, Naranjo V, Gortazar C, Kocan KM, et al. (2009) Gene expression profiles of European wild boar naturally infected with Mycobacterium bovis. Vet Immunol Immunopathol 129: 119–125.

49. Kottek M, Grieser j, Beck c, Rudolf b, Rubel F (2006) World map of the Köppen-Geiger climate classification updated. Meteorol Z 15: 259–263. DOI: 10.1127/0941-2948/2006/0130.

50. Jolles AE, Ezenwa VO, Etienne RS, Turner WC, Olff H (2008) Interactions between macroparasites and microparasites drive infection patterns in free-ranging African buffalo. Ecology 89: 2239–2250.

51. Lopez-Olvera JR, Hofle U, Vicente J, Fernandez-de-Mera IG, Gortazar C (2006) Effects of parasitic helminths and ivermectin treatment on clinical parameters in the European wild boar (Sus scrofa). Parasitol Res 98: 582–587.

52. Romero B, Aranaz A, Sandoval A, Alvarez J, de Juan L, et al. (2008) Persistence and molecular evolution of Mycobacterium bovis population from cattle and wildlife in Doñana national park revealed by genotype variation. Vet Microbiol 132: 87–95.

53. Duarte EL, Domingos M, Amado A, Botelho A (2008) Spoligotype diversity of Mycobacterium bovis and Mycobacterium caprae animal isolates. Vet Microbiol 130: 415–421.

54. Rodriguez S, Romero B, Bezos J, de Juan L, Alvarez J, et al. (2010) High spoligotype diversity within a Mycobacterium bovis population: Clues to understanding the demography of the pathogen in Europe. Vet Microbiol 141: 89–95.

55. Riordan P, Delahay RJ, Cheeseman C, Johnson PJ, Macdonald DW (2011) Culling-induced changes in badger (Meles meles) behaviour, social organisation and the epidemiology of bovine tuberculosis. PLoS One 6: e28904.

56. Van Campen H, Rhyan J (2010) The role of wildlife in diseases of cattle. Vet Clin North Am Food Anim Pract 26: 147–61, table of contents.

57. Gamelon M, Gaillard JM, Servanty S, Gimenez O, Toïgo C, et al. (2012) Making use of harvest information to examine alternative management scenarios: A body weight-structured model for wild boar. J Appl Ecol 49: 833–841.

58. Focardi S, Gaillard JM, Ronchi F, Rossi S (2008) Survival of wild boars in a variable environment: Unexpected life-history variation in an unusual ungulate. J Mammal 89: 1113–1123.

59. Radunz B (2006) Surveillance and risk management during the latter stages of eradication: Experiences from Australia. Vet Microbiol 112: 283–290.

60. Bieber C, Ruf T (2005) Population dynamics in wild boar Sus scrofa: Ecology, elasticity of growth rate and implications for the management of pulsed resource consumers. J Appl Ecol 42: 1203–1213.

61. Mentaberre G, Porrero MC, Navarro-Gonzalez N, Serrano E, Dominguez L, et al. (2012) Cattle drive Salmonella infection in the wildlife-livestock interface. Zoonoses Public Health.

# 4

# The Impact of Resources for Clinical Surveillance on the Control of a Hypothetical Foot-and-Mouth Disease Epidemic in Denmark

**Tariq Halasa\*, Anette Boklund**

Section of Epidemiology, the National Veterinary Institutes, Technical University of Denmark, Copenhagen, Denmark

## Abstract

The objectives of this study were to assess whether current surveillance capacity is sufficient to fulfill EU and Danish regulations to control a hypothetical foot-and-mouth disease (FMD) epidemic in Denmark, and whether enlarging the protection and/or surveillance zones could minimize economic losses. The stochastic spatial simulation model DTU-DADS was further developed to simulate clinical surveillance of herds within the protection and surveillance zones and used to model spread of FMD between herds. A queuing system was included in the model, and based on daily surveillance capacity, which was 450 herds per day, it was decided whether herds appointed for surveillance would be surveyed on the current day or added to the queue. The model was run with a basic scenario representing the EU and Danish regulations, which includes a 3 km protection and 10 km surveillance zone around detected herds. In alternative scenarios, the protection zone was enlarged to 5 km, the surveillance zone was enlarged to 15 or 20 km, or a combined enlargement of the protection and surveillance zones was modelled. Sensitivity analysis included changing surveillance capacity to 200, 350 or 600 herds per day, frequency of repeated visits for herds in overlapping surveillance zones from every 14 days to every 7, 21 and 30 days, and the size of the zones combined with a surveillance capacity increased to 600 herds per day. The results showed that the default surveillance capacity is sufficient to survey herds on time. Extra resources for surveillance did not improve the situation, but fewer resources could result in larger epidemics and costs. Enlarging the protection zone was a better strategy than the basic scenario. Despite that enlarging the surveillance zone might result in shorter epidemic duration, and lower number of affected herds, it resulted frequently in larger economic losses.

**Editor:** Mónica V. Cunha, INIAV, I.P.- National Institute of Agriculture and Veterinary Research, Portugal

**Funding:** This study was funded by the Danish Veterinary Authorities. The funders had no role in study design, data collection and analysis, decision to publish, or preparation of the manuscript.

**Competing Interests:** The authors have declared that no competing interests exist.

\* Email: tahbh@vet.dtu.dk

## Introduction

Foot-and-mouth disease (**FMD**) is a highly contagious viral disease affecting ruminants and pigs [1,2,3], and may have a large economic impact on FMD-free countries and regions, in case of an epidemic [4,5].

Following the FMD epidemic within the European Union (**EU**) in 2001, the European Commission updated a set of regulations and measures to control possible future epidemics of FMD in its member states [6,7]. The measures include, among others, depopulation of detected herds and establishing 3 km protection and 10 km surveillance zones around them, in which movement restrictions and surveillance of herds are performed. As these measures, however, may not be sufficient to control an expanding or already widespread epidemic, additional control measures must be considered, such as emergency vaccination [7] and/or pre-emptive depopulation [8].

For the national veterinary authorities, the application of protective emergency vaccination insures a public support compared to the mass killing of healthy animals, in case suppressive emergency vaccination or pre-emptive depopulation

is applied [6,9]. Nonetheless, from economic standpoint, protective emergency vaccination seems not to be a recommended control strategy in case of an epidemic in Denmark [10]. Thus the question remains to whether it is possible to minimize the economic loss due to an FMD epidemic in a large exporting country of livestock and livestock products such as Denmark, without the need to kill a large number of animals.

Clinical surveillance of herds within the protection and surveillance zones has the purpose to detect infected herds early, and thus limit the spread of the disease. The effect of enlargement of the zones must depend on whether the spread of disease is limited within the existing zones, or whether the disease is often spread to the area surrounding the zones. It has been shown that the disease can spread from one herd to another over distances longer than 10 km, which is the radius of the standard surveillance zone [11,12,13]. This means that enlargement of zones might limit the spread of the disease.

In order to model enlargements of zones and clinical surveillance properly, it is necessary to take into account the available resources for clinical surveillance. Resources can be a limitation, which is necessary to consider in a country that is densely populated with livestock herds, such as Denmark, where the daily number of herds to be surveyed might be larger than the surveillance capacity.

It is therefore important to model clinical surveillance properly, which will allow an assessment of whether the current surveillance capacity is sufficient to survey herds on time as required by the EU [7], and the Danish regulations [14], and to prevent delays that could result in extra economic losses The Danish regulations require all herds, within the surveillance zones, to be surveyed within the first 7 days following the establishment of the zone [14]. Modelling these processes will allow an assessment of whether enlargements of the protection and/or surveillance zones, could limit disease spread and the economic losses.

Simulation models are valuable tools that are used to assist the veterinary authorities in contingency planning [4,8,10,11,15,16,17,18]. They have also been used to study the potential spread of FMD and to evaluate the effectiveness of potential control strategies during an FMD outbreak [19]. To our knowledge, FMD models have not been used to assist whether surveillance capacity in a country is sufficient to survey herds without delays or whether extra resources are needed. Furthermore, the epidemiological and economic effects of enlarging the protection and/or surveillance zones and the impact of surveillance frequency of herds, in overlapping zones, on epidemic consequences have, to our knowledge, not been investigated before.

The objectives of this research were to assess: 1) whether the current surveillance capacity is sufficient to fulfill the EU and Danish regulations to control a hypothetical FMD epidemic in Denmark, 2) whether enlarging the surveillance and/or the protection zones could minimize the economic losses, using either default surveillance capacity, or extra resources for surveillance, and 3) to determine the impact of surveillance frequency of herds in overlapping surveillance zones on epidemic consequences.

## Materials and Methods

### Study area and population

The study consisted of all Danish cattle, swine, sheep and goat herds in the period from 1st October 2006 until 30th September 2007. This period was chosen to avoid possible influence from the outbreak of bluetongue in Denmark in October 2007. The data included 23,550 cattle herds, 11,473 swine herds and 15,830 sheep and goat herds. For each herd, the herd data included the Danish Herd ID System, referred to as CHR (central husbandry register) number, herd type, UTM geo-coordinates, number of animals, and rate of animal movements from the herd per day. Herds were categorized into 3 categories: cattle, swine, and sheep and goats. Cattle herds were categorized as dairy or non-dairy herds. Swine herds were categorized into 19 different types based on their production type and Specific Pathogen Free (SPF) status [20]. Sheep and goats were grouped and treated equally (referred to as sheep herds throughout the paper), because Denmark has a very limited number of goat herds, and because of the disease dynamics in goat herds are expected to be similar to sheep herds. When a farm included several animal species, each species was given a different ID and set as a different herd on the same location and with the same CHR number. Information about markets was also available, including the UTM geo-coordinates.

The input parameters of the model were based on Danish data, the literature and personal communication from experts, and are available in the supplementary materials of a recent publication [10].

## The simulation model

The model simulated hypothetical spread of FMD between herds in Denmark using the dynamic spatial simulation model DTU-DADS (version 0.140), that runs in the statistical software R (Version 3.0.2) [21], based on daily discrete time events. This is an updated version of the DTU-DADS model (version 0.100) [6,10,11], which incorporates changes necessary to model resources for surveillance.

The first change included modelling resources for surveillance of herds within the protection and surveillance zones and for traced herds. A queuing system was added to the model, and herds in the protection zone would be set to queue for surveillance two times, once directly following inclusion in the protection zone, and a second time 21 days later, while herds in the surveillance zones would be set to queue for surveillance one time only, directly after inclusion in the zone. For each day modelled, the daily resources for surveillance would determine the number of herds in the queue that would be surveyed. The rest of the queued herds would wait until resources are available. It was assumed that herds that are within multiple surveillance zones will be visited every 14 days, as long as they are in multiple surveillance zones. When a herd enters a new surveillance zone, while it was not anymore in any zone, 8 days must elapse before the herd would get a new surveillance visit. When a herd was in the queue for >7 days but ≤14 days, the second visit, for herds within the protection zone, was changed from 21 to 14 days after the first visit, while when a herd was in the queue for >14 days, the second visit, for herds in the protection zone, was changed to 7 days later. This was carried out to insure that herds are surveyed before lifting the zones [7], to keep the restrictions on movements from and to the herd, and to bind zones' duration to 30 days, in order to limit potential economic damage due to longer zones duration. Nonetheless, to insure that all herds are visited before lifting a zone, when any herd was in the queue for >21 days, the duration of all zones was extended by the longest time a herd was in the queue. For instance, as soon as a herd was in a queue for 22 days, the zone duration was extended from 30 to 52 days. In case a herd was set in the queue for a second visit, while it was already queuing from a previous visit, only the first visit would be executed.

A group of veterinarians and experts from the Danish Veterinary Authorities came together in 2013, in order to assess the available resources in case of an outbreak in Denmark (Personal communication, Maren Holm Johansen from the Danish Veterinary Authorities). Based on the available resources, it was estimated that it would be possible to survey, approximately, 450 herds per day. This number was used as the default surveillance resources capacity and was changed as explained bellow in the sensitivity analysis.

Detection of infected herds is carried out using 3 processes, which are detection of first infected herd, detection of herds by the farmer (basic detection) and finally detection through surveillance visits (as explained above). In the previous version of the model, detection of the first outbreak was always fixed to day 21 following the infection start [6,10,11]. Despite that this was based on actual detection data from the UK and the Dutch epidemics in 2001, variation is expected, and hence the detection of the first outbreak was set using a PERT (Program Evaluation and Review Technique) distribution with 18, 21, and 23 days as a minimum, most likely and maximum values, respectively, based on the sensitivity analysis from a previous study [6].

In the previous version of the DTU-DADS model, all infected herds would be eventually detected using the basic detection. This is not realistic as signs could pass undetected in small herds. Basic detection was therefore modelled based on our previous work using InterSpread Plus (version 2.001.11) [10]. Infected herds would be subjected to a probability of selection of 80%. The selected herds would then be subjected to a Bernoulli process of detection based on probabilities of detection that are based on the number of days following the appearance of clinical signs. These probabilities reflected the basic surveillance (farmers' awareness). Detection following surveillance in the zones was also dependent on the number of days following the appearance of clinical signs within the herd, for cattle and swine herds. Sheep herds were sampled for serological analysis as well, and hence probability of detection, in sheep herds, depended on number of days following infection [10]. Herds that were not detected would be recovered from the disease. Recovery was based on a mechanistic module of within-herd spread built in the DTU-DADS model [11,15]. When all animals in an un-detected herd were recovered, the herd was considered a recovered herd (infection was not detected).

## Disease spread

The simulation starts with one index herd, which is the first infected herd in the epidemic. Other studies have shown that the index herd does influence the size and duration of the epidemic [11,16,20]. To include the variation caused by different index herds, we randomly selected index herds of different herd type and when relevant from areas with different animal densities. The index herds were 1,000 cattle herds located in areas with high cattle density, 1,000 in areas with low cattle density, 1,000 swine herds located in areas with high swine density and 1,000 in areas with low swine density, and 1,000 sheep herds. In total 5,000 iterations were run per scenario.

Spread of infection between herds was simulated through 7 spread mechanisms: 1) direct animal movement between herds; 2) abattoir trucks; 3) milk tankers; 4) veterinarians, artificial inseminators, and/or a milk controllers (medium risk contact); 5) visitors, feedstuff and/or rendering trucks (low risk contact); 6) markets; and 7) local spread.

Based on actual movement data, a rate of movements per day was calculated for each herd. The individual daily movement rate was used as lambda in a Poisson distribution to represent the number of movements per day. Similarly, a rate of abattoir deliveries per day was calculated based on herds' actual data and used in a Poisson distribution to simulate the number of movements to the abattoir per day from the infectious herd. Thereafter, the number of herds visited by an abattoir truck on the way to the abattoir following visit to an infected herd was estimated from a Poisson distribution with a lambda depending on the herd type. Based on milk tank deliveries a lambda was calculated and used in a Poisson distribution, to represent the number of times milk is picked up in dairy herds [10]. Likewise, medium and low risk contacts were simulated, but with different lambdas and risks of infection as presented previously [10].

Because markets in Denmark are restricted to cattle only, an infection spreading from a market can initially affect only cattle herds. The spread via markets would be due to direct movements of infected animal to susceptible herds, or via people and vehicles that had been in contact with the infected animals, and then contacted susceptible herds.

Local spread was defined as infection of susceptible herds within a 3 km radius around the infected herd [10,17] due to unexplained reasons dependent or independent of human activities, such as rodents, birds and flies, machineries and equipment moved between neighbouring herds, and to a limited degree airborne spread. Herds located on the same farm had a daily chance of infection of 95%, when one herd was infected.

When a herd was infected, the disease would spread until the herd was detected, and hence was depopulated. The period from when a herd starts showing clinical signs until it was detected, with basic detection, was dependent on the herd type, e.g. cattle herds were detected faster than sheep herds, because some sheep do not show clinical signs.

## Basic control strategy

After detection of the first infected herd, a set of control measures were applied, representing the basic scenario. These included: 1) depopulation, cleaning and disinfection of detected herds; 2) a 3 days national stand still on direct animal movements in the country; 3) creation of a 3 km protection zone and a 10 km surveillance zone around the detected herds; in which movements between herds and out of the zone were restricted and herds were surveyed one (surveillance zone) or two (protection zone) times before lifting the zone; 4) backward and forward tracing of contacts from and to detected herds. When a herd had received animals from a detected herd, the receiving herd was also depopulated and disinfected, while in case of other kinds of contacts, the herd was surveyed. When a herd was subject to surveillance, the animals were inspected for clinical signs of FMD. Sheep herds were also sampled for serological analysis [10].

The daily animal depopulation capacity was set at 2,400 ruminants and 4,800 pigs [10]. Detected herds had higher priority for depopulation than traced herds. In case of several herds on the same farm, all herds on the farm were depopulated, when one herd was detected.

## Alternative scenarios

The alternative scenarios included enlargement of the protection and/or surveillance zones, with a surveillance capacity of 450 herds a day. The protection zone was enlarged to 5 km, while the surveillance zone was enlarged to 15 or 20 km in different scenarios. Furthermore, scenarios were run combining enlargement of the protection zone to 5 km and the surveillance zone to 15 or 20 km, simultaneously.

## Sensitivity analysis

Surveillance capacity was changed from 450 to 200, 350 or 600 herds per day, to study the impact of surveillance capacity on epidemic course and consequences. Furthermore, to study the impact of enlarging surveillance and protections zones with higher resources for surveillance, the zones were enlarged as explained in the previous section, and the surveillance capacities were increased from 450 to 600 herds per day.

Herds that are located in multiple surveillance zones would be surveyed every 14 days as long as they are in multiple surveillance zones, as explained earlier. A sensitivity analysis was conducted, in which herds were surveyed every 7, 21 or 30 days instead. Sensitivity analysis on other important parameters, such as detection time and risk of infection through the different mechanisms of disease spread, is presented in an earlier publication [10].

## Costs calculation

The costs and losses of the epidemics were calculated as presented previously [10]. Briefly, the direct costs consisted of surveillance, depopulation, cleaning and disinfection, empty stable, compensation, and national standstill costs. The indirect

**Table 1.** Median (5th and 95th percentiles) of epidemic duration, number of infected herds, number of surveillance visits, direct costs, export loss and the total costs of the epidemic, that were initiated in cattle herds in high (**highCat**) and low (**lowCat**) cattle density area, swine herds in high (**highPig**) and low (**lowPig**) swine density area and in sheep herds (**sheep**).

| | Epidemic duration (days)[1] | Infected herds | Surveillance visits | Direct Costs ($€×10^6$) | Export loss ($€×10^6$) | Total costs ($€×10^6$) |
|---|---|---|---|---|---|---|
| **highCat** | | | | | | |
| **Basic** | 45 (14–113) | 56 (10–192) | 11,122 (1,896–35,839) | 31 (10–103) | 491 (388–720) | 522 (400–829) |
| **PZ5** | 44 (13–110) | 56 (9–182) | 12,345*[2] (1,869–35,485) | 31 (10–97) | 487 (386–718) | 519 (398–800) |
| **SZ15** | 43 (13–95) | 51* (9–167) | 16,125*** (3,089–37,513) | 39*** (12–128) | 504 (386–743) | 544** (399–850) |
| **SZ20** | 41*** (13–92) | 48*** (9–165) | 17,225*** (3,304–38,697) | 44*** (13–193) | 506*** (395–842) | 551*** (408–1,036) |
| **PZ5+SZ15** | 43 (14–99) | 53 (10–175) | 16,606*** (3,042–39,932) | 39*** (12–139) | 502* (388–748) | 541*** (402–887) |
| **PZ5+SZ20** | 41*** (13–94) | 47*** (9–151) | 17,923*** (4,242–40,728) | 45*** (14–193) | 507*** (388–849) | 553*** (404–1,053) |
| **lowCat** | | | | | | |
| **Basic** | 57 (17–129) | 77 (13–269) | 12,746 (1,582–37,561) | 34 (10–105) | 522 (393–766) | 558 (405–858) |
| **PZ5** | 58 (18–131) | 77 (13–243) | 13,644* (1,928–38,532) | 33 (10–101) | 524 (394–748) | 558 (405–839) |
| **SZ15** | 50*** (16–119) | 70** (12–230) | 16,817*** (2,217–42,861) | 39*** (11–140) | 517 (392–793) | 556 (405–924) |
| **SZ20** | 50*** (15–113) | 65*** (12–223) | 19,609*** (2,675–45,737) | 45*** (12–193) | 525 (396–845) | 571*** (409–1,032) |
| **PZ5+SZ15** | 51*** (17–116) | 66** (12–238) | 17,412*** (2,573–44,438) | 38** (11–143) | 515 (400–800) | 553 (412–933) |
| **PZ5+SZ20** | 50*** (16–117) | 64*** (12–235) | 19,307*** (2,879–48,430) | 44*** (13–203) | 521 (399–893) | 564*** (415–1,101) |
| **highPig** | | | | | | |
| **Basic** | 33 (7–101) | 27 (4–129) | 4,852 (656–26,873) | 18 (8–72) | 451 (364–657) | 468 (372–726) |
| **PZ5** | 35 (7–98) | 28 (4–124) | 5,437* (837–26,347) | 19 (8–67) | 452 (360–659) | 469 (369–717) |
| **SZ15** | 32 (7–90) | 26 (4–114) | 8,074*** (1,283–30,486) | 24** (10–83) | 453 (366–661) | 477* (379–745) |
| **SZ20** | 33 (6–84) | 25 (4–102) | 10,867*** (1,529–33,674) | 28*** (11–104) | 466*** (366–700) | 494*** (378–802) |
| **PZ5+SZ15** | 33 (7–83) | 26 (4–112) | 8,513*** (1,281–31,010) | 24*** (10–82) | 455 (368–644) | 476*** (380–722) |
| **PZ5+SZ20** | 32* (7–85) | 26 (4–100) | 10,456*** (1,746–34,406) | 28*** (11–105) | 458** (372–699) | 486*** (385–803) |
| **lowPig** | | | | | | |
| **Basic** | 38 (7–113) | 32 (4–158) | 5,670 (588–25,611) | 18 (7–66) | 459 (364–679) | 477 (372–743) |
| **PZ5** | 39 (7–108) | 31 (4–151) | 5,996 (737–27,280) | 17 (7–65) | 460 (359–673) | 479 (367–732) |
| **SZ15** | 33*** (7–95) | 28*** (4–114) | 7,811*** (1,034–29,805) | 21*** (8–73) | 451 (361–656) | 472 (371–727) |
| **SZ20** | 33*** (8–94) | 27*** (4–114) | 10,452*** (1,631–34,370) | 25*** (8–93) | 461 (366–693) | 486 (376–770) |
| **PZ5+SZ15** | 33** (8–94) | 29*** (4–121) | 8,642*** (1,180–30,925) | 21*** (8–76) | 458 (362–639) | 479 (371–718) |
| **PZ5+SZ20** | 31*** (8–92) | 25*** (4–117) | 10,268*** (1,757–36,752) | 24*** (9–100) | 455 (371–704) | 479 (380–813) |
| **Sheep** | | | | | | |
| **Basic** | 30 (2–100) | 20 (2–138) | 3,341 (365–25,220) | 13 (6–70) | 435 (346–658) | 449 (354–722) |
| **PZ5** | 31 (2–97) | 21 (2–126) | 3,823* (410–26,260) | 14 (6–66) | 438 (345–641) | 450 (352–710) |
| **SZ15** | 30 (2–87) | 20 (2–121) | 5,692*** (571–31,770) | 17*** (7–81) | 440 (352–657) | 458* (360–729) |
| **SZ20** | 27 (3–83) | 18 (2–114) | 7,811*** (795–32,775) | 20*** (8–112) | 441* (350–710) | 463** (360–823) |
| **PZ5+SZ15** | 28 (2–96) | 17 (2–124) | 5,365*** (632–33,031) | 16*** (7–88) | 435 (349–683) | 452 (357–761) |
| **PZ5+SZ20** | 27* (3–83) | 19 (2–108) | 7,544*** (821–31,203) | 19*** (8–98) | 439 (354–680) | 460** (363–782) |

Basic control strategy as described by Danish and European legislation was modelled (**Basic**), and compared to alternative scenarios, with enlargements of the protection zone from 3 km to 5 km (**PZ5**) and surveillance zone from 10 km to 15 km (**SZ15**) or 20 km (**SZ20**), and a combination of these enlargements.
[1]Epidemic duration is calculated from detection of the first herd in the epidemic to the last herd is depopulated.
[2]Statistical significance level in comparison to the corresponding variable in the corresponding basic scenario (absence of a star represents a P-value ≥0.05, * represents a P-value <0.05, ** represents a P-value <0.01, and *** represents a P-value <0.001).

costs included losses incurred from restrictions on exports to EU and non-EU countries (export loss). Total costs were calculated per iteration and their summaries were thereafter calculated.

## Statistical analysis

The alternative scenarios were compared to the basic scenario using epidemiological and economic results. The epidemiological results were duration of epidemics, the numbers of infected herds, number of surveillance visits and the numbers of herds detected from surveillance visits, while economic results included the direct costs, export loss and the total costs.

To test the statistical differences between the scenarios, we used the Wilcoxon rank sum test run in the statistical software R (Version 3.0.2) [21].

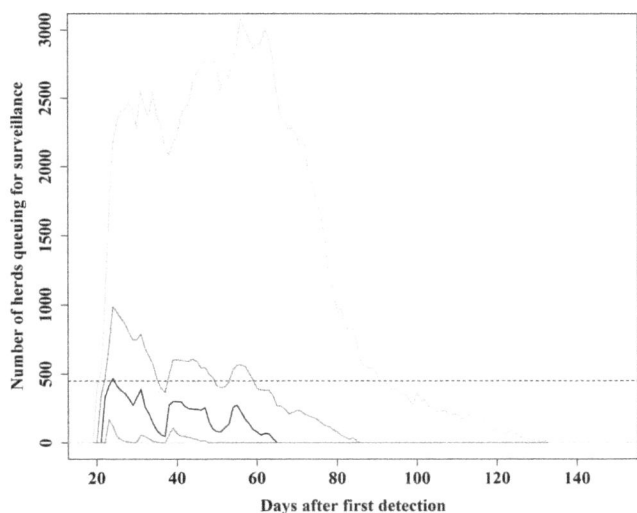

**Figure 1. Total number of herds queuing for surveillance visits, for each day, when epidemics were initiated in cattle herds located in areas with high cattle density.** A basic control strategy as described by Danish and European legislation was modelled. The black line represents the 50th percentile, the dark gray lines represent the 25th and 75th percentiles and the light gray lines represent the 5th and 95th percentiles. The interrupted line represents the daily surveillance capacity of 450 herds.

## Results

### Basic scenario

Out of the 5,000 iterations that represented the 5 different index herd types, there were 13 iterations in which the epidemics fade out before the disease was detected. All of these epidemics started in small sheep herds. In 11 out of the 5,000 iterations, the duration of the protection and surveillance zones were prolonged to more than 30 days, due to the lack of resources to survey herds within the time limit. Nine of these epidemics started in cattle herds. A large number of the herds that were in surveillance zones were actually in overlapping surveillance zones. For example, there were 1,701 (286–4,692, 5th and 95th percentiles (5–95%)) herds included in 2 or more surveillance zones in epidemics initiated in cattle herds in high cattle density areas, which is 55% (27–79%) of the total number of herds in the surveillance zones.

Epidemics initiated in cattle herds were larger, longer in duration and costlier than epidemics initiated in swine and sheep herds (Table 1). For example, when epidemics were initiated in cattle herds in high cattle density areas, the median epidemic duration was 45 days (14–113 days, 5–95%), the median number of infected herds was 56 (10–192, 5–95%), and the median total costs was €522 million, (€400–€829 million, 5–95%) (Table 1). In total, a median of 11,122 surveillance visits (1,896–35,839, 5–95%) were conducted in herds within the protection and surveillance zones and in traced contact herds.

For each day, the number of herds queuing for surveillance, in epidemics initiated in cattle herds in high cattle density areas, is shown in Figure 1. It shows that in a median size epidemic, the

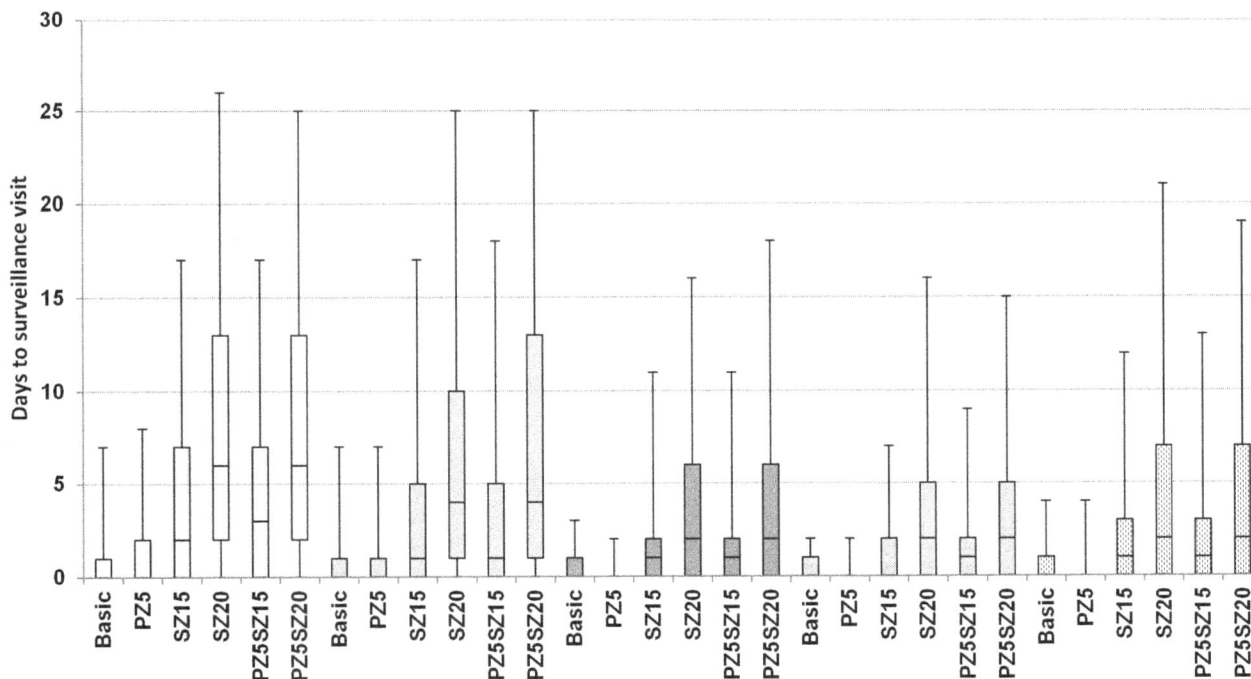

**Figure 2. Box plots of the waiting time before a scheduled surveillance visit is executed (days, between a herd was set for surveillance, and until the herd was actually surveyed), in epidemics that were initiated in cattle herds located in areas with high cattle density (empty boxes), cattle herds located in areas with low cattle density (light gray boxes), swine herds located in areas with high swine densities (dark gray boxes), swine herds located in areas with low swine densities (dotted boxes), and in sheep herds (vertical-dashed boxes).** A basic control strategy (Basic) as described by Danish and European legislation is compared to alternative scenarios, with enlargement of the protection zone from 3 km to 5 km (PZ5) and of the surveillance zone from 10 km to 15 km (SZ15) or 20 km (SZ20), and a combination of these enlargements. The middle line represents the median, the box represents the 25th and 75th percentiles and the whiskers represent the 5th and 95th percentiles.

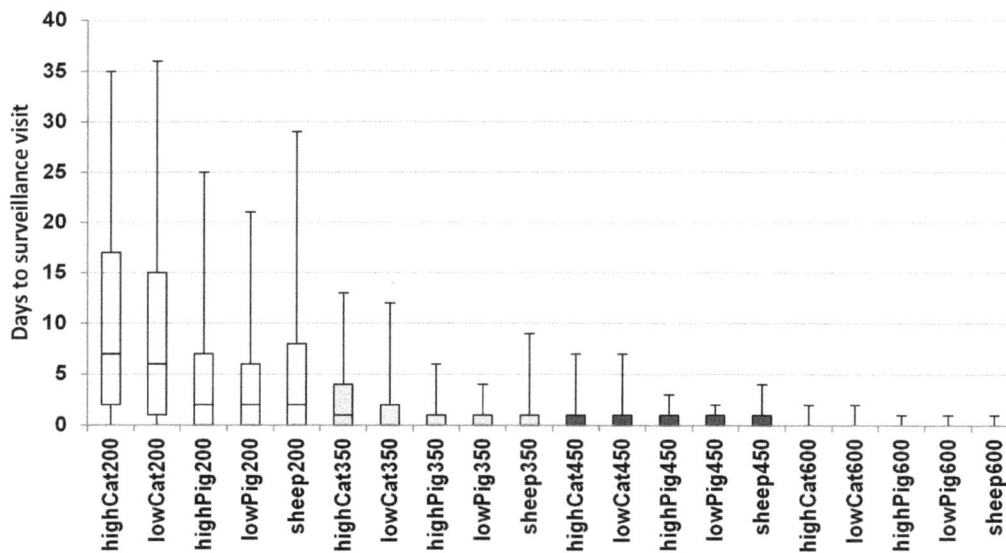

**Figure 3. Box plots of the waiting time before a scheduled surveillance visit is executed (difference, in days, between the day the herd was set for surveillance, and the day the herd was actually surveyed), in epidemics that were initiated in cattle herds in high cattle density areas (highCat), cattle herds in low cattle density areas (lowCat), swine herds in high swine density areas (highPig), swine herds in low swine density areas (lowPig), and in sheep herds (sheep).** The basic control strategy as described by Danish and European legislation (dark gray boxes) with a surveillance capacity of 450 herds per day is compared to scenarios with reduced or increased surveillance capacity to 200 (empty boxes), 350 (light gray boxes) or 600 (boxes do not appear) herds per day. The middle line represents the median, the box represents the 25th and 75th percentiles and the whiskers represent the 5th and 95th percentiles.

maximum number of herds queuing for surveillance is approximately 470 herds per day. This means that the available resources (450 herds per day) are sufficient, so that most often herds will be surveyed at the same day they were scheduled for surveillance. In epidemics corresponding to the 75th percentile, the maximum number of herds queuing for surveillance is approximately 990 herds, while in the 95th percentile situation, the maximum number is, approximately, 3,100 herds. In such extreme epidemics, the resources would still be sufficient for surveying herds on time (within 7 days from assignment to surveillance visit) (Figures 1 and 2). Figure 2, shows box plots of the delay time (days between when the herd was set for surveillance and when the herd was actually surveyed) before a scheduled surveillance visit is executed for the basic and alternative scenarios and the 5 different types of the index herds. For the basic scenario, generally, herds would be surveyed at the same day they were set for surveillance. Nevertheless, long delays can occur when epidemics are large, but herds would still be visited on time (Figure 2).

## Alternative scenarios

When the protection zone was enlarged from 3 to 5 km, in 10 of the 5,000 iterations that represented the 5 different types of index herd, the duration of the zones was increased to more than 30 days. When the surveillance zone was enlarged from 10 km to 15 km or 20 km, the number of iterations in which the zone duration was longer than 30 days were 97 and 315, respectively. When the protection zone was enlarged to 5 km and the surveillance zone was simultaneously enlarged to 15 or 20 km, the number of iterations, in which the zone duration was longer than 30 days were 98 and 328, respectively. Prolongation of the zone duration occurred, mainly, when epidemics where initiated in cattle herds.

Enlarging the protection zone from 3 km to 5 km did not change the epidemic duration, number of affected herds and the

total costs, regardless the type of index herd that was used to initiate the epidemics (Table 1). However, enlarging the protection zone resulted in the lowest total costs for the 5% worse epidemics (Table 1). Depending on the type of index herd, enlarging the surveillance zone from 10 to 15 km may reduce epidemic duration and the number of infected herds, compared to the corresponding basic scenario, but it would not reduce the economic damage (Table 1). Enlarging the surveillance zone from 10 to 20 km resulted frequently in shorter epidemic duration and fewer infected herds compared to the corresponding basic scenario, especially when epidemics were initiated in cattle herds (Table 1). However, in these situations, larger number of surveillance visits and higher costs were predicted (Table 1). Enlarging the protection zone to 5 km and the surveillance zone to 20 km resulted in the shortest epidemic duration and the lowest number of infected herds, regardless the type of index herd that was used to initiate the epidemics (Table 1). However, this scenario resulted in the largest number of surveillance visits and costs of the epidemics. When the surveillance zone is enlarged, longer delays occurred (Figure 2), due to the larger number of herds queuing for surveillance. This shows that the surveillance capacity would not be sufficient to survey herds on time for large epidemics, and hence extra resources would be needed.

Export losses are the driving force of the total economic losses in general (Table 1), but it also can be seen that the direct costs may increase, when the zones are enlarged, compared to the corresponding basic scenario (Table 1).

## Sensitivity analysis

Reducing surveillance capacity would result in longer delay time before a herd is surveyed, while increasing it would result in a shorter delay time (Figure 3). Reducing the capacity to 200 herds per day would result in fewer surveillance visits than the basic scenario (Table 2). However, it might result in longer epidemic

**Table 2.** Median with (5th and 95th percentiles) of epidemic duration, number of infected herds, number of surveillance visits and the total costs of the epidemic, using the basic scenario (**Basic**) that represent the EU and Danish control measures, when epidemics were initiated in cattle herds in high (**highCat**) and low (**lowCat**) cattle density area, swine herds in high (**highPig**) and low swine (**lowPig**) density area and in sheep herds (**sheep**); The influence of changes in the surveillance capacity (**Capacity**) from 450 herds per day to 200, 350 or 600 herds per day are compared.

| | Epidemic duration (days)[1] | Infected herds | Surveillance visits | Total costs ($\in \times 10^6$) |
|---|---|---|---|---|
| **highCat** | | | | |
| Basic | 45 (14–113) | 56 (10–192) | 11,122 (1,896–35,839) | 522 (400–829) |
| Capacity-200 herds/day | 47 (14–114) | 57 (10–201) | 8,822***[2] (1,785–22,250) | 523*** (393–1,030) |
| Capacity-350 herds/day | 45 (14–119) | 58 (9–197) | 11,449 (1,764–32,125) | 527 (395–856) |
| Capacity-600 herds/day | 46 (14–113) | 57 (10–183) | 11,171 (1,900–36,460) | 528 (400–809) |
| **lowCat** | | | | |
| Basic | 57 (17–129) | 77 (13–269) | 12,746 (1,582–37,561) | 558 (405–858) |
| Capacity-200 herds/day | 60 (17–144) | 79* (13–297) | 10,341*** (1,539–25,940) | 564*** (404–1,080) |
| Capacity-350 herds/day | 56 (17–133) | 76 (14–249) | 12,361*** (1,666–32,663) | 556 (405–873) |
| Capacity-600 herds/day | 57 (17–129) | 76 (13–244) | 12,514 (1,582–39,502) | 559 (402–832) |
| **highPig** | | | | |
| Basic | 33 (7–101) | 27 (4–129) | 4,852 (656–26,873) | 468 (372–726) |
| Capacity-200 herds/day | 36* (7–105) | 28* (4–146) | 4,822*** (678–19,267) | 473** (372–819) |
| Capacity-350 herds/day | 34 (7–106) | 27 (4–141) | 5,105 (646–25,614) | 469 (372–757) |
| Capacity-600 herds/day | 34 (7–103) | 28 (4–133) | 4,974 (656–27,233) | 473 (372–746) |
| **lowPig** | | | | |
| Basic | 38 (7–113) | 32 (4–158) | 5,670 (588–25,611) | 477 (372–743) |
| Capacity-200 herds/day | 38 (8–115) | 32 (4–156) | 5,425*** (581–19,628) | 479 (369–805) |
| Capacity-350 herds/day | 37 (7–108) | 31 (4–148) | 5,488** (580–24,048) | 477 (369–734) |
| Capacity-600 herds/day | 37 (7–106) | 30 (4–146) | 5,702** (588–25,128) | 474 (373–730) |
| **Sheep** | | | | |
| Basic | 30 (2–100) | 20 (2–138) | 3,341 (365–25,220) | 449 (354–722) |
| Capacity-200 herds/day | 29 (2–97) | 20 (2–142) | 3,045*** (343–16,811) | 446 (354–775) |
| Capacity-350 herds/day | 30 (2–104) | 20 (2–132) | 3,203 (365–24,355) | 451 (352–720) |
| Capacity-600 herds/day | 29 (2–101) | 21 (2–136) | 3,331 (365–26,558) | 448 (354–714) |

[1]Epidemic duration is calculated from detection of the first herd in the epidemic to the last herd is depopulated.
[2]Statistical significance level in comparison to the corresponding variable in the corresponding basic scenario (absence of a star represents a P-value ≥0.05, * represents a P-value <0.05, ** represents a P-value <0.01, and *** represents a P-value <0.001).

duration, larger number of infected herds, and larger economic damage, compared to the corresponding basic scenario (Table 2). Furthermore, it would result in a notably larger variation in the number of infected herds and in the total costs, compared to the corresponding basic scenario (Table 2). Reducing the capacity to 350 herds or increasing it to 600 herds per day did not result in extra economic losses compared to the corresponding basic scenario (Table 2).

When the frequency of surveying herds that are located in overlapping surveillance zones was changed from once every 14 days to once every 7, 21 or 30 days, the number and proportion of herds located in overlapping surveillance zones were close to those observed in the corresponding basic scenario. Changing the frequency to 7 or 30 days, increased or decreased the number of surveillance visits, respectively, while there were no changes to the number of infected herds, the number of diagnosed herds from surveillance and epidemic duration and costs (Table 3).

Increasing surveillance capacity from 450 to 600 herds per day and enlarging the protection and/or the surveillance zones would most often not affect epidemic duration, number of infected herds

and total costs (Table 4), compared to the corresponding scenario using the default surveillance capacity (Table 1). However, more herds would be surveyed when surveillance capacity is increased (Table 4).

## Discussion

Prior to the UK 2001 epidemic, the contingency plan of the Ministry of Agriculture, Forestry and Fisheries for notifiable diseases included that in case of a severe case scenario of spread of a specific exotic disease, the UK would need 235 veterinary officers. In a more extensive outbreak, the number of staff needed might rise to 300 [22]. Nonetheless, during the outbreak, 2,500 temporary veterinary inspectors were assigned, with nearly 70 from abroad, and a further 700 foreign government veterinarians and personnel assisted on temporary basis [22]. This reflects the importance of assessing whether available resources are sufficient to control an epidemic of FMD, in order to improve the contingency plan. The current study shows that the available resources for clinical surveillance, in case of an FMD outbreak in

**Table 3.** Median with (5th and 95th percentiles) of epidemic duration, number of infected herds, number of diagnosed herds from surveillance, number of surveillance visits and the total costs of the epidemic, using the basic scenario (**Basic**) that represent the EU and Danish control measures, when epidemics were initiated in cattle herds in high (**highCat**) and low (**lowCat**) cattle density area, swine herds in high (**highPig**) and low (**lowPig**) swine density area and in sheep herds (**sheep**); The influence of changing the frequency of surveying herds located in overlapping zones from every 14 days to every 7, 21 or 30 days is compared.

| | Epidemic duration (days)[1] | Infected herds | Diagnosed herds from surveillance | Surveillance visits | Total costs (€×10⁶) |
|---|---|---|---|---|---|
| **highCat** | | | | | |
| **Basic** | 45 (14–113) | 56 (10–192) | 7 (0–27) | 11,122 (1,896–35,839) | 522 (400–829) |
| **Survey every 7 days** | 46 (14–117) | 56 (9–197) | 7 (1–23) | 15,381***[2] (1,967–40,248) | 528 (397–822) |
| **Survey every 21 days** | 47 (14–113) | 59 (9–191) | 7 (1–24) | 10,298 (1,680–32,312) | 534 (399–817) |
| **Survey every 30 days** | 48 (14–110) | 59 (9–185) | 7 (1–24) | 9,989*** (1,575–29,301) | 536 (399–800) |
| **lowCat** | | | | | |
| **Basic** | 57 (17–129) | 77 (13–269) | 10 (1–36) | 12,746 (1,582–37,561) | 558 (405–858) |
| **Survey every 7 days** | 55 (17–126) | 75 (13–259) | 11 (1–37) | 16,585*** (2,007–44,861) | 548 (406–852) |
| **Survey every 21 days** | 57 (17–129) | 76 (14–259) | 10 (1–38) | 11,110** (1,489–33,343) | 557 (403–836) |
| **Survey every 30 days** | 61 (17–140) | 79 (14–271) | 10 (1–39) | 10,634*** (1,420–32,248) | 569 (403–882) |
| **highPig** | | | | | |
| **Basic** | 33 (7–101) | 27 (4–129) | 3 (0–17) | 4,852 (656–26,873) | 468 (372–726) |
| **Survey every 7 days** | 34 (7– 102) | 28 (4–121) | 3 (0–17) | 6,571*** (755–31,191) | 467 (372–719) |
| **Survey every 21 days** | 34 (7–98) | 28 (4–127) | 3 (0–15) | 4,549 (642–21,623) | 469 (372–712) |
| **Survey every 30 days** | 34 (7–97) | 27 (4–127) | 3 (0–15) | 4,066** (642–20,197) | 468 (372–710) |
| **lowPig** | | | | | |
| **Basic** | 38 (7–113) | 32 (4–158) | 4 (0–22) | 5,670 (588–25,611) | 477 (372–743) |
| **Survey every 7 days** | 37 (7–112) | 30 (4–146) | 4 (0–22) | 7,454*** (658–33,284) | 476 (370–753) |
| **Survey every 21 days** | 41 (7–112) | 33 (4–151) | 4 (0–22) | 5,276 (581–22,637) | 487 (372–756) |
| **Survey every 30 days** | 39 (7–113) | 32 (4–142) | 4 (0–18) | 4,575** (581–21,385) | 482 (372–748) |
| **Sheep** | | | | | |
| **Basic** | 30 (2–100) | 20 (2–138) | 2 (0–19) | 3,341 (365–25,220) | 449 (354–722) |
| **Survey every 7 days** | 28 (2–100) | 19 (2–134) | 2 (0–19) | 3,969** (382–31,743) | 445 (352–725) |
| **Survey every 21 days** | 30 (2–108) | 20 (2–140) | 2 (0–17) | 3,032*** (365–24,442) | 449 (354–753) |
| **Survey every 30 days** | 31 (2–105) | 21 (2–140) | 2 (0–18) | 2,781* (365–21,207) | 450 (354–734) |

[1]Epidemic duration is calculated from detection of the first herd in the epidemic to the last herd is depopulated.
[2]Statistical significance level in comparison to the corresponding variable in the corresponding basic scenario (absence of a star represents a P-value ≥0.05, * represents a P-value <0.05, ** represents a P-value <0.01, and *** represents a P-value <0.001).

Denmark, seem to be sufficient to survey herds within the protection and surveillance zones on time.

Regardless the type of index herd that was used to initiate the epidemics, reducing surveillance capacity did not change the epidemic duration and the number of infected herds. Nonetheless, it resulted in a larger costs and variability around the predicted costs in most situations, compared to the corresponding basic scenario. It also resulted in a fewer number of surveillance visits (Table 2). When surveillance capacity was reduced to 200 herds per day, a herd would have to wait few days before it could be surveyed (Figure 3). This delay would apparently not result in further spread of the disease, as the number of infected herds was not different from the corresponding basic scenario. Nonetheless, lower capacity might result in more variability in disease spread, and thus large epidemics might occur more frequently, as shown from the 95% percentiles (Table 2). At least, 8 days should elapse between two surveillance visits (see materials and methods). When resources were reduced to 200 herds per day, long delay time occurred (Figure 3), and therefore a herd could be set in the queue for a new surveillance visit, while the previous visit was not yet executed. In such cases, the model was set to execute only the first visit, which resulted in fewer number of surveillance visits (Table 2).

On the other hand, increasing surveillance capacity does not seem to affect the epidemic course (Table 2). This indicates that the estimated surveillance capacity in Denmark, under the modelled regulations, is sufficient to fulfill the EU and Danish regulations of surveying herds that are within the protection and surveillance zones without delays. However, when the surveillance zone was enlarged, the surveillance capacity was normally not sufficient to survey herds on time, when large epidemics occurred (Figure 2). Thus extra resources might be needed when the Veterinary Authorities consider enlarging the surveillance zone.

When the surveillance capacity was increased in scenarios with enlarged zones, more herds were surveyed, as a result of shorter waiting times for surveillance visits. Repeated visits that were not executed due to the lack of resources in the basic scenario were now executed, due to the availability of more resources. Nevertheless, enlargement of the zones combined with extra surveillance capacity, in most situations, did not minimize the economic losses of the simulated epidemics (Table 4).

**Table 4.** Median with (5th and 95th percentiles) of epidemic duration, number of infected herds, number of surveillance visits and the total costs of the epidemic, following enlargements of the protection zone from 3 km to 5 km (**PZ5**) and surveillance zone from 10 km to 15 km (**SZ15**) or 20 km (**SZ20**), and a combination of these enlargements, and increasing surveillance capacity from 450 herds per day to 600 herds per day, when epidemics were initiated in cattle herds in high (**highCat**) and low (**lowCat**) cattle density area, swine herds in high (**highPig**) and low (**lowPig**) swine density area and in sheep herds (**sheep**).

| | Epidemic duration (days)[1] | Infected herds | Surveillance visits | Total costs (€×10⁶) |
|---|---|---|---|---|
| **highCat** | | | | |
| PZ5 | 44 (13–106) | 55 (9–178) | 12,287 (1,868–40,073) | 525 (399–799) |
| SZ15 | 42 (13–99) | 52 (8–167) | 16,703*[2] (2,842–46,513) | 538 (399–852) |
| SZ20 | 40 (13–96) | 48 (9–169) | 19,941*** (3,569–51,503) | 544 (407–944) |
| PZ5+SZ15 | 43 (13–97) | 52 (10–162) | 18,201** (3,164–45,972) | 540 (404–823) |
| PZ5+SZ20 | 41 (13–89) | 48 (9–144) | 21,010*** (4,105–47,190) | 557 (408–855) |
| **lowCat** | | | | |
| PZ5 | 56 (18–136) | 76 (13–264) | 13,772 (1,904–45,936) | 552 (405–868) |
| SZ15 | 51 (16–114) | 68 (12–225) | 17,192 (2,129–48,082) | 557 (404–854) |
| SZ20 | 47* (15–106) | 63 (12–215) | 20,991* (2,747–53,332) | 559* (413–947) |
| PZ5+SZ15 | 53 (17–117) | 65 (12–242) | 18,789* (2,786–50,217) | 565 (412–860) |
| PZ5+SZ20 | 49 (16–115) | 64 (12–212) | 22,273*** (3,334–56,115) | 568 (412–944) |
| **highPig** | | | | |
| PZ5 | 35 (7–107) | 28 (4–129) | 5,715 (837–29,283) | 473 (372–751) |
| SZ15 | 33 (7–92) | 27 (4–108) | 8,363 (1,276–34,616) | 482 (376–734) |
| SZ20 | 32 (7–82) | 25 (4–93) | 10,647 (1,610–38,393) | 485 (379–762) |
| PZ5+SZ15 | 33 (7–86) | 26 (4–104) | 8,467 (1,343–34,282) | 480 (376–723) |
| PZ5+SZ20 | 32 (7–83) | 25 (4–98) | 11,121 (1,846–39,143) | 491 (381–751) |
| **lowPig** | | | | |
| PZ5 | 37 (7–110) | 30 (4–158) | 5,837 (737–30,835) | 473 (273–559) |
| SZ15 | 33 (7–91) | 28 (4–117) | 8,351 (1,090–31,455) | 474 (275–520) |
| SZ20 | 34 (7–89) | 28 (4–111) | 11,644* (1,610–39,374) | 488 (278–561) |
| PZ5+SZ15 | 35 (8–102) | 29 (4–129) | 8,928 (1,230–36,426) | 481 (275–566) |
| PZ5+SZ20 | 34 (8–90) | 28 (4–118) | 12,185** (1,772–38,772) | 489 (282–552) |
| **Sheep** | | | | |
| PZ5 | 30 (2–102) | 20 (2–124) | 3,740 (410–27,242) | 449 (352–725) |
| SZ15 | 29 (2–88) | 19 (2–116) | 5,409 (638–35,592) | 456 (360–715) |
| SZ20 | 28 (3–86) | 18 (2–104) | 7,896 (795–40,161) | 462 (361–763) |
| PZ5+SZ15 | 29 (2–88) | 18 (2–123) | 5,651 (702–36,926) | 454 (358–727) |
| PZ5+SZ20 | 28 (3–90) | 18 (2–116) | 7,954 (837–43,499) | 461 (363–792) |

[1]Epidemic duration is calculated from detection of the first herd in the epidemic to the last herd is depopulated.
[2]Statistical significance level in comparison to the corresponding variable and scenario in Table 1 (absence of a star represents a P-value ≥0.05, * represents a P-value < 0.05, ** represents a P-value <0.01, and *** represents a P-value <0.001).

Overlapping zones are expected to occur during an outbreak. It is important to determine, how often herds should be re-surveyed, in order to optimize FMD control, when new zones are created, including herds already in other zones. As explained earlier, we assumed that herds within overlapping surveillance zones would be surveyed every 14 days, as long as they are in overlapping zones. This assumption was based on expert knowledge from the Veterinary Authorities and their experience with other disease outbreaks. Nonetheless, a sensitivity analysis was conducted by changing this value to 7, 21 and 30 days. Increasing the surveillance frequency to every 7 days would not change the course of the epidemic, nor the number of detected herds through surveillance (Table 3). Furthermore, reducing it to every 21 or 30 days would not change the number of herds detected through

surveillance nor the total costs (Table 3). Generally, this indicates that the first surveillance visit seems to be important to detect herds early through surveillance. Repeated visits for these herds do not seem to be necessary, and thus can be minimized. It is important to mention though, that the model assumes that the surveillance teams are highly effective in finding clinical signs if present. During an outbreak, veterinarians will be very aware of the possibility of infection, and thus they will most likely find existing clinical signs. Given the availability of resources, the Veterinary Authorities would most likely re-survey herds as frequently as possible, in order to convince the World Organization of Animal Health (OIE) and EU member states of the sufficiency of the applied measures, to regain the free status as fast as possible.

Enlarging the protection zone was as good as the corresponding basic scenario, in terms of epidemic duration, number of affected herds and total epidemic costs. Although it resulted in larger number of surveillance visits compared to the corresponding basic scenario, the resources were usually sufficient to survey herds on time. Furthermore, enlarging the protection zone was a cheaper strategy than the corresponding basic scenario, in case of large epidemics as indicated by the $95^{th}$ percentile of the total costs of this scenario, regardless the index herd type that was used to initiate the epidemics (Table 1). Enlarging the protection zone was as good as the basic scenario in median size epidemics, but it included the advantage of minimizing economic losses in case of large epidemics, which makes it a better strategy than the basic scenario.

In certain situations, enlarging the surveillance zones resulted in shorter epidemic duration and lower number of infected herds (Table 1). However, it resulted frequently in larger number of surveillance visits (Table 1), and hence to extra delays, before herds can be visited (Figure 2). It also resulted in larger total costs compared to the corresponding basic scenario. This was due to the larger number of surveillance visits, which lead to higher direct costs (Table 1). Important to mention that it was assumed in the economic calculations that only herds outside the surveillance zones can export products to EU countries, without price reduction [10]. This means that enlargement of the surveillance zones would result in larger economic damage due to larger export loss to the EU countries (Table 1). Moreover, it was more often necessary to prolong the duration of the zones, when the surveillance zones were enlarged compared to the basic scenario. Longer zone duration means larger economic damage due to larger export loss. Generally, this means that the potential gain from shorter epidemic duration and fewer infected herds, caused by the enlarged surveillance zone, would not pay off the economic damage due to the higher costs. Shorter epidemic duration and fewer infected herds might actually include an advantage of reducing the risk of losing markets. In case of an epidemic, countries that import livestock and/or livestock products from Denmark might either find other suppliers and completely stop imports from Denmark, or might continue imports, following the end of the restriction on export, but with a lesser extent than before the epidemic. Although it is difficult to predict the reaction of foreign markets in case of an epidemic [10,23], the risk of losing markets would probably positively correlate with epidemic duration. Thus the economic outcomes might differ depending on the reaction of the importing countries.

The results shown in our study are influenced by the herd structure in Denmark and the large export of especially pigs and pig products. Therefore, the effect of enlarged zone sizes might be different in other countries. Furthermore, in this study we focused on zone size and surveillance capacity with the basic control strategy. In future work, it will be interesting to investigate the effect of changes on, for example, pre-emptive depopulation or emergency vaccination.

## Conclusions

The available resources for clinical surveillance, in case of an FMD outbreak in Denmark, are sufficient to survey herds in the protection and surveillance zones within the first week of the zones' establishment, under EU and Danish control regulations. However, when enlarging the surveillance zone is considered, extra resources may be needed, in order to survey herds on time. Generally, enlargement of the protection zone seems to be a better option than the basic scenario. Enlarging the surveillance zone may reduce epidemic duration and the number of affected herds. However, reduction of the economic losses would not be expected. Extra resources for clinical surveillance do not minimize the total costs of the epidemic when the protection and/or surveillance zones are enlarged. Fewer resources may result in larger and costlier epidemics.

## Acknowledgments

The Authors acknowledge Sten Mortensen and Maren Holm Johansen from the Danish Veterinary Authorities for feedback.

## Author Contributions

Conceived and designed the experiments: TH AB. Performed the experiments: TH. Analyzed the data: TH. Contributed reagents/materials/analysis tools: TH AB. Wrote the paper: TH AB.

## References

1. Halasa T, Boklund A, Cox S, Enøe C (2011) Meta-analysis on the efficacy of foot-and-mouth disease emergency vaccination. Prev Vet Med 98: 1–9.
2. Cox SJ, Barnett PV (2009) Experimental evaluation of foot-and-mouth disease vaccines for emergency use in ruminants and pigs: a review. Vet Res 40: 13–43.
3. Grubmann MJ, Baxt B (2004) Foot-and-mouth disease. Clin Microbiol Rev 17: 465–493.
4. Pendell DL, Leatherman J, Schroeder TC, Alward GS (2007) The economic impact of foot-and-mouth disease outbreak: a regional analysis. J Agr App Econ 39: 19–33.
5. Knight-Jones TJD, Rushton J (2013) The economic impact of foot-and-mouth disease: what are they, how big are they and where do they occur? Prev Vet Med 112: 161–173.
6. Halasa T, Willeberg P, Christiansen LE, Boklund A, AlKhamis M, et al. (2013) Decisions on control of foot-and-mouth disease informed using model predictions. Prev Vet Med 112: 194–202.
7. European Commission (2003) Council Directive 2003/85/EC on community measures for the control of foot-and-mouth disease repealing, Directive 85/511/EEC and amending directive 92/46/EEC. Official J Eur Union L306, 46, 22 November 2003.
8. Backer JA, Hagenaars TJ, Nodelijk G, van Roermund HJW (2012) Vaccination against foot-and-mouth disease I: Epidemiological consequences. Prev Vet Med 107: 27–40.
9. Hutber AM, Kitching RP, Phillipcinec E (2006) Predictions for the timing and use of culling or vaccination during a foot-and-mouth disease epidemic. Res Vet Sci 81: 31–36.
10. Boklund A, Halasa T, Christiansen LE, Enøe C (2013) Comparing control strategies against foot-and-mouth disease: Will vaccination be cost-effective in Denmark? Prev Vet Med 111: 206–219.

11. Halasa T, Boklund A, Stockmarr A, Enøe C, Christiansen LE (2014) A comparison between two models for spread of foot-and-mouth disease. PLoS ONE, DOI:10.1371/journalpone.0092521.
12. Gibbens JC, Sharpe CE, Wilesmith JW, Mansley LM, Michalopoulou E, et al. (2001) Descriptive epidemiology of the 2001 foot-and-mouth disease epidemic in Great Britain: the first five months. Vet Rec 149: 729–743.
13. Perez A, Ward MP, Carpenter TE (2004) Control of a foot-and-mouth disease epidemic in Argentina. Prev Vet Med 65: 217–226.
14. Danish Contingency Plan (2004) (Mund-og-klovesyge beredskabsplan), Operational manual, Husdyrsygdomskontoret, Fødevaredirektoratet, Mørkhøj Bygade 19, 2860 Søborg, June 2004.
15. Bates T, Thurmond MC, Carpenter TE (2003) Description of and epidemic simulation model for use in evaluating strategies to control an outbreak of foot-and-mouth disease. AJVR 64: 195–204.
16. Velthuis AGJ, Mourits MCM (2007) Effectiveness of movement prevention regulations to reduce the spread of foot-and-mouth disease in The Netherlands. Prev Vet Med 82: 262–281.
17. Martinez-Lopez B, Perez AM, Sanchez-Vizcaino JM (2010) A simulation model for the potential spread of foot-and-mouth disease in the Castile and Leon region of Spain. Prev Vet Med 96: 19–29.
18. Ward MP, Highfield LD, Vongseng P, Garner MG (2009) Simulation of foot-and-mouth disease spread within an integrated livestock system in Texas, USA. Prev. Vet. Med. 88, 286–297.
19. Keeling MJ, Woolhouse MEJ, Shaw DJ, Mathews L, Chase-Topping M, et al. (2001) Dynamics of the 2001 UK foot and mouth disease epidemic: Stochastic dispersal in heterogeneous landscape. Science 294: 813–817.

20. Boklund A, Alban L, Toft N, Uttenthal Å (2009) Comparing the epidemiological and economic effects of control strategies against classical swine fever in Denmark. Prev Vet Med 90: 180–193.

21. R Development Core Team (2013) R: A language and environment for statistical computing. R Foundation for Statistical Computing, Vienna, Austria. URL http://www.R-project.org/.

22. Anderson I (2002) Foot and Mouth Disease 2001: Lessons to be Learned Inquiry Report, Published by TSO (The Stationary Office), UK.

23. Junker F, Komorowska J, van Tongeren F (2009) Impact of Animal Disease Outbreaks and Alternative Control Practices on Agricultural Markets and Trade: The case of FMD. OECD Food, Agriculture and Fisheries Working Papers, No. 19, OECD Publishing, doi: 10.1787/221275827814.

# 5

# Transmission of Chronic Wasting Disease in Wisconsin White-Tailed Deer: Implications for Disease Spread and Management

Christopher S. Jennelle[1]*, Viviane Henaux[1], Gideon Wasserberg[2], Bala Thiagarajan[1], Robert E. Rolley[3], Michael D. Samuel[4]

1 Department of Forest and Wildlife Ecology, University of Wisconsin, Madison, Wisconsin, United States of America, 2 Biology Department, University of North Carolina, Greensboro, North Carolina, United States of America, 3 Wisconsin Department of Natural Resources, Madison, Wisconsin, United States of America, 4 U.S. Geological Survey, Wisconsin Cooperative Wildlife Research Unit, University of Wisconsin, Madison, Wisconsin, United States of America

## Abstract

Few studies have evaluated the rate of infection or mode of transmission for wildlife diseases, and the implications of alternative management strategies. We used hunter harvest data from 2002 to 2013 to investigate chronic wasting disease (CWD) infection rate and transmission modes, and address how alternative management approaches affect disease dynamics in a Wisconsin white-tailed deer population. Uncertainty regarding demographic impacts of CWD on cervid populations, human and domestic animal health concerns, and potential economic consequences underscore the need for strategies to control CWD distribution and prevalence. Using maximum-likelihood methods to evaluate alternative multi-state deterministic models of CWD transmission, harvest data strongly supports a frequency-dependent transmission structure with sex-specific infection rates that are two times higher in males than females. As transmissible spongiform encephalopathies are an important and difficult-to-study class of diseases with major economic and ecological implications, our work supports the hypothesis of frequency-dependent transmission in wild deer at a broad spatial scale and indicates that effective harvest management can be implemented to control CWD prevalence. Specifically, we show that harvest focused on the greater-affected sex (males) can result in stable population dynamics and control of CWD within the next 50 years, given the constraints of the model. We also provide a quantitative estimate of geographic disease spread in southern Wisconsin, validating qualitative assessments that CWD spreads relatively slowly. Given increased discovery and distribution of CWD throughout North America, insights from our study are valuable to management agencies and to the general public concerned about the impacts of CWD on white-tailed deer populations.

**Editor:** Roy Martin Roopll, East Carolina University School of Medicine, United States of America

**Funding:** Funding was provided by the Wisconsin Department of Natural Resources and U.S. Geological Survey. The University of Wisconsin Department of Forest and Wildlife Ecology provided assistance with publication costs. The funders had no role in study design, data collection and analysis, decision to publish, or preparation of the manuscript.

**Competing Interests:** The authors have declared that no competing interests exist.

* E-mail: chris.jennelle@dnr.iowa.gov

## Introduction

As in humans [1], chronic diseases constitute an important threat to wildlife because of the potential for demographic and evolutionary consequences [2] that negatively impact host populations. Detection and monitoring of these diseases can be difficult because prolonged epizootics can result in low, usually undetected, levels of infection, morbidity, or mortality [3]. Evaluating the incidence and spatial dynamics of chronic wildlife diseases requires long-term studies that may be difficult to conduct in natural populations due to financial and logistical constraints. These issues limit the ability of wildlife managers to understand and predict wildlife disease epizootics, assess their impacts on natural populations, and evaluate alternative control strategies. Because of such complexity, modeling disease dynamics may be the only practical way to quantify the spatial and temporal patterns of chronic diseases in wildlife, evaluate alternative transmission mechanisms, predict the spread of the infectious agents across the landscape, and identify viable management options.

Among transmissible spongiform encephalopathies (TSE), chronic wasting disease (CWD) is a fatal neurodegenerative disease of free-ranging and captive cervids. First recognized in captive mule deer (*Odocoileus hemionus*) in Colorado in the 1960s [4], CWD has subsequently been detected in wild and captive cervids of 21 states and two Canadian provinces. The uncertainty regarding long-term demographic impacts of CWD on cervid population health [5–7], possible human and domestic animal health concerns, and economic consequences of CWD have led management agencies to seek effective strategies to control CWD distribution and prevalence. In the absence of a treatment or vaccine for CWD, the main tool available for disease management in free-ranging populations is either selective harvest of infected individuals [8] or non-selective harvest of deer in known affected areas [9]. While selective harvest is impractical, the long-term efficacy of non-selective harvest is uncertain; only New York has officiated a CWD recovery phase after detecting two positive deer out of 32,000 sampled (NY Department of Environmental Conservation). Given a lack of clear understanding of CWD transmission dynamics in wild cervids, limited management tools, and finite financial resources, control or eradication of CWD is a tenuous and controversial undertaking.

An important tool in wildlife disease management is the mathematical model, which can be constructed to estimate important disease and population parameters, and predict the consequences of alternative management strategies [10]. A crucial issue in modeling host-pathogen dynamics is determining how infectious contact rate is affected by host density [6,11,12]. Two contrasting modes of transmission are typically considered: density-dependent transmission (DD) when infectious contacts increase monotonically with host density and frequency-dependent transmission (FD) when infectious contacts are independent of host density [11,12]. In addition, a variety of intermediate forms may be modeled as non-linear functions [11,13]. The theoretical implications of these contrasting forms of transmission on host population dynamics vary from stable host-pathogen coexistence for DD transmission to either host or pathogen extinction for FD transmission [14]; with an outcome that also depends on disease mitigating factors such as prophylactics or vaccines (see [15] for review). Consequently, effective management options depend on which transmission mode predominates [6,11] and what additional tools (e.g., sterilization [16]) are available.

Transmission of CWD has been assumed to be FD in mule deer [5,17], but little empirical research has been conducted and prior analysis of harvested Wisconsin white-tailed deer (*O. virginianus*) was inconclusive [18]. In Wisconsin, CWD was discovered in 2001 in three male white-tailed deer harvested in the south-central part of the state [19] from a core affected area (544 km²) of highest prevalence covering parts of Dane and Iowa counties, likely originating from a single introduction event followed by spatial spread [20]. In general, prevalence is higher in males and increases with age [21,22]. For CWD, and other wildlife diseases, rates of geographic spread are unknown or very difficult to determine despite new techniques for determining the spatial distribution of diseases [20,23,24]. Although there is evidence that infection rate in this core area has increased [25], modeling of hunter harvest data to determine temporal and spatial trends has proved challenging [22], likely because of low prevalence and slow spatial spread. Owing to low temporal heterogeneity in age-specific prevalence data, earlier modeling efforts of the Wisconsin system suggested that CWD was introduced at least 2–3 decades before it was discovered [18].

The hypothesis of FD transmission in deer is largely based on the assumption that female matrilineal social structure and site-fidelity limits infectious contact between female social groups [5,26,27]; a finding corroborated by Grear *et al.* [28]. Schauber and Woolf [6] challenged this notion on the grounds of insufficient empirical support and encouraged modeling CWD under a broader transmission framework. High CWD prevalence in captive deer herds [9,29], positive correlation between prevalence and deer abundance indices [20], and deer congregation on winter range, around bait-piles, or at mineral licks [30–32] suggest that DD transmission is also a feasible mechanism. Furthermore, behavioral and social differences between sexes or seasons (in both white-tailed and mule deer) may drive differences in CWD prevalence and transmission [7,21,22].

In this study, we investigated alternative modes of CWD transmission and evaluated the consequences of recreational harvest management on the dynamics and control of CWD in free-ranging white-tailed deer in south-central Wisconsin. Specif-ically, we built upon our previous work in this system [18] to test and compare seven transmission models accounting for DD, FD, and non-linear (NL) intermediate transmission functions. We also tested for sex-specific variation in infection rates, allowing for homogeneous or sex-specific model structure. We fit our matrix model to existing data in south-central Wisconsin using a maximum-likelihood approach to assess: (1) CWD infection rates with respect to host density vs. disease prevalence (i.e., transmission mode), and sex; (2) the time since CWD was introduced and rate of spatial spread in south-central Wisconsin, and (3) the implications of our results for recreational harvest strategies to manage the disease.

## Methods

### Ethics statement

As part of the requirement for mandatory registration of harvested deer in Wisconsin, regardless of whether the animal was obtained on public or private land, hunters were required to allow tissue collection by the Department of Natural Resources for CWD testing.

### Study area and data

The study area for our CWD analysis was focused on 544 km² in south-central WI (core area of proposed CWD origin [20]), characterized by the highest prevalence within the CWD management zone (≈23,310 km² [33]). We obtained data from the WI DNR in the south-central core area (hereafter core) of WI, using 15,136 records of hunter harvested white-tailed deer obtained between October and January 2002–2011 for parameter estimation, and 1,637 records between October and January 2011–2013 for validation of model predicted prevalence (Table S1). Of these samples, brain stem (obex) or retropharyngeal lymphatic tissue from 958 animals tested positive for CWD using immunohistochemistry or ELISA [34]. We classified each record by CWD status (positive/negative), sex, and five age groups; fawns, 1-year-olds, 2-year-olds, 3-year-olds, and >3 year-olds. Data from the core was used to evaluate the best supported transmission mode (next section). For analysis of spatial spread, we analyzed five surrounding regions, similar in size to the south-central core and each with 1,685 to 8,945 harvested deer, of which 18 to 298 tested CWD positive (with prevalence ranging from 2–4%). Although deer densities in the core area varied during the study, primarily in response to changes in harvest regulations and rates [33], there is no evidence that CWD-induced mortality was responsible for measureable variation in deer abundance.

### Model structure and selection

We used a multi-state non-spatial deterministic matrix model [18,35], which accounts for age, sex, infection-stage, and seasonal (i.e., semi-annual time step: summer-winter) heterogeneity with respect to demographic, epidemiologic, and harvest parameters. Full details are provided in the Methods S1 section with a model structure diagram (Figs. S1 & S2) and component matrices (Figs. S3, S4, S5). As CWD infections are always fatal [9], we used a projection matrix with no recovery from the four disease stages in our model [35–37]. Fecundity and non-hunting survival rates were provided by the Wisconsin Department of Natural Resources (WDNR) (see Table S2) and following the detection of CWD in 2001, after which our prevalence data begins, we used estimates of sex-specific harvest provided by the WDNR.

Historical information about changes in deer density in the study area is subject to considerable uncertainty and our best estimate (given harvest records from Iowa County, WI, which is located in the study area) is that deer density was near zero in the early 1940s, but reached 9.3 deer km$^{-2}$ just prior to CWD discovery in 2001. For simplicity, we simulated past deer population growth to achieve this density threshold using a logistic model (see Methods S1 for details).

We initiated population and disease dynamics based on a stable-age distribution obtained by using sustainable harvest rates of 48% and 26% for antlered and antlerless deer as per WDNR (see Methods S1). We assessed the potential sensitivity of model parameter estimates to the initial stable-age distribution by also using the sex-age structure from the harvest data to project the simulated deer population, but found negligible differences in model fit. For each model, we introduced CWD with one 2-year-old female into a simulated deer population that grew according to the demographic and harvest parameters available (see Methods S1). We simulated CWD potential introduction each year between 1945 and 2000 as historical records suggest that deer were effectively extirpated in southern Wisconsin prior to 1945. Based on previous simulations [18], models are not sensitive to the age or sex class initiating CWD in the population, however, increasing the initial number of infected deer results in lower time since disease introduction (TDI) estimates.

We evaluated seven alternative sex-specific transmission models and estimated infection coefficients ($\beta$s) and TDI under mixtures of density-dependent (DD) and frequency-dependent (FD) transmission. We also estimated infection coefficients for a non-linear (NL) model whose parameter values can specify a structure that is intermediate between DD and FD [11]. The mode of transmission or contact structure determines the formulation of the force-of-infection ($\lambda$, the instantaneous rate at which a susceptible acquires infection). Assuming homogeneous infectious contacts among and between each sex $i$: $\lambda_i = \beta_i \bullet I$ for DD-transmission [10] and $\lambda_i = \beta'_i \bullet (I/N)$ for FD-transmission [38], with infection coefficient $\beta_i$ or $\beta'_i$, number of infected individuals ($I$), and total number of individuals ($N$). For our non-linear function, $\lambda_i = (\beta_i \bullet I)/(1 - \varepsilon_i + (\varepsilon_i \bullet N))$ with scaling coefficient $\varepsilon$, which ranges from 0 to 1 [11]. As $\varepsilon \rightarrow 0$, $\lambda_i = \beta_i \bullet I$ and as $\varepsilon \rightarrow 1$, $\lambda_i = \beta'_i \bullet (I/N)$.

The form of our models do not control or specifically estimate directional transmission from the environment or model the dynamics of an environmental reservoir, thus our empirical infection rate estimates are likely a weighted combination of various direct and indirect transmission mechanisms which may depend on seasonal contacts among deer or with contaminated environments (see [39]). All age and sex groups are able to transmit and receive CWD, but for the most general model (i.e., with sex-specificity) the annual infection rate is constant across ages for each sex. For illustration, if we consider a WAIFW matrix (Who Acquires Infection From Whom; [10]) for male and female deer, where columns correspond to infectors and rows correspond to receivers of infection, our sex-specific transmission structure follows from:

$$\begin{array}{cc} & \begin{array}{cc} F & M \end{array} \\ \begin{array}{c} F \\ M \end{array} & \begin{bmatrix} \beta_f & \beta_f \\ \beta_m & \beta_m \end{bmatrix} \end{array}$$

Thus, our models assume females receive infection from females and males at the same rate (via the $\beta_f$ coefficient), while males receive infection from females and males with infection coefficient ($\beta_m$). Infection rates are derived by the expression $1 - \exp(-\beta_i \bullet \Delta t)$, where $\Delta t$ is equal to 0.5 year. In earlier modeling efforts, we attempted to estimate directional transmission coefficients (e.g., $\beta_{fm}$ or the transmission coefficient for females receiving infection

from males), but our data was not sufficient to support such complex model structures.

We used maximum-likelihood ($L$) profile analysis [40] with a binomial likelihood function based on annual CWD prevalence to estimate model parameters and compare relative fit (of model predicted prevalence) to observed prevalence data for hunter-harvested white-tailed deer from 2002 to 2010 in the CWD core area. The form of this likelihood function was:

$$L\big(\beta_i, TDI | n_{ij(t)}, y_{ij(t)}, N_{TDI}\big) = \binom{n_{ij(t)}}{y_{ij(t)}} p_{ij(t)}^{y_{ij(t)}} \big(1 - p_{ij(t)}\big)^{n_{ij(t)} - y_{ij(t)}} | N_{TDI},$$

where $n_{ij(t)}$ is the sample size of all hunter-harvested deer tested for CWD in year $t$ (2002–2010), age class $j$ (fawns, yearlings, 2, 3, and 4+ year olds), and sex $i$, $y_{ij(t)}$ is the number of hunter-harvested deer that tested positive for CWD in year $t$, age class $j$, and sex $i$, and $p_{ij(t)}$ is the model-predicted probability (given $\beta_i$ and TDI) that hunter-harvested deer in year $t$, age class $j$, and sex $i$ were CWD positive. $N_{TDI}$ is the simulated deer population vector distributed with stable age distribution in that year (TDI<2002), which corresponds with the estimated year of introduction of an index CWD infected (stage I) 2-year-old female. We evaluated goodness-of-fit of the most general model using Pearson's chi-squared test, and for each model, calculated Quasi-likelihood Akaike Information Criterion (QAIC) as $-(2 \bullet \ln(L)/\hat{c}) + 2n$, where $n$ = number of parameters and $\hat{c}$ is the variance inflation factor [41]. We made subsequent model comparisons using QAIC weights ($w$) [41] and used 2011 and 2012 harvest data (Oct 2011 to Jan 2013) to validate the predictive capability of our best supported model.

We note that deer density was not included in our Likelihood function; instead we used historic deer demographic, harvest, and density information to predict a plausible progression of deer density over time. Therefore, infection coefficients and TDI estimates were based solely on evaluation of observed and model predicted CWD prevalence (given the model simulated deer population) according to sex and age during the 2002 to 2010 harvest seasons. Optimally, it is preferable to incorporate both deer densities and prevalence into a Likelihood function for parameter estimation.

## Sensitivity analysis

We evaluated model sensitivity for predicted CWD prevalence and deer density 25 years after the last year of observed data (i.e., 2035) to variations in estimated model parameters TDI, $\beta$s, $\gamma$ (probability of advancing to brain infection over a 6-month period; Fig. S1), fecundity, and harvest using Latin Hypercube sampling [42]. We used a semipartial correlation coefficient ($SPC$) to measure the correlation between each model parameter and output variable, corrected for other correlated parameters [43].

## Rate of spread

To estimate the geographic rate of CWD spread across southern Wisconsin, we used the best supported transmission model from the core area (sex-specific FD model – see Results) to calculate sex-specific infection coefficients and TDI for five core-sized regions where data were sufficient to achieve model convergence (Fig. 1). We note that parameter convergence was not possible in other surrounding regions because of small sample sizes. Regions we considered ranged from $\approx$20–40 km from the center of the core area. We regressed the linear distance between the centers of the core and each region versus the respective difference in disease introduction time (TDI), thus the core area is represented by 0 distance and 0 $\Delta TDI$ relative to other areas. Available evidence suggests that the core contains the spatial introduction point of CWD in the study area [20,22,44], and no other published work suggests otherwise. Given this nexus for disease spread and initial arrival time, we used regression through the origin. The resulting slope of this distance-time relationship estimates the rate of CWD spread (km year$^{-1}$) from the core area. Our calculation also assumes that average disease spread has occurred uniformly outward and likely represents the rate of spread early in the CWD epizootic. This assumption appears reasonable for locations near the core area [44].

## CWD dynamics and alternative harvest strategies

With infection coefficients from the best supported model (sex-specific FD model – see Results), we investigated the effect of three sex-specific harvest strategies on predicted CWD prevalence and deer density. These represent a range of possible management actions to address sex-specific FD CWD transmission using recreational harvest. The strategies included a *female-focused* harvest (approximately 50% female and 25% male harvest rates), a *herd-control* harvest based on average harvest rates since CWD discovery in Wisconsin in 2002 (27.7% females, 21% males), and a *male-focused* harvest (25% females, 50% males). To accommodate differences between agency harvest goals and realized harvest (*RH*) by hunters [45], we assumed density-dependent harvest in year $t$, strategy $s$, and sex $i$ using a post-harvest societal tolerance level ($N_{tol}$) in the core area of 5,040 deer. We subjectively designated this regulatory effect of societal tolerance for deer ($N_{tol} = 9.3$ deer km$^{-2}$ or $9.3 \cdot 544$ km$^{-2} \approx 5040$ deer) because prior to CWD discovery in the study area, harvest registration data suggested this asymptotic level of deer density was maintained in the study area. Thus, $RH_{is(t)} = (N_{is(t)}/N_{tol}) \cdot h_{is(t)}$, where $h_{is(t)}$ is the nominal harvest rate with imposed constraints on $RH$, such that $10\% \leq RH_{is} \leq 50\%$. All projections were applied to a modeled deer population beginning in 2011 and followed for $\approx 50$ years.

We also projected CWD prevalence and deer density for a deer population where harvest is either precluded or substantially restricted such as in national parks, urban areas, or some private lands that restrict hunting. In this *no-harvest* scenario we imposed density-dependent fecundity ($f_{DD}$) at a deer carrying capacity ($K$) of $\approx 77$ deer km$^{-2}$; the expected carrying capacity in south-central Wisconsin (WDNR). The functional form we used was $f_{DD(t)} = f_{(t)} - ((N_{(t)}/K) \cdot f_{(t)})$, where $(N_{(t)}/K)$ is constrained to be $\leq 1$, such that values of $f_{DD}$ range from zero to values of nominal fecundity ($f$) at any time $t$ (see Methods S1). We initiated dynamics

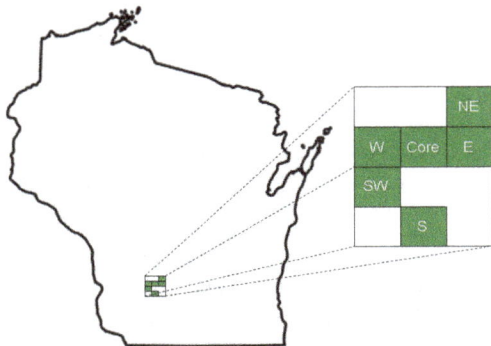

**Figure 1. Map of study area including the southwestern core (544 km² area of expected CWD origin in southwestern Wisconsin), and surrounding approximately core-sized regions used to estimate CWD spread.**

with a post-harvest deer population of 9.3 deer km$^{-2}$, assumed a stable age distribution, and introduced CWD into the simulated disease free population with a 2-year-old female. All matrix model calculations, likelihood calculations, sensitivity analysis, and projections were computed using MATLAB (Mathworks Inc., R2011a), while we used SAS v9.2 (SAS Institute Inc., Cary, NC, USA) for the rate of spread regression and diagnostics.

## Results

### Alternative transmission models

We found that sex-specific FD transmission was strongly supported by the data with $w = 0.99$ (next most parsimonious model had $\Delta QAIC$ of 10 units) (Table 1). Pure DD with equal sex infection coefficients was the least supported model with virtually no support from the data ($\Delta QAIC = 112$), while our non-linear function also had negligible support ($\Delta QAIC = 35$). The data were not sufficient to accommodate the sex-specific non-linear model. The infection coefficients ($\beta$s) for the best model (sex-specific FD) were 0.62 (95% CI: 0.56–0.67) for females and 1.20 (95% CI: 1.14–1.31) for males, with a *TDI* of 40 years (95% CI: 37–43) (Table 1).

For the sex-specific FD model, observed and model-predicted prevalence resulted in good fit for females ($\chi^2 = 47.73$, $df = 52$, $P = 0.64$), but poor fit for males ($\chi^2 = 204.44$, $df = 52$, $P < 0.001$) where there was significant divergence between observed and predicted prevalence for several years (Fig. 2A). Predicted deer density using observed harvest rates over the years of observed data differed less than 5% for the sex-specific FD and DD models, so we only show densities for the FD model (Fig. 2B). Using the goodness-of-fit statistics, we estimated a variance-inflation-factor ($\hat{c}$) of 2.43, indicating mild overdispersion likely due to spatial and/or temporal dependence of CWD prevalence in the study area. The estimated variance of infection coefficients and TDI parameters ($\theta$) were inflated accordingly by $\hat{c} \cdot var(\theta)$. Although this adjustment may account for all or part of the overdispersion in the data, precision of the model parameters may still be overestimated. We validated our sex-specific FD model predictions with data from 2011 and 2012, which resulted in good fit for adult females ($\chi^2 = 5.32$, $df = 5$, $P = 0.38$) and adult males ($\chi^2 = 9.32$, $df = 5$, $P = 0.10$).

We evaluated temporal autocorrelation of predicted prevalence by examining the 1$^{st}$ order autocorrelation of the residuals from the FD-sex model using a Durbin-Watson test for males and females separately. For females the test indicated positive 1$^{st}$ order autocorrelation with residuals ($d = 0.851$, $df = 1$, $P = 0.03$), while for males 1$^{st}$ order temporal autocorrelation in residuals was not detected ($d = 2.19$, $df = 1$, P = 0.10).

### Sensitivity analysis

The sensitivity analysis conducted on the sex-specific FD model showed that CWD prevalence in 25 years was negatively correlated to the harvest rate of antlered deer ($SPC = -0.64$) and tended to increase with harvest of antlerless deer ($SPC = 0.41$) (Table 2). Antlerless harvest had the most impact on deer density in 25 years, with abundance declining for increasing harvest of adult does and fawns ($SPC = -0.80$; Table 2). We found at best a weak influence of parameters $\beta$, $\gamma$, and *TDI* on future prevalence and deer density. We evaluated a range of starting deer population sizes in the core area for our simulations, ranging from 2 through 544 ($\leq 1$ deer km$^{-2}$). We found that starting population size did not affect the ability of the models to fit the data, and infection coefficient estimates and *TDI* varied <5% across different starting population sizes.

**Table 1.** Alternative CWD transmission models used to estimate infection coefficients ($\beta$) and time since disease introduction (*TDI*) of chronic wasting disease in white-tailed deer from south-central Wisconsin during the 2002–2010 harvest seasons.

| Model | $k^b$ | $\Delta QAIC$ | TDI | $\beta$ | |
|---|---|---|---|---|---|
| | | | | Male | Female |
| FD(F) FD(M) | 3 | 0 | 40 (37–43) | 1.20 (1.14–1.31) | 0.62 (0.56–0.67) |
| FD(M) DD(F) | 3 | 10 | 45 (44–55) | 1.36 (1.31–1.43) | $1.19\times10^{-4}$ ($1.08$–$1.27\times10^{-4}$) |
| NL(F = M)$^c$ | 2 | 35 | 34 (31–37) | 0.83 (0.0122–0.93) | |
| FD(F = M) | 2 | 36 | 34 (32–35) | 0.90 (0.89–0.92) | |
| FD(F) DD(M) | 3 | 38 | 42 (28–69) | $2.08\times10^{-4}$ ($1.98$–$2.27\times10^{-4}$) | 0.88 (0.85–0.90) |
| DD(F) DD(M) | 3 | 109 | 29 (27–31) | $2.31\times10^{-4}$ ($2.15$–$2.50\times10^{-4}$) | $1.82\times10^{-4}$ ($1.71$–$1.91\times10^{-4}$) |
| DD(F = M) | 2 | 112 | 29 (28–30) | $2.00\times10^{-4}$ ($1.99$–$2.00\times10^{-4}$) | |

[a]Akaike weight [41] for second best model was <0.01, while other models had support near zero.
[b]Number of model parameters.
[c]For the scaling coefficient $\varepsilon$ of the non-linear model structure, the MLE was 0.94 with 95% CI of 0.23 to 1.0.
We used Quasi-likelihood Akaike Information Criterion (*QAIC*) for model comparison, with the best model having a *QAIC* of 223.11 and Akaike weight = 0.99[a]. These models evaluate transmission modes including density-dependent (DD), frequency-dependent (FD), and non-linear transmission (NL) as a function of sex specificity. Estimated parameters include 95% confidence intervals.

## Rate of spread

For areas west and southwest of the core, infection coefficients were significantly greater than in the core for male deer (Table 3). For regions outside the core, *TDI* estimates were significantly lower indicating later CWD establishment, with the exception of an area east of the core where sparse data resulted in an unidentifiable upper confidence bound (Table 3). A zero-intercept linear regression of distance from the core versus difference in *TDI* had a significant adjusted $R^2 = 0.87$ ($F_{1,4} = 26.82$, $P = 0.007$) with slope parameter of 1.13 ($SE = 0.22$), indicating an average geographic rate of spread of CWD in the vicinity of the western core of south-central Wisconsin of 1.13 km year$^{-1}$ (Fig. 3).

## Harvest strategies

Of the three harvest strategies, male-focused harvest resulted in eventual decline of CWD prevalence to under 5% by 2060 (and 2.5% by 2110; not shown) and stable post-harvest deer density of $\approx 9$ deer km$^{-2}$ after 20 years (Fig. 4), resulting in a female-dominated population compared to other strategies (Fig. 5). Average realized harvest rates under this scenario were close to nominal rates at 24% and 49% for females and males, respectively. For both the herd-control and female-focused harvest strategies, projected CWD prevalence increased to 26% and 30%, while total post-harvest deer densities stabilized at $\approx 7$ and 4 deer km$^{-2}$, respectively (Fig. 4). The reduction in deer density resulted in average harvest rates that were considerably lower than nominal levels for females and males, respectively, with realized harvest rates of 20% and 16% for the herd-control, and 20% and 10% for the female-focused strategies. For a naïve population with no hunting, density-dependent fecundity as a regulatory population mechanism, and one introduced infectious individual, prevalence increased to 57% for adult males after 40 years (Fig. 6). Total deer density reached an asymptote of $\approx 46$ deer km$^{-2}$ after 40 years, although adults declined by as much as 50% during the near-exponential phase of CWD prevalence increase (years 25–40) (Fig. 6).

## Discussion

### CWD Transmission

Using white-tailed deer harvest data from south-central Wisconsin, we show that FD CWD transmission is the best supported model for both sexes (with higher infection rates for males) at a broad spatial scale, whereas our earlier efforts to model this system could not discriminate between FD and DD transmission [18]. It has been suspected that FD was a dominant transmission mechanism in mule deer [5,17; but see 6], and more recently in white-tailed deer [28,46]. Furthermore, our modeling results suggest a more recent and biologically plausible time since CWD introduction in south-central Wisconsin compared with earlier analysis [18]. As demonstrated in previous work in this CWD system [21,22,25] and in Colorado [7,47], adult males have higher CWD infection rates than females. Although the mechanism for higher CWD infection and prevalence in males is unknown, these differences may be driven by sex-specific social behavior [7,21]. Males typically have larger home ranges, longer dispersal distances, interactions with other males, or rut-related behavior [48] that could result in more contacts with infectious deer. In contrast, females generally interact within a much smaller matrilineal group [27,28,49], and only briefly with males during rut [47].

Given the simplicity of our model, our estimated infection coefficients are likely a function of several different (and largely unknown) mechanisms that may vary between/among sexes, seasons, and the environment. These infection rates represent a weighted average of many potential drivers as summarized by Potapov et al. [39]. Our models do not account explicitly for indirect transmission from the environment where prions can persist for years [50,51], although our infection rates implicitly subsume both direct and indirect routes of infection. The importance of environmental transmission has been demonstrated in captive mule deer [52,53] and theoretical modeling indicates that population impacts can be driven by the length of time that prions remain infectious in the environment [54]. In the long term, the potential accumulation of an environmental reservoir of infectious prions may become an increasingly important component of CWD transmission; however, the relative contribution of direct and indirect transmission in wild deer populations remains

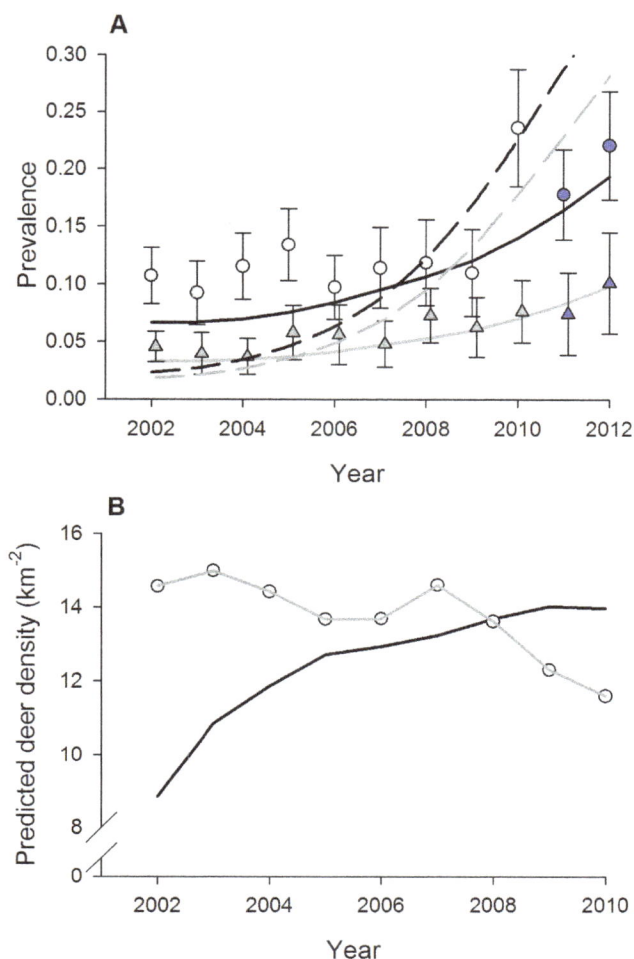

**Figure 2. A) Observed female (grey △) and male (○) prevalence (95% CI) using data from the south-central core area (544 km²) of Wisconsin from the 2002–2010 harvest seasons including sex-specific model predictions under frequency- (FD) or density-dependent (DD) transmission: FD female (solid grey), FD male (solid black), DD female (dashed grey), and DD male (dashed black). B) Predicted deer density of females (grey) and males (black) over the years of observed data using observed harvest rates.** Note that observed data for the 2011–2012 harvest seasons (blue-filled icons) in panel A were not used in parameter estimation, and are presented here to support validation of the predicted model.

unknown and requires further research. Although we expect infectious contact likely varies by sex and season, harvest data were insufficient to account for intra-annual complexity in sex-specific transmission. Additional insights for CWD management given directional sex-specific transmission (i.e., female-to-male, female-to-female) may require focal research studies that determine differences in infectious contact between and among sexes [49,55–57] and how these influence the risk of disease transmission [28]. In particular, understanding the mechanisms that lead to rates of male infection twice as high as females could provide crucial insights on management strategies designed to reduce male CWD prevalence as an alternative to high male harvest.

Assuming CWD originated in the core area and environmental accumulation of prions contributes significantly to transmission, we would expect higher infection rate estimates in the core

compared with surrounding areas. We are uncertain why infection rate is apparently greater in males for some areas to the west and southwest of the core. These surrounding areas have similar habitat characteristics with the core, and we would not expect deer abundance to vary significantly prior to CWD discovery. Heterogeneous harvest management conducted among areas may be one potential explanation. However, this difference also suggests that unidentified environmental characteristics or management actions may influence the current and future trends in CWD prevalence. Regardless, these patterns suggest that our model predictions for the core area may underestimate the rate of CWD increase in other areas. Future research is needed to understand the drivers of CWD transmission, how these vary spatially, and their influence on future patterns of infection. The identification of potential environmental reservoirs (e.g., common feeding areas, mineral licks) and evaluation of the significance of indirect transmission in free-ranging deer populations would also enhance our ability to predict future trends in infection and allow a better evaluation of alternative control strategies.

In concept QAIC should help account for overdispersion in our data, which might result from missing covariates in the model and/or a lack of independence in the data (e.g., [58]). Such lack of independence may be due to spatial and/or temporal autocorrelation, and while we do not explicitly account for such effects, we rely on QAIC to generally accommodate a portion of these impacts. While we detected significant temporal autocorrelation in residuals for predicted female prevalence, other research in the same study area [44,46] found no spatial autocorrelation in model residuals using a 93.6 km² or 2.6 km² spatial frame, respectively. We caution that despite use of QAIC, our model parameter estimates may still be overly precise.

## Rate of spread

Several studies indicate that the southwestern core area of WI is the likely point of origin for CWD in our study area, with an inverse relationship between distance-to-core and prevalence as would be expected from an introduced disease spreading across the landscape [20,22,44]. To our knowledge, we present the first empirical estimate of CWD geographic spread, based on sex-specific FD transmission, which indicated a low average rate (1.13 km year$^{-1}$) during initial phases of the epizootic. There is no current evidence to suggest that CWD spread in our study area was facilitated by humans (via movements of infectious animals between game farms or preserves); however, the anecdotal evidence of such events warrants further investigation. Though DD transmission was not supported by our data, the estimated rate of geographic spread was similar for this model structure. Our results suggest that in the south-central Wisconsin endemic area, CWD has slowly moved across the landscape and is probably not a recent development. Clearly this estimated rate of spread must be considered unique to the outbreak in south-central Wisconsin.

Rates of CWD spread in other regions are likely influenced by a number of factors including habitat features [44,59], mode of disease transmission, host species (e.g., white-tailed or mule deer), population structure, host movements [60], dispersal [61], and possibly the environment [54]. For example, recent analyses [44] indicate that CWD may be spreading faster from the outbreak in eastern Wisconsin and northern Illinois than from south-central Wisconsin. Our simple estimate also assumes an average uniform diffusion from the point of origin and ignores potential disease movement via longer distance dispersal [60], although recent discovery of CWD in north-west Wisconsin does not appear to be linked to long-distance dispersal from southern Wisconsin based on genetic analysis (S. Robinson Pers. Comm.). In addition, our

**Table 2.** Sensitivity of primary model parameters on predicted prevalence of CWD infection and deer density after 25 years (2035).

| Input parameters | Distribution[a] | Prevalence[b] | Deer density[b] |
|---|---|---|---|
| *TDI* | | 0.09±0.08 (0.72) | −0.02±0.04 (0.92) |
| $\beta_{male}$ | $N(\{40,1.20,0.62\},\sum)^c$ | 0.20±0.09 (0.40) | −0.05±0.04 (0.82) |
| $\beta_{female}$ | | 0.22±0.10 (0.34) | −0.07±0.04 (0.78) |
| $\gamma$ | $N(0.5,0.08^2)^d$ | −0.01±0.08 (0.96) | 0.01±0.05 (0.98) |
| Harvest antlered deer | $N(0.5,0.009)^e$ | **−0.64±0.10** (0.003) | 0.15±0.05 (0.53) |
| Harvest antlerless deer | $N(0.25,0.01)^e$ | 0.41±0.11 (0.07) | **−0.80±0.08** (<0.001) |

[a]We used Latin Hypercube Sampling for each parameter with $S = 20$ equal probability intervals and one random value from each interval. Values for each parameter were paired randomly with values from all other parameters.
[b]Mean *SPC* ± *SE* between input parameters and prevalence or deer density in 2035; stochastic analysis based on $S = 20$ replications. Probability of a *t*-statistic (with $S$-2 df; [43]) that evaluates *SPC* = 0 provided in parentheses.
[c]Because $\beta_{male}$, $\beta_{female}$, and time since disease introduction (*TDI*) are correlated, we used a trivariate normal distribution, $N(\{TDI,\beta_{male},\beta_{female}\}, \sum)$, where $\sum$ = variance-covariance matrix, calculated for parameter combinations within the 95% confidence region [69]; *TDI* rounded to closest integer.
[d]Transition ($\gamma$) from lymph-node positive (I) to obex-positive (C) represents differences in CWD progression among deer genotypes in terms of CWD susceptibility; standard error (*SE*) derived from 95% CI bounds = 8–16 months (e.g., representing transition to Obex infection for the two common genotypes).
[e]Gaussian distributions for harvest rates of antlered and antlerless deer are based on mean hunting rates and coefficients of variation (0.18 and 0.15, respectively) during 2002–2010 in the core area.
We used Latin Hypercube Sampling and a semi-partial correlation coefficient (*SPC*) to measure the relative influence of model parameters; significant coefficients are bolded.

analysis does not account for habitat heterogeneity and physical barriers (natural or anthropogenic) that influence landscape scale movement and interaction of deer populations [62,63] or CWD distribution [44,63]. We also note that despite a highly significant $R^2$ value, our simple regression utilizes only six data points (including the core, which we assume is the origin of the epizootic), with uncertainty that is not accounted for in the regression. As such, there is likely higher variance associated with our estimated rate of spread.

Despite these limitations, our estimate provides a starting place to conceptualize early CWD spread across the southern Wisconsin landscape. In the context of CWD, we believe the areas surrounding the core are currently in relatively early stages of the epizootic with low, but increasing prevalence. Under FD transmission and barring effective management efforts, CWD prevalence is predicted to increase over time, and we suspect that the rate of spread may also increase because more young males will become infected prior to dispersal [46]. As such, we consider our spread estimate as a lower bound that is likely to increase as the epizootic progresses.

## Harvest strategies

As a consequence of FD transmission, our simulations predict that in the next decade CWD prevalence can increase to relatively high levels (25% in females and 50% in males) in the absence of significant management actions to reduce infection rates. Of the three harvest strategies we evaluated, only male-focused harvest succeeded in reducing CWD prevalence below current levels. Prevalence is reduced because this strategy removes animals from the highest prevalence class (reducing infection rates), while allowing dilution of population-level CWD prevalence by recruitment of more females [64]. In contrast, CWD increased under female-focused and herd-control harvest strategies. By focusing harvest on the portion of the population with highest prevalence and infection rates, our simulation suggests that harvest management can effectively reduce prevalence despite FD disease transmission. Although disease eradication may not be possible, prevalence reduction (especially in higher risk groups), which reduces force of infection, is the key to mediating disease impacts on host populations in the long term. Effective disease manage-

**Table 3.** Maximum-likelihood estimates (and 95% confidence intervals) for infection coefficients ($\beta$) and time since disease introduction (*TDI*) of chronic wasting disease in white-tailed deer in core-sized regions ($\approx$544 km²) surrounding the south-central core in Wisconsin from 2002–2010.

| Direction (distance)[a] | $\beta$ Male | $\beta$ Female | *TDI* |
|---|---|---|---|
| North-East (27 km)[b] | 1.29 (0.70–2.05) $P = 0.795$ | 1.08 (0.66–1.70) $P = 0.085$ | **8 (3–32) $P < 0.001$** |
| East (19 km)[c] | 1.49 (1.08–1.91) $P = 0.192$ | 0.48 (0.24–0.74) $P = 0.307$ | 36 (23-NA)[d] |
| South (39 km)[b] | 1.58 (1.11–2.16) $P = 0.162$ | 0.79 (0.46–1.19) $P = 0.368$ | **12 (5–32) $P < 0.001$** |
| South-West (27 km)[c] | **1.64 (1.28–2.04) $P = 0.033$** | 0.57 (0.35–0.81) $P = 0.691$ | **25 (10–38) $P = 0.042$** |
| West (19 km)[c] | **1.55 (1.31–1.78) $P = 0.011$** | 0.77 (0.61–0.91) $P = 0.087$ | **19 (13–29) $P < 0.001$** |

[a]Direction and distance from the center of the core to the center of a given region.
[b]no $\hat{c}$ correction; North-East: $\chi^2 = 5.64$, $df = 8$, $P = 0.69$; South: $\chi^2 = 7.07$, $df = 13$, $P = 0.90$.
[c]$\hat{c}$ correction; East: $\chi^2 = 22.53$ $df = 14$, $P = 0.07$, $\hat{c} = 1.61$; South-West: $\chi^2 = 29.63$, $df = 16$, $P = 0.02$, $\hat{c} = 1.85$; West: $\chi^2 = 27.85$, $df = 16$, $P = 0.03$, $\hat{c} = 1.74$.
[d]The 95% CI upper bound was not estimable.
The transmission model assumes sex-specific FD transmission. *P* are the z-test probabilities evaluating the null hypothesis that parameter values are equal between the core and a given region; bold values indicate $\alpha \leq 0.05$.

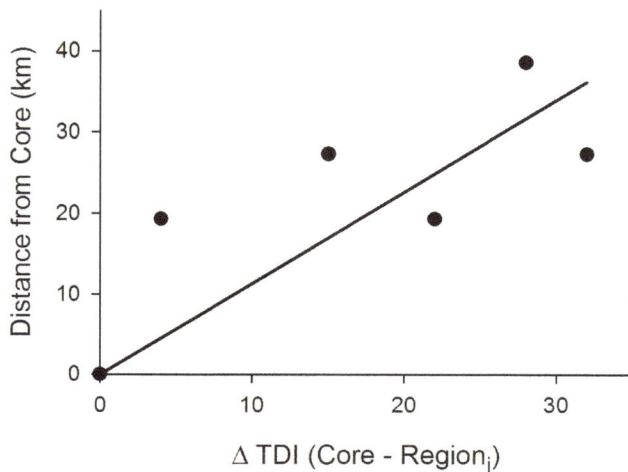

**Figure 3. Plot of points for zero-intercept linear regression of distance from the core versus difference in TDI (Core – Region$_i$) in years.** The estimated slope with adjusted $R^2 = 0.87$ ($F_{1,4} = 26.82$, $P = 0.007$) was 1.13 ($SE = 0.22$), suggesting CWD spread across the south-central core area of Wisconsin was on average approximately 1.13 km yr$^{-1}$.

ment by sex-specific differential harvest has also been explored for bovine tuberculosis in deer [55].

The density-dependent harvest structure we imposed produced much lower average realized harvest (RH) rates for the female-focused and herd-control strategies, compared with male-focused harvest. High female harvest reduces population size, which requires lower realized harvest rates to maintain stable population goals (based on societal tolerance for deer). While this density-dependent harvest structure is artificial, it is intended to represent hunter effort in response to perceived deer densities. In the absence of such a mechanism, static harvest rates over the simulated time frame of 50 years resulted in host and disease extinction, as predicted in theoretical models of FD disease transmission [14]. In addition, our results show that deer demography and CWD dynamics are sensitive to changes in harvest. Estimation of unbiased harvest rates requires accurate information on both the distribution of harvested animals and the distribution of the underlying population. Although harvest-based estimates for deer populations have various limitations [9,65], the importance of this parameter for monitoring the performance of CWD management programs suggests future research to improve estimation procedures should be considered.

The demographic implications of alternative harvest strategies for disease management are also important as they affect deer densities, recreational opportunities (e.g., hunting or observation), and potential disease spread. While male-focused harvest reduces CWD prevalence in the long term, it results in lower densities of adult males (compared with herd-control), which are usually of primary interest to deer hunters. For the herd-control harvest strategy (current deer management goals) nearly 50% of adult males and 25% of adult females are expected to become infected within another decade. Even worse, for female-focused harvest not only are deer densities expected to be low, but more than 50% of surviving adult males and 30% of adult females would be infected. In general, these harvest strategies are characterized by accelerating rates of infection in all deer, and higher prevalence, particularly in males. Considering the constraints of our model the tradeoff between strategies is clear; CWD can eventually be

reduced with fewer opportunities to harvest healthy adult bucks, or more adult bucks may be available for harvest, but with higher rates of CWD infection. Given that quality deer management practices focus on production of older bucks with large antlers, management agencies could face difficult alternatives from these competing interests. However, if an efficacious CWD vaccine was available and cost-effectively distributed to broad segments of a deer population (particularly males), managers would have more flexibility to employ a disease control strategy combining harvest and vaccination to provide adequate recreational opportunities to harvest CWD-free deer.

The mechanism for density-dependent population regulation in deer is not well known, but one hypothesis is that deer reduce body size and maintain survival rates while lowering reproduction [66]. Therefore, we used density-dependent fecundity to regulate population size in our *no-harvest* simulations. The goal of these

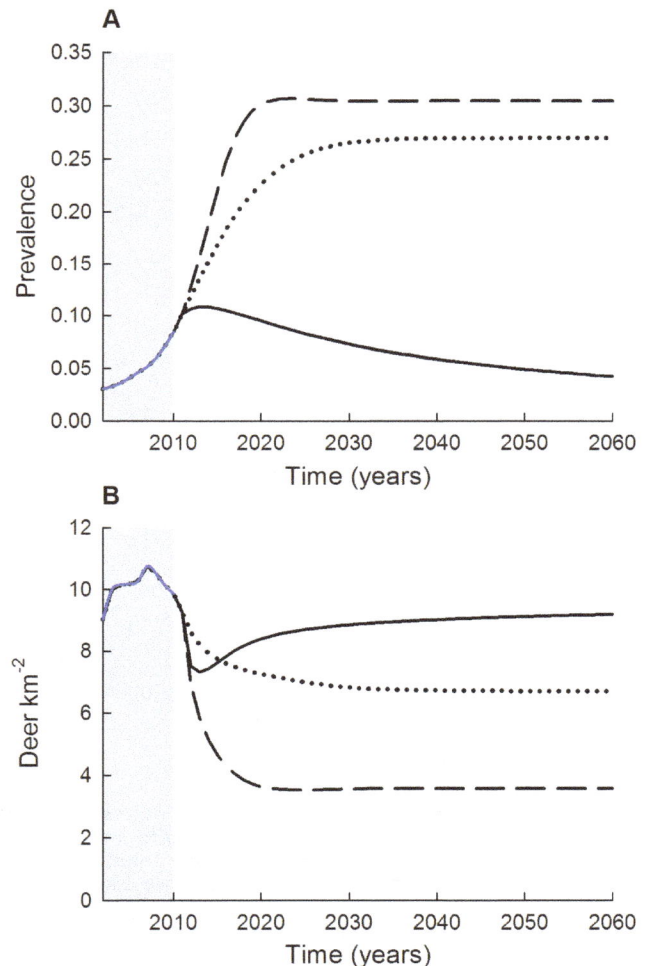

**Figure 4. Predicted CWD population prevalence (A) and deer density (B) using transmission estimates from the best supported sex-specific frequency-dependent model.** Three strategies were considered including male-focused harvest rates (solid line; female = 25%, male = 50%), herd-control harvest (dotted line; female = 28%, male = 22%), and female-focused harvest (dashed line; female = 50%, male = 25%). Note that the herd-control harvest strategy represents an average of the existing harvest conditions in the south-central core of WI during the 2002–2010 harvest seasons (blue shaded area).

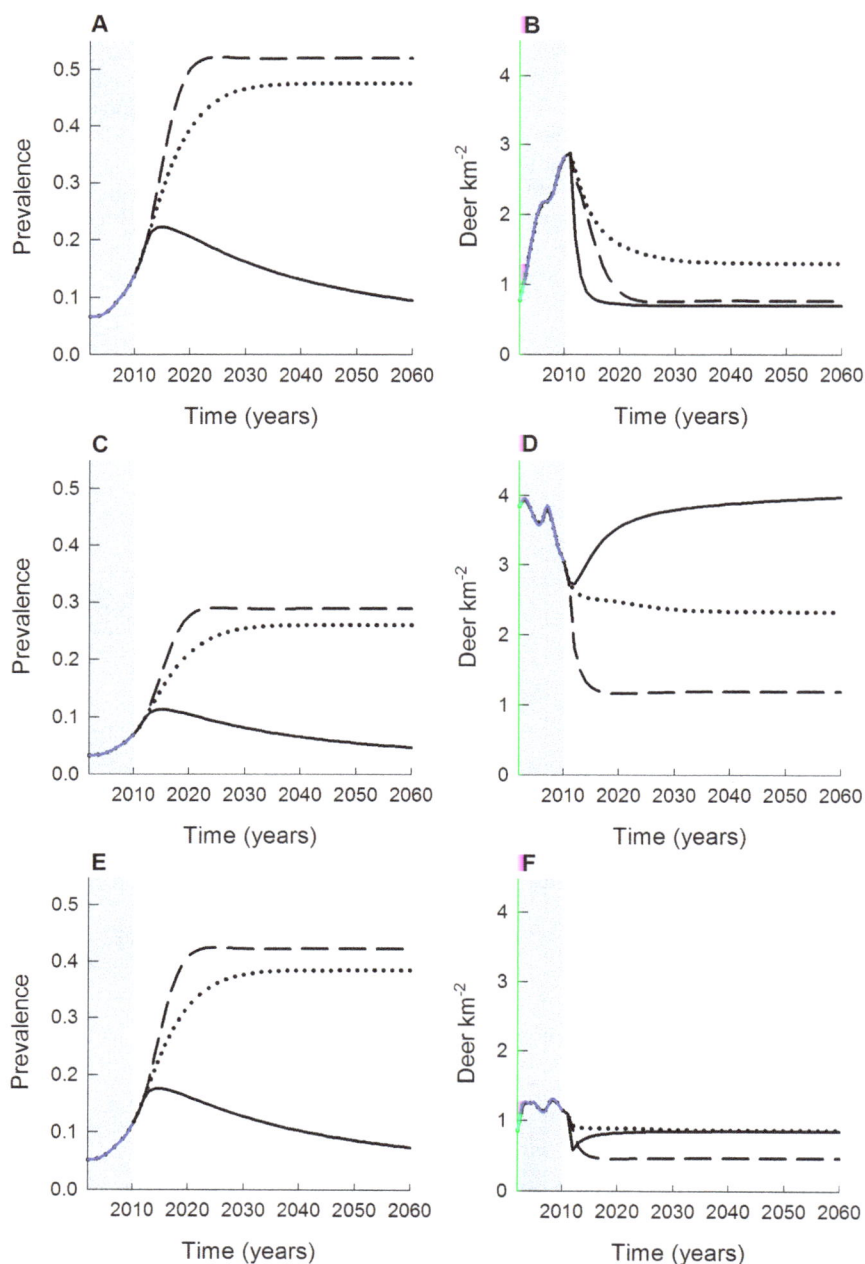

**Figure 5. Predicted CWD prevalence (A, C, E) and respective deer density (B, D, F) for three harvest strategies using transmission estimates from the best supported sex-specific frequency-dependent model: male-focused harvest (solid line; female = 25%, male = 50%), herd-control harvest (dotted line; female = 28%, male = 22%), and female-focused harvest (dashed line; female = 50%, male = 25%).** Panels A and B show adult males, panels C and D show adult females, and panels E and F show yearling males. Note that the herd-control harvest strategy represents an average of the existing harvest conditions in the south-central core of WI during the 2002–2010 harvest seasons. The areas shaded in blue represent the observed data years, and FD-sex model predictions are based on observed harvest rates.

simulations was to illustrate the rapid increase in CWD prevalence and eventual impact on deer populations in the absence of harvest or other factors that remove infected animals prior to mortality from CWD. Such situations might be likely in high density urban deer populations, national parks, captive deer farms, or other areas where deer harvest or removal is limited. This simulation is not designed to represent current conditions in Wisconsin, and we consider this a worst-case disease scenario in areas without harvest. However, we also note that CWD transmission rates and

prevalence are much higher in captive deer farms than has been reported in wild populations [67].

## Caveats

We highlight that our models do not specifically account for potentially important mechanisms such as environmental transmission, differences in Prnp genotypes [2] or infectious contact within matrilineal social groups [27,28], which could contribute to future infection rates, and affect future predictions of CWD

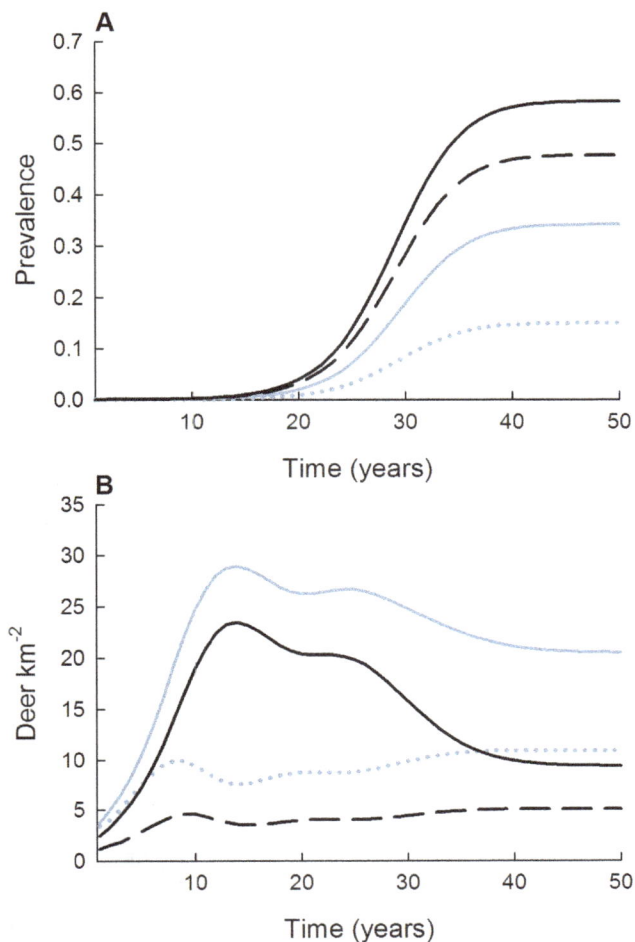

**Figure 6. Predicted CWD prevalence (A) and deer density (B) for fawns (dotted), male yearlings (dashed), female adults (solid blue), and male adults (solid black) using transmission estimates from the best supported sex-specific frequency-dependent model.** This scenario represents a no-harvest strategy, initiating CWD in a deer population with initial density of $\approx 9$ deer km$^{-2}$ with density-dependent fecundity as a population regulation mechanism ($K \approx 77$ deer km$^{-2}$).

Unfortunately, our data was collected in one season (winter) each year, making it impossible to estimate seasonal, environmental, or between/among sex infection rates without assumptions about the infectious contact structure between/among males and females, and with the environment. Spatial heterogeneity, deer aggregation, and the broad spatial scale of our study area could impact our estimated CWD transmission mode and infection rates. Although DD transmission could operate at finer spatial scales, a recent study of transmission in yearlings at a 2.6 km$^2$ scale also indicates transmission is primarily FD [46]. Given the sparse data available at a fine scale, such analysis within our modeling framework was not possible. The purpose of this paper was not to fully describe the many different potential transmission mechanisms on CWD dynamics (which is a very desirable, but challenging goal). Rather, our goal was to evaluate relatively broad-scale dynamics of the disease and implications for disease management, given the available data for harvested deer in Wisconsin.

## Conclusions

Given our model structure and data, our results provide strong support for FD transmission of CWD with the force of infection driven by changes in prevalence, which we suggest is a vital metric for focused control efforts. Generally as prevalence increases, as found in Wisconsin, infection rate also increases in the absence of intervention, producing an accelerating pattern of infection. Assuming that frequency-dependent transmission predominates (as our evaluation indicates), management to reduce prevalence will mediate potential CWD population impacts. The higher rate of infection and prevalence in males, thus, provides the basis for effective CWD management using deer harvest focused on this sex. Management to reduce prevalence might be accomplished through the synergistic effects of targeted harvest and vaccination of males. Unfortunately, we know little about the mechanisms for male infection and further research is needed before alternative management strategies to reduce male infection rates can be developed. Spatial differences in CWD infection rates, despite similar habitat and pre-CWD deer abundance, suggest that unidentified environmental or management factors may also influence disease dynamics and future trends in prevalence. Future research to understand the drivers of CWD transmission, how these vary spatially, and the relative importance of environmental and direct transmission is critical to understanding future CWD dynamics in wild deer.

Our results also indicate that even with high deer densities CWD has been spreading at a relatively slow rate across the landscape; in agreement with larger scale spatial patterns for prevalence [44]. However, as disease prevalence continues to increase, the rate of infection in yearling bucks will also increase [46]. Because dispersing bucks may be an important source of disease spread, these patterns suggest that CWD prevalence outside the core area will continue to grow and the disease may spread at an increasing rate. Although the drivers of CWD spatial spread are not generally known (see [44] for identification of landscape features that affect spread), management efforts to reduce both local prevalence and deer abundance will likely reduce dispersal of infected yearling bucks. However, the relative impact of reducing deer abundance versus prevalence in lowering the number of infected yearling bucks likely depends on disease prevalence and deer density [46]. Further research is needed to determine the factors that affect spatial spread and develop effective management strategies.

dynamics. For instance, infectious prions may accumulate in the environment causing increased future rates of environmental transmission. Our projections of CWD dynamics are limited because we cannot account for these unknown, but potentially important, effects on transmission due to accumulation of infectious prions in the environment over time. Two recent evaluations of the potential effects of soil characteristics (specifically clay content) on CWD transmission to yearling deer and on spatial patterns of CWD prevalence in Wisconsin [44,46] failed to show an association between soil characteristics and CWD, unlike a similar study from Colorado [68]. While there is no current evidence supporting a significant role for environmental CWD transmission in Wisconsin, we cannot discount the possible influence this may have on future CWD dynamics in our study system. The relative importance of environmental and direct transmission is critical to understanding future CWD dynamics in wild deer.

## Supporting Information

**Figure S1** Compartmental model structure of the CWD study system. CWD stages are based on disease progression using 0.5 year time-steps. All individuals are assumed to be born susceptible (S). Infection is first detectable in retropharyngeal lymph-nodes when animals are assumed to be infectious (I). The sex-specific S-to-I transition probability is $\pi_i$. Infection of the brain stem is the next detectable infection stage (O) and usually takes up to 6 months after prion detection in the alimentary lymph-nodes. The I-to-O transition probability ($\gamma$) is, hence, assumed to be equal to one. The final stage of infection is brain vacuolization which occurs 10–12 months after initial brain infection and is commonly associated with clinical signs (C). Accordingly, the O-to-C transition probability ($\varphi$) is assumed to be 0.5. From this stage most animals die within 6 months. Therefore, the disease-induced mortality probability ($\alpha$) is assumed to equal one. Deer survive within and between compartments with age-sex survival probabilities $s_{ij}$ for the $j^{\text{th}}$ age of sex $i$ and reproduce with age-specific fecundity probabilities $f_j$.

**Figure S2** General matrix structure organization. The general hierarchical structure of the model where age-specific sub-matrices (20 6-month steps) of demographic, epidemiologic, and harvest parameters are nested within matrices accounting for four disease stages and both sexes. These matrices are further nested within season (summer and winter). Disease stages include S (Susceptible), I (Infectious), O (Obex brain positive), and C (Clinical) with F and M representing female and male deer, respectively.

**Figure S3** Seasonal demographic matrices. Each seasonal demographic matrix accounts for four disease stages for each sex, and is composed of eight sub-matrix elements. Panels A and B contain the summer $\mathbf{D^{(s)}}$ and winter $\mathbf{D^{(w)}}$ demographic matrices, respectively and are composed of the following sub-matrix elements: sex-specific (indexed f or m) transition from Susceptible to Infectious stages ($\mathbf{\Pi_i}$), transition from Infectious to Obex positive stages ($\mathbf{\Gamma}$), transition from Obex positive to Clincial stages ($\mathbf{\Phi}$), transition from Clinical stage to death ($\mathbf{A}$),

sex-specific survival ($\mathbf{S}$), fecundity ($\mathbf{F}$), identity ($\mathbf{I}$), and zero sub-matrices ($\mathbf{0}$).

**Figure S4** Seasonal epidemiological matrices. Each seasonal epidemiological matrix accounts for four disease stages for each sex and is composed of five sub-matrix elements. Panels A and B contain the summer $\mathbf{E^{(s)}}$ and winter $\mathbf{E^{(w)}}$ epidemiological matrices, respectively and are composed of the following sub-matrix elements: sex-specific (indexed f or m) transition from Susceptible to Infectious stages ($\mathbf{\Pi_i}$), transition from Infectious to Obex positive stages ($\mathbf{\Gamma}$), transition from Obex positive to Clincial stages ($\mathbf{\Phi}$), sex-specific survival ($\mathbf{S}$), and zero sub-matrices ($\mathbf{0}$).

**Figure S5** Seasonal harvest matrices. Each seasonal harvest matrix accounts for four disease stages for each sex and is composed of three sub-matrix elements. Panels A and B contain the summer $\mathbf{H^{(s)}}$ and winter $\mathbf{H^{(w)}}$ harvest matrices, respectively and are composed of the following sub-matrix elements: sex-specific (indexed f or m) harvest ($\mathbf{H}$), identity ($\mathbf{I}$), and zero sub-matrices ($\mathbf{0}$).

**Methods S1** Additional details regarding the harvest data utilized and methodology provided in distinct sections including *Deer Demography and Harvest*, *Disease Stages and Transition Probabilities*, and *Model Structure*. Also included are the harvest data and demographic parameter estimates used in this study.

## Acknowledgments

We thank the numerous volunteers and WDNR staff who dedicated themselves to collecting deer tissue samples, and the Wisconsin hunters who provided them. We thank D. Grear, E. Merrill, and anonymous reviewers for helpful comments on earlier drafts. Note that any use of trade, product or firm names is for descriptive purposes, and does not imply endorsement by the US Government.

## Author Contributions

Conceived and designed the experiments: CSJ VH GW MDS. Performed the experiments: CSJ VH BT GW. Analyzed the data: CSJ VH BT. Contributed reagents/materials/analysis tools: CSJ VH BT RER MDS. Wrote the paper: CSJ VH MDS GW RER. Provided critical data and information for modelling: RER.

## References

1. Ewald PW (2011) Evolution of virulence, environmental change, and the threat posed by emerging and chronic diseases. Ecol Res 26: 1017–1026. doi:10.1007/s11284-011-0874-8

2. Robinson SJ, Samuel MD, Johnson CJ, Adams M, McKenzie DI (2012) Emerging prion disease drives host selection in a wildlife population. Ecol Appl 22: 1050–1059.

3. Wobeser GA (2007) Disease in wild animals. Berlin; New York: Springer. 393 p.

4. Williams ES (2005) Chronic Wasting Disease. Vet Pathol 42: 530–549. doi:10.1354/vp.42-5-530

5. Gross JE, Miller MW (2001) Chronic wasting disease in mule deer: Disease dynamics and control. J Wildl Manag 65: 205–215.

6. Schauber EM, Woolf A (2003) Chronic wasting disease in deer and elk: A critique of current models and their application. Wildl Soc Bull 31: 610–616.

7. Miller MW, Conner MM (2005) Epidemiology of chronic wasting disease in free-ranging mule deer: spatial, temporal, and demographic influences on observed prevalence patterns. J Wildl Dis 41: 275–290.

8. Wolfe LL, Miller MW, Williams ES (2004) Feasibility of "test-and-cull" for managing chronic wasting disease in urban mule deer. Wildl Soc Bull 32: 500–505. doi:10.2193/0091-7648(2004)32[500:FOTFMC]2.0.CO;2

9. Williams ES, Miller MW, Kreeger TJ, Kahn RH, Thorne ET (2002) Chronic wasting disease of deer and elk: A review with recommendations for management. J Wildl Manag 66: 551–563.

10. Anderson RM, May RM (1991) Infectious diseases of humans: dynamics and control. Oxford; New York: Oxford University Press. 757 p.

11. McCallum H, Barlow N, Hone J (2001) How should pathogen transmission be modelled? Trends Ecol Evol 16: 295–300.

12. Begon M, Bennett M, Bowers RG, French NP, Hazel SM, et al. (2002) A clarification of transmission terms in host-microparasite models: numbers, densities and areas. Epidemiol Infect 129: 147–153.

13. Roberts MG (1996) The Dynamics of Bovine Tuberculosis in Possum Populations, and its Eradication or Control by Culling or Vaccination. J Anim Ecol 65: 451–464.

14. Getz WM, Pickering J (1983) Epidemic Models: Thresholds and Population Regulation. Am Nat 121: 892–898. doi:10.1086/284112

15. Cross ML, Buddle BM, Aldwell FE (2007) The potential of oral vaccines for disease control in wildlife species. Vet J 174: 472–480. doi:10.1016/j.tvjl.2006.10.005

16. Barlow ND (1996) The ecology of wildlife disease control: Simple models revisited. J Appl Ecol 33: 303–314.

17. Miller MW, Williams ES, McCarty CW, Spraker TR, Kreeger TJ, et al. (2000) Epizootiology of chronic wasting disease in free-ranging cervids in Colorado and Wyoming. J Wildl Dis 36: 676–690.

18. Wasserberg G, Osnas EE, Rolley RE, Samuel MD (2009) Host culling as an adaptive management tool for chronic wasting disease in white-tailed deer: a modelling study. J Appl Ecol 46: 457–466. doi:10.1111/j.1365-2664.2008.01576.x

19. Joly DO, Ribic CA, Langenberg JA, Beheler K, Batha CA, et al. (2003) Chronic wasting disease in free-ranging Wisconsin White-tailed Deer. Emerg Infect Dis 9: 599–601.

20. Joly DO, Samuel MD, Langenberg JA, Blanchong JA, Batha CA, et al. (2006) Spatial epidemiology of chronic wasting disease in Wisconsin white-tailed deer. J Wildl Dis 42: 578–588.

21. Grear DA, Samuel MD, Langenberg JA, Keane D (2006) Demographic Patterns and Harvest Vulnerability of Chronic Wasting Disease Infected White-Tailed Deer in Wisconsin. J Wildl Manag 70: 546–553. doi:10.2193/0022-541X(2006)70[546:DPAHVO]2.0.CO;2

22. Osnas EE, Heisey DM, Rolley RE, Samuel MD (2009) Spatial and temporal patterns of chronic wasting disease: fine-scale mapping of a wildlife epidemic in Wisconsin. Ecol Appl 19: 1311–1322.

23. Conner MM, Miller MW (2004) Movement patterns and spatial epidemioology of a prion disease in mule deer population units. Ecol Appl 14: 1870–1881. doi:10.1890/03-5309

24. Blanchong JA, Samuel MD, Scribner KT, Weckworth BV, Langenberg JA, et al. (2008) Landscape genetics and the spatial distribution of chronic wasting disease. Biol Lett 4: 130–133. doi:10.1098/rsbl.2007.0523

25. Heisey DM, Osnas EE, Cross PC, Joly DO, Langenberg JA, et al. (2010) Linking process to pattern: estimating spatiotemporal dynamics of a wildlife epidemic from cross-sectional data. Ecol Monogr 80: 221–240. doi:10.1890/09-0052.1

26. Cross PC, Drewe J, Patrek V, Pearce G, Samuel MD, et al. (2009) Wildlife Population Structure and Parasite Transmission: Implications for Disease Management. In: Delahay RJ, Smith GC, Hutchings MR, editors. Management of Disease in Wild Mammals. Tokyo: Springer. pp. 9–29.

27. Magle SB, Samuel MD, Van Deelen TR, Robinson SJ, Mathews NE (2013) Evaluating spatial overlap and relatedness of white-tailed deer in a chronic wasting disease management zone. PloS One 8: e56568. doi:10.1371/journal.pone.0056568

28. Grear DA, Samuel MD, Scribner KT, Weckworth BV, Langenberg JA (2010) Influence of genetic relatedness and spatial proximity on chronic wasting disease infection among female white-tailed deer. J Appl Ecol 47: 532–540. doi:10.1111/j.1365-2664.2010.01813.x

29. Keane DP, Barr DJ, Bochsler PN, Hall SM, Gidlewski T, et al. (2008) Chronic wasting disease in a Wisconsin white-tailed deer farm. J Vet Diagn Invest 20: 698–703.

30. Van Deelen TR, Campa III H, Hamady M, Haufler JB (1998) Migration and Seasonal Range Dynamics of Deer Using Adjacent Deeryards in Northern Michigan. J Wildl Manag 62: 205–213.

31. Van Deelen TR (1999) Deer-cedar interactions during a period of mild winters: implications for conservation of conifer swamp deeryards in the Great Lakes region. Nat Areas J 19: 263–274.

32. Dunkley L, Cattet MRL (2003) A comprehensive review of the ecological and human social effects of artificial feeding and baiting of wildlife. Saskatoon, Saskatchewan: Canadian Cooperative Wildlife Health Centre.

33. Wisconsin Department of Natural Resources (2010) Wisconsin's chronic wasting disease response plan: 2010–2025. Madison, Wisconsin.

34. Keane DP, Barr DJ, Keller JE, Hall SM, Langenberg JA, et al. (2008) Comparison of retropharyngeal lymph node and obex region of the brainstem in detection of chronic wasting disease in white-tailed deer (Odocoileus virginianus). J Vet Diagn Invest 20: 58–60.

35. Caswell H (2001) Matrix population models: construction, analysis, and interpretation. 2nd ed. Sunderland, Mass: Sinauer Associates. 722 p.

36. Oli MK, Venkataraman M, Klein PA, Wendland LD, Brown MB (2006) Population dynamics of infectious diseases: A discrete time model. Ecol Model 198: 183–194. doi:10.1016/j.ecolmodel.2006.04.007

37. Klepac P, Caswell H (2011) The stage-structured epidemic: linking disease and demography with a multi-state matrix approach model. Theor Ecol 4: 301–319. doi:10.1007/s12080-010-0079-8

38. Rudolf VHW, Antonovics J (2005) Species coexistence and pathogens with frequency-dependent transmission. Am Nat 166: 112–118. doi:10.1086/430674

39. Potapov A, Merrill E, Pybus M, Coltman D, Lewis MA (2013) Chronic wasting disease: Possible transmission mechanisms in deer. Ecol Model 250: 244–257. doi:10.1016/j.ecolmodel.2012.11.012

40. Hilborn R, Mangel M (1997) The Ecological Detective: Confronting Models with Data. Princeton: Princeton University Press. 330 p.

41. Burnham KP, Anderson DR (1998) Model selection and inference: a practical information-theoretic approach. New York: Springer-Verlag. 353 p.

42. McKay MD, Beckman RJ, Conover WJ (1979) Comparison of Three Methods for Selecting Values of Input Variables in the Analysis of Output from a Computer Code. Technometrics 21: 239–245. doi:10.1080/00401706.1979.10489755

43. Manache G, Melching CS (2004) Sensitivity Analysis of a Water-Quality Model Using Latin Hypercube Sampling. J Water Resour Plan Manag 130: 232–242. doi:10.1061/(ASCE)0733-9496(2004)130:3(232)

44. Robinson SJ, Samuel MD, Rolley R, Shelton P (2013) Using landscape epidemiological models to understand factors affecting the distribution of chronic wasting disease in the Midwestern USA. Landsc Ecol 28: 1923–1935.

45. Holsman RH, Petchenik J (2006) Predicting Deer Hunter Harvest Behavior in Wisconsin's Chronic Wasting Disease Eradication Zone. Hum Dimens Wildl 11: 177–189. doi:10.1080/10871200600669916

46. Storm DJ, Samuel MD, Rolley RE, Shelton P, Keuler NS, et al. (2013) Deer density and disease prevalence influence transmission of chronic wasting disease in white-tailed deer. Ecosphere 4: 10. doi:10.1890/ES12-00141.1

47. Farnsworth ML, Wolfe LL, Hobbs NT, Burnham KP, Williams ES, et al. (2005) Human land use influences chronic wasting disease prevalence in mule deer. Ecol Appl 15: 119–126. doi:10.1890/04-0194

48. Halls LK (1984) White-tailed deer: ecology and management. Harrisburg, PA: Stackpole Books. 870 p.

49. Habib TJ, Merrill EH, Pybus MJ, Coltman DW (2011) Modelling landscape effects on density–contact rate relationships of deer in eastern Alberta: Implications for chronic wasting disease. Ecol Model 222: 2722–2732. doi:10.1016/j.ecolmodel.2011.05.007

50. Brown P, Gajdusek D (1991) Survival of scrapie virus after 3 years' interment. The Lancet 337: 269–270. doi:10.1016/0140-6736(91)90873-N

51. Johnson CJ, Phillips KE, Schramm PT, McKenzie D, Aiken JM, et al. (2006) Prions Adhere to Soil Minerals and Remain Infectious. PLoS Pathog 2: e32. doi:10.1371/journal.ppat.0020032

52. Miller MW, Williams ES, Hobbs NT, Wolfe LL (2004) Environmental Sources of Prion Transmission in Mule Deer. Emerg Infect Dis 10: 1003–1006. doi:10.3201/eid1006.040010

53. Miller MW, Hobbs NT, Tavener SJ (2006) Dynamics of prion disease transmission in mule deer. Ecol Appl 16: 2208–2214.

54. Almberg ES, Cross PC, Johnson CJ, Heisey DM, Richards BJ (2011) Modeling Routes of Chronic Wasting Disease Transmission: Environmental Prion Persistence Promotes Deer Population Decline and Extinction. PLoS ONE 6: e19896. doi:10.1371/journal.pone.0019896

55. Fenichel EP, Horan RD (2007) Gender-Based Harvesting in Wildlife Disease Management. Am J Agric Econ 89: 904–920. doi:10.1111/j.1467-8276.2007.01025.x

56. Kjær LJ, Schauber EM, Nielsen CK (2008) Spatial and Temporal Analysis of Contact Rates in Female White-Tailed Deer. J Wildl Manag 72: 1819–1825. doi:10.2193/2007-489

57. Silbernagel ER, Skelton NK, Waldner CL, Bollinger TK (2011) Interaction among deer in a chronic wasting disease endemic zone. J Wildl Manag 75: 1453–1461. doi:10.1002/jwmg.172

58. Richards SA (2008) Dealing with overdispersed count data in applied ecology. J Appl Ecol 45: 218–227. doi:10.1111/j.1365-2664.2007.01377.x

59. Palmer MV, Waters WR, Whipple DL (2004) Shared feed as a means of deer-to-deer transmission of Mycobacterium bovis. J Wildl Dis 40: 87–91.

60. Oyer AM, Mathews NE, Skuldt LH (2007) Long-Distance Movement of a White-Tailed Deer Away From a Chronic Wasting Disease Area. J Wildl Manag 71: 1635–1638. doi:10.2193/2006-381

61. Long ES, Diefenbach DR, Rosenberry CS, Wallingford BD, Grund MD (2005) Forest cover influences dispersal distance of white-tailed deer. J Mammal 86: 623–629. doi:10.1644/1545-1542(2005)86[623:FCIDDO]2.0.CO;2

62. Lang KR, Blanchong JA (2012) Population genetic structure of white-tailed deer: Understanding risk of chronic wasting disease spread. J Wildl Manag 76: 832–840. doi:10.1002/jwmg.292

63. Robinson SJ, Samuel MD, Lopez DL, Shelton P (2012) The walk is never random: subtle landscape effects shape gene flow in a continuous white-tailed deer population in the Midwestern United States. Mol Ecol 21: 4190–4205. doi:10.1111/j.1365-294X.2012.05681.x

64. Potapov A, Merrill E, Lewis MA (2012) Wildlife disease elimination and density dependence. Proc R Soc B Biol Sci 279: 3139–3145. doi:10.1098/rspb.2012.0520

65. Roseberry JL, Woolf A (1991) A Comparative Evaluation of Techniques for Analyzing White-Tailed Deer Harvest Data. Wildl Monogr 117: 3–59.

66. Gaillard J-M, Festa-Bianchet M, Yoccoz NG (1998) Population dynamics of large herbivores: variable recruitment with constant adult survival. Trends Ecol Evol 13: 58–63. doi:10.1016/S0169-5347(97)01237-8

67. Williams ES, Young S (1980) Chronic wasting disease of captive mule deer: a spongiform encephalopathy. J Wildl Dis 16: 89–98.

68. Walter WD, Walsh DP, Farnsworth ML, Winkelman DL, Miller MW (2011) Soil clay content underlies prion infection odds. Nat Commun 2: 200. doi:10.1038/ncomms1203

69. Bolker BM (2008) Ecological models and data in R. Princeton, NJ: Princeton University Press. 396 p.

# 6

# Reverse Zoonotic Disease Transmission (Zooanthroponosis): A Systematic Review of Seldom-Documented Human Biological Threats to Animals

**Ali M. Messenger[1,2], Amber N. Barnes[1], Gregory C. Gray[1,2]***

1 College of Public Health and Health Professions, University of Florida, Gainesville, Florida, United States of America, 2 Emerging Pathogens Institute, University of Florida, Gainesville, Florida, United States of America

## Abstract

***Background:*** Research regarding zoonotic diseases often focuses on infectious diseases animals have given to humans. However, an increasing number of reports indicate that humans are transmitting pathogens to animals. Recent examples include methicillin-resistant *Staphylococcus aureus*, influenza A virus, *Cryptosporidium parvum*, and *Ascaris lumbricoides*. The aim of this review was to provide an overview of published literature regarding reverse zoonoses and highlight the need for future work in this area.

***Methods:*** An initial broad literature review yielded 4763 titles, of which 4704 were excluded as not meeting inclusion criteria. After careful screening, 56 articles (from 56 countries over three decades) with documented human-to-animal disease transmission were included in this report.

***Findings:*** In these publications, 21 (38%) pathogens studied were bacterial, 16 (29%) were viral, 12 (21%) were parasitic, and 7 (13%) were fungal, other, or involved multiple pathogens. Effected animals included wildlife (n = 28, 50%), livestock (n = 24, 43%), companion animals (n = 13, 23%), and various other animals or animals not explicitly mentioned (n = 2, 4%). Published reports of reverse zoonoses transmission occurred in every continent except Antarctica therefore indicating a worldwide disease threat.

***Interpretation:*** As we see a global increase in industrial animal production, the rapid movement of humans and animals, and the habitats of humans and wild animals intertwining with great complexity, the future promises more opportunities for humans to cause reverse zoonoses. Scientific research must be conducted in this area to provide a richer understanding of emerging and reemerging disease threats. As a result, multidisciplinary approaches such as One Health will be needed to mitigate these problems.

**Editor:** Bradley S. Schneider, Metabiota, United States of America

**Funding:** This work was supported by the US Armed Forces Health Surveillance Center - Global Emerging Infections Surveillance Operations (multiple grants to GCG) and a supplement from the National Institute of Allergy and Infectious Diseases (R01 AI068803 to GCG). The funders had no role in study design, data collection and analysis, decision to publish, or preparation of the manuscript.

**Competing Interests:** The authors have declared that no competing interests exist.

* E-mail: gcgray@phhp.ufl.edu

## Introduction

With today's rapid transport systems, modern public health problems are growing increasingly complex. A pathogen that emerges today in one country can easily be transported unnoticed in people, animals, plants, or food products to distant parts of the world in less than 24 hours [1]. This high level of mobility makes tracking and designing interventions against emerging pathogens exceedingly difficult, requiring close international and interdisciplinary collaborations. Fundamental to these efforts is an understanding of the ecology of emerging diseases. Published works often cite the large proportion of human emerging pathogens that originate in animals [2,3,4,5]. However, scientific reports seldom mention human contributions to the variety of emerging diseases that impact animals. The focus of this review is to examine and summarize the scientific literature regarding such zoonoses transmission. A comprehensive table of the results is included in this document.

## Methods

For the purpose of this review several terms require definitions. Despite the fact that the term "zoonosis" usually refers to a disease that is transmitted from animals to humans (also called "anthropozoonosis") [6], in this paper, "zoonosis" was defined as any disease that is transmitted from animals to humans, or vice versa [6], There are two related terms ("zooanthroponosis" and "reverse zoonosis") that refer to any pathogen normally reservoired in humans that can be transmitted to other vertebrates [6]. Acknowledging that the terms "reverse zoonosis" or "zooanthroponosis" are seldom used, and that the term "zoonosis" can have several meanings, search methods were designed to

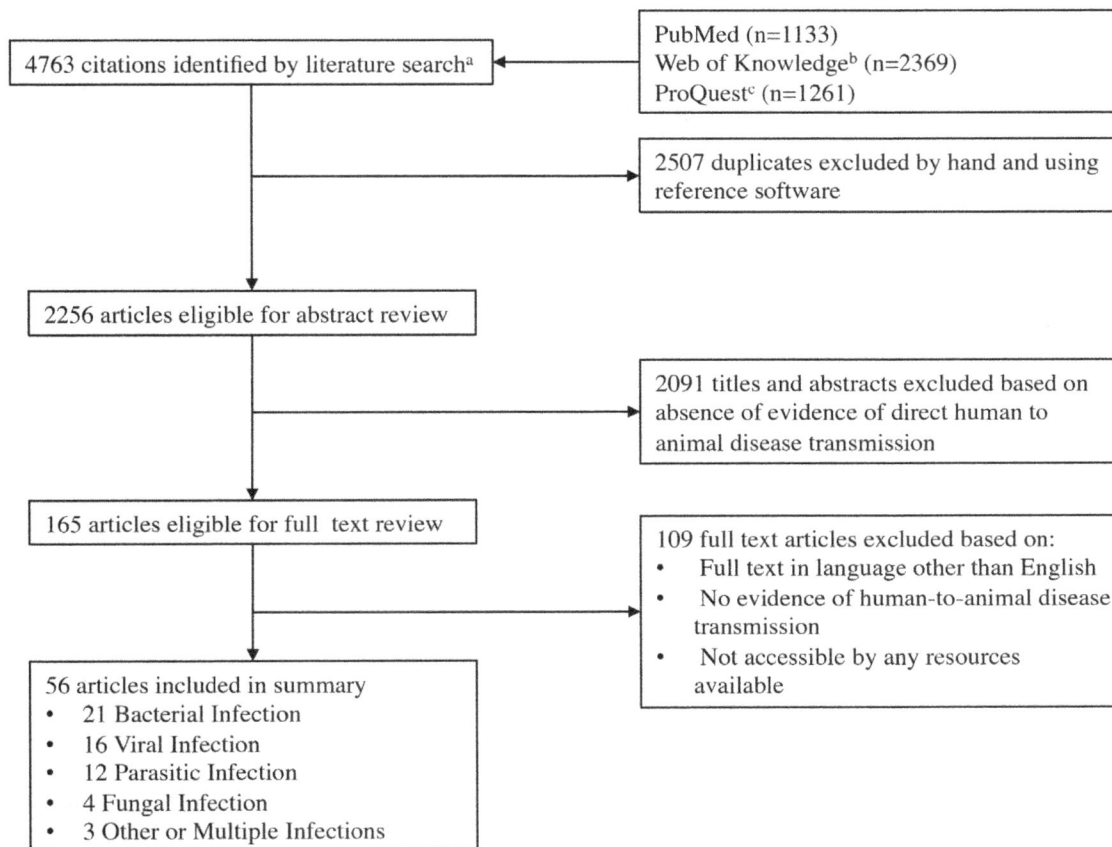

**Figure 1. Flowchart demonstrating the identification and selection process for publications included in this review.**

include all of these terms in an effort to capture the widest possible subset of publications with documented human-to-animal transmission.

## Literature search

In June 2012, we searched PubMed in addition to several databases within Web of Knowledge and ProQuest to find articles documenting reverse zoonoses transmission. Search terms included: *reverse zoonosis, bidirectional zoonosis, anthroponosis, zooanthroponosis, anthropozoonosis,* and *human-to-animal disease transmission.* Articles were limited to clinical and observational type studies and were restricted to English only. Review articles were not included as they did not demonstrate a specific account of transmission. Letters to editors or similar correspondence were also excluded. Only publications with documented human-to-animal transmission were included. No time period was stipulated.

Four search strings were used for the PubMed database: ((bidirectional OR reverse) AND (zoono* or "disease transmission")) OR anthropono* OR "human-to-animal"), ((bidirectional OR reverse OR "human-to-animal") AND (zoono* or "disease transmission")) OR anthropono*), ("reverse zoonoses" OR " bidirectional zoonoses" OR "reverse zoonosis" OR " bidirectional zoonosis" OR "reverse zoonotic" OR " bidirectional zoonotic" OR anthropono* OR ("human-to-animal" AND disease* AND transmi*)), and (((bidirectional OR reverse OR "human-to-animal") AND (zoonoses[majr] OR "Disease Transmission, Infectious"[majr] OR zoonosis[tiab] OR zoonoses[tiab] OR zoonotic[tiab])) OR Anthroponos*[tiab] OR Zooanthroponos*[-

tiab] OR Anthropozoonos*[tiab]). In the ProQuest and Web of Knowledge databases, we only used one string: ((bidirectional OR reverse) AND (zoonosis OR zoonoses OR zoonotic)) OR anthropono* OR Zooanthropono* OR anthropozoono* OR "human-to-animal" OR "human to animal"). The lack of additional search strings for the latter databases was due to less comprehensive search capabilities. Duplicate articles were removed.

## Literature analyses

Titles and abstracts were reviewed and articles were retained when there was evidence of disease transmission from humans to animals. During full text review, some citations proved straightforward in distinguishing transmission from humans to animals (e.g. via direct contact), while others were selected based on strong author suggestion or research implications toward reverse zoonotic transmission. In an effort to highlight trends in an otherwise diverse set of articles, citations were grouped by pathogen type and year of publication. To further clarify relationships, we also pictorially displayed the study locations and animal types discussed in the various articles.

## Results

This comprehensive literature review yielded 4763 titles, 2507 of which were excluded as duplicates (Figure 1). During the review of abstracts, 2091 studies were excluded due to a lack of evidence of human-to-animal disease transmission. After consideration of the 165 eligible for full text review, 109 studies were excluded

**Table 1.** Descriptors of reports included in review with documented human-to-animal transmission.

| Publications | Study Location | Specimen Source | Pathogen Name | Animal(s) Infected |
|---|---|---|---|---|
| **Bacteria** | | | | |
| Cosivi et al (1995) [7] | Morocco | Assorted | *Mycobacterium tuberculosis, Mycobacterium bovis*[1] | Wildlife |
| Seguin et al (1999) [8] | United States | Veterinary hospital | *Methicillin-resistant Staphylococcus aureus* (MRSA)[1,2] | Livestock |
| Donnelly et al (2000) [9] | United States | 4H project livestock | *Streptococcus pneumonia*[1] | Livestock |
| Nizeyi et al (2001) [10] | Uganda | National park | *Campylobacter* spp., *Salmonella* spp., *Shigella sonnei, Shigella boydii, Shigella flexneri*[1,3] | Wildlife |
| Michel et al (2003) [11] | South Africa | Zoo | *M. tuberculosis*[1,3] | Wildlife |
| Hackendahl et al (2004) [12]; also see Erwin et al (2004) [13] | United States | Veterinary hospital | *M. tuberculosis*[1,4] | Companion |
| Prasad et al (2005) [14] | India | Veterinary hospital | *M. tuberculosis*[3,4] | Livestock |
| Weese et al (2006) [15] | Canada, United States | Household; Veterinary hospital | MRSA[1] | Companion |
| Morris et al (2006) [16] | United States | Household; Veterinary hospital | MRSA[1] | Companion |
| Kwon et al (2006) [17] | Korea | Slaughterhouse | MRSA[1,3] | Companion; Livestock |
| Rwego et al (2008) [18] | Uganda | National park | *Escherichia coli*[1,3] | Livestock; Wildlife |
| Hsieh et al (2008) [19] | Taiwan | Livestock farm | *Oxacillin-resistant Staphylococcus aureus* (ORSA) | Livestock |
| Berg et al (2009) [20] | Ethiopia | Slaughterhouse | *M. tuberculosis*[3] | Livestock |
| Heller et al (2010) [21] | United Kingdom | Household; Veterinary hospital | MRSA[1,2] | Companion |
| Kottler et al (2010) [22] | United States | Household; Veterinary hospital | MRSA[1] | Companion |
| Ewers et al (2010) [23] | Germany, Italy, Netherlands, France, Spain, Denmark, Austria & Luxembourg | Veterinary hospital | *Escherichia coli* | Companion; Livestock |
| Every et al (2011) [24] | Australia | University zoology department | *Helicobacter pylori*[1] | Wildlife |
| Lin et al (2011) [25] | United States | Veterinary hospital | MRSA[1] | Companion; Livestock |
| Rubin et al (2011) [26] | Canada | Veterinary hospital; Human hospital | MRSA[1] | Companion |
| Price et al (2012) [27] | Austria, Belgium, Canada, Switzerland, China, Germany, Denmark, Spain, Finland, France, French Guiana, Hungary, Italy, the Netherlands, Peru, Poland, Portugal, Slovenia, and United States | Animal meat for sale | MRSA[1] | Livestock |
| **Virus** | | | | |
| Meng et al (1998) [28] | United States | Veterinary laboratory; Human sample | Hepatitis E[5] | Wildlife |
| Willy et al (1999) [29] | United States | Veterinary laboratory | Measles[1,4] | Wildlife |
| Kaur et al (2008) [30] | Tanzania | National park | Human metapneumovirus (hMPV)[1,4] | Wildlife |
| Feagins et al (2008) [31] | United States | Commercially sold laboratory animals | Hepatitis E[5] | Livestock |
| Song et al (2010) [32] | South Korea | Livestock farm | Influenza A (2009 pandemic H1N1)[1] | Livestock |
| Swenson et al (2010) [33] | United States | Household; Veterinary hospital | Influenza A (2009 pandemic H1N1)[1,4] | Companion |
| Tischer et al (2010) [34] | Various; Unspecified | Unknown (previous reports cited) | Human herpesvirus 1, human herpesvirus 4[1,3,4] | Companion; Wildlife |
| Abe et al (2010) [35] | Japan | Wildlife | Rotavirus[1,3] | Wildlife |
| Berhane et al (2010) [36] | Canada, Chile | Livestock farm | Influenza A (2009 pandemic H1N1)[1,4,5] | Livestock |
| Poon et al (2010) [37] | Hong Kong | Slaughterhouse | Influenza A (2009 pandemic H1N1) | Livestock |
| Forgie et al (2011) [38] | Canada | Veterinary laboratory | Influenza A (2009 pandemic H1N1) | Livestock |
| Holyoake et al (2011) [39] | Australia | Livestock farm | Influenza A (2009 pandemic H1N1)[4] | Livestock |

**Table 1.** Cont.

| Publications | Study Location | Specimen Source | Pathogen Name | Animal(s) Infected |
|---|---|---|---|---|
| Scotch et al (2011) [40] | Mexico, United States, Canada, Australia, United Kingdom, France, Ireland, Argentina, Chile, Singapore, Norway, China, Italy, Thailand, South Korea, Indonesia, Germany, Japan, Russia, Finland, and Iceland | Unknown (previous reports cited) | Influenza A (2009 pandemic H1N1) | Companion; Livestock; Wildlife |
| Trevennec et al (2011) [41] | Vietnam | Livestock farm; Slaughterhouse | Influenza A (2009 pandemic H1N1)[1,2] | Livestock |
| Wevers et al (2011) [42] | Cameroon, Democratic Republic of the Congo, Gamiba, Côte d'Ivoire, Republic of Congo, Rwanda, Tanzania, Uganda, Germany (initial samples in Asia and South America) | Wildlife; Zoo | Human adenovirus A-F[1,3] | Wildlife |
| Crossley et al (2012) [43] | United States | Private zoo | Influenza A (2009 pandemic H1N1)[2,3] | Wildlife |
| **Parasite** | | | | |
| Sleeman et al (2000) [44] | Rwanda | National park | *Chilomastix mesnili, Endolimax nana, Stronglyoides fuelleborni, Trichuris trichiura*[1,3] | Wildlife |
| Graczyk et al (2001) [45] | Uganda | National park | *Cryptosporidium parvum* | Wildlife |
| Graczyk et al (2002) [46] | Uganda | National park | *Encephalitozoon intestinalis*[1,3] | Wildlife |
| Graczyk et al (2002) [47] | Uganda | National park | *Giardia duodenalis*[1,3] | Wildlife |
| Guk et al (2004) [48] | Korea | Laboratory | *C. parvum*[5] | Livestock; Wildlife |
| Noël et al (2005) [49] | Singapore, Pakistan, Japan, Thailand, United States, France, Czech Republic | N/A | *Blastocystis* spp | Livestock; Wildlife |
| Coklin et al (2007) [50] | Canada | Livestock farm | *G. duodenalis, C. parvum*[1,3] | Livestock |
| Adejinmi et al (2008) [51] | Nigeria | Zoo | *Ascaris lumbricoides, T. trichiura*[1] | Wildlife |
| Teichroeb et al (2009) [52] | Ghana | Wildlife | *Isospora* spp., *Giardia duodenalis*[1,3] | Wildlife |
| Ash et al (2010) [53] | Zambia; Namibia; Australia | Wildlife; Zoo | *G. duodenalis*[1] | Wildlife |
| Johnston et al (2010) [54] | Uganda | National park | *G. duodenalis*[1,3] | Livestock; Wildlife |
| Dixon et al (2011) [55] | Canada | Livestock farm | *G. duodenalis, C. parvum*[1,3] | Livestock |
| **Fungus** | | | | |
| Jacobs et al (1988) [56] | Unspecified | Assorted | *Microsporum* spp., *Trichophyton* spp.[1] | Assorted |
| Pal et al (1997) [57] | India | Household | *Trichophyton rubrum*[1] | Wildlife |
| Wrobel (2008) [58] | United States | Veterinary hospital | *Candida albicans*[3] | Companion; Livestock; Wildlife |
| Sharma et al (2009) [59] | India | Household; Veterinary hospital | *Microsporum gypseum*[1] | Wildlife |
| **Other** | | | | |
| Epstein et al (2009) [60][+] | Assorted | Wildlife; Livestock farm; Zoo; Laboratory | Herpes simplex 1, influenza A, parasite spp, Measles, MRSA, *M. tuberculosis*[1,2,3,4,6] | Assorted |
| Guyader et al (2000) [61][&] | France | Shellfish-growing waters | Astrovirus, enterovirus, hepatitis A, Norwalk-like (norovirus), rotavirus[1,3] | Wildlife |
| Muehlenbein et al (2010) [62][^] | Malaysia | Wildlife | Assorted illnesses[1,6] | Wildlife |

**Other assorted pathogen types:**
[+]**virus; parasite/bacteria,**
[&]**virus/bacteria,**
[^]**assorted.**
**Modes of transmission as indicated by authors:**
[1]**direct contact,**
[2]**fomite,**
[3]**oral,**
[4]**aerosol,**
[5]**inoculation,**
[6]**other.**

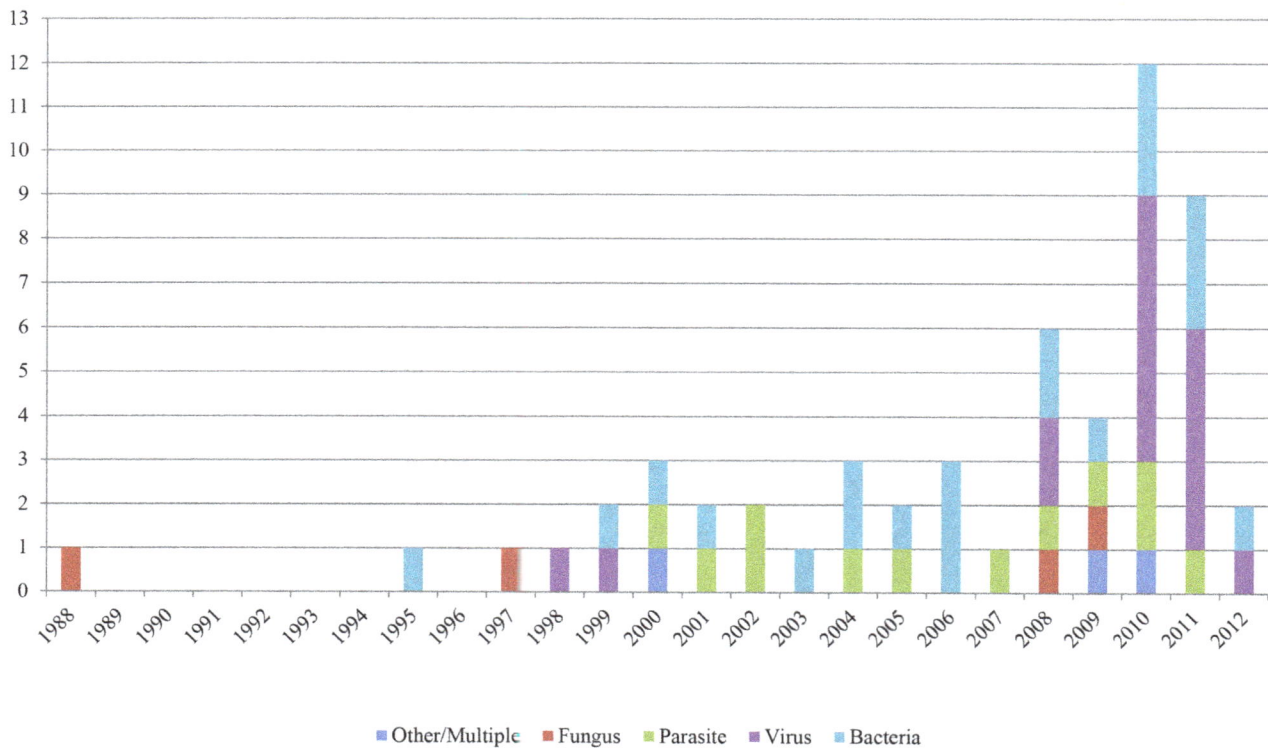

**Figure 2. Timeline and frequency of reverse zoonoses publications included in this review shown by pathogen type.**

based on full texts being written in a language other than English, absence of human-to-animal disease transmission, or full texts being unavailable. After all exclusions, 56 articles were considered for this review (Table 1).

Included reports were based in 56 different countries. Although the reports spanned three decades, there seems to be an increasing number of studies published in recent years (Figure 2). Twenty eight percent of the studies were conducted in the United States

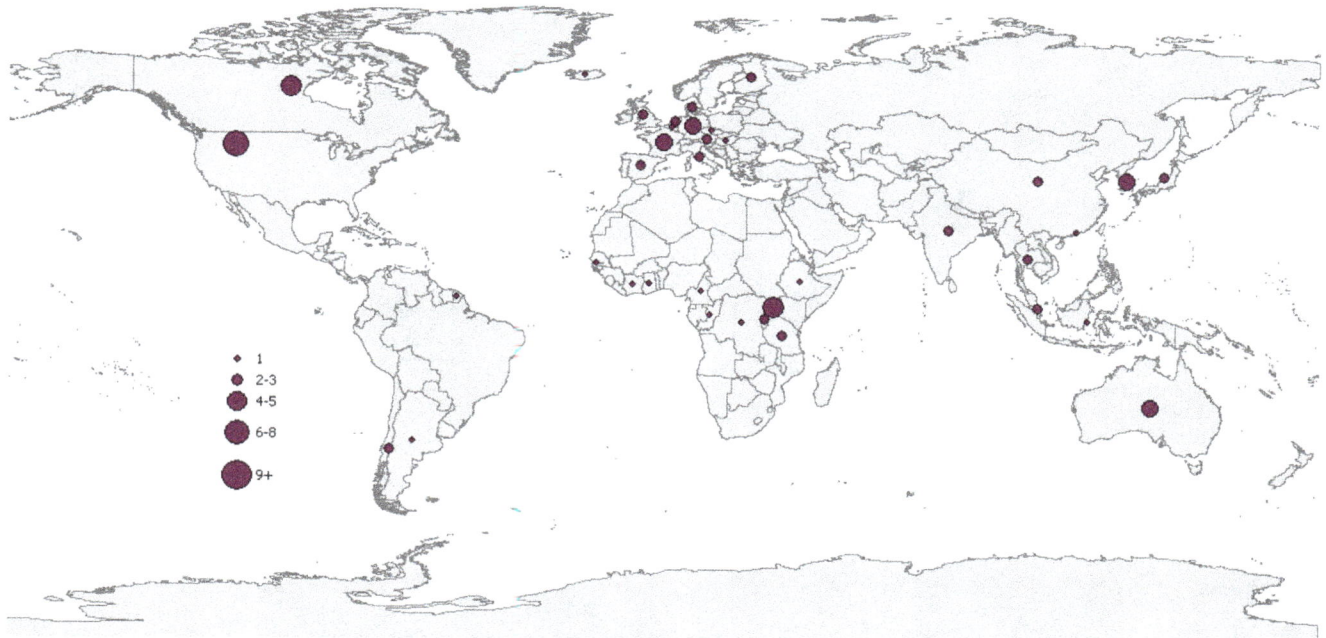

**Figure 3. Proportion of reverse zoonoses scientific reports included in review as illustrated by study location.** Note: Many reports identified several countries therefore each country in this figure does not necessarily represent a single corresponding publication.

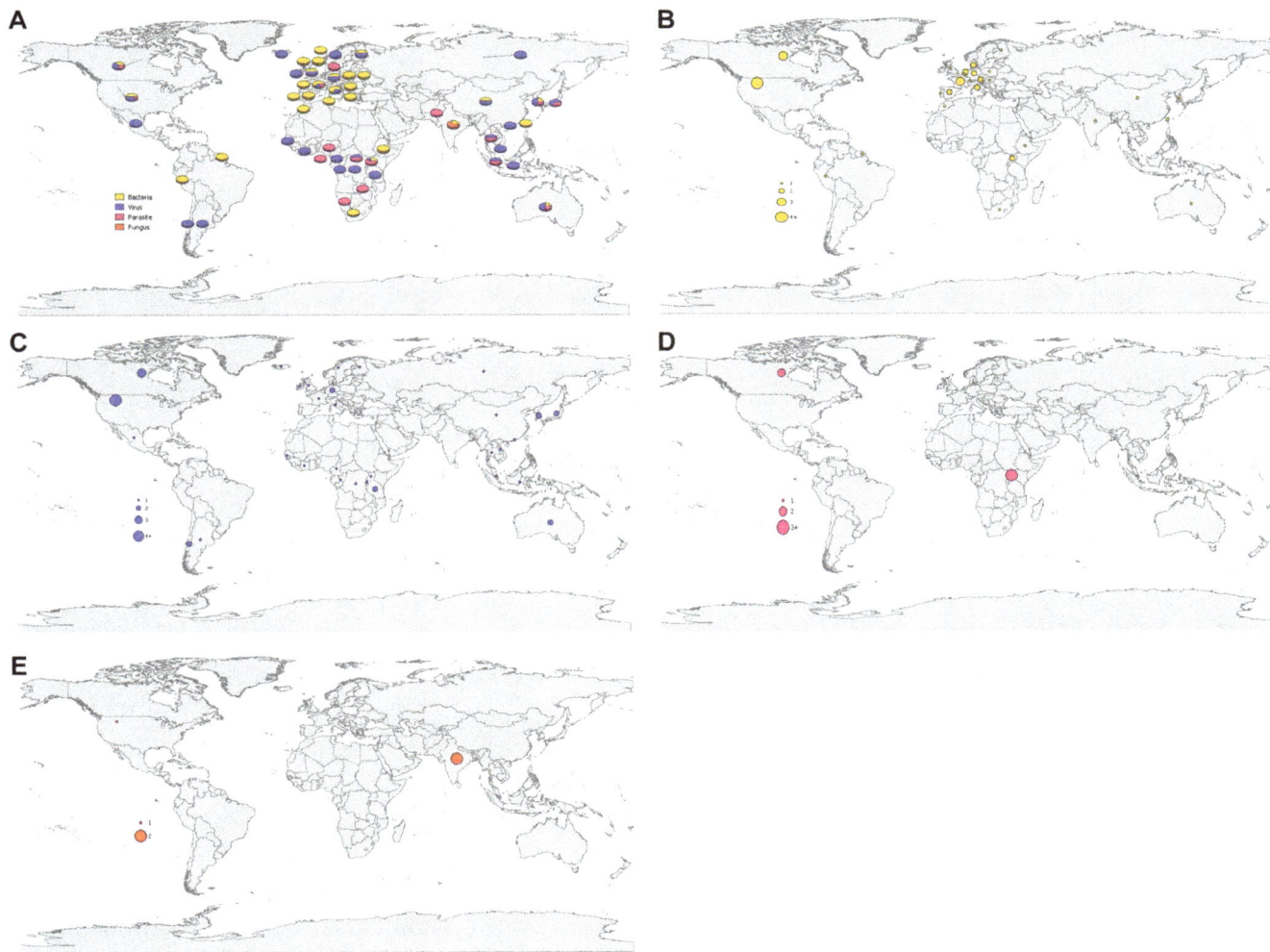

**Figure 4. Study locations for literature included in review.** A. Proportion of reverse zoonoses scientific reports as illustrated by study location and pathogen type; B. Proportion of reverse zoonoses scientific reports on bacterial pathogens as illustrated by study location; C. Proportion of reverse zoonoses scientific reports on viral pathogens as illustrated by study location; D. Proportion of reverse zoonoses scientific reports on parasitic pathogens as illustrated by study location; E. Proportion of reverse zoonoses scientific reports on fungal pathogens as illustrated by study location.

(n = 16), 14% in Canada (n = 8), and 13% in Uganda (n = 7) (Figure 3). Within the study results, 21 publications discussed human-to-animal transmission of bacterial pathogens (38%); 16 studies discussed viral pathogens (29%); 12 studies discussed human parasites (21%); and seven studies discussed transmission of fungi, other pathogens, or diseases of multiple etiologies (13%). Bacterial pathogen reports were centered in North America and Europe. Viral studies were well-distributed globally. Parasitic disease reports were conducted chiefly in Africa. Fungal studies were conducted almost exclusively in India (Figure 4).

Animals with reported infection or inoculation with human diseases included wildlife (n = 28, 50%), livestock (n = 24, 43%), companion animals (n = 13, 23%), and other animals or animals not explicitly mentioned (n = 2, 4%). The majority of companion and livestock animals were studied in North America and Europe, while wildlife studies were most prevalent in Africa (Table 1, Figure 5). Typically, diagnostic specimens were collected at veterinary hospitals (n = 15, 27%), national parks (n = 8, 14%) and livestock farms (n = 8, 14%). Direct contact was the suggested transmission route 71% of the time (n = 40). Other transmission routes included fomite, oral contact, aerosols, and inoculation.

As early as 1988, zoonoses research focusing on fungal pathogens was being conducted. Initial studies implied human transmission of *Microsporum* (n = 2) and *Trichophyton* (n = 2) to various animal species, with a later article centered on *Candida albicans* (n = 1) (Figure 2). These publications were set in India (n = 2) and the United States (n = 1).

Since 1988, research with implications of reverse zoonoses has been largely focused on infections of bacterial origin, beginning in 1995. The majority of articles in this review focused on methicillin-resistant *Staphylococcus aureus* (MRSA) (n = 9) and *Mycobacterium tuberculosis* (n = 5). Reports regarding these bacteria were primarily conducted in the United States (n = 8) among livestock (n = 10) or companion animals (n = 9).

Viruses were the second most common pathogen associated with human-to-animal transmission. Reverse zoonoses reports regarding viral pathogens began in 1998 and have since been focused primarily on influenza with great interest surrounding the 2009 H1N1 pandemic (n = 9). These studies were conducted largely in the United States (n = 6) in livestock (n = 8) and wildlife (n = 8).

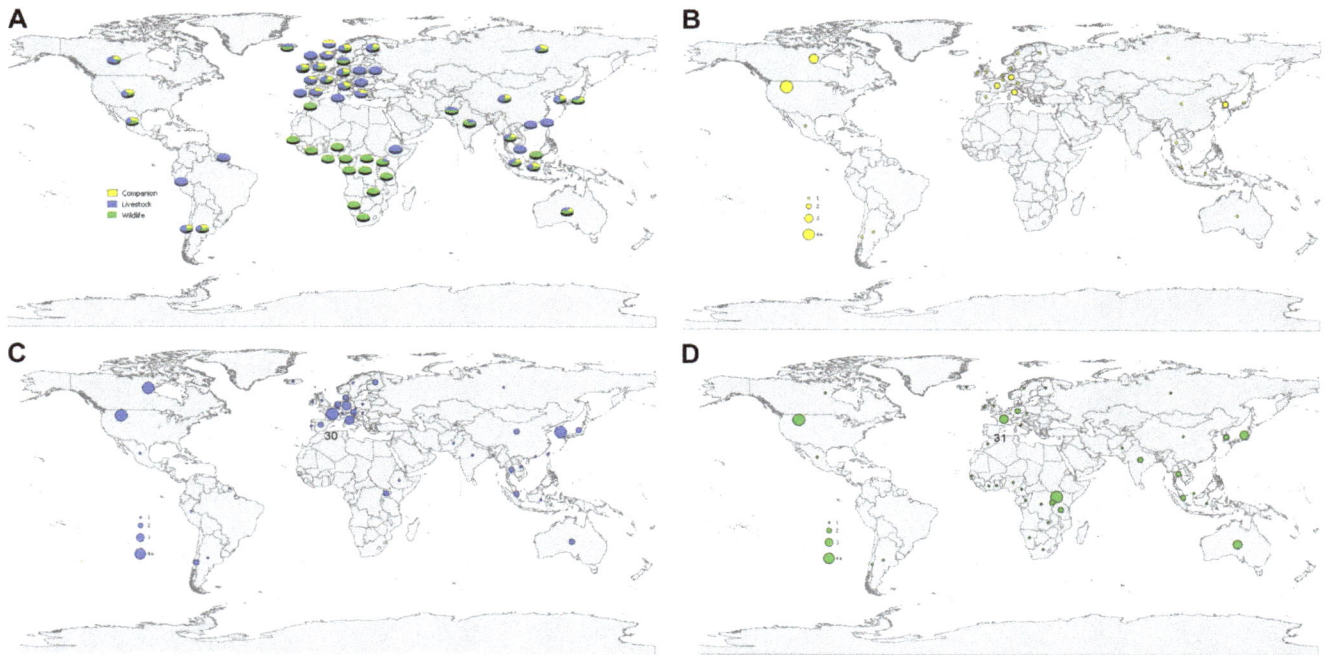

**Figure 5. Animal type and study location included in review literature.** A. Proportion of reverse zoonoses scientific reports as illustrated by study location and animal(s) infected; B. Proportion of reverse zoonoses scientific reports on companion animals as illustrated by study location; C. Proportion of reverse zoonoses scientific reports on livestock as illustrated by study location; D. Proportion of reverse zoonoses scientific reports on wildlife as illustrated by study location.

Studies suggestive of transmission of human parasites to animals were first published in 2000. The most commonly reported parasitic agents to be transmitted from humans to animals were *Giardia duodenalis* (n = 6) and *Cryptosporidium parvum* (n = 4). Parasitic research has been carried out most frequently in Uganda (n = 4) and Canada (n = 2). The authors investigated human parasitic infections chiefly in wildlife (n = 10) and livestock (n = 5).

Human-to-animal transmission is plausible for a large number of diseases because the pathogens concerned are known to infect multiple species [3]. For instance, 77.3% of the pathogens infecting livestock are considered "multiple species pathogens [3]." However, this review only found 24 reports which considered reverse zoonoses disease transmission as a potential threat to livestock, underscoring a need for further research in this area [3]. Similarly, in companion animals this review found even fewer studies (n = 13) that implied reverse zoonoses as a possible cause of infection, despite the fact that 90% of known pathogens for domestic carnivores are recognized as "multiple species pathogens [3]." The majority of publications in this reverse zoonoses review involved studies documenting human-to-wildlife transmission (n = 28). Unfortunately, they too were severely lacking in comparison to the research need. Each type of animal- livestock, companion, or wildlife, represents a unique set of risk factors for reverse zoonoses through their specific routes of human contact.

## Discussion

Human and animal relationships are likely to continue to intensify worldwide over the next several decades due in part to animal husbandry practices, the growth of the companion animal market, climate change and ecosystem disruption, anthropogenic development of habitats, and global travel and commerce [2]. As the human-animal connection escalates, so does the threat for

pathogen spread [1,63]. This review notes a number of factors that influence the risk of disease transmission from humans to animals.

For instance, human population growth and expansion encourages different species to interact in ways and at rates previously not encountered, and to do so in novel geographical areas [4]. The term "pathogen pollution" refers to the process of bringing a foreign disease into a new locality due to human involvement [64]. In the case of the endangered African painted dog, wild dogs have been infected with human strains of *Giardia duodenalis*, leading researchers to believe that pathogen pollution occurred through open defecation in and around national parks by tourists and local residents [53]. Anthropogenic changes in the ecosystem increase the amount of shared habitats between humans and animals thus exposing both to new pathogens. Researchers discovered the human strain of pandemic *Escherichia coli* strain 025:H4-ST131 CTX-M-15 in many different species of animals indicating inter-species transmission from humans to pets and livestock [23]. This particular human strain found to be infecting animals was documented across Europe.

In addition to habitat change, growth, and/or destruction, there is the ever-increasing global movement of products and travelers that extends to both humans and animals. During the pandemic of 2009 H1N1 influenza, the novel virus was able to travel across the globe and from humans to swine in less than two months [32]. One driving force behind the movement of animals and animal products is the worldwide shipment of meat. This phenomenon is a relatively new event as developing countries adjust their diets to include more meat- and dairy-based products [4]. While food and animal safety guidelines attempt to keep up with the speed of global trade, international efforts appear to be outpaced by product demand. For example, it has been estimated that five tons of illegal bushmeat pass through Paris' main Roissy-Charles de Gaulle airport each week in personal luggage [65]. However, overt retail systems of animal and animal products can also contribute to the danger of zoonoses and reverse zoonoses transmission. Many animals are sold in markets which allow humans and a myriad of animal species to interact in conditions that are known to trigger emerging diseases [66]. Specifically, this is true for live animal markets and warehouses for exotic pets [4].

The pet industry is an enormous global business that now expands from domestic to exotic animals. A 2011–2012 national pet owners survey found that in the United States alone, 72.9 million homes or 62% of the population have a pet [67]. Of these pets, the majority of animals are dogs (78.2 million) or cats (86.4 million), but a large number of pets are birds (16.2 million), reptiles (13 million), or small animals (16 million) [67]. As pet ownership seems to be increasing worldwide and more exotic pets are being introduced to private homes, the potential for disease transmission between humans and animals will continue to increase. Veterinarians must more fervently protect animals under their care from human disease threats [68]. Adopting a One Health strategy for emerging disease surveillance and reporting will benefit both humans and animals and produce a more collaborative response plan.

Veterinarians, animal health workers, and public health professionals are not the only ones who should recognize the threat of reverse zoonoses. Increased awareness must also be communicated to the general public. Worldwide, there are 1,300 zoos and aquariums that sustain more than 700 million visitors each year [69]. The potential for pathogen spread to animals can come from a visitor with an illness, contamination of a shared environment or food, and the spread of disease through relocation of animals for captivity or educational purposes. In Tanzania, a fatal outbreak of human metapneumovirus in wild chimpanzees is believed to be the result of researchers and visitors viewing the animals in a national park that was once the great apes' territory [30]. Public education and awareness should be augmented to include the potential health threats inflicted on a susceptible animal by an unhealthy human.

This report has limitations. As demonstrated in this review paper, the trend for reporting pathogen spread of human-to-animal is increasing. However the route of human transmission to animal disease manifestation is often unknown in these reports and not well documented in this review. Also the report did not examine articles that did not document human-to-animal transmission. We acknowledge that many additional works that have recorded the existence of human pathogens in animals were not evaluated. However, this review was designed to summarize only the publications that document reverse zoonotic transmission.

Many common and dangerous pathogens have not, to the authors' knowledge, been researched as reverse zoonoses threats to animals representing a significant gap in the scientific literature. Future investigations of reverse zoonoses should take into account both transmission routes and disease prevalence. Prospective research should also include a wider variety of etiological agents and animal species. Scientific literature must document the presence and transmission of human diseases in animals such that the wealth of literature on this subject will become defined and accessible across multiple disciplines. A wider knowledge and understanding of reverse zoonoses should be sought for a successful One Health response. We recommend that future research be conducted on how human disease can, and does, affect the animals around us.

## Acknowledgments

The authors especially thank Nancy Schaffer and Jennifer Lyon from the University of Florida Library Sciences for their research assistance.

## Author Contributions

Analyzed the data: AM AB GG. Wrote the paper: AM AB GG.

## References

1. Wilson ME (2003) The traveller and emerging infections: sentinel, courier, transmitter. J Appl Microbiol 94 Suppl: 1S–11S.
2. Worldbank (2010) People, pathogens and our planet: Volume 1: Towards a one health approach for controlling zoonotic diseases.
3. Cleaveland S, Laurenson MK, Taylor LH (2001) Diseases of humans and their domestic mammals: pathogen characteristics, host range and the risk of emergence. Philos Trans R Soc Lond B Biol Sci 356: 991–999.
4. Brown C (2004) Emerging zoonoses and pathogens of public health significance–an overview. Rev Sci Tech 23: 435–442.
5. World Health Organization (2010) The FAO-OIE-WHO Collaboration: Tripartite Concept Note: Sharing responsibilities and coordinating global activities to address health risks at the animal-human-ecosystems interfaces. Food and Agriculture Organization, World Organization for Animal Health, World Health Organization.
6. Hubalek Z (2003) Emerging human infectious diseases: anthroponoses, zoonoses, and sapronoses. Emerg Infect Dis 9: 403–404.
7. Cosivi O, Meslin FX, Daborn CJ, Grange JM (1995) Epidemiology of Mycobacterium bovis infection in animals and humans, with particular reference to Africa. Rev Sci Tech 14: 733–746.
8. Seguin JC, Walker RD, Caron JP, Kloos WE, George CG, et al. (1999) Methicillin-resistant Staphylococcus aureus outbreak in a veterinary teaching hospital: potential human-to-animal transmission. J Clin Microbiol 37: 1459–1463.
9. Donnelly TM, Behr MJ, Nims LJ (2000) What's your diagnosis? Septicemia in La Mancha goat kids - Apparent reverse zoonotic transmission of Streptococcus pneumoniae. Lab Animal 29: 23–25.
10. Nizeyi JB, Innocent RB, Erume J, Kalema G, Cranfield MR, et al. (2001) Campylobacteriosis, salmonellosis, and shigellosis in free-ranging human-habituated mountain gorillas of Uganda. J Wildl Dis 37: 239–244.
11. Michel AL, Venter L, Espie IW, Coetzee ML (2003) Mycobacterium tuberculosis infections in eight species at the National Zoological Gardens of South Africa, 1991–2001. J Zoo Wildl Med 34: 364–370.
12. Hackendahl NC, Mawby DI, Bemis DA, Beazley SL (2004) Putative transmission of Mycobacterium tuberculosis infection from a human to a dog. J Am Vet Med Assoc 225: 1573–1577.
13. Erwin PC, Bemis DA, Mawby DI, McCombs SB, Sheeler LL, et al. (2004) Mycobacterium tuberculosis transmission from human to canine. Emerg Infect Dis 10: 2258–2210.
14. Prasad HK, Singhal A, Mishra A, Shah NP, Katoch VM, et al. (2005) Bovine tuberculosis in India: potential basis for zoonosis. Tuberculosis (Edinb) 85: 421–428.
15. Weese JS, Dick H, Willey BM, McGeer A, Kreiswirth BN, et al. (2006) Suspected transmission of methicillin-resistant Staphylococcus aureus between domestic pets and humans in veterinary clinics and in the household. Vet Microbiol 115: 148–155.
16. Morris DO, Mauldin EA, O'Shea K, Shofer FS, Rankin SC (2006) Clinical, microbiological, and molecular characterization of methicillin-resistant Staphylococcus aureus infections of cats. Am J Vet Res 67: 1421–1425.
17. Kwon N, Park K, Jung W, Youn H, Lee Y, et al. (2006) Characteristics of methicillin resistant Staphylococcus aureus isolated from chicken meat and hospitalized dogs in Korea and their epidemiological relatedness. Vet Microbiol 117: 304–312.
18. Rwego IB, Isabirye-Basuta G, Gillespie TR, Goldberg TL (2008) Gastrointestinal bacterial transmission among humans, mountain gorillas, and livestock in Bwindi Impenetrable National Park, Uganda. Conserv Biol 22: 1600–1607.
19. Hsieh J, Chen R, Tsai T, Pan T, Chou C (2008) Phylogenetic analysis of livestock oxacillin-resistant Staphylococcus aureus. Vet Microbiol 126: 234–242.
20. Berg S, Firdessa R, Habtamu M, Gadisa E, Mengistu A, et al. (2009) The Burden of Mycobacterial Disease in Ethiopian Cattle: Implications for Public Health. PLoS One 4: e5068–e5068.
21. Heller J, Kelly L, Reid SWJ, Mellor DJ (2010) Qualitative Risk Assessment of the Acquisition of Methicillin-Resistant Staphylococcus aureus in Pet Dogs. Risk Anal 30: 458–472.

22. Kottler S, Middleton JR, Perry J, Weese JS, Cohn LA (2010) Prevalence of *Staphylococcus aureus* and Methicillin-Resistant *Staphylococcus aureus* Carriage in Three Populations. J Vet Intern Med 24: 132–139.

23. Ewers C, Grobbel M, Stamm I, Kopp PA, Diehl I, et al. (2010) Emergence of human pandemic O25:H4-ST131 CTX-M-15 extended-spectrum-beta-lactamase-producing *Escherichia coli* among companion animals. J Antimicrob Chemother 65: 651–660.

24. Every AL, Selwood L, Castano-Rodriguez N, Lu W, Windsor HM, et al. (2011) Did transmission of *Helicobacter pylori* from humans cause a disease outbreak in a colony of Stripe-faced Dunnarts (*Sminthopsis macroura*)? Vet Res 42: 26.

25. Lin Y, Barker E, Kislow J, Kaldhone P, Stemper ME, et al. (2011) Evidence of multiple virulence subtypes in nosocomial and community-associated MRSA genotypes in companion animals from the upper midwestern and northeastern United States. Clin Med Res 9: 7–16.

26. Rubin JEJ, Chirino-Trejo MM (2011) Antimicrobial susceptibility of canine and human *Staphylococcus aureus* collected in Saskatoon, Canada. Zoonoses Public Health 58: 454–462.

27. Price LB, Stegger M, Hasman H, Aziz M, Larsen J, et al. (2012) *Staphylococcus aureus* CC398: host adaptation and emergence of methicillin resistance in livestock. MBio 3.

28. Meng X, Halbur PG, Shapiro MS, Sugantha G, Bruna JD, et al. (1998) Genetic and experimental evidence for cross-species infection by swine hepatitis E virus. J Virol 72: 9714–9721.

29. Willy ME, Woodward RA, Thornton VB, Wolff AV, Flynn BM, et al. (1999) Management of a measles outbreak among Old World nonhuman primates. Lab Anim Sci 49: 42–48.

30. Kaur T, Singh J, Tong SX, Humphrey C, Clevenger D, et al. (2008) Descriptive epidemiology of fatal respiratory outbreaks and detection of a human-related metapneumovirus in wild chimpanzees (*Pan troglodytes*) at Mahale Mountains National Park, western Tanzania. Am J Primatol 70: 755–765.

31. Feagins AR, Opriessnig T, Huang YW, Halbur PG, Meng XJ (2008) Cross-species infection of specific-pathogen-free pigs by a genotype 4 strain of human hepatitis E virus. J Med Virol 80: 1379–1386.

32. Song M, Lee J, Pascua PNQ, Baek Y, Kwon H, et al. (2010) Evidence of human-to-swine transmission of the pandemic (H1N1) 2009 influenza virus in South Korea. J Clin Microbiol 48: 3204–3211.

33. Swenson SL, Koster LG, Jenkins-Moore M, Killian ML, DeBess EE, et al. (2010) Natural cases of 2009 pandemic H1N1 Influenza A virus in pet ferrets. J Vet Diagn Invest 22: 784–788.

34. Tischer BK, Osterrieder N (2010) Herpesviruses–a zoonotic threat? Vet Microbiol 140: 266–270.

35. Abe N, Yamasaki A, Ito N, Mizoguchi T, Asano M, et al. (2010) Molecular characterization of rotaviruses in a Japanese raccoon dog (*Nyctereutes procyonoides*) and a masked palm civet (*Paguma larvata*) in Japan. Vet Microbiol 146: 253–259.

36. Berhane Y, Ojkic D, Neufeld J, Leith M, Hisanaga T, et al. (2010) Molecular characterization of pandemic H1N1 influenza viruses isolated from turkeys and pathogenicity of a human pH1N1 isolate in turkeys. Avian Dis 54: 1275–1285.

37. Poon LL, Mak PW, Li OT, Chan KH, Cheung CL, et al. (2010) Rapid detection of reassortment of pandemic H1N1/2009 influenza virus. Clin Chem 56: 1340–1344.

38. Forgie SE, Keenliside J, Wilkinson C, Webby R, Lu P, et al. (2011) Swine outbreak of pandemic influenza A virus on a Canadian research farm supports human-to-swine transmission. Clin Infect Dis 52: 10–18.

39. Holyoake PK, Kirkland PD, Davis RJ, Arzey KE, Watson J, et al. (2011) The first identified case of pandemic H1N1 influenza in pigs in Australia. Aust Vet J 89: 427–431.

40. Scotch M, Brownstein JS, Vegso S, Galusha D, Rabinowitz P (2011) Human vs. animal outbreaks of the 2009 swine-origin H1N1 influenza A epidemic. Ecohealth 8: 376–380.

41. Trevennec K, Leger L, Lyazrhi F, Baudon E, Cheung CY, et al. (2011) Transmission of pandemic influenza H1N1 (2009) in Vietnamese swine in 2009–2010. Influenza Other Respi Viruses.

42. Wevers D, Metzger S, Babweteera F, Bieberbach M, Boesch C, et al. (2011) Novel adenoviruses in wild primates: a high level of genetic diversity and evidence of zoonotic transmissions. J Virol 85: 10774–10784.

43. Crossley B, Hietala S, Hunt T, Benjamin G, Martinez M, et al. (2012) Pandemic (H1N1) 2009 in captive cheetah. Emerg Infect Dis 18: 315–317.

44. Sleeman JM, Meader LL, Mudakikwa AB, Foster JW, Patton S (2000) Gastrointestinal parasites of mountain gorillas (*Gorilla gorilla beringei*) in the Parc National des Volcans, Rwanda. J Zoo Wildl Med 31: 322–328.

45. Graczyk TK, DaSilva AJ, Cranfield MR, Nizeyi JB, Kalema G, et al. (2001) *Cryptosporidium parvum* Genotype 2 infections in free-ranging mountain gorillas (*Gorilla gorilla beringei*) of the Bwindi Impenetrable National Park, Uganda. Parasitol Res 87: 368–370.

46. Graczyk TK, Bosco-Nizeyi J, da Silva AJ, Moura IN, Pieniazek NJ, et al. (2002) A single genotype of *Encephalitozoon intestinalis* infects free-ranging gorillas and people sharing their habitats in Uganda. Parasitol Res 88: 926–931.

47. Graczyk TK, Bosco-Nizeyi J, Ssebide B, Thompson RCA, Read C, et al. (2002) Anthropozoonotic *Giardia duodenalis* genotype (assemblage) a infections in habitats of free-ranging human-habituated gorillas, Uganda. J Parasitol 88: 905–909.

48. Guk S, Yong T, Park S, Park J, Chai J (2004) Genotype and animal infectivity of a human isolate of *Cryptosporidium parvum* in the Republic of Korea. Korean J Parasitol 42: 85–89.

49. Noel C, Dufernez F, Gerbod D, Edgcomb VP, Delgado-Viscogliosi P, et al. (2005) Molecular phylogenies of Blastocystis isolates from different hosts: implications for genetic diversity, identification of species, and zoonosis. J Clin Microbiol 43: 348–355.

50. Coklin T, Farber J, Parrington L, Dixon B (2007) Prevalence and molecular characterization of *Giardia duodenalis* and *Cryptosporidium* spp. in dairy cattle in Ontario, Canada. Vet Parasitol 150: 297–305.

51. Adejinmi OJ, Ayinmode AB (2008) Preliminary investigation of zooanthroponosis in a Nigerian Zoological Garden. Vet Res (Pakistan) 2: 38–41.

52. Teichroeb JA, Kutz SJ, Parkar U, Thompson RCA, Sicotte P (2009) Ecology of the Gastrointestinal Parasites of *Colobus vellerosus* at Boabeng-Fiema, Ghana: Possible Anthropozoonotic Transmission. Am J Phys Anthropol 140: 498–507.

53. Ash A, Lymbery A, Lemon J, Vitali S, Thompson RCA (2010) Molecular epidemiology of *Giardia duodenalis* in an endangered carnivore - The African painted dog. Vet Parasitol 174: 206–212.

54. Johnston AR, Gillespie TR, Rwego IB, McLachlan TL, Kent AD, et al. (2010) Molecular epidemiology of cross-species *Giardia duodenalis* transmission in western Uganda. PLoS Negl Trop Dis 4: e683.

55. Dixon B, Parrington L, Cook A, Pintar K, Pollari F, et al. (2011) The potential for zoonotic transmission of *Giardia duodenalis* and *Cryptosporidium* spp. from beef and dairy cattle in Ontario, Canada. Vet Parasitol 175: 20–26.

56. Jacobs PHP (1988) Dermatophytes that infect animals and humans. Cutis; cutaneous medicine for the practitioner 42: 330–331.

57. Pal M, Matsusaka N, Chauhan P (1997) Zooanthroponotic significance of *Trichophyton rubrum* in a rhesus monkey (*Macaca mulatta*). Verh. ber. Erkrg. Zootiere 38: 355–358.

58. Wrobel L, Whittington JK, Pujol C, Oh S-H, Ruiz MO, et al. (2008) Molecular Phylogenetic Analysis of a Geographically and Temporally Matched Set of *Candida albicans* Isolates from Humans and Nonmigratory Wildlife in Central Illinois. Eukaryot Cell 7: 1475–1486.

59. Sharma DK, Gurudutt J, Singathia R, Lakhotia RL (2009) Zooanthroponosis of *Microsporum gypseum* infection. Haryana Veterinarian 48: 108–109.

60. Epstein JH, Price JT (2009) The significant but understudied impact of pathogen transmission from humans to animals. Mt Sinai J Med 76: 448–455.

61. Guyader Fl, Haugarreau L, Miossec L, Dubois E, Pommepuy M (2000) Three-year study to assess human enteric viruses in shellfish. Appl Environ Microbiol 66: 3241–3248.

62. Muehlenbein MP, Martinez LA, Lemke AA, Ambu L, Nathan S, et al. (2010) Unhealthy travelers present challenges to sustainable primate ecotourism. Travel Med Infect Dis 8: 169–175.

63. DeHart RL (2003) Health issues of air travel. Annu Rev Public Health 24: 133–151.

64. Daszak P, Cunningham AA, Hyatt AD (2000) Emerging infectious diseases of wildlife–threats to biodiversity and human health. Science 287: 443–449.

65. Chaber A-L, Allebone-Webb S, Lignereux Y, Cunningham AA, Marcus Rowcliffe J (2010) The scale of illegal meat importation from Africa to Europe via Paris. Conservation Letters 3: 317–321.

66. Fournie G, Pfeiffer DU (2013) Monitoring and controlling disease spread through live animal market networks. Vet J 195: 8–9.

67. American Pet Products Association Pet Industry Market Size & Ownership Statistics.

68. Leighton FA (2004) Veterinary medicine and the lifeboat test: a perspective on the social relevance of the veterinary profession in the 21st century. Can Vet J 45: 259–263.

69. World Association of Zoos and Aquariums (2013) Zoos and Aquariums of the World.

# 7

# Spatial and Temporal Pattern of Rift Valley Fever Outbreaks in Tanzania; 1930 to 2007

Calvin Sindato[1,2,3]*, Esron D. Karimuribo[2,3], Dirk U. Pfeiffer[4], Leonard E. G. Mboera[5], Fredrick Kivaria[6], George Dautu[7], Bett Bernard[8], Janusz T. Paweska[9,10]

1 National Institute for Medical Research, Tabora, Tanzania, 2 Department of Veterinary Medicine and Public Health, Sokoine University of Agriculture, Morogoro, Tanzania, 3 Southern Africa Centre for Infectious Disease Surveillance, Morogoro, Tanzania, 4 Royal Veterinary College, London, United Kingdom, 5 National Institute for Medical Research, Dar es Salaam, Tanzania, 6 Food and Agriculture Organization of the United Nations, Dar es Salaam, Tanzania, 7 Department of Disease Control, University of Zambia, Lusaka, Zambia, 8 International Livestock Research Institute, Nairobi, Kenya, 9 Center for Emerging and Zoonotic Diseases, National Institute for Communicable Diseases, of the National Health Laboratory Service, Sandringham, South Africa, 10 School of Pathology, Faculty of Health Sciences, University of the Witwatersrand, Johannesburg, South Africa

## Abstract

***Background:*** Rift Valley fever (RVF)-like disease was first reported in Tanzania more than eight decades ago and the last large outbreak of the disease occurred in 2006–07. This study investigates the spatial and temporal pattern of RVF outbreaks in Tanzania over the past 80 years in order to guide prevention and control strategies.

***Materials and Methods:*** A retrospective study was carried out based on disease reporting data from Tanzania at district or village level. The data were sourced from the Ministries responsible for livestock and human health, Tanzania Meteorological Agency and research institutions involved in RVF surveillance and diagnosis. The spatial distribution of outbreaks was mapped using ArcGIS 10. The space-time permutation model was applied to identify clusters of cases, and a multivariable logistic regression model was used to identify risk factors associated with the occurrence of outbreaks in the district.

***Principal Findings:*** RVF outbreaks were reported between December and June in 1930, 1947, 1957, 1960, 1963, 1968, 1977–79, 1989, 1997–98 and 2006–07 in 39.2% of the districts in Tanzania. There was statistically significant spatio-temporal clustering of outbreaks. RVF occurrence was associated with the eastern Rift Valley ecosystem (OR = 6.14, CI: 1.96, 19.28), total amount of rainfall of >405.4 mm (OR = 12.36, CI: 3.06, 49.88), soil texture (clay [OR = 8.76, CI: 2.52, 30.50], and loam [OR = 8.79, CI: 2.04, 37.82]).

***Conclusion/Significance:*** RVF outbreaks were found to be distributed heterogeneously and transmission dynamics appeared to vary between areas. The sequence of outbreak waves, continuously cover more parts of the country. Whenever infection has been introduced into an area, it is likely to be involved in future outbreaks. The cases were more likely to be reported from the eastern Rift Valley than from the western Rift Valley ecosystem and from areas with clay and loam rather than sandy soil texture.

**Editor:** Tetsuro Ikegami, The University of Texas Medical Branch, United States of America

**Funding:** This study received financial support from the Wellcome Trust Grant [WT087546MA] to the Southern African Centre for Infectious Disease Surveillance (www.sacids.org). The funder had no role in study design, data collection and analysis, decision to publish, or preparation of the manuscript.

**Competing Interests:** The authors have declared that no competing interests exist.

* E-mail: kndato@yahoo.co.uk

## Introduction

Rift Valley fever (RVF) is an arthropod-borne viral zoonotic disease caused by RVF virus (RVFV) belonging to the genus *Phlebovirus* of family *Bunyaviridae* [1,2]. The disease is endemic in sub-Saharan Africa [3–5], but it has been reported outside this region [6–8] and it is considered to have potential for global spread [9–11]. The disease affects primarily domestic ruminants and humans [12]. The capacity of RVFV to cause large and severe outbreaks in animal and human populations and to cross significant natural geographic barriers, as exemplified by the virus spread over the Indian Ocean, Sahara desert, and the Red Sea in the past 3 decades, is of great concern for veterinary and public health authorities worldwide. RVFV is one of the most important emerging zoonotic threats, particularly to vulnerable African communities with low resilience to economic and environmental challenges [11–15].

There are significant differences in the ecology and transmission patterns of RVFV in endemic regions. In eastern and southern Africa large outbreaks of RVF occur at irregular intervals of up to 15 years, after heavy rainfall and floods [13–15]. After flooding of aedine mosquitoes breeding habitats (dambos), they are succeeded by *Culex* spp., which if infected upon feeding on viraemic vertebrate hosts further disperse the virus.

Recent molecular epidemiology studies indicate ongoing RVFV activity and evolution during the inter-epidemic period (IEP) in endemic areas and highlight the importance of a cryptic enzootic transmission cycle that allows for the establishment of RVFV endemicity and to precipitate explosive outbreaks [16,17]. The RVFV transmission during IEP without noticeable outbreak or clinical cases has been reported in different species of African wildlife [18–20], in cattle in Mayotte [21], in sheep and goats in Mozambique [22], in humans in Tanzania [23], Kenya [15], and Gabon [24]. It has been postulated that during IEP, the virus persists in eggs of floodwater *Aedes* mosquito species or via low-level transmission between mosquitoes and vertebrates [12].

Host susceptibility depends on age and animal species. Young lambs, calves and kids are highly susceptible to infection with RVFV. In young lambs, the common signs include sudden rise of body temperature to 40.5–42.2°C, followed by death within 36 hours. Clinical signs in adult sheep and goats are not consistent but may include rise in body temperature, vomiting, mucopurulent nasal discharge, unsteady gait and high abortion rate up to 100% amongst pregnant ewes as well as haemorrhages manifestations. Clinical signs in adult cattle include high temperature, salivation, anorexia, general weakness, fetid diarrhoea, a rapid decrease in lactation and abortion. Abortion may be the only marked sign in cattle and mortality in adult cattle is usually less than 10% (25). The majority of infections in humans are unapparent or associated with moderate to severe, non-fatal, flu-like febrile illness with headache, nausea, myalgia and arthralgia [12]. Less than one percent of human patients develop the haemorrhagic and/or encephalitic forms of the disease. The overall case fatality ratio is estimated to range from 0.5% to 2%, but it appears to be higher in recent outbreaks of the disease in East Africa and South Africa [26–28]. In a minority of patients the disease is complicated by the development of ocular lesions [12].

Diagnosis of RVF is commonly carried out using enzyme linked immunosorbent assay (ELISA) methods that detects type-specific anti-RVFV immunoglobulins [29–33] and polymerase chain reaction (PCR) that detects RVFV nucleic acid [12] in blood. There is no specific treatment for RVFV infection in humans and animals and therefore management of clinical cases is only through supportive therapy [34].

Unpublished records available at the Ministry of Livestock and Fisheries Development (MoLFD) in Tanzania indicate that RVF-like disease in domestic ruminants occurred for the first time in 1930. RVF was added to the list of notifiable diseases under the Tanzanian Animal Disease Act in 1980 [35] and to the Integrated Disease Surveillance and Response (IDSR) Guidelines of the Tanzania Ministry of Health and Social Welfare in June 2011 [36]. RVF outbreaks have severe socio-economic impacts in Tanzania [37,38]. For instance the last disease outbreak in 2006–07 had major adverse effects on rural household livelihoods, food security and nutrition [37]. In addition to pastoralists, the disease threatened the livelihoods of those who depend on livestock products and related activities for labour opportunities [37]. Past disease outbreaks in the country led to cessation of trade in ruminants. This resulted in serious economic losses for the sections of the population which were dependent on this source of income. Animals dropped in monetary value by 34%; the monthly internal market flow of livestock reduced by 37% and the annual external market flow by 54%. Loss due to death of domestic ruminants was estimated to be more than US$ 6 million. The Government spent about US$ 4 million for the control of the disease in 2006/2007 [37].

Despite the long presence of RVF in Tanzania, its spatial and temporal pattern has not been analysed. The objective of this study is to describe RVF outbreaks that have occurred in Tanzania between 1930 and 2007 and investigate the potential presence of clustering of cases during past outbreaks. We also aimed at investigating the association of the various environmental risk factors with the occurrence of reported outbreaks at district level during the last outbreak wave in 2006/2007.

## Materials and Methods

### Ethics Statement

This study was approved by the Tanzania Medical Research Coordinating Committee of the National Institute for Medical Research (NIMR/HQ/R.8a/Vol.IX/1296).

### Description of the Study Area

The United Republic of Tanzania, made up of Tanzania Mainland and Zanzibar, is located between longitude 29° and 41° East and latitude 1° and 12° South. The country experiences two major rainy seasons, namely a long rainy season during the months of March through to May and a short rainy season during the months of October through to January. The total annual rainfall ranges from 750–1400 mm. The dry season is mainly from July to September. A large central plateau makes up most of the mainland, at between 900 m and 1800 m above sea level.

Pastoralism is mainly concentrated in the northern zone (Arusha and Manyara regions) and agro-pastoralism in the western zone (Tabora region), Lake Victoria zone (Shinyanga and Mwanza regions) and central zones (Dodoma and Singida regions) [39,40]. The plateaus of the northern and lake zones are comprised of relatively higher livestock density; cattle ≥50, goats ≥45 and sheep≥14 heads per square kilometre (Figure 1). Spatial data for the past outbreaks was available at district and village resolutions. For administrative purposes each region in Tanzania is subdivided into districts which are further sub-divided into divisions, wards and villages. Districts are the smallest administrative units responsible for human and livestock disease management. To allow an analysis across the whole period, outbreaks were geo-referenced according to the administrative arrangement consisting of 21 regions, 120 administrative districts and 9504 villages during the latest disease outbreak in 2006/2007 [41].

RVF is associated with the Great Rift Valley system which is a long depression in the earth that runs down the eastern side of Africa. It extends from Syria in the Middle East, right down to Mozambique in south-eastern Africa. The well-expressed Eastern branch (flunk) traverses Ethiopia (Main Ethiopian Rift), Kenya (Kenya or Gregory Rift) and reaches north Tanzania, where it forms the north Tanzania divergence (Figure 1). Tanzania is the only country with two branches of this system forming the eastern and western ecosystems with one flunk branching at the south-western tip of Tanzania and running through the western, periphery of both Tanzania and Uganda. This is the one in which Lakes Tanganyika and Nyasa are found. The eastern branch runs through the centre of both Kenya and Tanzania dividing each country into two halves forming important internal drainage ecosystem basins [42]. The eastern branch finally rejoins the western branch in Mbeya region fading progressively towards Lake Nyasa (Figure 1).

### Case, Outbreak and Outbreak Wave Definition

**RVF case definition in domestic ruminants.** A RVF case was suspected in domestic ruminants whenever there was a report within herd/village/district of high mortality in neonatal animals and abortion and/or stillbirths in pregnant animals. Other clinical features that were considered included reports of mucopurulent nasal discharge, bloody diarrhoea and vomiting in domestic ruminants. A probable case was considered to be a suspected case if it occurred during periods with above normal rainfall and involved widespread abortion and high mortality in neonatal

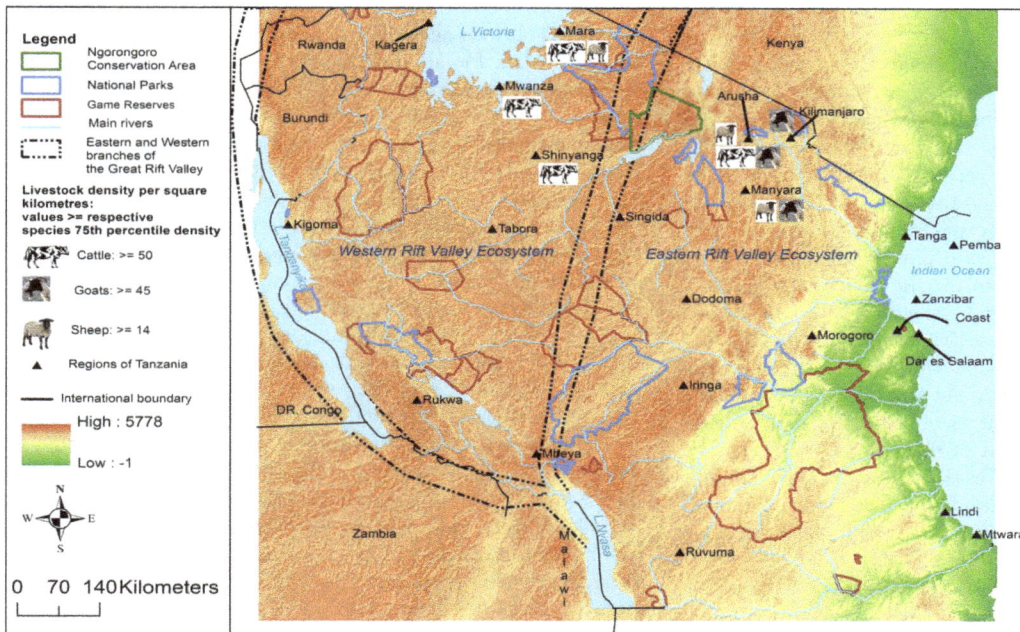

**Figure 1. Digital elevation map of Tanzania and main features.** Map of Tanzania showing the elevation (metres above sea level), Eastern and Western Great Rift Valley ecosystems (dashed-dot lines), main regions, main rivers, National Parks, Game Reserves, Ngorongoro Conservation Area, international borders and neighbouring countries. Rift Valley fever occurrence is associated with the Great Rift Valley. The animal symbols on the map indicate the areas where the density is equal to and above the threshold mentioned in the legend. Livestock density is higher in the plateau of the northern and lake zones of the country.

domestic ruminants. In addition, the presence of haemorrhages in the internal organs of affected animals would have been reported on post-mortem.

A confirmed case was any case with laboratory confirmation of RVF by detection of specific immunoglobulin G (IgG) and/or immunoglobulin M (IgM) antibodies by ELISA. Reports on other specific tests for confirmation of RVF cases in domestic ruminants in the country were not available. In this study, both probable and confirmed cases of RVF in domestic ruminants were used collectively in the data analysis.

**RVF case definition in humans.** A confirmed case was any suspected or probable case with laboratory confirmation of RVF by detection of specific IgM antibodies by ELISA or detection of viral RNA by real-time reverse transcriptase PCR or detection of viral antigens in biopsy tissues by immunohistochemistry. No probable or suspected human cases of RVF, which fulfil clinical criteria without laboratory confirmation being done, have been identified in our data.

**Outbreak definition.** In this study, RVF outbreak was defined as occurrence in a specific location of multiple related cases likely to be caused by RVFV (both confirmed and probable cases characterized in the case definition) affecting domestic ruminants and/or humans.

**Outbreak wave definition.** A RVF outbreak wave referred to sequential reports of the outbreaks at various locations within Tanzania from date of onset of the first outbreak during a particular time period of the year until outbreaks were no longer reported in the country.

## Sources of Data

For the years 2000 to 2012, information on RVF outbreaks was gathered from the databases at MoLFD, Zonal Veterinary Investigation Centres (VICs), Ministry of Health and Social Welfare (MoHSW) and National Institute for Medical Research (NIMR) in Tanzania. Comparable records for the years 1930 to 2012 were collated from the files archived at MoLFD, zonal VICs, MoHSW and NIMR that included case report forms, laboratory registers/investigation forms, field surveillance forms, monthly and annual reports, and Food and Agriculture Organization reports. The small number of available published articles and reports describing the epidemiology and trend of RVF outbreaks in Tanzania were also used as a data source [35]. In addition, expert opinions on the historical occurrence of RVF outbreaks were obtained from NIMR, MoHSW and MoLFD. Historical weather data (monthly rainfall and mean minimum and maximum temperatures) for the years 1977 to 2008 were obtained from the Tanzania Meteorological Agency (TMA). The weather data were aggregated by seasons adapted from the TMA; 1 = October-December, 2 = January-February, 3 = March-May and 4 = June-September. The district and village-specific geo-coordinates were obtained from the local digital maps developed by the Institute of Resource Assessment, of the University of Dar es Salaam, Tanzania. Data on soil types and texture were obtained from the Mlingano Agricultural Research Institute in Tanga, Tanzania and were classified by their physical and chemical properties using the Food and Agriculture Organization (FAO) scheme [43].

## Data Preparation and Analysis

The month, year and geographical location of the districts and villages that reported RVF outbreaks between January 1930 and June 2007 were entered into a Microsoft Excel spreadsheet. Since data were obtained from various sources, location names were standardized before data were sorted and checked for consistency and duplication. The district and village-specific geo-coordinates were used to identify the locations that had similar names. Only one entry was retained for those villages with multiple entries for a particular month.

The data analysis focused on a spatial and temporal description of outbreaks at district/village and year/month resolution, respectively. Shapiro-Wilk and Shapiro-Francia tests were used to assess normality of continuous variables. Summary statistics were reported by using STATA version 12 (Statacorp, College Station, TX, USA). The study period was divided into two periods to identify potential changes in the reporting of the disease over time and space. Period one referred to time period prior to 1980 when RVF was not yet added into the list of notifiable diseases under the Ministry responsible for livestock in Tanzania. Period two referred to the time period from 1980 onwards after RVF had been added into the list of notifiable diseases. The dataset was stratified annually in order to carry out separate analysis of each year and explore the temporal patterns of outbreak waves. Disease frequency was expressed as counts of disease cases per outbreak wave and cumulative number of cases between period one and period two. Outbreak curves were plotted in relation to rainfall and temperature to identify the monthly temporal pattern of cases throughout the study period.

**Spatio-temporal cluster analysis of RVF cases.** In order to identify high risk districts and villages, the location of most likely spatio-temporal clusters was investigated using the space-time permutation model [44]. In the current study we used presence-only data as no investigational surveys that could provide absence data had been conducted. The space-time permutation model only requires case data (presence-only data) for which the spatial location and time is known, but no information is needed about controls or a background population at risk [44]. The model parameters for maximum spatial and temporal window sizes were set such that a cluster could include a maximum of 50% of all cases. The number of Monte Carlo replications was set to 9999, so that the minimum detectable p-value would be 0.0001. This analysis was implemented using the SatScan 9.1 software (Information Management Services, Inc, Boston, MA, USA).

The distribution of areas that reported cases and buffering of the clusters (in kilometres) were mapped using ArcGIS 10 (ESRI East Africa). For the purpose of this study the districts that had reported RVF cases were assigned specific identification numbers before projecting them onto the map as follows: 1, Babati; 2, Dodoma; 3, Bariadi; 4, Bunda; 5, Hai; 6, Hanang; 7, Handeni; 8, Igunga; 9, Iringa-Urban; 10, Iringa-Rural; 11, Kahama; 12, Karatu; 13, Kibaha; 14, Kilindi; 15, Kilombero; 16, Kilosa; 17, Kiteto; 18, Kondoa; 19, Kongwa; 20, Korogwe; 21, Kwimba; 22, Lushoto; 23, Magu; 24, Manyoni; 25, Maswa; 26, Mbulu; 27, Meatu; 28, Monduli; 29, Moshi Rural, 30, Mpwapwa; 31, Mufindi; 32, Muheza; 3, Ngorongoro; 34, Njombe; 35, Nzega; 36, Pangani; 37, Rombo; 38, Same; 39, Serengeti; 40, Simanjiro; 41, Singida Rural; 42, Iramba; 43, Tanga Rural; 44, Ulanga; 45, Urambo; Morogoro Urban; 46 and Mvomero; 47.

**Multivariable analysis.** Logistic regression was used to analyse the association between various risk factors and the risk of outbreak occurrence at the district level. From descriptive data analysis of this study it was found that there was major temporal heterogeneity with respect to reporting of RVF in Tanzania. It was concluded that the latest outbreak wave in 2006/07 was likely to have the lowest reporting bias, and it was therefore used in the multivariable analysis. The outcome variable of interest was whether at least one outbreak involving domestic ruminants had been reported within each district during the 2006/07 outbreak wave. The risk factors included in this analysis have been suggested to be associated with occurrence of RVF [28,45–50].

Data for 106 districts (88.33% of all districts) were used in this analysis. Fourteen (all urban) districts were excluded as they did not have data for all risk factors. To take account of possible nonlinear effects of continuous-scale risk factors on the logit form of the outcome variable, these variables were grouped into three contiguous categories, each representing a third of the observations. The analysis was conducted in two steps. First, all potential risk factors were screened for statistical significance at a p-value of $\leq 0.20$ in a univariable logistic regression analysis. In the second step, these statistically significant variables were included in a multivariable logistic regression analysis based on a forward variable selection approach utilising the likelihood ratio statistic and a p-value $\leq 0.05$. Variables not statistically significant in the univariable analysis, but with known association with RVFV activity were also included in the multivariable analysis. The variables included in the model were limited to those that did not show significant collinearity using a diagnostic cut-off value for tolerance $>0.1$ and variance inflation factor $<10$. The Mantel-Haenszel method was used to identify the effect of confounding factors. A factor was considered to have potential confounding effect if its magnitude of change was $\geq 25\%$ in the coefficient estimates of other predictors. The Hosmer and Lemeshow test was used to assess the goodness of fit of the final model [51]. The discrimination ability of the final model was assessed using receiver operating characteristic curves (ROC), based on area under the curve (AUC) [52].

## Results

### Exploratory Data Analysis

From 1930 when RVF-like disease was reported for the first time in Tanzania, further outbreaks were reported in 1947, 1957, 1960, 1963, 1968, 1977/1978, 1989, 1997/1998 and 2006/2007. During this time interval a total of 10 outbreak waves (one outbreak wave in a year) of varying size and location were reported with average inter-epidemic period (IEP) of 7.9 years (range = 3–17 years). During these past outbreaks a total of 194,750 domestic ruminant cases (cattle = 54.01%; goats = 22.78% and sheep = 23.21%) were reported. A total of 309 human cases were reported during the latest outbreak in 2006/2007 and there was no documentation on cases in humans prior to 2006.

Of the 194,750 domestic ruminant cases, 140,377 (72.08%) had information about month and district of occurrence and, 55,415 (28.45%, n = 194,750) had information about month and village of occurrence been recorded. A total of 5,197 domestic ruminant cases had information on only the year and district of occurrence. A total of 63 domestic ruminant cases had information on only the year and region of occurrence. A total of 49,113 (25.22%, n = 194,750) domestic ruminant cases had information on the year without location of occurrence been recorded. All 309 human cases reported had information about month and district and 292 (94.50%) of these had information about month and village of occurrence. Of the 198 villages that were included in this study we were unable to identify the geographical coordinates for two and 16 of those that reported cases in domestic ruminants and humans, respectively. In these instances, the results were summarized at district and village and, year and month resolutions.

Out of 145,637 domestic ruminant cases that had the information on the location and time of occurrence been recorded, 14,990 (10.29%) and 130,637 (89.71%) were reported in period one and two respectively with significantly higher proportion of cases (73.11%) been reported in the eastern Rift Valley ecosystem (p = 0.03). About half (53.93%) of domestic ruminant cases were confirmed in the laboratory and 46.07% were the probable cases. All 309 humans cases were confirmed in the laboratory and nearly all (99.35%) were reported in the eastern Rift Valley ecosystem. Out of 120 districts of the Tanzania mainland, 47 (39.17%) had reported at least an outbreak involving livestock and/or humans during the study period.

The spatial distribution of the RVF cases in Tanzania varied throughout the study period. During period one (from 1930 to 1979), the cases were persistently reported in four districts in northern Tanzania. In contrast, during period two (from 1980 to 2007), spatial progression of the spread of cases from north to east-central and southern parts of the country was observed (Figure 1). Over the subsequent years, there was an increase in the number of villages that reported cases from 2 villages in 1930 to 175 villages in 2006/2007 (Table 1; Figure 2). Once the disease had been introduced into the district/village, it was likely to be involved in future outbreaks.

From 1930 to 2007 there was a remarkable trend of increased number of ruminant cases that were reported with stability in the proportion of each animal species affected through the study period (Table 1). From 1930 to 1978 there was a 11-folds increase in the number of cases and from 1978 to 2007 there was a 12-folds further increase in the number of cases reported (Table 1). Generally during the past outbreaks, RVF cases were reported between December and June. For each of the outbreak waves from 1930 to 2007, the space-time permutation model identified statistically significant most likely and secondary clusters of cases.

According to Shapiro-Wilk and Shapiro-Francia tests, the continuous variables included into this study were not normally distributed, and therefore the median and ranges (instead of mean and standard deviation) of these variables are reported. Overall between 1930 and 2007 the number of cases per outbreak wave ranged from 1,026–136,570 with the median number of cases of 7,458.5 ($25^{th}$ percentile = 1.402; $75^{th}$ percentile = 40, 835; CI = 1063.6, 126996.5). During the study period the monthly number of cases ranged from 108 to 44,367 with the median number of monthly cases of 2,281 ($25^{th}$ percentile = 841; $75^{th}$ percentile = 9,814; CI = 1067.4, 6141.7). The elevation of the districts that reported RVF cases ranged from 57–1,864 m above sea level with the median elevation of 1,190 m ($25^{th}$ percentile = 943; $75^{th}$ percentile = 1,445; CI = 1122, 1115).

## The Pattern of Rainfall and RVF Outbreaks

The total annual rainfall ranged from 369.1–1,562.9 mm with the median total annual rainfall of 777.8 mm ($25^{th}$ percentile = 665.8; $75^{th}$ percentile = 914.6; CI = 691.4, 826.1). The rainfall was not significantly different between the eastern and western Rift valley ecosystems (p = 0.52). As shown in figure 3 (arrows) the onset of past outbreaks occurred following an

increased total annual rainfall compared to the previous year. The onset of the latest two outbreak waves in 2006–07 and 1997–98 occurred when the average total annual rainfall had increased by 69.97% and 51.83% respectively compared to the previous year. The onset of the 1989 and 1977–78 outbreak waves occurred when the average total annual rainfall had increased by 15.21% and 13.91% respectively compared to the previous year (Figure 3). There were other periods when the average total annual rainfall had increased by at least 22.24% compared to the previous year however, outbreaks were not reported. These year periods (together with their percentage increase in the average total annual rainfall) were; the 2003/2004 (50.77%), 2001/2002 (30.38%), 1981/1982 (28.07%), 1980/1981 (22.45%) and 1993/1994 (22.24%).

As shown in figure 4 the onset of the 1977/1978 RVF outbreak wave in December 1977 coincided with the total maximum monthly rainfall of 147.17 mm in season 1. The peak of this outbreak wave coincided with the maximum total monthly rainfall of 195.98 mm in April 1978 (season 2). The onset of the 1997/1998 outbreak wave in December 1997 coincided with the total maximum monthly rainfall of 275.55 mm in season 1. Although the peak of this outbreak wave in March 1998 (season 3) did not coincide with maximum total monthly rainfall, there was a tendency for the outbreak to cease as the rainfall faded-out in June 1998 (season 4). The onset of the 2006/2007 outbreak wave (in livestock and humans) in January 2007 (season 2) was preceded by the maximum total monthly rainfall of 201.45 mm in December 2006 (season 1). The peak of the livestock outbreak wave in April 2007 was preceded by the maximum total monthly rainfall of 122.33 mm in March 2007 (season 3) that coincided with the peak of human outbreak wave (Figure 4). The odds of clustering of cases was higher in season 2 (OR = 2.64, CI: 0.35, 19.88) than season 3 (OR = 1.97, CI: 0.27, 14.19) and season 4 (OR = 1.4, CI: 0.14, 13.57) although not at the 0.05 level of significance (p = 0.56).

## The Pattern of Average Annual/Monthly Maximum/Minimum Temperature and RVF Outbreaks

There was no clearly defined pattern of the average annual maximum and minimum temperatures and the RVF outbreaks (data not shown). As shown in figure 4, the optimal values of maximum and minimum monthly temperatures preceded the onset of outbreaks by at least one month. There was no clear pattern on the timing for optimal values of temperatures and the peaks of outbreaks. However, the outbreaks showed the tendency to cease as the maximum and minimum monthly temperatures declined (Figure 4).

**Table 1.** Number of RVF cases (%) per outbreak wave by number of villages and animal species.

| Species | Number of RVF cases (%) per outbreak wave [No. villages affected] | | | | | |
| | 1930 [2] | 1947 [2] | 1957 [2] | 1977/1978 [9] | 1997/1998 [44] | 2006/2007 [175] |
|---|---|---|---|---|---|---|
| Cattle | 546 (53.22) | 699 (49.86) | 1,174 (33.37) | 4,796 (42.00) | 21,619 (52.94) | 76,346 (55.90) |
| Goats | 200 (19.49) | 378 (26.96) | 1,007 (28.62) | 2,459 (21.57) | 8,616 (21.10) | 31,704 (23.21) |
| Sheep | 280 (27.29) | 325 (23.18) | 1,337 (38.00) | 4,144 (36.35) | 10,600 (25.96) | 28,520 (20.88) |
| Total per outbreak wave (100%) | 1,026 | 1,402 | 3,518 | 11,399 | 40,835 | 136,570 |

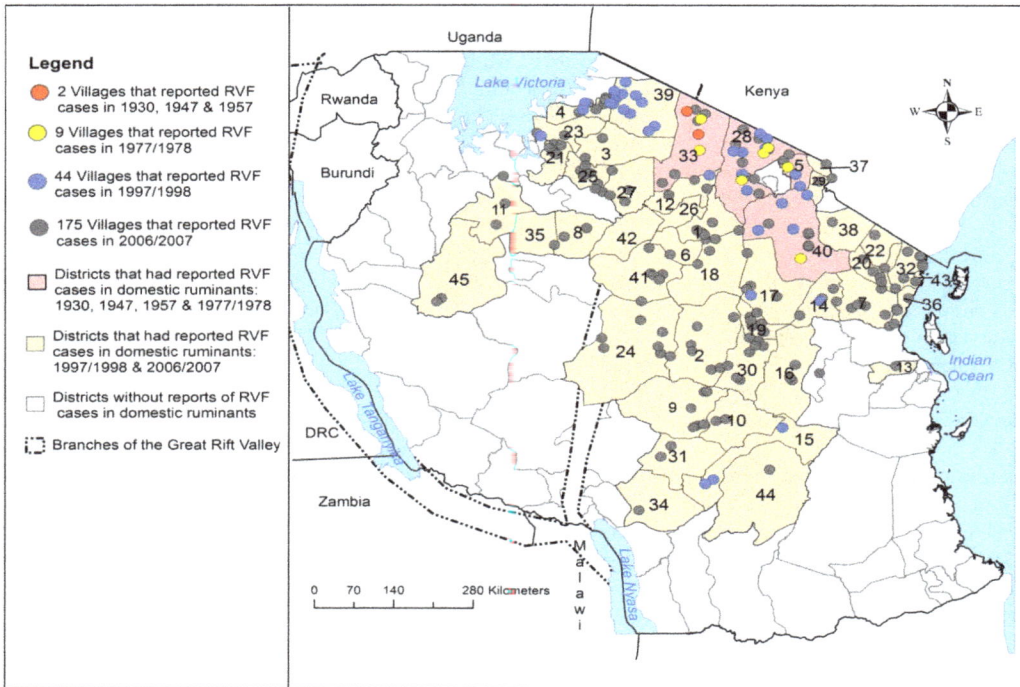

**Figure 2. The space-time progression of Rift Valley fever outbreaks by district and villages; 1930 to 2007.** Ngorongoro, Simanjiro, Monduli and Hai are the only districts in the eastern Rift Valley ecosystem that were involved in the outbreaks from 1930 to 1978. These four districts were persistently involved in subsequent outbreaks from 1997 to 2007 that had expanded progressively to east-south and western parts of the country.

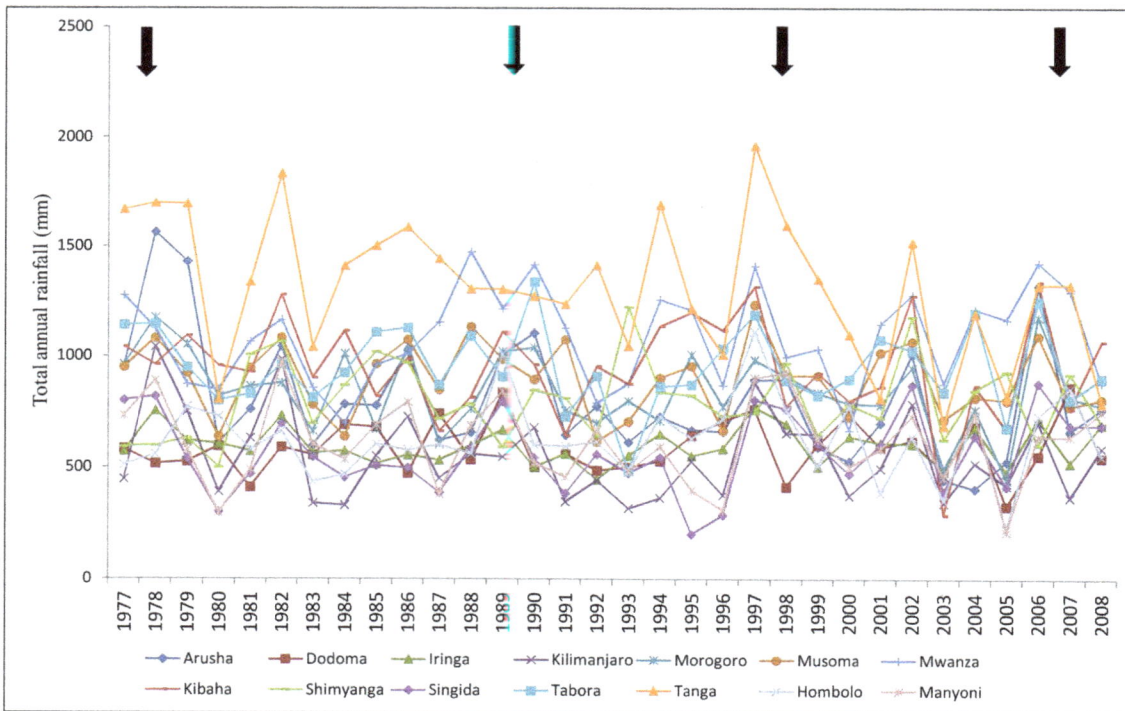

**Figure 3. Rainfall curves showing annual total rainfall in millimetres for the zones in Tanzania.** The zones represented by regions (in parenthses) are: The Northeastern zone (Arusha, Kilimanjaro, Tanga, Morogoro and Kibaha stations); Central zone (Dodoma, Hombolo, Singida and Manyoni stations); Western zone (Tabora station); Lake zone (Mwanza, Shinyanga and Musoma stations); Southern highland zone (Iringa station). The arrows indicate the years of RVF outbreak waves in Tanzania from 1977 to 2008.

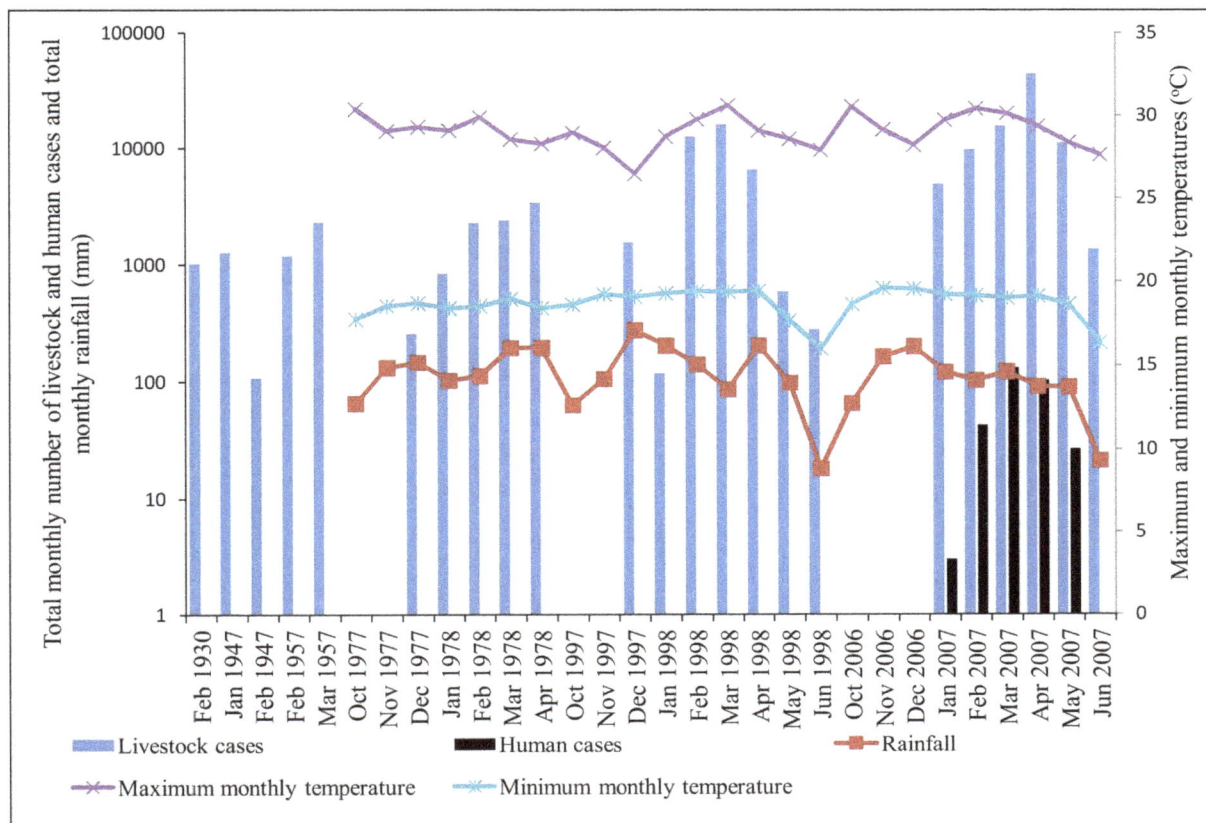

**Figure 4. Curves showing the pattern of total monthly rainfall, temperature and RVF outbreaks waves.** The onset of outbreaks in domestic ruminants [1977 to 2006/2007] and humans [2006/2007] were preceded by about two months rainful surplus. Clear pattern between the monthly tempearure and onset of outbreaks was not observed. The outbreaks had a tendency to cease as the rainfall faded-off. Left Y axis corresponds to total monthly rainfall in millimetres (mm) and total monthly number of livestock and humans cases. The right Y axis corresponds to the maximum and minimum monthly temperatures. The X axis corresponds to the months and years of RVF outbreak waves.

## Spatial and Temporal Clustering of RVF Cases

From 1930 to 2007 the clustering of RVF cases was persistently and predominantly detected in the eastern Rift Valley ecosystem of the country compared to the western ecosystem (Figure 5, 6, 7 and 8). The odds of clustering of RVF cases was higher in the eastern Rift Valley ecosystem than the western ecosystem (OR = 1.76, CI: 0.89, 3.47), although not at the 0.05 level of significance (p = 0.10). Out of 46 districts that had reported outbreaks in domestic ruminants in the past, 32 (69.57%) had reported at least one cluster of cases and 13 (28.26%) had no clustering of cases. Ngorongoro district in northern Tanzania was persistently involved in the clustering of cases throughout the study period. The spatio-temporal overlapping of the primary and secondary livestock and human clusters was observed during the study period (Figure 5, 6, 7 and 8). The space-time clustering of livestock and human cases showed a tendency to spread from the north to east-central and western parts of the country (Figure 5, 6, 7 and 8).

## District-level Clustering of Cases

The outbreak waves of 1930, 1947 and 1957 were reported in Ngorongoro district. During the 1977–788 and 1997–98 outbreak waves the district-level primary clusters were detected in Monduli in Arusha region with respective relative risk of 8.36 (in January 1978) and 3.77 (in May 1998) (Figure 5). During the 1997–98

outbreak wave a total of four secondary clusters were detected in Arusha, Kilimanjaro, Mara, and Morogoro regions (Figure 5). During the 2006–07 outbreak wave a larger livestock primary cluster (diameter of 495.66 km) was detected between January and March 2007. A total of 10 districts (including the district that was the primary cluster during the 1977–78 and 1997–98 outbreak waves) formed the primary cluster of the 2006/2007 outbreak wave (Figure 5). A relatively smaller human primary cluster (diameter of 255.72 km) was detected within the livestock primary cluster between January and February 2007 with a relative risk of 6.57 (Figure 5). During this outbreak wave one secondary human cluster with a diameter of 191.42 km and a relative risk of 4.60 was detected within the relatively bigger secondary cluster of livestock (diameter = 566.18 km; relative risk = 2.41) and both were detected in May 2007 (Figure 5).

## Village-level Clustering of Cases

Three village-level primary clusters were detected in one district in northern Tanzania during the 1930, 1947 and 1957 outbreak waves (Figure 6). Two primary clusters were detected in the same region during the 1997–98 (relative risk of 17.33) and 2006/2007 (relative risk of 2.18) outbreak waves (Figure 7). The primary cluster that was detected during 1997/1998 outbreak wave became part of the relatively larger primary cluster that was detected during 2006–07 outbreak wave (Figure 7). This figure indicate further that, two of the secondary clusters that were

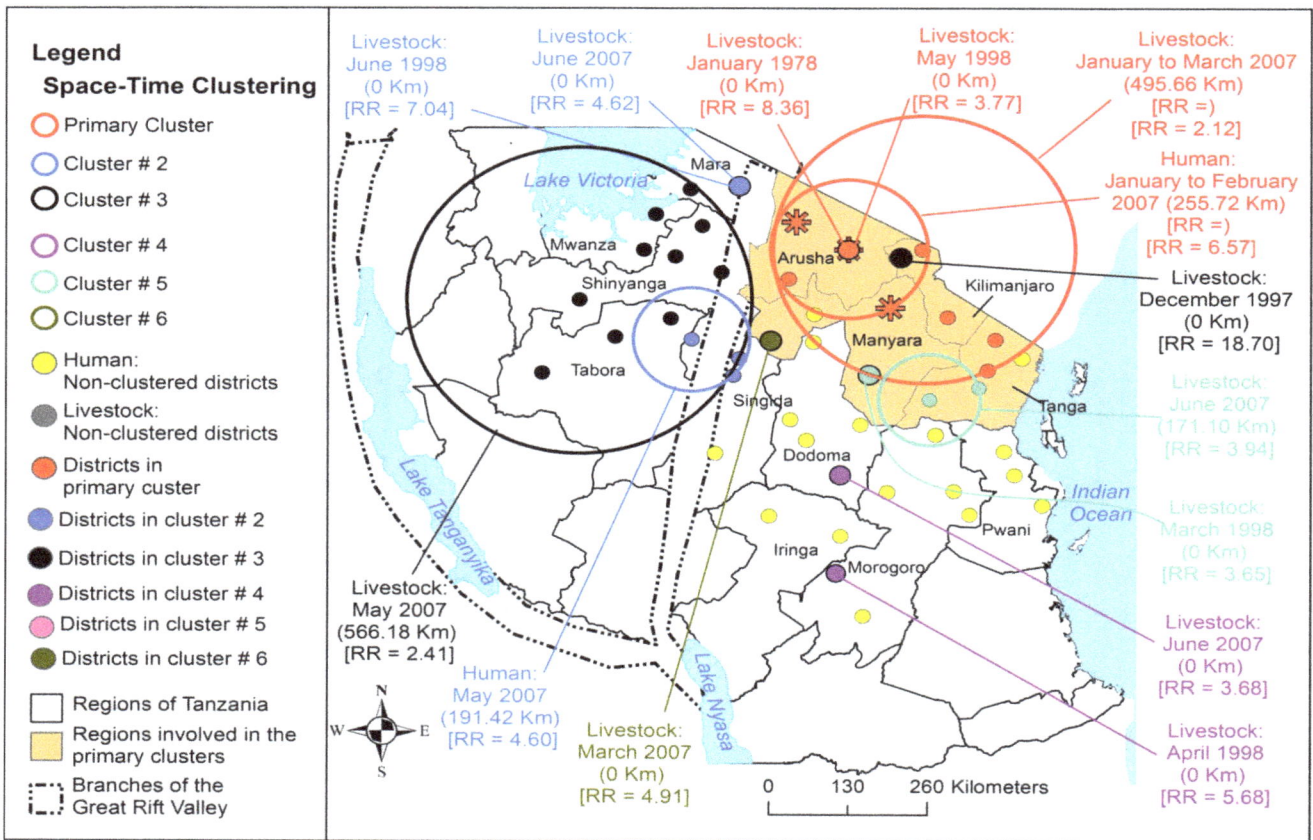

**Figure 5. Distribution of district level space-time clusters of RVF cases in domestic ruminants and humans.** The outbreak waves in 1930, 1947 and 1957 were persistently reported in one district in Arusha region. This figure indicates the persistence spatiotemporal overlapping of the livestock and human primary clusters. During the latest outbreak in 2006/2007, the primary and secondary human clusters had occurred within the respective primary and secondary livestock clusters. Asterisks correspond to districts that were included within the human primary cluster; relative risk for each cluster is displayed (RR) along with the buffer (circle) size in kilometres (km).

detected during 1997–98 outbreak wave were included in the primary cluster detected during 2006–07 outbreak wave.

## Descriptive Analysis of Specific RVF Outbreak Waves

**RVFV activity during the 1930 outbreak wave.** During this outbreak wave a total of 1,026 (0.53%, n = 194,750) domestic ruminant cases were reported in two villages in 1/120 (0.83%) districts of Tanzania Mainland. Ngorongoro was the only district that reported cases during this outbreak wave (Figure 2) in February (Figure 4). Clustering of cases was not detected during this period (Figure 5 and 6). Relatively larger proportion of cattle (53.22%) was affected followed by sheep (27.29%) and goats (19.49%) (Table 1).

**RVFV activity during the 1947 outbreak wave.** During this outbreak wave a total of 1,402 (0.72%, n = 194, 750) domestic ruminant cases were reported in two villages (the same that had reported cases during the 1930 outbreak wave) in Ngorongoro district (Figure 2) from January to February with peak in January (Figure 4). The monthly median number of cases was 688.5 (range: 108–1269; 25th percentile = 108; 75th percentile = 1,269). A primary cluster was detected in one village in Ngorongoro district in February with a relative risk of 3.82 (Figure 6). A relatively larger proportions of cattle (49.86%) was affected followed by goats (29.96%) and sheep (23.18%) [Table 1].

**RVFV activity during the 1957 outbreak wave.** During this outbreak wave a total of 3,518 (1.81%, n = 194,750) domestic ruminant cases were reported in two villages (the same that had reported cases during the 1947 outbreak wave) in Ngorongoro district (Figure 2) from February to March with peak in March (Figure 4). The monthly median number of cases was 1,740 (range: 1184–2,296; 25th percentile = 1,184; 75th percentile = 2,296). A primary cluster was detected in one village in Ngorongoro district in February with a relative risk of 3.61 (Figure 5). Relatively larger proportion of sheep (38.00%) was affected followed by cattle (33.37%) and goats (28.62%) (Table 1).

**RVFV activity during the 1960, 1963, 1968 and 1989 outbreak waves.** Limited information available in a consultancy report from a field mission of the Food and Agriculture Organization of the United Nations indicated that, RVFV had been isolated in Tanzania in 1960, 1963, 1968 and 1989. This report did not provide details on the specific outbreak wave, number of cases per month, year and districts or villages affected. It however, indicates that these outbreaks mainly affected exotic breeds of cattle and sheep where it resulted in abortion storms, mortality in young animals and drop in milk production associated with fever. The report indicate further that, RVFV was isolated from these animals in Ngorongoro, Mpwapwa, Morogoro Rural, Mufindi, Moshi Rural, Hai and Iringa Rural districts without

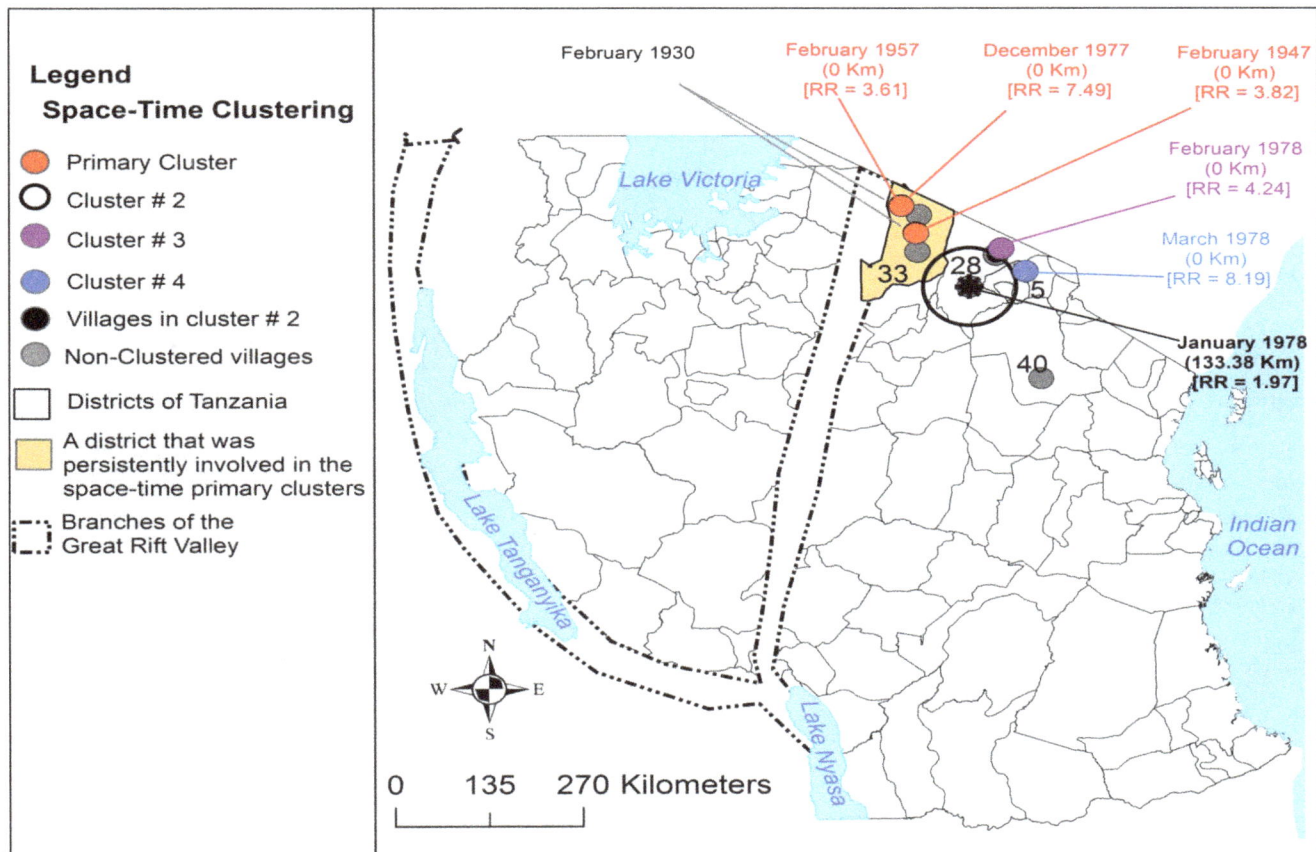

**Figure 6. Distribution of village-level space-time clusters of RVF cases from 1947 to 1978.** There were no clusters detected in 1930; from 1947 to 1978 three primary clusters were persistently detected in Ngorongoro district, each involving one village. An asterisk represents the centre of cluster that involved more than one village; relative risk for each cluster is displayed (RR) along with the buffer (circle) size in kilometres (km).

details of number of isolates. These outbreaks are reported in our study but were not included in the analysis.

**RVFV activity during the 1977/1978 outbreak wave.** Exploration of available data for 1977/1978 indicated that the outbreak had spread to include nine villages (number of villages in parentheses) in 4/120 (3.33%) districts; Ngorongoro (4), Monduli (3), Simanjiro (1) districts and Hai district (1) (Figure 2). In 1977 cases were reported in December and in 1978 cases were reported from January to March with the peak in January (Figure 4). During this outbreak wave a total of 11,399 (5.85%, n = 194,750) domestic ruminant cases were reported (Table 1). The monthly median number of cases was 2,281 (range: 257–3,413; 25th percentile = 841; 75th percentile = 2,389). The two villages that had previously reported cases were also involved in this outbreak. The district-level most likely cluster was detected in Monduli in January 1978 with a relative risk of 8.36 (Figure 5). The village-level most likely cluster was detected in one village in Ngorongoro district in December 1977 with a relative risk of 7.49 (Figure 6). Three statistically significant village-level secondary clusters were detected during this outbreak wave (Figure 6). Relatively larger proportion of cattle (42.00%) was affected followed by sheep (36.35%) and goats (21.57%) (Table 1).

**RVFV activity during the 1997/1998 outbreak wave.** A relatively large outbreak wave in 1997/1998 involved 44 villages (number of villages in parentheses) in 9/120 (7.50%) districts; Serengeti (11), Monduli (11), Ngorongoro (6), Simanjiro (4) and

Kiteto (2), Bunda (3), Hai (3), Kilombero (3) and Magu (1) (Figure 2). In 1997, RVF cases were reported in December and in 1998 cases were reported from January to June with the outbreak reaching its peak in March 1998 (Figure 4). During this outbreak wave a total of 40,835 (29.90%, n = 194,750) domestic ruminant cases were reported (Table 1). The monthly median number of cases during the wave of this outbreak was 1,554 (range: 119–16,175; 25th percentile = 281; 75th percentile = 12,612). The four districts and nine villages that had previously reported cases during the 1977/1978 outbreak wave were also involved in this outbreak. The most likely district-level cluster of domestic ruminant cases was detected in Monduli in May 1998 with a relative risk of 3.77. A total of four statistically significant district-level secondary clusters were detected in Serengeti, Hai, Kilombero and Kiteto (Figure 5). At village level, the most likely cluster of domestic ruminant cases was detected in one village in Serengeti district in May 1998 with a relative risk of 17.33 (Figure 7). A total of seven statistically significant village-level secondary clusters were detected during this outbreak wave (Figure 7). Relatively larger proportion of cattle (52.94%) was affected followed by sheep (25.96%) and goats (21.10%) (Table 1).

**RVFV activity during the 2006/2007 outbreak wave.** During this outbreak wave, documentation on RVF cases in domestic ruminants and humans was available and some villages had concurrently reported RVF in livestock and human populations.

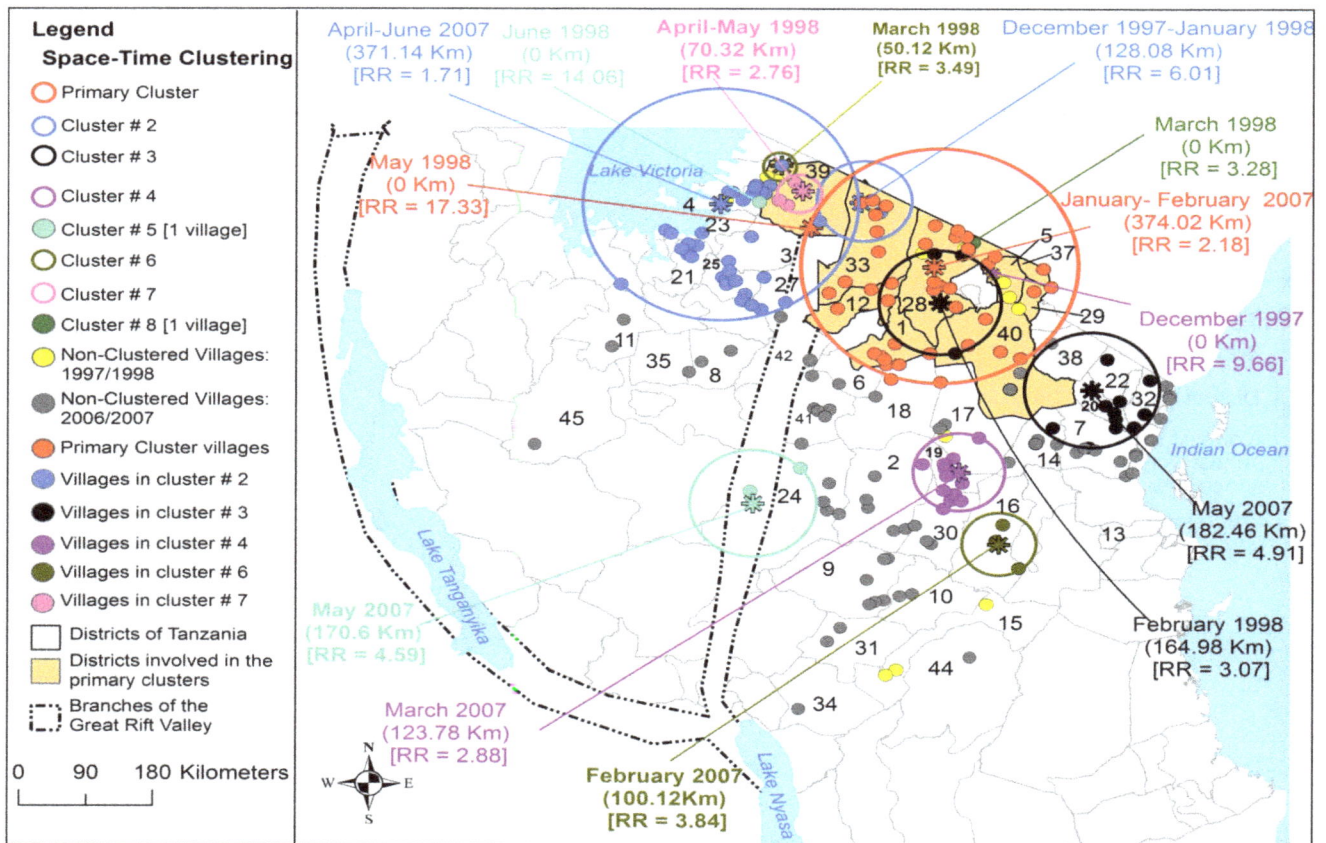

**Figure 7. Distribution of village-level space-time clusters of RVF cases in domestic ruminants from 1997 to 2007.** Asterisks represent the centre of clusters; relative risk for each cluster is displayed (RR) along with the buffer (circle) size in kilometres (km). The primary cluster was detected within the epicentre district (Ngorongoro) in the northern zone during the 1997/1998 outbreak wave. Nine districts formed the primary cluster including the epicentre district during the 2006/2007 outbreak wave that had expanded towards the south-west.

The widely spread outbreak wave in 2006/2007 in domestic ruminants involved 175 villages in 45/120 (37.50%) districts in north-eastern and central Tanzania (Figure 2). Seven districts and twenty one villages that had reported cases during the previous outbreak waves were also involved in this outbreak (Figure 2). RVF cases were reported from January to June with a peak in April (Figure 4). A total of 136, 570 (70.13%, n = 194, 750) domestic ruminant cases were reported during this outbreak wave (Table 1). The monthly median number of domestic ruminant cases during the wave of this outbreak was 10,513 (range: 1,356–44,367,175; $25^{th}$ percentile = 4,932; $75^{th}$ percentile = 15,726). Relatively larger proportion of cattle (55.90%) was affected followed by goats (23.21%) and sheep (20.88%) (Table 1).

The district-level most likely cluster of domestic ruminant cases was detected between January and March 2007 with 21, 092 cases. This cluster had involved 10 districts namely Simanjiro, Monduli, Ngorongoro, Karatu, Kiteto, Rombo, Same, Korogwe, Lushoto, and Babati with a diameter of 495.66 km and relative risk of 2.12. A total of 5 statistically significant district-level secondary clusters were detected during this outbreak wave (Figure 5). The village-level most likely cluster of domestic ruminant cases involved 44 villages and was detected between January and February 2007 with 9,704 cases, a diameter of 374 km and relative risk of 2.18 (Figure 7). The primary cluster that was detected during the 1997/1998 outbreak wave became part of the 2006/2007 primary cluster (Figure 7). A total of five statistically significant village-level

secondary clusters were detected (Figure 7). Two secondary clusters that were detected in December to January in 1997/1998 and February 1998 were embedded within the 2006/2007 primary cluster (Figure 7).

During 2006/2007 outbreak wave, a total of 309 human cases were reported in 210 villages in 28/120 (23.33%) districts of which 21 (75.00%) districts concurrently had reported cases in humans and domestic ruminants. A total of 163 (52.75%) human cases were reported in Dodoma region with relatively larger number of cases been reported in Dodoma Rural (43.56%) and Dodoma Urban (36.81%) districts. Generally human RVF cases were spatially concentrated in the central zone of the country (Figure 8). The monthly median number of human cases during the wave of this outbreak was 43 (range: 3–132; $25^{th}$ percentile = 27; $75^{th}$ percentile = 104). The human cases were reported from January to May with the peak in March and no cases were reported beyond May (Figure 4). During this outbreak wave the most likely cluster of human cases included seven districts and 16 villages. This cluster was detected between January and February 2007 with 17 cases, diameter of 369.8 km and relative risk of 6.3.

It was interestingly to observe that, the primary clusters of human and domestic ruminant cases were detected in the same location and time during the 2006/2007 outbreak wave (Figure 5 and 8). One district-level and two village-level statistically significant secondary clusters were detected (Figure 5 and 8). The secondary human and livestock space-time clusters showed a

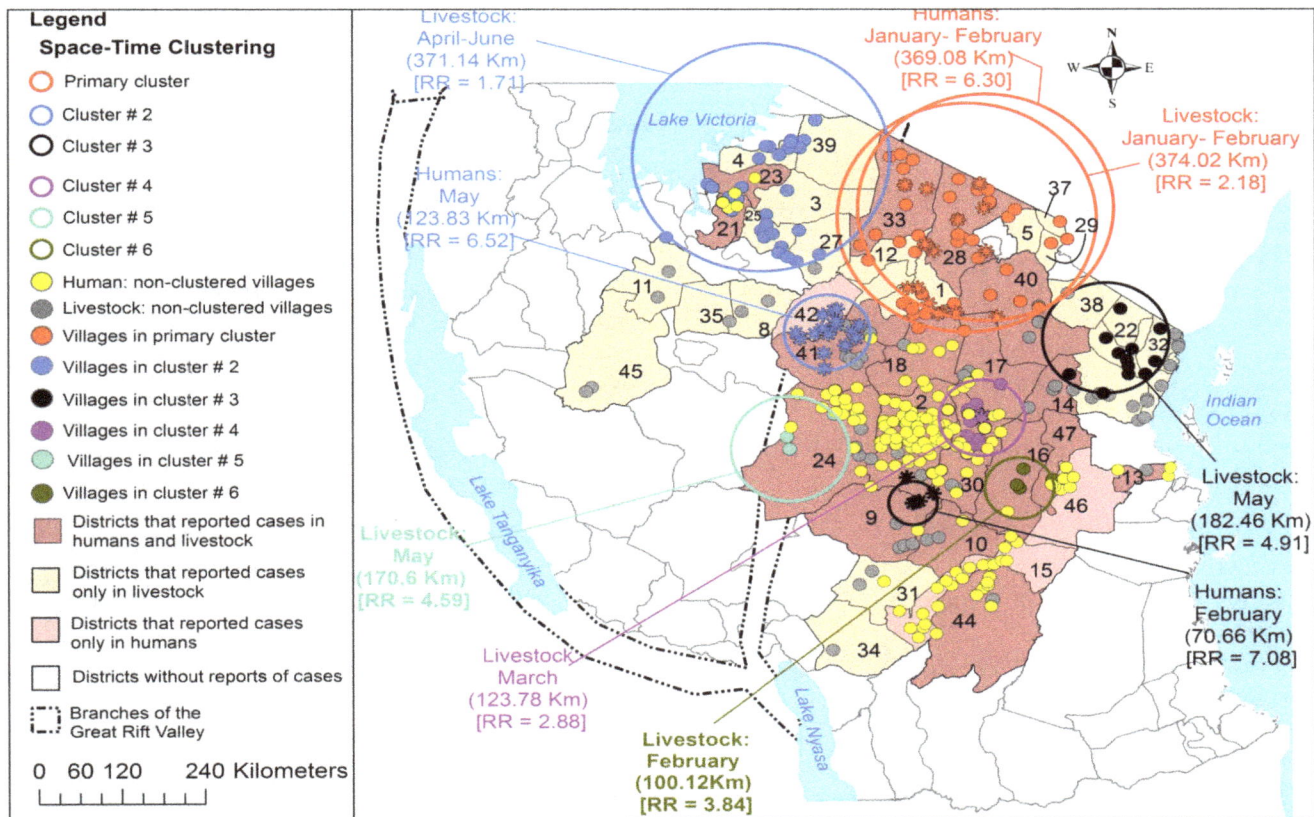

**Figure 8. Distribution of village-level space-time clusters of RVF cases in humans and domestic ruminants.** During the 2006/2007 outbreak wave the analysis of clustering of cases was made separately for humans and domestic ruminants. Between January and February 2007 there was an overlap of livestock and human primary clusters in the same location. Asterisks correspond to villages that were included within human space-time clusters; Relative risk for each cluster is displayed (RR) along with the buffer (circle) size in kilometres (km).

tendency to spread from north to western and east-central parts of the country (Figure 5 and 8). The onset of outbreaks in both the livestock and humans occurred in January with human to livestock case ratio of 1 to 1644. During this outbreak wave the overall ratio of human to livestock cases was 1 to 442.

## Risk Factor Analysis

**Univariable logistic regression analysis.** The univariable data analysis showed that the districts that experienced a bimodal rainfall pattern were more likely to report RVF cases than other districts (Table 2). This analysis suggested further that reports of cases within the districts were positively associated with cattle density of >13.5 heads per $km^2$; sheep density of >6.17 heads per $km^2$; goat density of >6.3 heads per $km^2$; pastoral livelihood zone; close to open grassland cover, clay and loam soil texture (Table 2). Outbreak occurrence was more likely to be preceded by a total monthly rainfall of >176.4 mm during each of the previous two months and total monthly rainfall of >133.8 mm during the previous month. Total amounts of rainfall during the previous 2 months >405.4 mm and during the previous 3 months of > 313.4 mm were associated with outbreak occurrence in the district.

**Multivariable logistic regression analysis.** Results of the multivariable logistic regression analysis are summarized in Table 3. Three of 15 variables were included in the final multivariable logistic regression model; eastern Rift Valley ecosystem versus western Rift Valley ecosystem in Tanzania

(OR = 6.14, CI: 1.96, 19.28), a total amount of rainfall during the previous two months >405.4 mm (OR = 12.36, CI: 3.06, 49.88), soil texture (clay [OR = 8.76, CI: 2.52, 30.50] and loam [OR = 8.79, CI: 2.04, 37.82]). There was no statistical evidence of collinearity between these risk factors. Confounding factors were not observed during the model building process. The Hosmer-Lemeshow statistic suggested a good fit to the data (chi2 = 7.29, 8 df, p = 0.51). The assessment of the predictive accuracy of the multivariable model based on the area under the curve (AUC) derived from the receiver operating characteristic curve analysis (AUC = 0.84) suggested that the final model provided good discrimination.

## Discussion

The spatial and temporal pattern of RVF outbreaks has not previously been described in Tanzania. It is interesting to note that the circumstances that allow the onset of sequential RVF outbreaks often prevail simultaneously throughout the eastern and southern African countries [28,45–50]. Although epidemiological features of RVF in Tanzania do not seem to be fundamentally different compared with the neighbouring countries, it is unique that, this is the only country with the two branches of the Great Rift Valley (that is associated with RVF occurrence). The Great Rift Valley branches in the north of the country as it traverses from Kenya forming the important eastern

**Table 2.** Results from univariable logistic regression analysis of potential risk factors for Rift Valley fever outbreak occurrence in domestic ruminants at district level in Tanzania, during the 2006/2007 outbreak wave.

| Variable | OR | 95% CI | P-value | Variable | OR | 95% CI | P-Value |
|---|---|---|---|---|---|---|---|
| **Livestock density (number per km$^2$)** | | | | **Cumulative rainfall (mm)** | | | |
| Cattle | | | | Sum of last two months | | | |
| ≤13.5 | Ref. | | | ≤257.7 | Ref. | | |
| >13.5–39.82 | 4.37 | 1.52, 12.64 | 0.006 | >257.7–405.4 | 2.38 | 0.86, 6.64 | 0.096 |
| >39.82 | 5.52 | 1.91, 15.99 | 0.002 | >405.4 | 7.00 | 2.41, 20.37 | 0.002 |
| Sheep | | | | Sum of last three months | | | |
| ≤1.22 | Ref. | | | ≤313.4 | Ref. | | |
| >1.22–6.17 | 2.07 | 0.73, 5.87 | 0.172 | >313.4–501 | 3.22 | 1.22, 8.48 | 0.018 |
| >6.17 | 7.64 | 2.64, 22.07 | 0.002 | >501.1 | 6.13 | 1.90, 19.76 | 0.002 |
| Goats | | | | **Elevation (metres above sea level)** | | | |
| ≤6.3 | Ref. | | | ≤887 | Ref. | | |
| >6.3–28.63 | 3.18 | 1.16, 8.67 | 0.024 | >887–1187 | 1.27 | 0.49, 3.31 | 0.626 |
| >28.63 | 3.18 | 1.16, 8.67 | 0.024 | >1187 | 1.43 | 0.55, 3.70 | 0.467 |
| **Rift Valley ecosystem** | | | | **Livelihood zones** | | | |
| Western Rift Valley | Ref. | | | Others | Ref. | | |
| Eastern Rift Valley | 2.08 | 0.92, 4.73 | 0.078 | cotton-paddy-cattle midlands | 2.24 | 0.73, 6.86 | 0.157 |
| **Rainfall pattern** | | | | Pastoral zone | 7.17 | 1.84, 28.06 | 0.004 |
| Unimodal | Ref. | | | **Soil types** | | | |
| Bimodal | 2.66 | 1.16, 6.10 | 0.021 | Others | Ref | | |
| **Total monthly rainfall (mm)** | | | | Acrisols | 2.54 | 0.59, 10.95 | 0.211 |
| Three months ago | | | | Cambisols | 0.56 | 0.22, 1.37 | 0.200 |
| ≤12.2 | Ref. | | | Ferralsols | 0.13 | 0.57, 1.94 | 0.876 |
| >12.2–55.7 | 0.21 | 0.07, 0.64 | 0.006 | **Soil texture** | | | |
| >55.7 | 1.79 | 0.69, 4.65 | 0.231 | Sandy | Ref. | | |
| Two months ago | | | | Clay | 9.20 | 2.81, 30.12 | 0.001 |
| ≤102 | Ref. | | | Loam | 6.19 | 1.63, 23.42 | 0.007 |
| >102–176.4 | 1.41 | 0.52, 3.84 | 0.498 | **Land cover** | | | |
| >176.4 | 4.23 | 1.55, 11.55 | 0.005 | Others | Ref. | | |
| One month ago | | | | Closed broadleaved deciduous forest | 2.32 | 0.53, 10.04 | 0.262 |
| ≤133.8 | Ref. | | | Closed to open grassland | 8.25 | 1.45, 46.86 | 0.017 |
| >133.8–210 | 8.06 | 2.72, 23.90 | 0.000 | Mosaic Vegetation/Croplands | 2.85 | 0.70, 11.54 | 0.142 |
| >210 | 3.98 | 1.29, 12.30 | 0.016 | | | | |

and western internal drainage ecosystems in Tanzania before finally rejoining in the southern highland of the country.

Results of our analysis indicate that most of the districts and villages that were involved in past outbreaks were located in northern Tanzania, the eastern wing of the Great Rift Valley, and that transmission was seasonal. In this study, a general trend of RVF outbreaks spreading from north to east-central and southern parts of the country was observed between 1930 and 2007. During the first 27 years following the first report of RVF-like disease in Tanzania, the disease was only reported from two villages in the Ngorongoro district where livestock are raised in proximity to wildlife. Subsequent outbreak waves included an increasing number of villages, districts and regions in Tanzania which had never reported outbreaks. The low numbers of reported cases of

RVF in the early years (1930 to 1978) before the disease was added in the list of notifiable diseases) could be attributed to poor awareness about the disease, inefficient recording/reporting systems and lack of diagnostic capacity. The surveillance activities were more comprehensive during the last outbreak in 2006–07 than during the previous outbreaks. These findings should therefore be interpreted cautiously due to the fact that the disease might have been present for some years before it was first diagnosed and may not have been detected in other potentially affected areas. It seems reasonable to assume, however, that initial amplification in the northern zone of Tanzania generated a source of risk which resulted in progressive infiltration of the disease to the rest of the country. Although the mechanisms of the spatial spread are not known, they are likely to include active and passive

**Table 3.** Final multivariable logistic regression model for Rift Valley fever occurrence at district level in Tanzania during the 2006/2007 outbreak wave.

| Rift Valley ecosystem | Odd Ratio | 95% CI | P-value |
|---|---|---|---|
| Western Rift Valley | Ref. | | |
| Eastern Rift Valley | 6.14 | 1.96, 19.28 | 0.002 |
| **Cumulative rainfall (mm)** | | | |
| Sum of last two months | | | |
| ≤257.7 | Ref. | | |
| >257.7–405.4 | 2.38 | 0.76, 7.48 | 0.137 |
| >405.4 | 12.36 | 3.06, 49.88 | 0.001 |
| **Soil texture** | | | |
| Sandy | Ref. | | |
| Clay | 8.76 | 2.52, 30.50 | 0.001 |
| Loam | 8.79 | 2.04, 37.82 | 0.004 |

movement of infected mosquitoes and uncontrolled livestock movements within the country. However, data on the distribution of potential vectors and livestock movement pattern is Tanzania is scarce.

The spatiotemporal progression of RVF outbreaks described in this study had a similar trend to that in neighbouring country Kenya [49]. In Tanzania, between 1930 and 1957 only less than 1% of the districts were constantly involved in the outbreaks. The 1977–78 outbreak wave had involved 4/120 (3.33%) districts. A relatively larger outbreak wave in 1997–98 involved 7.70% of the districts and the widely spread outbreak wave in 2006–07 involved humans and domestic ruminants in 39.17% of the districts in the country. The outbreak wave of 1951 in Kenya involved 8/69 (12%) administrative districts. Between 1961 and 1964 the outbreaks had expanded to include 32% districts across six provinces including all of the districts that had reported cases previously. The latest outbreak in 2006/2007 was most extensive and had involved 48% of the districts in Kenya [49].

Our findings indicate that the outbreak waves of 1977/1978, 1989, 1997/1998 and 2006/2007 were preceded with periods of positive surplus rainfall. Furthermore, the findings suggest that the outbreak waves were likely to end as the rainfall and warm temperatures faded-out. Compared to the eastern Rift Valley ecosystem; the western Rift Valley ecosystem received the unimodal rainfall and was less likely to report outbreaks and clustering of cases. The relationship between RVF outbreaks and rainfall has been indicated before [45–50]. However, there was no significant difference in the amount of rainfall between the two ecosystems during the study period. Furthermore, there were instances where no outbreaks were recorded following the seasons of exceptionally above normal rainfall. These observations suggest that while rainfall might be the major determinant for the onset and switch-off of an outbreak, it is likely to be not the only factor responsible for the spread and clustering of RVF cases. A causal association between local environmental factors, livestock density and movement, encroachment of mosquitoes into new areas and occurrence of RVF has been suggested in the previous studies [53–56]. Anecdotal reports also suggest that levels of herd immunity might be responsible for modifying temporal patterns of RVFV occurrence.

The multivariable model demonstrates the collective effect of the Rift Valley ecosystem, cumulative effect of the amount of

rainfall and soil texture on the RVF occurrence within districts. Previous studies had reported the association of some of these factors and RVF outbreaks [45–50]. Probably the eastern Rift Valley ecosystem provides suitable ecological features necessary for livestock keeping and survival of RVFV. This ecosystem experiences the bimodal rainfall pattern. It seems plausible to suggest that the occurrence of RVF outbreaks is associated with certain amount of rainfall. The increased rainfall preceding the onset of an outbreak provides an environment for *Aedes* and other mosquito species to emerge in large numbers with the resulting extensive transmission of the virus to animals and humans. The clay and loam soil texture support long period retention of water contributing to flooding and wetness habitat suitable for breeding and survival of the mosquito vectors. Uncontrolled livestock movement might have been responsible for the observed spatio-temporal spread of the outbreaks from north to east-central and southern parts of the country. These hypothesized mechanisms of disease occurrence and spread in the study areas need further investigation.

On the other hand, the district outbreak reporting status might be affected by the temporal dependence of the risk factors and implementation of surveillance and control activities. Heterogeneity was observed in the reporting of cases between districts over time. Although extensive surveillance and control measures were implemented during the last outbreak wave of 2006–07, it is not possible to account for variations and extent of surveillance activities between districts that might influence the disease reporting status of the district. The increased risk of RVF occurrence in the eastern Rift Valley ecosystems reported in this study is supported by the findings of the recent inter-epidemic sero-surveillance demonstrating higher prevalence of antibodies to RVFV in the eastern than the western Rift Valley ecosystem (C. Sindato et al., unpublished data). Past RVF outbreaks in Tanzania tend to cease as the rainfall faded-off, consequently it is difficult to conclude on the success of emergency vaccination programmes usually implemented too late during RVF outbreaks. Therefore, specific studies should be carried out to monitor and evaluate the effectiveness of the vaccination strategies.

Our findings further suggest that, once RVFV had been introduced to a new geographical area, it becomes endemic. These newly established endemic areas constitute a source for future outbreaks once favourable environmental conditions allow for re-activation of large scale virus transmission. A similar observation was reported in Kenya [49]. In this study we identified areas with persistence risk and clustering of RVF cases in humans and livestock. The onset of outbreaks in both the livestock and humans in 2006/07 occurred in January with human to livestock case ratio of 1 to 1644. This suggests that, for a single human case to be reported, a certain level of disease incidence in livestock may be necessary. The pattern of RVF outbreak waves in livestock and human populations and spatio-temporal overlapping of both populations' primary clusters, suggest that there is a strong relationship between human and livestock outbreaks. A similar observation was reported in Kenya where the clustering of human RVF cases occurred around livestock cases that was preceded by the onset of outbreak in the latter [50]. In our study, concluding whether the onset of outbreak in livestock preceded the outbreak in humans or the *vice versa* is however, limited since the specific date of the onset of livestock outbreak was rarely recorded. Likewise, largely the district and village of outbreak origin were not recorded, and the specific onset of human outbreaks was difficult to determine from data passively captured by health facilities. Although the human clusters were of relatively smaller size and were likely to be detected within the relatively bigger livestock clusters, the overlapping of the primary clusters in the same location and time period make it difficult to determine the exact interval between the onset of outbreaks in livestock and humans. Improved surveillance and inter-sectoral collaboration during outbreak investigation would improve the quality of data in future.

Based on the reported data for the last disease outbreak in 2006–07, it appears that in central Tanzania humans were more likely to be affected compared with other areas of the country. This is a surprising observation for a zone in which no RVF outbreaks have ever been reported before. While the reasons are not known, it is likely that RVFV persisted in transovarially infected eggs of floodwater *Aedes* mosquito species or circulated at sub-epidemic levels between vectors and susceptible animals until anomalous high rainfalls leading to massive flooding and the resultant swarms of competent mosquito vectors triggered transmission of the virus to a wide range of susceptible vertebrate species [12]. Other factors that might have contributed to amplification of cases in central Tanzania could have been introduction of infected animals and behavioural risk practices including the human consumption of meat from carcasses that had not been inspected or were from dead animals (L.E.G. Mboera *et al.* unpubl. data). Given that the majority of human RVF cases are caused by animal-human transmission there is a need to examine the social and economic factors that may differentiate these sites from others. Furthermore, the observed spatial RVF outbreaks in humans coincide with malaria outbreaks reported previously in northern (Ngorongoro, Babati, Hanang and Mbulu Districts) and central (Dodoma, Mpwapwa and Kongwa Districts) Tanzania [57] suggesting that RVF cases might have been misdiagnosed. For instance, during the latest outbreak in 2006–07 the majority of cases in central Tanzania were initially admitted as malaria or psychiatric cases but later confirmed to be RVF cases (L. E. G. Mboera *et al.* unpubl. data).

Our findings suggest that there is continuous endemicity of RVFV in some areas making them vulnerable to periodic outbreaks, an observation that collaborate with results from previous studies in Kenya [49] and South Africa [58]. For example, Ngorongoro district was involved in the outbreak wave of 1930 and it was involved in all the subsequent outbreaks that had occurred in the country. Our results suggest that there has been the recurrence of disease in this district and that the district has remained the index foci during outbreaks before the disease is reported elsewhere in the country. RVF cases were reported only in this district between 1930 and 1957. Ngorongoro district borders Kenya in the north and humans, wild and domestic animals are able to mix freely in this district. Available data on the role of wildlife in the epidemiology of RVF is limited. Serological evidence of RVFV activity has been reported in wildlife in Zimbabwe and Kenya [59,60]. Of recently the RVF activity has been detected in limited samples of African buffalo and elephant collected during the IEP in Tanzania [61]. The role of wildlife in the maintenance and transmission of RVFV in the country therefore requires further investigation.

The observed geographical spread of RVF over the period from 1930 until 2007 examined in this study provides evidence that the next outbreak may well spread rapidly to large populations of humans and domestic animals, potentially even involving the entire country. The reported clusters defined as high risk areas should be targeted with strategic control measures including targeted livestock vaccination and public health education especially during the IEP. The priority for strategic control programme should target the recent human and livestock overlapping primary and secondary space-time clusters. This strategy would allow more cost-effective usage of limited resources that can help to control future outbreaks/spread and the associated disease health and socio-economic impacts. The currently in use live attenuated veterinary vaccine based on the Smithburn neurotropic strain (SNS) of the virus strain should not be used once the outbreak starts to minimize the risk of needle spread of outbreak virus [62]. It is worth mentioning that recent results of molecular study by Grobbelaar et al. [13] suggest that the natural history of RVFV and its pathogenicity to humans might be influenced by massive vaccination of ruminants in Africa with the live attenuated SNS vaccine.

This study has some important limitations. First, although under-reporting and misdiagnosis of cases during the past outbreaks might have contributed to the observed pattern, we are unable to unveil a possibility of more cases to have been reported during the latest outbreak wave due to increased levels of awareness, surveillance and advocacy. For example in the 2006/07 outbreak, there was more extensive livestock surveillance than in any of the previous outbreaks. Second, even though our study has shown a non-random distribution of cases, data from some surveillance systems can manifest significant non-random geographic distribution because of variability not only in disease incidence, but also in diagnosis and reporting, factors which are strongly affected by human socioeconomic activities/behaviour and could not be measured or controlled for in our analyses. Furthermore, RVF cases in domestic ruminants were not always confirmed in the laboratory during past outbreaks and this may have resulted in over-reporting of the number of cases per district/village. However, while investigating the epidemiological trend of outbreaks in Tanzania, the focus was made to the years that corresponded to periods of past outbreaks that had occurred in the neighbouring country Kenya. We believe that the findings of this study illustrate the need to improve inter-sectoral collaboration, diagnosis, reporting and recording of disease events in the country as well as cross-border surveillance. This study offers a useful baseline description of apparent spread of RVF risk in the country. Despite its limitations, our investigation provides important findings which should be used to influence research priorities, policy development and allocation of disease control/management resources.

## Conclusion

The RVF outbreaks were found to be distributed heterogeneously and transmission dynamics appeared to vary even between areas within a few kilometres apart. The sequence of outbreak waves, continuously cover more parts of the country. Whenever infection has been introduced into an area, it is likely to be involved in future outbreaks. During the 2006/07 outbreak wave, cases were more likely to be reported from the eastern Rift Valley than the western Rift Valley ecosystem and in areas with clay and loam soil than sandy soil texture. The findings demonstrate the value of retrospective spatio-temporal analysis for informing the planning and implementation of strategic control measures.

## Acknowledgments

The authors acknowledge the Ministry of Livestock and Fisheries Development, Ministry of Health and Social Welfare, zonal Veterinary Investigation Centres, National Institute for Medical Research, Tanzania Meteorological Agency and Mlingano Agricultural Research Institute in Tanzania for making data available for this study. Mark Rweyemamu (Southern African Centre for Infectious Disease Surveillance) is thanked for his technical and logistical support during the design and implementation of this study. Abisalom Omolo and Jasper Kiplimo (International Livestock Research Institute, Kenya), Grades Stanley (National Institute for Medical

Research, Tanzania) and Robert Sumaye (Ifakara Health Institute, Tanzania) are thanked for sharing their expertise in the ArcGIS. Kim Stevens (The Royal Veterinary College, United Kingdom) is thanked for her support during the space-time permutation analysis of clusters. Sharadhuli Kimera (Sokoine University of Agriculture) is thanked for his critical review of the earlier version of the manuscript. We also wish to thank for all the constructive inputs received when the earlier version of this manuscript was shared with the public at the Faculty of Veterinary Medicine, Sokoine University of Agriculture, Tanzania. Three anonymous reviewers are thanked for their constructive comments, which helped greatly to improve the manuscript.

## Author Contributions

Conceived and designed the study: CS EDK DUP LEGM FK GD JTP. Led the study: CS. Analyzed the data: CS. Wrote the first draft of the manuscript: CS. Revised the manuscript critically for important intellectual content: CS EDK DUP LEGM FK GD BB JTP. This study was carried out as part of a PhD thesis by: CS. Provided the final approval of the version to be published: CS EDK DUP LEGM FK GD BB JTP.

## References

1. Flick R, Bouloy R (2005) Rift Valley Fever Virus. Curr. Mol. Med 5: 827–834.
2. Murphy FA, Gibbs EPJ, Horzinek MC, Studdert MJ (1999) Veterinary Virology. USA: Elsevier 469–475.
3. Rich KM, Wanyoike F (2010) An assessment of the regional and national socioeconomic impacts of the 2007 Rift Valley fever outbreak in Kenya. Am J Trop Med Hyg 83: 52–57.
4. Dar O, McIntyre S, Hogarth S, Heymann D (2013) Rift Valley fever and a new paradigm of research and development for zoonotic disease control. Emerg Infect Dis. 19(2): 189–193.
5. Chevalier V, Lancelot R, Thiongane Y, Sall B, Diaite A, et al. (2005) Rift Valley fever in small ruminants, Senegal, 2003. Emerg Infect Dis 11: 1693–1700.
6. Morvan J, Rollin PE, Laventure S, Rakotoarivony I, Roux J (1992) Rift Valley fever epizootic in the central highlands of Madagascar. Res Virol 143: 407–415.
7. Shoemaker T, Boulianne C, Vincent MJ, Pezzanite L, Al-Qahtani MM, et al. (2002) Genetic analysis of viruses associated with emergence of Rift Valley fever in Saudi Arabia and Yemen, 2000–2001. Emerg Infect Dis 12: 1415.
8. Balkhy HH, Memish ZA (2003) Rift Valley fever: an uninvited zoonosis in the Arabian Peninsula. International Journal of Antimicrobiological Agents 21: 153–7.
9. Hartley DM, Rinderknecht JL, Nipp TL, Clarke NP, Snowder GD (2011) National Centre for Foreign Animal and Zoonotic Disease Defense Advisory Group. Potential effects of Rift Valley fever in the United States. Emerg Infect Dis 17. Available: http://dx.doi.org/10.3201/eid1708.101088. Accessed 13 May 2013.
10. European Food Safety Authority (2005) Opinion of the Scientific Panel on Animal Health and Welfare on a request from the commission related to the risk of a Rift Valley fever incursion and its persistence within the community. European Food Safety Authority Journal 238: 1–128.
11. Versteirt V, Ducheyne E, Schaffner F, Hendrickx G (2013) Systematic literature review on the geographic distribution of Rift Valley Fever vectors in the Europe and the neighbouring countries of the Mediterranean Basin. Supporting Publications. Available: www.efsa.europa.eu/publications. Accessed 13 May 2013.
12. Pepin M, Bouloy M, Bird B, Kemp A, Paweska J (2010) Rift Valley fever virus (Bunyaviridae: Phlebovirus): an update on pathogenesis, molecular epidemiology, vectors, diagnostics and prevention, Veterinary Research 41: 61 DOI: 10.1051/vetres/2010033.
13. Grobbelaar AA, Weyer J, Leman PA, Kemp A, Paweska JT, et al. (2011) Molecular epidemiology of Rift Valley fever virus. Emerg Infect Dis. 12: 2270–76.
14. Murithi RM, Munyua P, Ithondeka PM, Macharia JM, Hightower A, et al (2011) Rift Valley fever in Kenya: history of epizootics and identification of vulnerable districs. Epidemiol Infect. 139: 372–80.
15. LaBeaud AD, Ochiai Y, Peters CJ, Muchiri EM, King CH (2007) Spectrum of Rift Valley fever virus transmission in Kenya: insight from three distinct regions. J Trop Med Hyg. 76: 795–800.
16. Bird BH, Githinji JWK, Macharia JM, Kasiiti JL, Muriithi RM, et al (2008) Multiple virus lineages sharing recent common ancestry were associated with a large Rift Valley fever outbreak among livestock in Kenya during 2006–2007. J Virol. 111: 52–66.
17. Nderitu L, Lee JS, Omolo J, Omulo S, O'Guinn ML, et al (2011) Sequential Rift Valley fever outbreaks in Eastern Africa caused by multiple lineages of the virus. J Infect Dis. 203: 655–65.
18. Evans A, Gakuya F, Paweska JT, Rostal M, Akoolo L, et al. (2008) Prevalence of antibodies against Rift Valley fever virus in Kenyan wildlife. Epidemiol Infect 136: 1261–1269. doi: 10.1017/S0950268807009806.
19. Desirée LaBeaud A, Bashir F, King CH (2011) Measuring the burden of arboviral diseases: the spectrum of morbidity and mortality from four prevalent infections. Population Health Metrics 9: 1.
20. Britch SC, Binepal YS, Ruder MG, Karithi HM, Linthicum KJ, et al. (2013) Rift Valley fever risk map model and seroprevalence in selected wild ungulates and camels from Kenya. PLoS ONE. 8(6): e66626.
21. Cêtre-Sossah C, Pédarrieu A, Guis H, Defernez C, Bouloy M, et al. (2012) Prevalence of Rift Valley Fever among Ruminants, Mayotte. Emerging Infectious Diseases 18: 6. DOI: 10.3201/eid186.111165.
22. Fafetine J, Neves L, Thompson PN, Paweska JT, Rutten VPMG, et al. (2013) Serological Evidence of Rift Valley Fever Virus Circulation in Sheep and Goats in Zambézia Province, Mozambique. PLoS Negl Trop Dis 7(2): e2065. doi:10.1371/journal.pntd.0002065.
23. Heinrich N, Saathoff E, Weller N, Clowes P, Kroidl I, et al. (2012) High Seroprevalence of Rift Valley Fever and evidence for endemic circulation in Mbeya Region, Tanzania, in a cross-sectional study. PLoS Negl Trop Dis 6(3): e1557. doi:10.1371/journal.pntd.0001557.
24. Poourrut X, Nkoghe D, Souris M, Paupy C, Paweska J, at al (2010) Rift Valley fever seroprevalence in human rural populations of Gabon. PLoS Negl Trop Dis. 4: e763.
25. Swanepoel RCJ (1994) Rift Valley fever in JAW Coetzer GR, Thompson RD Tustin (eds.), Infectious diseases of Livestock with special reference to southern Africa. 688–717, Oxford University Press, Cape Town.
26. Archer BN, Thomas J, Weyer J, Cengimbo A, Essoya LD, et al. (2013) Epidemiological investigations into outbreaks of Rift Valley fever in humans, South Africa, 2008–2011. Emerg Infect Dis 19(2): 1918–25.
27. Mohamed M, Mosha F, Mghamba J, Zaki SR, Shieh W-J, et al. (2010) Epidemiologic and clinical aspects of a Rift Valley fever outbreak in humans in Tanzania, 2007. Am J Trop Med Hyg 83 (Suppl. 2): S22–7.
28. Nguku P, Sharif SK, Mutonga D, Amwayi S, Omolo J, et al. (2010) An investigation of a major outbreak of Rift Valley fever in Kenya: 2006–2007. Am J Trop Med Hyg 83 (Suppl. 2): S5–13.
29. Paweska JT, Burt FJ, Swanepoel R (2005) Validation of IgG-sandwich and IgM-capture ELISA for the detection of antibody to Rift Valley fever virus in humans. Journal of Virological Methods 124: 173–181.
30. Paweska JT, Van Vuren PJ, Swanepoel R (2007) Validation of an indirect ELISA based on a recombinant nucleocapsid protein of Rift Valley fever virus for the detection of IgG antibody in humans. Journal of Virology Methods, 146: 119–124.
31. Paweska JT, Burt FJ, Anthony F, Smith SJ, Grobbelaar AA, et al. (2003) IgG sandwich and IgM-capture enzyme-linked immunosorbent assay for the detection of antibody to Rift Valley fever virus in domestic ruminants. J Virol Methods 113: 103–112.
32. Paweska JT, Smith SJ, Wright IM, Willliams R, Cohen AS, et al. (2003b) Indirect enzyme-linked immunosorbent assay for the detection of antibody against Rift Valley Fever virus in domestic and wild ruminant sera. Onderstepoort J. Vet. Res., 70: 49–64.
33. Paweska JT, Mortimer E, Leman PA, Swanepoel R (2005) An inhibition enzyme-linked immunosorbent assay for the detection of antibody to Rift Valley fever virus in humans, domestic and wild ruminants. Journal of Virology Methods 127: 10–18.
34. Paweska JT, Jansen van Vuren P (2013) Rift Valley fever virus: a virus with potential for global emergence. In: Johnson N. The role of Animals in emerging viral diseases, editor. Elsevier, Academic Press. 169–200.
35. United Republic of Tanzania; The Animal Diseases Act No. 17 of 2003. Government Printer, Dar-es-Salaam.
36. Ministry of Health and Social Welfare United Republic of Tanzania (2011) The National Integrated Disease Surveillance and Response (IDSR) Guidelines, 2nd edition.
37. Mlozi MRS, Mtambo MMA (2008) Socio-economic impact analysis of the recent Rift Valley fever outbreak in Tanzania. FAO consultancy report.
38. Sindato C, Karimuribo E, Mboera LEG (2011) The epidemiology and socio-economic impact of rift valley fever epidemics in Tanzania: a review. Tanzania Journal of Health Research 13 (Suppl 1) DOI: http://dx.doi.org/10.4314/thrb.v13i5.1.
39. United republic of Tanzania; National sample census of agriculture, small holder agriculture volume III 2007/2008.
40. Food and Agriculture Organization; Livestock Information, sector analysis and policy branch, United Republic of Tanzania.
41. NBS (2002) United Republic of Tanzania, Population and Housing Census.
42. Morley CK (1999) Tectonic evolution of the East African Rift System and the modifying influence of magmatism: a review. Acta Vulcanologia 11: 1–19.
43. FAO (1988) FAO/UNESCO Soil Map of the World, Revised Legend with Corrections and Updates. World Soil Resources Report 60. Rome, Italy: FAO, Rome.
44. Kulldorff M, Heffernan R, Hartman J, Assunçao RM, Mostashari F (2005) A space-time permutation scan statistic for the early detection of disease outbreaks. PLoS Medicine 2: 216–224.

45. Anyamba A, Chretien JP, Small J, Tucker CJ, Formenty P, et al. (2009) Prediction of Rift Valley fever outbreak in the horn of Africa 2006–2007. Proceedings of the National Academy of Sciences of the United Staes of America USA 106: 955–959.

46. Anyamba A, Linthicum KJ, Tucker CJ (2001) Climate-disease connections: Rift Valley fever in Kenya. Cadernos de Saude Publica 17: 133–140.

47. Nguku PM, Sharif SK, Mutonga D, Amwayi S, Omolo J, et al. (2010) An Investigation of a Major Outbreak of Rift Valley Fever in Kenya: 2006–2007. Am. J. Trop. Med. Hyg. (Suppl 2): 5–13. doi:10.4269/ajtmh.2010.09-0288.

48. Hightower A, Kinkade C, Nguku PM, Anyangu A, Mutonga D, et al. (2012) Relationship of Climate, Geography, and Geology to the Incidence of Rift Valley Fever in Kenya during the 2006–2007 Outbreak. Am. J. Trop. Med. Hyg. 86(2): 373–380 doi:10.4269/ajtmh.2012.11–0450.

49. Murithi RM, Munyua P, Ithondeka PM, Macharia JM, Hightower A, et al (2010) Rift Valley fever in Kenya: history of epizootics and identification of vulnerable districts. Epidemiology and Infectious Diseases 18: 1–9.

50. Munyua P, Murithi RM, Wainwright J, Githinji J, Hightower A, et al. (2010) Rift Valley Fever Outbreak in Livestock in Kenya, 2006–2007. Am J Trop Med Hyg 83: 58–64.

51. Hosmer DW, Lemeshow S (2002) Applied logistic regression. 2nd ed. New York: John Wiley & Sons.

52. Balk D, Deichmann U, Yetman G, Pozzi F, Hay S, et al. (2006) Determining global population distribution: methods, applications and data. Advances in parasitology 62: 119–156.

53. Chevalier V, Lancelot R, Thiongane Y, Sall B, Diaite A, et al. (2005) Rift Valley fever in small ruminants, senegal, 2003. Emerg Infect Dis 11: 1693–1700.

54. Pfeffer M, Dobler G (2010) Emergence of zoonotic arboviruses by animal trade and migration. Parasites and Vectors 3: 35.

55. Gubler DJ (2002) The global emergence/resurgence of arboviral diseases as public health problems. Archives of Medical Research 33: (4) 330–342.

56. LaBeaud AD, Muchiri EM, Ndzovu M, Mwanje MT, Muiruri S (2005) Interepidemic Rift Valley fever virus seropositivity, northeastern Kenya. Emerg Infect Dis 14: 1240–1246.

57. Mboera LE, Kitua AY (2001) Malaria epidemics in Tanzania: An overview. African Journal of Health Scinces 8: 17–23.

58. Pienaar NJ, Thompson PN (2013) Temporal and spatial history of Rift Valley fever in South Africa: 1950 to 2011. Onderstepoort Journal of Veterinary Research 80: (1), Art. #384. Available: http://dx.doi.org/10.4102/ojvr.v80i1.384. Accessed 9 September 2013.

59. Anderson EC, Rowe LW (1998) The prevalence of antibody to the viruses of bovine virus diarrhea, bovine herpes virus 1, Rift Valley fever, ephemeral fever and bluetongue and to Leptospira sp. in free-ranging wildlife in Zimbabwe. Epidemiol. Infect. 121: 441–449.

60. Evans A, Gakuya F, Paweska JT, Rostal M, Akoolo L, et al. (2008) Prevalence of antibodies against Rift Valley fever virus in Kenyan wildlife. Epidemiol. Infect. 136: 1261–1269. doi:10.1017/S0950268807009806).

61. Sindato C, Swai ES, Karimuribo ED, Dautu G, Pfeiffer DU, et al. (2013) Spatial distribution of non-clinical Rift Valley fever viral activity in domestic and wild ruminants in northern Tanzania. Tanzania Veterinary Journal (Special) 28: 21–38.

62. Turell MJ, Rossi CA (1991) Potential for mosquito transmission of attenuated strains of Rift Valley fever virus. Am J Trop Med Hyg 44: 278–282.

# 8

# Detection and Characterization of *Leishmania* (*Leishmania*) and *Leishmania* (*Viannia*) by SYBR Green-Based Real-Time PCR and High Resolution Melt Analysis Targeting Kinetoplast Minicircle DNA

**Marcello Ceccarelli[1], Luca Galluzzi[1]\*, Antonella Migliazzo[2], Mauro Magnani[3]**

[1] Department of Biomolecular Sciences, University of Urbino "Carlo Bo", Fano (PU), Italy, [2] Istituto Zooprofilattico Sperimentale della Sicilia, Palermo (PA), Italy, [3] Department of Biomolecular Sciences, University of Urbino "Carlo Bo", Urbino (PU), Italy

## Abstract

Leishmaniasis is a neglected disease with a broad clinical spectrum which includes asymptomatic infection. A thorough diagnosis, able to distinguish and quantify *Leishmania* parasites in a clinical sample, constitutes a key step in choosing an appropriate therapy, making an accurate prognosis and performing epidemiological studies. Several molecular techniques have been shown to be effective in the diagnosis of leishmaniasis. In particular, a number of PCR methods have been developed on various target DNA sequences including kinetoplast minicircle constant regions. The first aim of this study was to develop a SYBR green-based qPCR assay for *Leishmania (Leishmania) infantum* detection and quantification, using kinetoplast minicircle constant region as target. To this end, two assays were compared: the first used previously published primer pairs (qPCR1), whereas the second used a nested primer pairs generating a shorter PCR product (qPCR2). The second aim of this study was to evaluate the possibility to discriminate among subgenera *Leishmania (Leishmania)* and *Leishmania (Viannia)* using the qPCR2 assay followed by melting or High Resolution Melt (HRM) analysis. Both assays used in this study showed good sensitivity and specificity, and a good correlation with standard IFAT methods in 62 canine clinical samples. However, the qPCR2 assay allowed to discriminate between *Leishmania (Leishmania)* and *Leishmania (Viannia)* subgenera through melting or HRM analysis. In addition to developing assays, we investigated the number and genetic variability of kinetoplast minicircles in the *Leishmania (L.) infantum* WHO international reference strain (MHOM/TN/80/IPT1), highlighting the presence of minicircle subclasses and sequence heterogeneity. Specifically, the kinetoplast minicircle number per cell was estimated to be $26,566 \pm 1,192$, while the subclass of minicircles amplifiable by qPCR2 was estimated to be $1,263 \pm 115$. This heterogeneity, also observed in canine clinical samples, must be taken into account in quantitative PCR-based applications; however, it might also be used to differentiate between *Leishmania* subgenera.

**Editor:** Joao Inacio, National Institute for Agriculture and Veterinary Research, IP (INIAV, I.P.), Portugal

**Funding:** Funds used to support the authors throughout the study period and manuscript preparation were from Department of Biomolecular Sciences of University of Urbino. The funder had no role in study design, data collection and analysis, decision to publish, or preparation of the manuscript.

**Competing Interests:** The authors have declared that no competing interests exist.

\* E-mail: luca.galluzzi@uniurb.it

## Introduction

Leishmaniasis is a neglected disease of the Old and New Worlds with a broad clinical spectrum encompassing asymptomatic infection and three main clinical syndromes: visceral leishmaniasis (VL), cutaneous leishmaniasis (CL), and mucosal leishmaniasis (ML). Worldwide, at least 15 *Leishmania* species are pathogenic for *Homo sapiens*. They are primarily transmitted by phlebotomine sandflies, although infection may also occur sporadically through blood transfusion, contaminated needles, and organ transplantation [1]. *Leishmania donovani* complex (including *L. infantum* and *L. donovani*) belongs to the subgenus *Leishmania (Leishmania)* and it is the etiological agent of VL, while the species belonging to the subgenus *Leishmania (Viannia)* are the etiological agents of CL and ML. The leishmaniasis is still a public health problem in 98 countries, affecting both rural and urban areas. Worldwide there are an estimated 0.2–0.4 million new cases of VL and 0.7–1.2 million new cases of CL annually, while 12 million people are currently affected by the disease [2]. The VL mortality is second only to malaria among parasitic diseases [3].

In zoonosis caused by *L. (L.) infantum*, dogs are the main reservoir for the disease and canine visceral leishmaniasis (CVL) is considered to be a major problem in veterinary medicine [4,5]. Cases of canine leishmaniasis have been reported in over 50% of the countries where human leishmaniasis is endemic, and the Mediterranean Basin is one of the most affected areas [6]. Moreover, many infected dogs are asymptomatic [7,8].

In this context, efficient and reliable diagnostic approaches in veterinary medicine are very important in the treatment of symptomatic and asymptomatic dogs. Moreover, the definition of the subgenus/complex in humans may be useful in helping physicians to choose the appropriate therapeutic protocols and in gaining insights into the disease evolution [9].

To this end, many diagnostic systems have been developed. Among the serological methods, the indirect fluorescence antibody test (IFAT) is considered by the World Organization for Animal Health (OIE-Office International des Epizooties) as a reference serologic method [10]. Nevertheless, serological methods are not always reliable when dealing with prepatent periods, remission stages, and the appearance of non-specific cross-reactions or latent forms of the disease like in "cryptic leishmaniasis" [11]. Moreover, in endemic areas, a significant number of animals display antibody titres ranging from 1:40 to 1:80 (below the positivity threshold: titre ≥1:160), referred to as uncertain titres or "borderline titres" [12].

Molecular techniques can lead to improvements in the diagnosis of leishmaniasis; in particular quantitative PCR (qPCR) could play an important role in *Leishmania* detection and the monitoring of therapy [13,14] in humans and animals. Several PCR methods have been developed on various *Leishmania* target sequences. The conserved region of *Leishmania* kinetoplast DNA (kDNA) minicircles has been used as a specific target for conventional or quantitative PCR assays [15–17]. In fact, *Leishmania* belongs to the Kinetoplastida order, Trypanosomatidae family, in which all the members contain a kinetoplast situated at the base of the flagellum. The kinetoplast contains a concatenated network of circular DNA molecules [18], i.e. mitochondrial DNA, composed of minicircles and maxicircles. The minicircles, which encode for guide RNAs (gRNAs) required for editing the mRNA from maxicircles, have been reported to be present in about 10,000 copies per parasite [19,20]. Structurally, the kDNA minicircle is organized into one to four conserved regions representing approximately 10% of the molecule and an equal number of variable regions [21].

In this study, we compared two SYBR green–based qPCR assays (named qPCR1 and qPCR2), targeting the kDNA minicircle constant region, for the detection and estimation of the *Leishmania* parasites in canine clinical samples. Then, we evaluated the possibility to discriminate among the subgenera *Leishmania* (*Leishmania*) and *Leishmania* (*Viannia*) using a high resolution melt (HRM) approach. Moreover, the number of kDNA minicircles and their genetic variability were also investigated in an attempt to characterize the *L. (L.) infantum* WHO reference strain and gain insight the minicircle heterogeneity in veterinary clinical samples.

## Materials and Methods

### Ethical Statement

Approval of the study was obtained on July 31st 2012 from the Ethical Committee for Animal Experiments of the University of Urbino (CESA). The study's title was "Diagnosi biomolecolare della leishmaniosi attraverso l'uso di campioni clinici non invasivi e loro utilizzo per il monitoraggio terapeutico" (Prot. CESA 2/2012).

### *Leishmania* DNA

A Chelex-purified DNA from promastigotes of *L. (L.) infantum* MHOM/TN/80/IPT1 (WHO international reference strain), used in Italy as the national reference strain, was obtained from

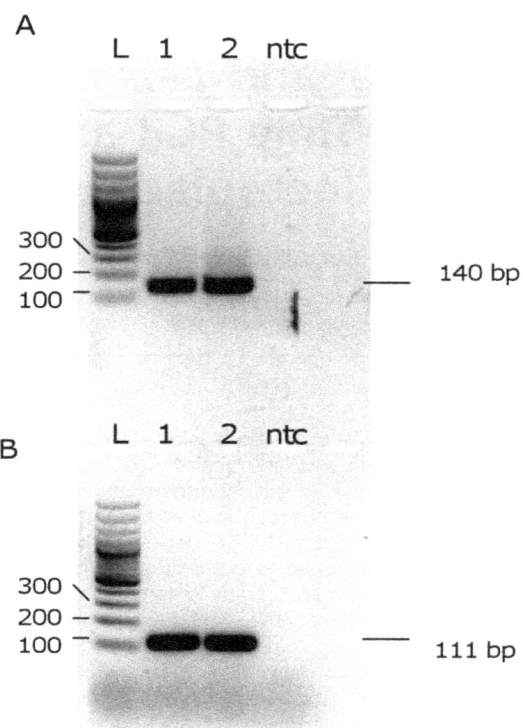

**Figure 2. Electrophoretic analysis of PCR products.** Agarose gel analysis of PCR products obtained with primers MaryF-MaryR (A) and MLF-MLR (B). 1,2: PCR products obtained with *L. (L.) infantum* MHOM/TN/80/IPT1 DNA as template; L: ladder; ntc: no template control.

the Institute of Experimental Preventive Veterinary Medicine (Istituto Zooprofilattico Sperimentale) (IZS) of Sicily, the National Italian Reference Centre for leishmaniasis located in Palermo, Italy. The equivalent concentration of reference sample was $10^8$ parasites/ml. DNA quantification was performed by fluorimetric analysis using the Qubit 2.0 Fluorometer (Invitrogen).

The DNA concentration was 23.5 ng/μl, and the content of DNA per cell was calculated to be 235 fg/parasite, in agreement with literature data [22,23]. This value confirmed the accuracy of parasite concentration in the DNA reference sample, and supported the accuracy of the subsequent determinations and quantifications.

Chelex-purified DNA from New World Leishmanias *L. (L.) amazonensis*, *L. (V.) guyanensis*, *L. (V.) panamensis*, *L. (V.) braziliensis* were also obtained from the same Institution. These strains were isolated from clinical samples in Argentina and typed at the species level at the Institute of Biomedicine and molecular immunology, CNR (Palermo, Italy). The DNA concentration of the New World *Leishmania* species was also analyzed, and the following results were

```
  1   AATGGTCAAAAATAGCCCAAAATTCCAAACTTTTCTGGTCCTCCGGGTAGGGGCGTTCTG

 61   CGAAAACCGAAAAATGGGTGCAGAAATCCCGTTCAAAAAATGGCTGAAAATGCCGAAAAT

121   CGGCTCCGGGGCGGGAAACTGGGGGTTGGTGTAAAATAGGGCCGGGTGGTGGCTGGAAAT
```

**Figure 1. *L. (L.) infantum* kDNA minicircle DNA partial sequence (acc. n. Z35272) and primer localization.** The underlined bold sequences represent the MaryF-MaryR primers; the boxed sequences represent MLF-MLR primers.

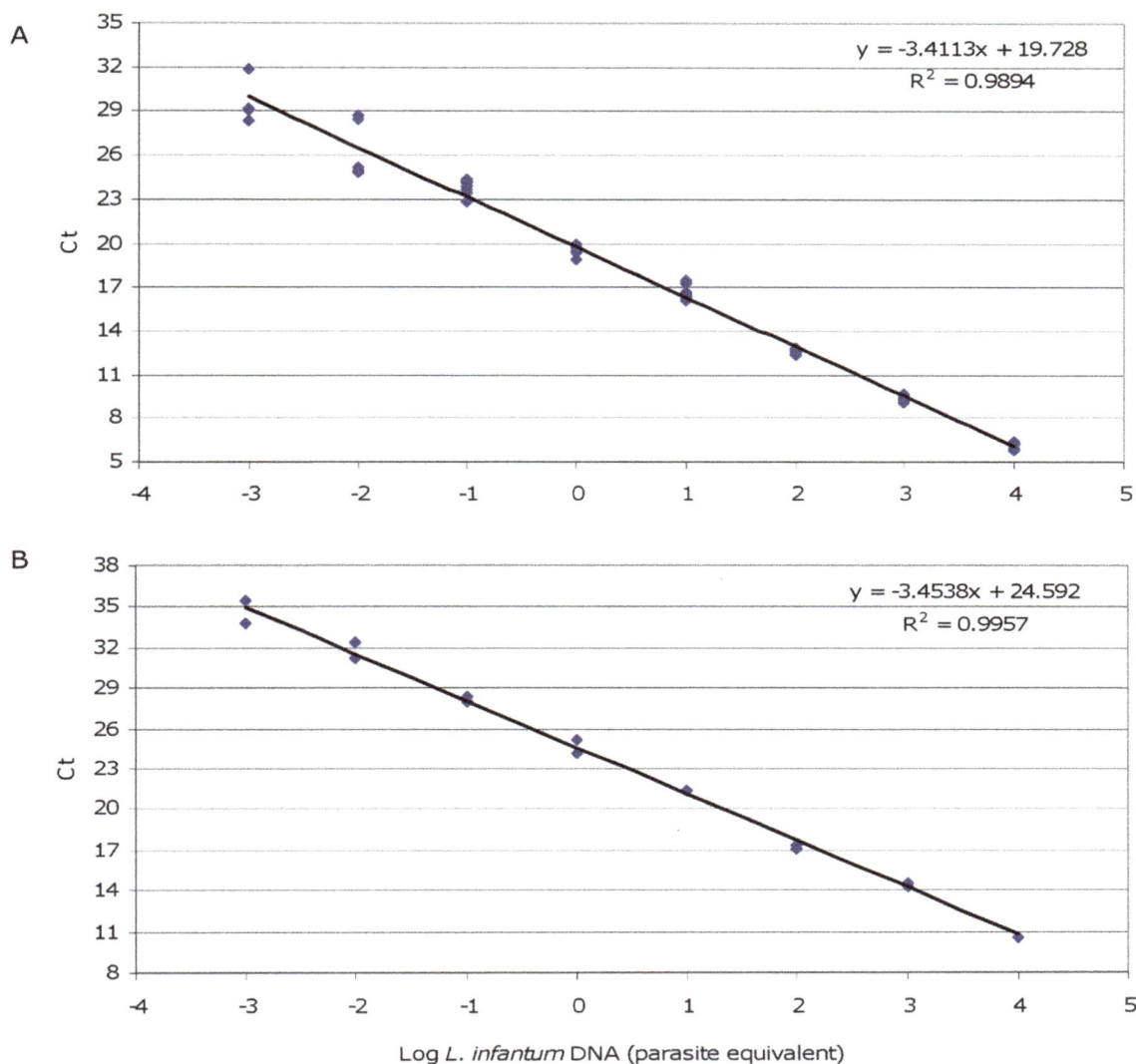

**Figure 3. Calibration curves constructed with serial dilutions of *L. (L.) infantum* DNA.** Standard curves obtained from serial dilutions of *L. (L.) infantum* MHOM/TN/80/IPT1 DNA with primers MaryF-MaryR and MLF-MLR are represented in panel A and B, respectively. The standard curves were obtained with serial dilutions ranging from 10,000 to 0.001 parasites equivalent/tube.

obtained: *L. (L.) amazonensis* 0.98 ng/µl, *L. (V.) guyanensis* 2.31 ng/µl, *L. (V.) panamensis* 1.79 ng/µl and *L. (V.) braziliensis* 1.32 ng/µl.

## Canine Samples

Canine peripheral blood and conjunctival swabs samples were provided by the veterinary clinic "S. Teresa" (Fano, Italy) as part of samples used for routine clinical tests. Sixty-two animals were selected and grouped on the basis of IFAT test results and clinical signs reported by veterinary practitioners (i.e. lymphadenopathy, alopecia, skin ulceration, weight loss, onychogryposis, ocular lesions, epistaxis, lameness). IFAT was performed on serum samples, obtained from both symptomatic and asymptomatic dogs, with an in-house assay validated and provided by IZS of Sicily.

The buffy-coat samples (100 to 320 µl) were obtained after centrifugation of 1 ml peripheral blood at 1500 rpm for 10 minutes. The DNA was extracted from these samples using the DNeasy Blood & Tissue kit (Qiagen) following the manufacturer's protocol with some slight modifications. In particular, the

incubation time with proteinase K was prolonged to 2 h, and the elution was repeated twice with the same 200 µl elution buffer. Conjunctival swabs were collected from the right and left conjunctivas using sterile cotton swabs. The swabs were transferred into 1.5 ml sterile tubes, immersed in 200 µl lysis buffer (10 mM Tris-HCl pH 8.3, 50 mM KCl, 0.5% Nonidet P40, 0.5% Tween 20, 0.1 mg/ml proteinase K), and incubated 2 h at 56°C. After swabs elimination, the samples were incubated for 10 min at 95°C and centrifuged at 14,000 rpm for 10 min. Supernatants were used as template in PCR reactions.

## PCR Assays

The primers used to amplify a 140 bp conserved region of the *Leishmania* kDNA minicircle were from Mary *et al.* [15] (defined in this paper as MaryF and MaryR). Two new primers (forward MLF: 5′-CGTTCTGCGAAAACCGAAA-3′; and reverse MLR: 5′-CGGCCCTATTTTACACCAACC-3′) were designed to target a 111 bp fragment of the same region of *L. (L.) infantum* kDNA minicircle (acc. n. Z35272) using the Primer Express software

A

$y = -3.3598x + 34.854$
$R^2 = 0.9907$

Log plasmid 1 copy number

B

$y = -3.457x + 34.822$
$R^2 = 0.9986$

Log plasmid 3 copy number

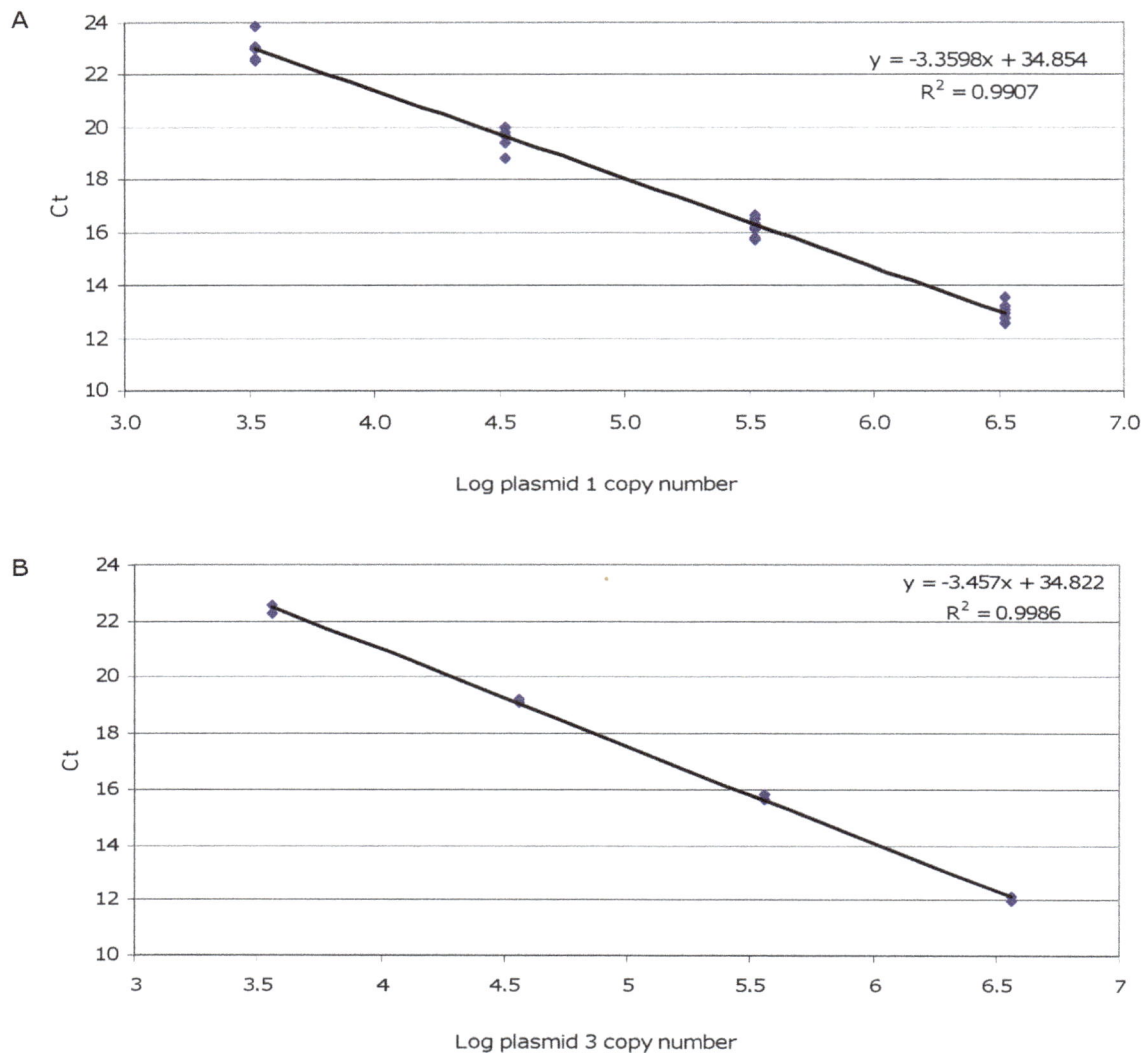

**Figure 4. Calibration curves constructed with plasmid serial dilutions.** Standard curves were obtained from serial dilutions of plasmid 1 (A) and plasmid 3 (B) with primers MaryF-MaryR and MLF-MLR, respectively. Each point derived from duplicates of 3 independent experiments.

(Applied Biosystems). The positions of MLF-MLR primers as well as MaryF-MaryR primers along the kDNA minicircle sequence are depicted in Fig. 1.

Conventional PCR using both primer pairs was carried out in a 50 µl volume with 25–50 ng template DNA, containing 200 µM dNTPs, 2.5 mM MgCl$_2$, 200 nM of each primer and 1U Hot-Rescue DNA Polymerase (Diateva). The amplification was performed in a GeneAmp® PCR System 2700 (Applied Biosystems). The thermal cycling profile was as follows: 94°C for 7 min, followed by 35 cycles at 94°C for 30 s, 60°C for 20 s and 72°C for 20 s, with a final extension at 72°C for 5 min. Each sample was amplified in duplicate. Amplified fragments were analyzed by electrophoresis in a 1.8% agarose gel containing Gel Red (1:10,000) (Sichim, Italy). The gels were visualized under UV light using a gel doc apparatus (Bio-Rad).

Two qPCR assays were named as qPCR1 and qPCR2 and were performed using MaryF-MaryR primers and MLF-MLR primers, respectively. Both qPCR were carried out in a 25 µl volume with 1 µl template DNA and 24 µl SYBR green PCR master mix (Diatheva srl, Italy) containing 1U Taq Polymerase and 200 nM of

each primer. The PCR reactions were performed in a Rotor-Gene 6000 instrument (Corbett life science, Australia). The amplification profile was: 94°C for 10 min, followed by 40 cycles at 94°C for 30 s, 60°C for 20 s and 72°C for 20 s. At the end of each run, a melting curve analysis was performed from 55°C to 95°C to monitor primer dimers or non-specific product formation. The reactions were performed in duplicate or triplicate.

A standard curve was established using Chelex-purified L. (L.) infantum DNA; 1 µl of serial dilutions, ranging from 100 to 0.001 parasites, was introduced into reaction tubes. The standard curve concentration was expressed as parasite/µl (par/µl).

In order to evaluate the potential interference of host DNA as background in the qPCR analysis, we spiked the qPCR reactions, containing L. (L.) infantum DNA from 100 to 0.001 parasites, with 100 ng or 30 ng of human or canine DNA, respectively. The amount of canine DNA approximately reflected the median amount of DNA from clinical samples used as templates. All quantification analyses were performed with the Rotor-Gene 6000 software. Primer sequence specificity was confirmed in silico by BLAST searches in the subset database order Kinetoplastida. The

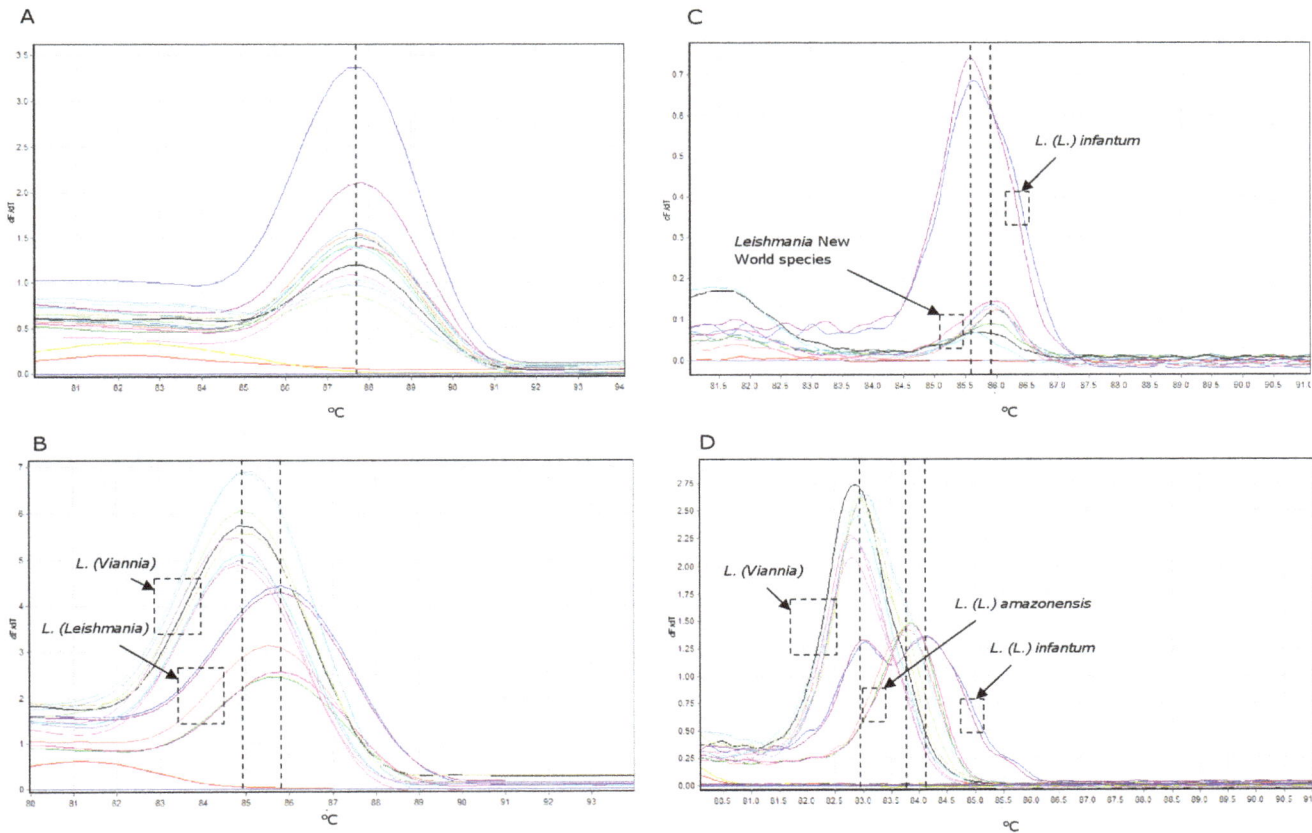

**Figure 5. Melting analyses of PCR products.** Representative melting profiles of amplicons obtained with primers MaryF-MaryR (A, C) and MLF-MLR (B, D). Panels A and B show results of standard melting analysis, while panels C and D show results of HRM analysis. The species tested were *L. (L.) infantum, L. (L.) amazonensis, L. (V.) guyanensis, L. (V.) panamensis, L. (V.) braziliensis*. Each species was tested in duplicate or triplicate. The melting curves which did not show a melting peak represent the no template controls.

assay specificities were also tested with DNA purified from *Trypanosoma cruzi*, obtained from the Institute of Biomedicine and Molecular Immunology, CNR (Palermo, Italy). To exclude false-negative results due to low DNA extraction efficiency or the presence of PCR inhibitors, a random subset (approximately 24%) of canine DNA samples which resulted qPCR-negative were tested for the quantitative amplification of the beta-2-microglobulin (B2M) gene using primers B2Mcanis_F (5′-GTCCCACA-GATCCCCCAAAG-3′) and B2Mcanis_R (5′- CTGGTGGA-

**Table 1.** HRM analysis with MLF-MLR primers of different *Leishmania* species.

| Species | subgenus | Tm peak 1 (°C) | Tm peak 2 (°C) |
|---------|----------|----------------|----------------|
| *L. infantum* | *Leishmania* | 83.20±0.47 | 84.32±0.34 |
| *L. amazonensis* | *Leishmania* | | 84.09±0.26 |
| *L. guyanensis* | *Viannia* | 83.21±0.27 | |
| *L. panamensis* | *Viannia* | 83.07±0.09 | |
| *L. braziliensis* | *Viannia* | 83.08±0.21 | |
| *L. infantum* Plasmid 3 | *Leishmania* | | 84.02±0.12 |
| *L. infantum* Plasmid 17 | *Leishmania* | 83.34±0.30 | |

Tm values are ± SD.

TGGAACCCTGAC-3′) with qPCR conditions as reported above.

## High Resolution Melt (HRM) Analysis

HRM curves acquisition was performed after PCR amplification on a Rotor-Gene 6000 instrument (Corbett life science, Australia). HRM range was set from 75°C to 92°C, with a slope of 0.1°C/s, and 2 s at each temperature. Each sample was run in duplicate or triplicate and gain was optimized before melt on all tubes. HRM curve analysis was performed with the derivative of the raw data, after smoothing, with the Rotor-Gene 6000 software.

To analyze intra-assay variation, the standard curve ranging from 100 to 0.01 *L. (L.) infantum* parasites, and spiked with 30 ng of canine DNA, was tested with 3 replicates within one run, and the coefficient of variation (CV) was calculated.

## Cloning and Sequencing

The PCR product amplified with primers MaryF-MaryR from the *L. (L.) infantum* MHOM/TN/80/IPT1 strain was cloned in the plasmid pCR®2.1 using the TA cloning Kit (Qiagen) and *E. coli* Top10 F competent cells. The recombinant plasmids were purified from five colonies (1, 2, 3, 4, 17) using QIAprep mini kit (Qiagen). The plasmid concentration was estimated using a gel doc apparatus (Biorad) by 1.8% agarose gel electrophoresis and λDNA/HinDIII marker (Thermo Scientific) as a reference. Plasmid copy number was calculated using the molar

**Table 2.** Intra-assay reproducibility of the qPCR2 HRM analysis.

| Parasite equivalents/reaction | Average Ct | Average Tm peak 1 (°C) ± SD | %CV | Average Tm peak 2 (°C) ± SD | %CV |
|---|---|---|---|---|---|
| 100 | 20.86 | 83.04±0.05 | 0.03 | 84.14±0.05 | 0.06 |
| 10 | 23.99 | 83.09±0.05 | 0.06 | 84.13±0.09 | 0.11 |
| 1 | 27.44 | 83.15±0.11 | 0.13 | 84.23±0.03 | 0.03 |
| 0.1 | 31.10 | 83.24±0.10 | 0.11 | 84.49±0.08 | 0.09 |
| 0.01 | 33.77 | 83.72±0.47 | 0.56 | 84.42±0.70 | 0.83 |

concentration and the molecular mass of the plasmid and the insert. The five clones were sequenced with M13 primers.

The PCR products obtained with MaryF-MaryR primers from canine clinical samples and New World Leishmanias were purified using the Minelute PCR purification kit (Qiagen) and directly sequenced using MaryF and MaryR primers.

All sequences were performed on a ABI PRISM 310 Genetic Analyzer (Applied Biosystems).

### kDNA Minicircle Quantification

The number of minicircles per parasite was determined in the *L. (L.) infantum* MHOM/TN/80/IPT1 strain by qPCR. Two standard curves were constructed with serial dilutions of plasmid 1 (ranging from $3.36 \times 10^6$ to $3.36 \times 10^3$ copies/PCR tube) or plasmid 3 (ranging from $3.59 \times 10^6$ to $3.59 \times 10^3$ copies/PCR tube) for amplification with primers MaryF-MaryR, or MLF-MLR, respectively.

### Statistical Analysis

Statistical analysis to evaluate differences among Tm values was performed using a Mann-Whitney test on GraphPad InStat (GraphPad Software, San Diego, CA).

## Results

### Specificity and Sensitivity of PCR Assays

Initially, to test the primers performance on DNA from *L. (L.) infantum* MHOM/TN/80/IPT1, 2.3 ng of template DNA were amplified by conventional PCR either with MaryF-MaryR primers and MLF-MLR primers. The electrophoretic analysis of the PCR mixtures showed the amplicons at the expected size (140 bp and 111 bp, respectively) and the absence of non-specific products or primer dimers (Fig. 2).

Subsequently, qPCR conditions with SYBR green were optimized with MaryF-MaryR and MLF-MLR primers: the results showed specific amplicons having melting temperatures of about 87°C and 85°C, respectively, without non-specific products or primer dimers (Fig. S1). Both qPCR assays showed a sensitivity of $1 \times 10^{-3}$ parasites per PCR tube using calibration curves constructed with serial dilutions of *L. (L.) infantum* MHOM/TN/80/IPT1 DNA. Moreover, the PCR efficiencies were also similar (95% and 96%) (Fig. 3).

The specificity of both pairs of primers was tested with genomic human and canine DNA from healthy donors and with chelex-purified DNA from *L. (L.) infantum*, *L. (L.) amazonensis*, *L. (V.) guyanensis*, *L. (V.) panamensis*, *L. (V.) braziliensis*, and *Trypanosoma cruzi*. Human, canine or *T. cruzi* DNA did not show any amplification product (not shown). Both pairs of primers were able to amplify all the *Leishmania* species tested, including the New World species; however, in these species the Ct in the qPCRs were

strongly delayed compared to *L. (L.) infantum* DNA, using comparable template DNA amounts (not shown). To exclude non-specific amplification, the same PCRs were performed with the annealing temperature at 65°C. The amplification products were also obtained under these more stringent conditions with both primer pairs (Fig. S2), indicating the existence of a subpopulation of kDNA minicircles matching primer sequences.

In order to exclude possible interference of background DNA derived from clinical specimens in qPCR assays, different amounts of *L. (L.) infantum* DNA (down to $1 \times 10^{-3}$ parasites equivalent) were amplified in the presence of 100 ng of human DNA or 30 ng of canine DNA as background. Although the PCR efficiencies were affected by the presence of background DNA, $1 \times 10^{-3}$ parasites were detected and the sensitivity of the assays remained unchanged (Fig. S3 and S4).

The qPCR2 sensitivities for *L. (L.) amazonensis*, *L. (V.) guyanensis*, *L. (V.) panamensis*, *L. (V.) braziliensis* were $1.0 \times 10^{-2}$, $2.3 \times 10^{-3}$, $2.0 \times 10^{-4}$, $1.3 \times 10^{-3}$ ng/PCR tube, respectively.

### kDNA Minicircle Quantification

kDNA minicircle quantification was first performed using MaryF-MaryR primers (qPCR1 assay). Serial dilutions of the PCR product cloned into a plasmid (plasmid 1), ranging from $3.36 \times 10^6$ to $3.36 \times 10^3$ copies, were used to construct the calibration curve. The kDNA minicircles were quantified in chelex-purified DNA equivalent to 10 and 1 par/μl. The quantification was performed in three independent experiments. The three standard curves were gathered, showing good correlation (Fig. 4A) and reproducible quantification results. We found $26,566 \pm 1,192$ kDNA minicircles amplifiable by MaryF-MaryR primers in *L. (L.) infantum* MHOM/TN/80/IPT1.

The plasmid 1 was not amplifiable using MLF-MLR primers (data not shown). In fact, the cloned DNA sequence showed two mismatches with the MLF primer (see below). However, these primers successfully amplified a different cloned sequence (plasmid 3). Hence, serial dilutions of recombinant plasmid 3, ranging from $3.59 \times 10^6$ to $3.59 \times 10^3$ plasmid copies, were used in the construction of the calibration curve for kDNA minicircle quantification by MLF-MLR primers (fig. 4B). Dilutions of 100 and 10 par/μl were tested in duplicate obtaining an average of $1,263 \pm 115$ kDNA minicircles per parasite amplifiable by MLF-MLR primers. Since the MLF-MLR primers are nested to MaryF-MaryR primers, we hypothesized that the $1,263 \pm 115$ copies of this amplicon per cell, could represent a subclass of minicircles amplifiable by MaryF-MaryR primers.

### Melting Analysis

Melting analysis of PCR products obtained with MaryF-MaryR primers (qPCR1) did not show significant Tm differences for the two subgenera *Leishmania (Leishmania)* (average Tm $87.62 \pm 0.18$;

**Table 3.** Results from canine clinical samples.

| | | | qPCR1 | qPCR2 | | |
| | | | Parasite load (par/ml | Parasite load (par/ml | | |
| Clinical status | Sample ID | IFAT titre | blood) | blood) | Tm HRM peak 1 | Tm HRM peak 2 |
|---|---|---|---|---|---|---|
| Diagnosed Leishmaniasis | 1 | 1:80 | 0.35 | 0.27 | – | 84.73±0.07 |
| | 2 | n.a. | 0.10 | 0.14 | 83.62±0.14 | 84.54±0.23 |
| | 3 | ≥1:160 | 1.72 | 12.24 | – | 83.87±0.05 |
| | 4 | ≥1:160 | 8.00 | 2.40 | – | 83.95±0.04 |
| | 5 | ≥1:160 | 20.58 | 1.27 | 83.82±0.23 | 84.80±0.10 |
| | 8 | ≥1:160 | 1.40 | 5.00 | 83.95±0.25 | 84.68±0.25 |
| | 9 | ≥1:160 | 3.18 | 26.91 | 84.07±0.12 | 84.80±0.04 |
| | 21 | ≥1:160 | 0.52 | 19.88 | – | 84.23±0.07 |
| | 22 | ≥1:160 | neg | n.a. | n.a. | n.a. |
| | 23 | ≥1:160 | neg | n.a. | n.a. | n.a. |
| | 24 | ≥1:160 | neg | n.a. | n.a. | n.a. |
| | 25 | ≥1:160 | neg | n.a. | n.a. | n.a. |
| | 28 | ≥1:160 | neg | neg | – | – |
| | 29 | ≥1:160 | 0.88 | 4.94 | – | 84.21±0.13 |
| | 30 | ≥1:160 | 1.66 | 19.20 | 84.22 * | 85.40±0.04 |
| | 31 | ≥1:160 | 0.25 | 1.41 | 84.68±0.14 | 85.37 * |
| | 32 | ≥1:160 | 0.56 | 4.68 | 84.1±0.08 | 84.83±0.08 |
| Asymptomatic Leishmaniasis | 6 | neg | 22.27 | 10.40 | 83.03±0.07 | 83.94±0.08 |
| | 7 | neg | 4.26 | 6.45 | 83.71±0.06 | 84.45±0.11 |
| | 10 | neg | neg | neg | – | – |
| | 11 | neg | neg | neg | – | – |
| | 12 | neg | neg | neg | – | – |
| | 13 | neg | neg | n.a. | n.a. | n.a. |
| | 33 | neg | neg | n.a. | n.a. | n.a. |
| | 49 | neg | neg | n.a. | n.a. | n.a. |
| | 50 | neg | neg | n.a. | n.a. | n.a. |
| | 51 | neg | neg | n.a. | n.a. | n.a. |
| | 52 | neg | neg | n.a. | n.a. | n.a. |
| | 53 | neg | neg | n.a. | n.a. | n.a. |
| | 54 | neg | neg | n.a. | n.a. | n.a. |
| | 55 | neg | neg | n.a. | n.a. | n.a. |
| | 56 | neg | neg | n.a. | n.a. | n.a. |
| | 57 | neg | neg | n.a. | n.a. | n.a. |
| | 58 | neg | neg | n.a. | n.a. | n.a. |
| | 59 | neg | neg | n.a. | n.a. | n.a. |
| | 60 | neg | neg | n.a. | n.a. | n.a. |
| | 61 | neg | neg | n.a. | n.a. | n.a. |
| | 62 | neg | neg | n.a. | n.a. | n.a. |
| Suspected Leishmaniasis | 14 | 1:40 | neg | n.a. | n.a. | n.a. |
| | 15 | 1:40 | neg | n.a. | n.a. | n.a. |
| | 16 | 1:80 | neg | n.a. | n.a. | n.a. |
| | 17 | 1:80 | neg | n.a. | n.a. | n.a. |
| | 34 | 1:40 | neg | n.a. | n.a. | n.a. |
| | 35 | 1:80 | neg | n.a. | n.a. | n.a. |
| | 36 | 1:40 | neg | n.a. | n.a. | n.a. |
| | 37 | 1:40 | neg | n.a. | n.a. | n.a. |
| | 38 | 1:40 | neg | n.a. | n.a. | n.a. |

**Table 3.** Cont.

| Clinical status | Sample ID | IFAT titre | qPCR1 Parasite load (par/ml blood) | qPCR2 Parasite load (par/ml blood) | Tm HRM peak 1 | Tm HRM peak 2 |
|---|---|---|---|---|---|---|
| | 39 | 1:80 | neg | neg | – | – |
| | 40 | 1:40 | neg | n.a. | n.a. | n.a. |
| | 41 | 1:40 | neg | n.a. | n.a. | n.a. |
| | 42 | 1:80 | neg | neg | n.a. | n.a. |
| | 43 | 1:40 | neg | n.a. | n.a. | n.a. |
| Monitored after therapy | 18 | ≥1:160 | neg | neg | – | – |
| | 19 | ≥1:160 | neg | neg | – | – |
| | 20 | ≥1:160 | neg | neg | – | – |
| | 26 | ≥1:160 | 1.29 | 26.21 | 83.30±0.71 | 84.23±0.81 |
| | 27 | ≥1:160 | 1.21 | neg | – | – |
| | 44 | ≥1:160 | neg | neg | – | – |
| | 45 | 1:80 | neg | n.a. | n.a. | n.a. |
| | 46 | ≥1:160 | neg | n.a. | n.a. | n.a. |
| | 47 | ≥1:160 | neg | n.a. | n.a. | n.a. |
| | 48 | ≥1:160 | neg | n.a. | n.a. | n.a. |

*only one replicate showed the melting peak.
neg: negative.
n.a.: not available.

n = 10) and *Leishmania* (*Viannia*) (average Tm 87.67±0.16; n = 9), while PCR products obtained with MLF-MLR primers (qPCR2) showed two significantly different Tm values for the subgenera *Leishmania* (*Leishmania*) (average Tm 85.74±0.25; n = 16) and *Leishmania* (*Viannia*) (average Tm 85.01±0.24; n = 26) (Mann-Whitney test p<0.0001) (Fig. 5AB). This observation was further strengthened by performing HRM analysis on the same samples (Fig. 5CD): the Tm analysis performed with MaryF-MaryR primers was still unable to efficiently discriminate among the different subgenera, while the assay with MLF-MLR primers showed significantly different HRM profiles for species belonging to subgenus *Leishmania* (*Viannia*), for *L. (L.) amazonensis*, and for *L.*

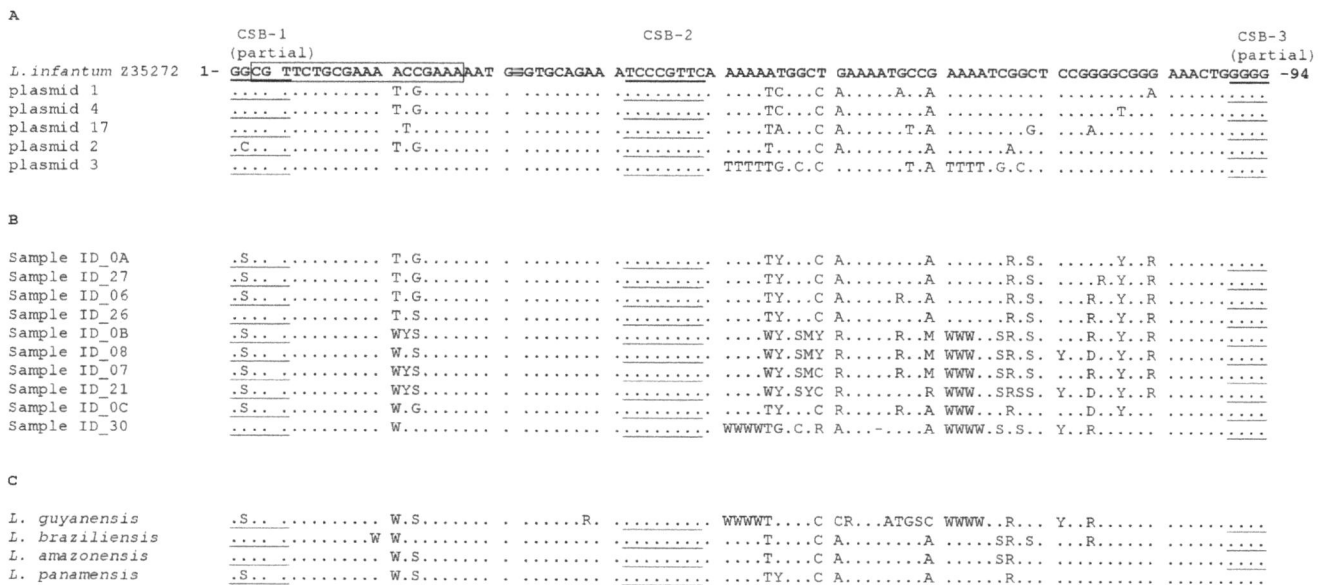

**Figure 6. Sequence alignment of kDNA minicircle conserved region amplified with primers MaryF-MaryR.** Panel A: alignment of five clones derived from *L. (L.) infantum* MHOM/TN/80/IPT1 strain. Panel B: alignment of PCR products from canine clinical samples. Panel C: alignment of PCR products obtained from New World *Leishmania* species. The boxed sequence represents the MLF primer. Underlined sequences represent CSBs box.

*(L.) infantum* MHOM/TN/80/IPT1 (Mann-Whitney test p< 0.0001). Average Tm values obtained with HRM analysis from 32 replicates are shown in Table 1. These results suggest that it is possible to discriminate between *Leishmania* (*Viannia*) and *Leishmania* (*Leishmania*) subgenera by performing real-time PCR followed by melt or HRM analysis, corroborating similar results previously obtained by Pita-Pereira *et al.* [24], obtained with Brazilian strains. Moreover, using HRM analysis we were also able to discriminate between the reference strain *L. (L.) infantum* MHOM/TN/80/IPT1, showing a characteristic double peak, and *L. (L.) amazonensis*, showing a single peak (Fig. 5D) (Table 1). The HRM intra-assay analysis showed good reproducibility up to 0.1 parasite equivalent/reaction (average Ct ~31) in samples containing 30 ng canine DNA as background (Table 2). Below this parasite concentration, the CV values were sensibly higher and the Tm of the peaks appeared slightly shifted.

## Canine Clinical Sample Analysis

A total of 62 different canine blood samples from the Marches region (Central Italy), where *L. (L.) infantum* is present as a veterinary parasite, were analyzed with IFAT and qPCR assays (Table 3). These samples were divided into 4 groups: diagnosed Leishmaniasis (17 samples); asymptomatic Leishmaniasis (21 samples); suspected Leishmaniasis (14 samples); monitored after therapy (10 samples). The samples showing IFAT titres ≥1:160 were defined positive. All samples from dogs diagnosed with Leishmaniasis also showed positive results in qPCR assays, with the exception of 5 samples (22, 23, 24, 25, 28). The qPCRs were subsequently repeated in conjunctival swabs from these dogs, showing positive results (data not shown). Samples from dogs monitored after therapy showed a positive IFAT titre but qPCR did not reveal any parasites, except for samples 26, 27, which showed a low parasite load. Moreover, two samples (6 and 7) from IFAT negative asymptomatic dogs resulted positive in both qPCR assays. Approximately 24% of the canine samples which resulted negative in qPCR assays were tested for the amplification of the B2M gene. The B2M Ct values ranged from 24.13 to 25.07 (average was 24.42±0.34), showing amplifiability and homogeneity of the DNA amount in all the tested samples.

HRM analyses using MLF-MLR primers were also performed in 15 canine clinical samples, always using *L. (L.) infantum* MHOM/TN/80/IPT1 DNA as reference. Despite some variability, the results allowed us to confirm the presence of the subgenus *Leishmania* (*Leishmania*) in all the samples tested. However, the presence of an HRM profile comparable to *L. (L.) infantum* MHOM/TN/80/IPT1 (double peak) was confirmed in 10 of 15 samples (Table 3). Representative melting profiles of clinical samples are depicted in Fig. S5.

## Genetic Variability of kDNA Minicircles

To investigate the genetic variability in the kDNA minicircle sequences amplified by qPCR1 assay, 5 cloned sequences obtained from *L. (L.) infantum* MHOM/TN/80/IPT1 were bidirectionally sequenced. Moreover, 10 amplicons obtained from canine clinical samples were directly sequenced. Comparing these nucleotide sequences by CLUSTALW2 [25], numerous polymorphic *loci* were highlighted both on plasmidic clones and on clinical samples (fig. 6AB). Interestingly, we also found a single base polymorphism G/C in the conserved sequence block 1 (CSB-1).

Regarding the New World species, the sequences of Mary's amplicons were similar to *L. (L.) infantum* (fig. 6C), suggesting that Mary's primers amplify a subclass of minicircles conserved among different subgenera or species.

## Discussion

A singular characteristic of the Kinetoplastida order is the mitochondrial DNA network organized in 20–50 maxicircles and 10,000–20,000 kDNA minicircles [21,26]. With respect to the *Leishmania* genus, about 10,000 kDNA minicircles are estimated per parasite [19]. The conserved region of these minicircles has been used as a diagnostic PCR target since the 1990s [27]. Several genomic targets, other than the kDNA minicircle conserved region, have allowed species or complex differentiation in qPCR [28–30]. However, these assays may be less sensitive due to the lack of multiple copies of target sequence per cell.

The primers designed by Mary et al [15] have been widely used for *L. (L.) infantum* detection with the Taqman probe [31,32]. We used these primers and a new primer pair (MLF-MLR) in a quantitative real-time PCR assay based on SYBR green chemistry. Good sensitivity, specificity and efficiency were obtained with both pairs of primers, although some inhibition was noted using an elevated amount (100 ng) of human DNA as background. Nevertheless, this inhibition did not affect the sensitivity of both assays.

These assays were used to make diagnoses in several canine blood samples, generally confirming the qualitative results obtained with IFAT. The discrepancies observed between IFAT and qPCR in samples from dogs diagnosed with Leishmaniasis (22, 23, 24, 25, 28) may be due to the low parasite content in blood compared to that which is found in bone marrow, lymphnodes or ocular conjunctiva [33]. In fact, a subsequent qPCR in conjunctival swabs from those dogs yielded positive results. On the contrary, the case of two samples that were qPCR positive and IFAT negative from asymptomatic dogs highlights the sensitivity of molecular methods, making this approach also useful for blood donor screening.

The discrepancies in quantification results between qPCR1 and qPCR2 may be explained by kDNA minicircle variability, in terms of number and sequence heterogeneity, in clinical samples. In fact, quantifications were performed using a standard curve obtained with DNA from the *L. (L) infantum* MHOM/TN/80/IPT1 strain.

Parasite quantification could be useful in follow-up, disease relapse or therapy monitoring. Parasite quantification by qPCR can be performed using standard curves obtained either with parasite serial dilutions or with dilutions of a cloned target sequence [34]. In this last case it is very important to know the amount of the PCR target per cell [35]. We attempted to quantify the amount of kDNA minicircles in *L. (L.) infantum* MHOM/TN/80/IPT1 WHO international reference strain with MaryF-MaryR primers and MLF-MLR primers using a cloned sequence as reference standard, resulting in about 26,000 and 1,200 copies per cell, respectively. The value obtained with MaryF-MaryR primers is greater than the value usually reported in literature [19,34]. This may be due to the variability in kDNA minicircle number observed among different strains [15]. On the other hand, the value obtained with MLF-MLR primers represents a subclass of minicircles matching the primer sequences, as demonstrated by sequencing data. In fact, the heterogeneity of the kDNA minicircle conserved region was shown by sequencing five cloned sequences amplified with Mary's primers (clones n. 1, 2, 3, 4, 17). The sequences were aligned, revealing several variations. Only clone n. 3 showed a perfect match with MLF-MLR primers, indicating that the kDNA minicircle sequence amplified by these primers was a subclass of the total kDNA minicircle population. This variability could make absolute quantification of *Leishmania* parasites in clinical samples difficult to achieve; however, the qPCR assays could still be useful for monitoring the relative changes of parasite loads during disease and/or therapy in clinical specimens from single patients.

The GC content in the Mary's amplicons varied between 53.2% (clone n. 3) and 48.9% (clone n. 17), accounting for the two melting peaks observed in HRM analysis. Direct sequencing of qPCR1 amplicons from clinical samples confirmed the heterogeneity of these samples (Fig. 6B). It is worth noting the presence of a yet-to-be-described polymorphic site (G/C) in the conserved block 1 (CSB-1), which was confirmed with direct sequencing of PCR products from clinical samples. Due to the observed variability, SYBR green-based assays seem to be preferable to probe-based assays, unless the probe is designed on the 27 conserved nucleotides encompassing the CSB-2 region (Fig. 6) or it overlaps one of the primers.

These PCR assays were also used to test New World *Leishmania* species: *L. (L.) amazonensis*, *L. (V.) guyanensis*, *L. (V.) panamensis* and *L. (V.) braziliensis*. As represented in Fig. S2, primers MaryF-MaryR and MLF-MLR amplified all these New World species. However, a BLAST search highlighted the lack of sequence homology for MaryF-MaryR primers in *L. (V.) guyanensis*, *L. (V.) panamensis* and *L. (V.) braziliensis* kDNA minicircle sequences, and 4–7 mismatches in *L. (L.) amazonensis* kDNA minicircle sequences. In addition, MLF-MLR primers showed from 1 to 6 mismatches with these species' sequences in Genbank database. Nevertheless, the kDNA minicircle sequences belonging to these species were also amplifiable under very stringent conditions (annealing temperature up to 65°C), indicating the presence of a subpopulation of minicircles with sequences matching the primers used. The fact that Mary's primers can amplify New World species has recently been confirmed [36]. Taken together, these data suggest that Mary's primers amplify a subclass of minicircles conserved among different subgenera or species. However, this does not explain the differences in Tm observed with MLF-MLR primers since the target of these primers belongs to a different subclass of minicircles.

When New World species DNA was used as a template, the qPCR2 assay resulted in lower Ct values than those found with the qPCR1 assay. Hence, it could be hypothesized that these New World species have more kDNA minicircles amplifiable (perfectly matching) by MLF-MLR primers respect to MaryF-MaryR primers.

The early characterization of the infecting parasite is important for appropriate treatment and evolution of the disease [9]. The ability to discriminate between the subgenera *Leishmania* (*Leishmania*) and *Leishmania* (*Viannia*) using real-time PCR and melt analysis targeting kinetoplast DNA has already been demonstrated in Brazilian *Leishmania* strains [24]. Here we confirmed that it is possible to discriminate between *Leishmania* (*Leishmania*) and *Leishmania* (*Viannia*) subgenera using MLF-MLR primers. The assays were performed on the *L. (L.) infantum* WHO reference strain and *L. (L.) amazonensis*, *L. (V.) guyanensis*, *L. (V.) panamensis*, *L. (V.) braziliensis* isolates (Fig. 5B).

Saturating fluorescent dyes such as LC Green, SYTO9 or Eva Green were generally considered necessary for HRM analysis [37]. However, also SYBR Green has proven to be a very successful dye for HRM analysis using the Rotor-Gene 6000 [38,39], probably due to the technical features of this instrument (i.e. high thermal precision, short optical path, multiple readings for each thermal point). Therefore, performing HRM analysis with SYBR green, we were able to further confirm the Tm differences and to discriminate, in the subgenus *Leishmania* (*Leishmania*), between *L. (L.) infantum* WHO reference strain and *L. (L.) amazonensis* (Fig. 5D). These results were also confirmed in 15 canine clinical samples from Central Italy: although clinical samples showed a greater variability in Tm, it was always possible to confirm the presence of *Leishmania* (*Leishmania*) DNA or to exclude the presence of *Leishmania* (*Viannia*) DNA. Moreover, in 10 of 15 samples, the HRM profile typical of the *L. (L.) infantum* WHO reference strain was also confirmed. The fact that five clinical samples did not show the first peak may be due to kDNA minicircle variability in the parasite. Samples that amplify late (Ct>30) or fail to reach a plateau in the PCR phase can result in inconclusive or low-resolution HRM data [40]. In our experience, reproducible Tm profiles were obtained when amplicons Ct values were approximately from 20 to 30. Out of this range, it should be difficult to compare Tm profiles (Table 2) and this could be a limit of the method when clinical samples with low parasite load are analyzed.

The fact that clinical sample DNA was in low-salt buffer and DNA from *L. (L.) infantum* MHOM/TN/80/IPT1 (used as positive control in all qPCR and HRM analyses) was Chelex-purified did not affect the analyses since chelex-purified DNA was diluted at least 1:10,000 prior to be used as template and proved not to induce PCR inhibition.

In conclusion, the new SYBR green-based assay developed using MLF-MLR primers was shown to reliably detect *L. (L.) infantum* in canine clinical samples. Moreover, the kDNA minicircle constant region in the *L. (L.) infantum* WHO international reference strain was quantified and several polymorphic sites were highlighted. The qPCR2 followed by HRM analysis has shown to be able to discriminate between subgenera *Leishmania* (*Leishmania*) and *Leishmania* (*Viannia*), confirming the results previously obtained in Brazilian strains, and to differentiate the *L. (L) infantum* WHO reference strain from *L. (L.) amazonensis*.

## Supporting Information

**Figure S1 Melting analysis of PCR products.** Melting temperature analysis of amplicons generated with primers MaryF-MaryR (A) and MLF-MLR (B) are shown. The Tm were 87.0°C and 85.3°C, respectively. Moreover, no dimers or non-specific products were detected.

**Figure S2 Conventional PCR under stringent conditions.** The PCR was conducted under stringent conditions (annealing temperature 65°C) with primers MaryF-MaryR (A) and MLF-MLR (B). 1: *L. (L.) infantum* ($2.3 \times 10^{-4}$ ng DNA/tube) (positive control); 2: *L. (L.) amazonensis* (1 ng DNA/tube); 3: *L. (V.) guyanensis* (2.3 ng DNA/tube); 4: *L. (V.) panamensis* (1.8 ng DNA/tube); 5: *L. (V.) braziliensis* (1.3 ng DNA/tube). All samples were tested in duplicate. A 100 bp-DNA ladder and a marker 9 (Fermentas) were used as reference in panel A and B, respectively.

**Figure S3 Standard curves with human DNA as background.** Standard curves were obtained from serial dilutions of *L. (L.) infantum* MHOM/TN/80/IPT1 DNA with primers MaryF-MaryR (A) and MLF-MLR (B) in the presence of 100 ng of human DNA per PCR tube. *L. (L.) infantum* DNA scalar dilutions were equivalent to 100, 0.1, 0.01 and 0.001 parasites/tube.

**Figure S4 Standard curves with canine DNA as background.** Standard curves were obtained from serial dilutions of *L. (L.) infantum* MHOM/TN/80/IPT1 DNA with primers MaryF-MaryR (A) and MLF-MLR (B) in the presence of 30 ng of canine DNA per PCR tube. *L. (L.) infantum* DNA scalar dilutions were equivalent to 100, 10, 1, 0.1, 0.01 and 0.001 parasites/tube.

**Figure S5 Representative HRM profiles of amplicons obtained with MLF-MLR primers (qPCR2) in clinical samples.** All samples are shown in duplicates. The melting profile of *L. (L.) infantum* MHOM/TN/80/IPT1 was always included as reference. The samples 3 and 4 show a single peak, corresponding to peak 2 of *L. (L.) infantum* (A). The samples 2, 6, 7, 8 show two peaks corresponding to peak 1 and 2 of *L. (L.) infantum* (B, C, D). Tm values are indicated in Table 3.

## Acknowledgments

We would like to thank Dr. Fabrizio Vitale, Dr. Tiziana Lupo, Dr. Stefano Reale from IZS Palermo and Dr. Mirella Ciaccio from CNR Palermo for providing *Leishmania* strains and isolates. We also wish to thank the Veterinary Clinic "S. Teresa", Fano (PU) Italy, for providing canine clinical samples; Dr. Mirco Fanelli, Dr. Stefano Amatori and Dr. Elena Bertozzini from the Biotechnology section of University of Urbino for technical assistance.

## Author Contributions

Conceived and designed the experiments: MC LG. Performed the experiments: MC. Analyzed the data: MC LG MM. Contributed reagents/materials/analysis tools: AM MM. Wrote the paper: MC LG.

## References

1. Murray HW, Berman JD, Davies CR, Saravia NG (2005) Advances in leishmaniasis. Lancet 366: 1561–1577.
2. Alvar J, Velez ID, Bern C, Herrero M, Desjeux P, et al. (2012) Leishmaniasis worldwide and global estimates of its incidence. PLoS One 7: e35671.
3. Desjeux P (2004) Leishmaniasis: current situation and new perspectives. Comp Immunol Microbiol Infect Dis 27: 305–318.
4. Marty P, Le FY, Giordana D, Brugnetti A (1992) Leishmanin reaction in the human population of a highly endemic focus of canine leishmaniasis in Alpes-Maritimes, France. Trans R Soc Trop Med Hyg 86: 249–250.
5. Semiao-Santos SJ, el HA, Ferreira E, Pires CA, Sousa C, et al. (1995) Evora district as a new focus for canine leishmaniasis in Portugal. Parasitol Res 81: 235–239.
6. Alvar J, Canavate C, Molina R, Moreno J, Nieto J (2004) Canine leishmaniasis. Adv Parasitol 57: 1–88.
7. Cabral M, O'Grady JE, Gomes S, Sousa JC, Thompson H, et al. (1998) The immunology of canine leishmaniosis: strong evidence for a developing disease spectrum from asymptomatic dogs. Vet Parasitol 76: 173–180.
8. Sideris V, Papadopoulou G, Dotsika E, Karagouni E (1999) Asymptomatic canine leishmaniasis in Greater Athens area, Greece. Eur J Epidemiol 15: 271–276.
9. Goto H, Lindoso JA (2010) Current diagnosis and treatment of cutaneous and mucocutaneous leishmaniasis. Expert Rev Anti Infect Ther 8: 419–433.
10. Gradoni L, Gramiccia M (2000) Leishmaniasis. OIE manual of standards for diagnostic tests and vaccine, Office International des Epizooties, pp. 802–812.
11. Iniesta L, Fernandez-Barredo S, Bulle B, Gomez MT, Piarroux R, et al. (2002) Diagnostic techniques to detect cryptic leishmaniasis in dogs. Clin Diagn Lab Immunol 9: 1137–1141.
12. Gradoni L, Gramiccia M, Khoury C, Maroli M (2004) Guidelines for the control of the canine reservoir of zoonotic visceral leishmaniasis in Italy. Rapporti ISTISAN 04/12. Istituto Superiore di Sanità, Rome, Italy.
13. Sudarshan M, Weirather JL, Wilson ME, Sundar S (2011) Study of parasite kinetics with antileishmanial drugs using real-time quantitative PCR in Indian visceral leishmaniasis. J Antimicrob Chemother 66: 1751–1755.
14. Manna L, Reale S, Vitale F, Picillo E, Pavone LM, et al. (2008) Real-time PCR assay in *Leishmania*-infected dogs treated with meglumine antimoniate and allopurinol. Vet J 177: 279–282.
15. Mary C, Faraut F, Lascombe L, Dumon H (2004) Quantification of *Leishmania infantum* DNA by a real-time PCR assay with high sensitivity. J Clin Microbiol 42: 5249–5255.
16. Lachaud L, Chabbert E, Dubessay P, Reynes J, Lamothe J, et al. (2001) Comparison of various sample preparation methods for PCR diagnosis of visceral leishmaniasis using peripheral blood. J Clin Microbiol 39: 613–617.
17. Lachaud L, Marchergui-Hammami S, Chabbert E, Dereure J, Dedet JP, et al. (2002) Comparison of six PCR methods using peripheral blood for detection of canine visceral leishmaniasis. J Clin Microbiol 40: 210–215.
18. Shlomai J (2004) The structure and replication of kinetoplast DNA. Curr Mol Med 4: 623–647.
19. Degrave W, Fernandes O, Campbell D, Bozza M, Lopes U (1994) Use of molecular probes and PCR for detection and typing of *Leishmania*-a mini-review. Mem Inst Oswaldo Cruz 89: 463–469.
20. Simpson L (1986) Kinetoplast DNA in trypanosomid flagellates. Int Rev Cytol 99: 119–179.
21. Simpson L (1997) The genomic organization of guide RNA genes in kinetoplastid protozoa: several conundrums and their solutions. Mol Biochem Parasitol 86: 133–141.
22. Vergel C, Walker J, Saravia NG (2005) Amplification of human DNA by primers targeted to *Leishmania* kinetoplast DNA and post-genome considerations in the detection of parasites by a polymerase chain reaction. Am J Trop Med Hyg 72: 423–429.

23. Harris E, Kropp G, Belli A, Rodriguez B, Agabian N (1998) Single-step multiplex PCR assay for characterization of New World *Leishmania* complexes. J Clin Microbiol 36: 1989–1995.
24. Pita-Pereira D, Lins R, Oliveira MP, Lima RB, Pereira BA, et al. (2012) SYBR Green-based real-time PCR targeting kinetoplast DNA can be used to discriminate between the main etiologic agents of Brazilian cutaneous and visceral leishmaniases. Parasit Vectors 5: 15.
25. Larkin MA, Blackshields G, Brown NP, Chenna R, McGettigan PA, et al. (2007) Clustal W and Clustal X version 2.0. Bioinformatics 23: 2947–2948.
26. Simpson L, Da SA (1971) Isolation and characterization of kinetoplast DNA from *Leishmania tarentolae*. J Mol Biol 56: 443–473.
27. Rodgers MR, Popper SJ, Wirth DF (1990) Amplification of kinetoplast DNA as a tool in the detection and diagnosis of *Leishmania*. Exp Parasitol 71: 267–275.
28. Schulz A, Mellenthin K, Schonian G, Fleischer B, Drosten C (2003) Detection, differentiation, and quantitation of pathogenic *Leishmania* organisms by a fluorescence resonance energy transfer-based real-time PCR assay. J Clin Microbiol 41: 1529–1535.
29. Tupperwar N, Vineeth V, Rath S, Vaidya T (2008) Development of a real-time polymerase chain reaction assay for the quantification of *Leishmania* species and the monitoring of systemic distribution of the pathogen. Diagn Microbiol Infect Dis 61: 23–30.
30. Tsukayama P, Nunez JH, De Los SM, Soberon V, Lucas CM, et al. (2013) A FRET-based real-time PCR assay to identify the main causal agents of New World tegumentary leishmaniasis. PLoS Negl Trop Dis 7: e1956.
31. Aoun O, Mary C, Roqueplo C, Marie JL, Terrier O, et al. (2009) Canine leishmaniasis in south-east of France: screening of *Leishmania infantum* antibodies (western blotting, ELISA) and parasitaemia levels by PCR quantification. Vet Parasitol 166: 27–31.
32. Martin-Ezquerra G, Fisa R, Riera C, Rocamora V, Fernandez-Casado A, et al. (2009) Role of *Leishmania* spp. infestation in nondiagnostic cutaneous granulomatous lesions: report of a series of patients from a Western Mediterranean area. Br J Dermatol 161: 320–325.
33. Gramiccia M, Di MT, Fiorentino E, Scalone A, Bongiorno G, et al. (2010) Longitudinal study on the detection of canine *Leishmania* infections by conjunctival swab analysis and correlation with entomological parameters. Vet Parasitol 171: 223–228.
34. Quaresma PF, Murta SM, Ferreira EC, da Rocha-Lima AC, Xavier AA, et al. (2009) Molecular diagnosis of canine visceral leishmaniasis: identification of *Leishmania* species by PCR-RFLP and quantification of parasite DNA by real-time PCR. Acta Trop 111: 289–294.
35. Galluzzi L, Bertozzini E, Penna A, Perini F, Garcés E, et al. (2010) Analysis of rRNA gene content in the Mediterranean dinoflagellate *Alexandrium catenella* and *Alexandrium taylori*: implications for the quantitative real-time PCR-based monitoring methods. J Appl Phycol 22: 1–9.
36. Cruz I, Millet A, Carrillo E, Chenik M, Salotra P, et al. (2013) An approach for interlaboratory comparison of conventional and real-time PCR assays for diagnosis of human leishmaniasis. Exp Parasitol 134: 281–289.
37. Reed GH, Kent JO, Wittwer CT (2007) High-resolution DNA melting analysis for simple and efficient molecular diagnostics. Pharmacogenomics 8: 597–608.
38. Price EP, Smith H, Huygens F, Giffard PM (2007) High-resolution DNA melt curve analysis of the clustered, regularly interspaced short-palindromic-repeat locus of *Campylobacter jejuni*. Appl Environ Microbiol 73: 3431–3436.
39. Pornprasert S, Phusua A, Suanta S, Saetung R, Sanguansermsri T (2008) Detection of alpha-thalassemia-1 Southeast Asian type using real-time gap-PCR with SYBR Green1 and high resolution melting analysis. Eur J Haematol 80: 510–514.
40. White H, Potts G (2006) Mutation scanning by high resolution melt analysis. Evaluation of RotorGene™ 6000 (Corbett Life Science), HR1™ and 384 well LightScanner™ (Idaho Technology). Technology Assessment. National Genetics Reference Laboratory (Wessex), Salisbury, UK.

# 9

# Using Auxiliary Information to Improve Wildlife Disease Surveillance When Infected Animals Are Not Detected: A Bayesian Approach

**Dennis M. Heisey[1]\*, Christopher S. Jennelle[2]¤, Robin E. Russell[1], Daniel P. Walsh[1]**

**1** United States Geological Survey, National Wildlife Health Center, Madison, Wisconsin, United States of America, **2** Department of Forest and Wildlife Ecology, University of Wisconsin, Madison, Wisconsin, United States of America

## Abstract

There are numerous situations in which it is important to determine whether a particular disease of interest is present in a free-ranging wildlife population. However adequate disease surveillance can be labor-intensive and expensive and thus there is substantial motivation to conduct it as efficiently as possible. Surveillance is often based on the assumption of a simple random sample, but this can almost always be improved upon if there is auxiliary information available about disease risk factors. We present a Bayesian approach to disease surveillance when auxiliary risk information is available which will usually allow for substantial improvements over simple random sampling. Others have employed risk weights in surveillance, but this can result in overly optimistic statements regarding freedom from disease due to not accounting for the uncertainty in the auxiliary information; our approach remedies this. We compare our Bayesian approach to a published example of risk weights applied to chronic wasting disease in deer in Colorado, and we also present calculations to examine when uncertainty in the auxiliary information has a serious impact on the risk weights approach. Our approach allows "apples-to-apples" comparisons of surveillance efficiencies between units where heterogeneous samples were collected.

**Editor:** James M. McCaw, University of Melbourne, Australia

**Funding:** The support for this study was provided by the United States Geological Survey-National Wildlife Health Center. The funders had no role in study design, data collection and analysis, decision to publish, or preparation of the manuscript.

**Competing Interests:** The authors have declared that no competing interests exist.

\* E-mail: dheisey@usgs.gov

¤ Current address: Iowa Department of Natural Resources, Boone, Iowa, United States of America

## Introduction

Managing a harmful contagious disease in either domestic animals or wildlife can typically result in expensive and unpopular actions such as culling and quarantine. For free-ranging wildlife populations subject to hunting, restrictions on carcass transportation and hunting over bait are other examples of common but unpopular disease management tools. If a management unit (or population) can be declared "disease-free", these actions can be avoided. Demonstrating "freedom from disease" in an animal population is rooted in regulatory requirements pertaining to national and international domestic animal trade [1], although the phrase can be conceptually and legally ambiguous [2],[3]. The only way to demonstrate an area is truly disease-free is to conduct a complete census, which is almost always impractical. Instead, a sample of animals from a population must be tested to obtain a probabilistic statement about disease level. Sampling methods to achieve this goal have been investigated for several decades (see [4] for review), and management agencies are increasingly tasked with developing sampling programs in free ranging wildlife [5],[6].

Although the term freedom-from-disease is commonly used in this sampling setting [7],[8],[9], it is a misnomer from the statistical point of view. What is usually actually meant is that disease prevalence $\pi$ is ascertained to be below some designated target threshold $\pi_t$ with some level of "assurance" (we elaborate on

what this means later). Indeed, policy may allow an area to be declared "free from disease" even if disease is observed to be present, but at an acceptably low level $\pi < \pi_t$ (e.g., [7]). Determining what target prevalence level $\pi_t$ is acceptably low for an area to be deemed disease-free is a case-by-case policy issue (see [3]) which we do not address; our concern is in efficiently determining whether the true prevalence $\pi$ is less than the target threshold $\pi_t$ with an appropriate degree of statistical assurance.

Sampling to ascertain freedom-from-disease is often referred to as surveillance. Surveillance in free-ranging wildlife is typically very expensive financially and logistically. While easy to design, popular simple random sampling (SRS) may also be the least efficient for heterogeneous populations and will in general require the greatest number of samples to determine $\pi < \pi_t$ with the degree of prescribed assurance. Large gains over SRS in terms of information per sample can often be realized with some type of stratified, targeted, or weighted sampling.

We use surveillance for chronic wasting disease (CWD) for illustration. Chronic wasting disease is a prion disease of free-ranging and captive cervids (deer, elk, moose), and although there is no evidence that it has been transmitted to humans, it is concerning because prion diseases also include bovine spongiform encephalopathy (BSE), or "mad cow" disease, known to be transmissible to humans. CWD has been discovered in 15 states in the United States of America, and negatively affects cervid populations in those regions. Additionally, its known extent continues to spread [10]. For such diseases, it is desirable to detect their presence while the prevalence is still very low and hopefully amenable to management, hence the target thresholds $\pi_t$ are typically quite low, and potentially very challenging to assess. We show the value in using what is known about individual-specific infection risk factors obtained from outside the surveillance area but reasonably generalizable to the surveillance area. This work was initially motivated to facilitate the design of efficient surveillance. However, our approach also provides a valuable tool for evaluating the effectiveness of surveillance already conducted; in fact we would argue an approach such as ours is really the only valid way to make "apples-to-apples" comparisons of the effectiveness of multiple surveillance efforts (either in space or time) involving heterogeneous samples.

Several papers have considered the SRS designs of CWD surveillance programs for free-ranging wild animal populations [11],[12]. Nusser et al. [13] explored sampling designs in a simulated CWD system and highlighted the shortcomings of convenience sampling, proposing alternatives based on probability sampling. Diefenbach, Rosenberry and Boyd [14] considered CWD surveillance protocols in Pennsylvania and called for an expanded surveillance stream beyond sole reliance on hunter harvested deer. More recently, to exploit auxiliary information about CWD risk, Walsh and Miller (WM; [15]) developed a surveillance design incorporating a points-based risk factor weighting system (also see [16]). By focusing on high value (high risk) animals, statistical assurance of freedom-from-disease can be achieved with substantially fewer animals than SRS.

Like stratified sampling designs, weighted surveillance programs such as WM's promise great increases in efficiency when there is substantial population heterogeneity in the measured response (e.g. infected or not) associated with observable risk factors. Typically two sample sets are required: 1) a "learning sample" from an area where the disease is present, and 2) the "surveillance sample" from the area to be evaluated. The learning sample is used to determine what factors, such as age and sex, put animals at different risks for infection. In essence, this is a regression problem, where the risk weights are estimated by (potentially transformed) regression coefficients from the learning sample. In contrast to the learning sample, it is typical to not observe any diseased animals in the surveillance sample. But even in the absence of positive animals in the surveillance sample, risk weights from the learning set can increase the assurance that $\pi < \pi_t$ in the surveillance population, which forms the basis of the WM approach. As with regression coefficients in general, the precision and accuracy of these estimated weights depends on the quality and quantity of data used to estimate them. Taking these regression coefficients or weights at face-value without accounting for their uncertainty can result in a considerably over-optimistic assessment of the assurance of $\pi < \pi_t$.

Some background seems desirable before we present our method. We first present how the goal of disease surveillance is equivalent to applying a confidence or credible bound on $\pi$. This task has historically been a statistical challenge; when none of $N$ samples are positive it amounts to putting a confidence bound on an estimate of zero. Special techniques are required, and there are both frequentist confidence bound and Bayesian credible bound procedures that perform well for the $0/N$ situation. However, because of the nature of the calculations, frequentist confidence bounds appear to troublesome when auxiliary data (a learning set) exists, while Bayesian procedures appear to generalize naturally. Therefore, we propose a Bayesian approach that automatically propagates uncertainty about risk factors and weights sampled

individuals appropriately. The development of our approach is as follows:

1) We first show SRS surveillance as traditionally designed and conducted can be productively framed as a traditional one-sided hypothesis test.

2) Then, we note the equivalence of one-sided hypothesis tests and confidence bounds.

3) Frequentist confidence bounds work fine in the SRS context, but Bayesian credible bounds prove more useful for extension to auxiliary information. So, we develop a Bayesian credible bound that has good frequentist coverage properties using a "prior matching" approach. Prior matching involves identifying Bayesian posterior probabilities that also have interpretations as frequentist confidence intervals [17].

4) We briefly consider various concepts of "statistical assurance"; although confidence and credible bounds "look" similar, they have very different substantive interpretations with respect to what they tell us about $\pi < \pi_t$.

5) We show how a learning and surveillance sample can be combined into a single augmented regression analysis containing data set-specific intercepts, and how statements about the assurance of $\pi < \pi_t$ in the surveillance sample can then be formulated in terms of either confidence or credible bounds on the surveillance sample-specific intercept. This is readily accomplished in a Bayesian setting using the software WinBUGS [18], which generalizes the credible bounds from the SRS situation. We present a hypothetical example, and distinguish between what we call "nominal" and "real" weights. The rationale for the specific regression models structure is presented in Appendix S1 (Weight Models).

6) We compare real weights, which accommodate uncertainty in the learning data set, to nominal weights, which are unadjusted point estimates of sample weights. We demonstrate that real weights should be preferred when the learning data set is small to moderate in size. We compare our real and nominal weights to the WM's weights obtained for Colorado mule deer (*Odocoileus hemionus*).

7) We discuss the application of our ideas from both surveillance design and surveillance evaluation perspectives. We advocate real weights as a heuristic surveillance design tool; that is, various sample compositions can be evaluated by totaling up their real weight point scores. To evaluate a surveillance program after it has been performed, we advocate an exact posterior bound approach.

We provide the software code that we used for our examples in the Supplement.

## Model Background

### Freedom-from-disease surveillance as a traditional hypothesis test

Frequentist hypothesis tests are usually designed such that the Type I error rate ($\alpha$) is controlled at some prescribed level. The Type I error rate is the probability that the alternate hypothesis ($H_A$) is declared true when in fact the null hypothesis ($H_0$) is true. Statistical hypothesis tests should be structured such that the Type I error is the scientifically more important because hypothesis tests generally do not control the Type II error rate [19]. Regardless of whether our focus is on wildlife, domestic animal, or human health, in freedom-from-disease testing, we want to control the probability ($\alpha$) we incorrectly declare units disease-free, especially when the consequences of mistakenly concluding a unit is disease-free are serious. If $\pi_t$ is the disease-free policy target (or threshold) prevalence, with freedom-from-disease really meaning $\pi < \pi_t$, then these considerations lead to the appropriate hypothesis test structure:

$$H_0 : \pi \geq \pi_t$$

$$H_A : \pi < \pi_t$$

This hypothesis structure reflects that the burden of proof rests on the declaration that a unit is disease-free (e.g., [19], [20], [21]).

Let $C$ be the number of positive animals observed in a sample of size $N$. For a declaration of freedom-from-disease to be credible, $C = 0$ (this might not be the case for all diseases, but few would question this for CWD) prescribes the critical region for this test (probability of rejecting $H_0$), which means the total sample size $N$ must be manipulated to achieve $\alpha$ (this is a little different from most typical testing setups in which $N$ is fixed and the critical region is manipulated to achieve $\alpha$, but this is of no particular significance otherwise). The Type I error rate $\alpha$ is the maximum probability of observing the critical region $C = 0$ when $H_0$: $\pi \geq \pi_t$ is true. Assuming a large population with SRS, this is generally given as $\Pr(C > 0) = (1 - \pi)^N$ under $H_0$, which is maximized at $\alpha = (1 - \pi_t)^N$. If for example we set $\alpha = 0.05$ and $\pi_t = 0.01$, we obtain $N(\alpha = 0.05, \pi_t = 0.01) = 298$ (for small populations, this approach gives conservative results).

These calculations are at the core of most wildlife disease surveillance sampling designs, although they are often not explicitly framed in terms of hypothesis tests. Because the probability of observing at least one positive subject is $\Pr(C > 0) = 1 - (1 - \pi)^N$, solving $\beta = 1 - (1 - \pi)^N$ for $N$ with fixed $\beta$ and $\pi_t$ is sometimes described as a surveillance design that achieves a "confidence of $\beta$" that disease would be detected $\Pr(C > 0)$ if prevalence is greater than or equal to $\pi_t$ (e.g., [11]). While this terminology appears to be blending aspects of hypothesis testing and confidence intervals, the intent and effect appear to be essentially the same as our hypothesis test framing.

## The Equivalence of hypothesis tests and confidence bounds

There is a one-to-one correspondence between one-sided hypothesis tests and confidence bounds (e.g., [19]), and an $\alpha$-level one-sided hypothesis test can always be inverted to obtain a $1 - \alpha$ confidence bound (we address confidence intervals/bounds and the notion of coverage probability in more detail later). Thus confidence bounds lead to a unifying interpretation of disease surveillance in terms of supported prevalence values (values consistent with the observation $0/N$), rather than disease detection in a hypothesis testing framework. Disease surveillance can be reframed in terms of a confidence bound: $N$ should be large enough that if $C = 0$ was observed, only prevalence values less than $\pi_t$ are supported at confidence level $1 - \alpha$. This confidence bound view of disease surveillance is implicit in [21].

Thus, disease surveillance objectives can be viewed "simply" as a problem of constructing narrow enough confidence bounds for the situation when $C = 0$ positives out of $N$ samples is observed. Although simple in statement, this problem is not so simple in solution. Most confidence intervals involved in the analysis of binary (0–1) data involve large sample theory (asymptotic) approximations. When $C = 0$, the maximum likelihood estimate

(MLE) of prevalence is 0 and the estimate is on the boundary of the parameter space. At this boundary, Brown, Cai and DasGupta ([22]; BCD) show asymptotic approximations break down and a popular solution is to invert the binomial exact test used in the hypothesis test above, referred to as the "exact" or Clopper-Pearson procedure (BCD). Cai [23] and BCD criticize the Clopper-Pearson procedure because it is conservative; it never produces confidence bounds with coverage less than $1 - \alpha$, and sometimes coverage can be substantially greater. For freedom-from-disease surveillance, conservative coverage seems reasonable as the method should always perform at least as advertised (e.g., [24]) and we adopt the Clopper-Pearson confidence bound as the standard to emulate as closely as reasonably possible.

## Bayesian Credible Intervals; Reverse Engineering to Achieve Good Coverage

Many Bayesians acknowledge the usefulness of the frequentist notion of confidence interval (or bound) coverage probabilities as a performance metric, and employ it to evaluate Bayesian credible intervals (or bounds). Alternatively, a Bayesian perspective often suggests ways in which frequentist confidence intervals can be improved (e.g., [17], [25]).

As noted by Cai [23], exact binomial Clopper-Pearson confidence bounds correspond to $Beta_{1-\alpha}(1, N)$, meaning the $(1 - \alpha) * 100$ percentile of a $Beta(a = 1, b = N)$ distribution. When viewed in a Bayesian context as a posterior credible bound given the observations $C = 0|N$, it is reasonable to ask what prior distribution was imposed on $\pi$ to achieve this posterior. To achieve this posterior for a binomial likelihood with $0|N$, it can be seen that this corresponds to assigning the prior $Beta(1, b \to 0)$ to $\pi$ (Appendix S1; Prior Matching). This is a curiously pessimistic prior that puts all the prior mass at $\pi = 1$; it expresses the prior belief that all animals are infected. This pessimism is consistent with the observed conservatism of Clopper-Pearson bounds. BCD advocate the Jeffreys prior Beta(0.5, 0.5) on the basis that resulting confidence intervals are "more accurate" and "less wasteful" than Clopper-Pearson, but this produces coverage that may be considerably less than $1 - \alpha$ (See [25] for a discussion of Jeffreys and other priors). Our initial analyses indicated that Jeffreys priors can produce coverages substantially less than $1 - \alpha$ for small $\pi$, which is a particular problem for freedom-from-disease surveillance studies which should never be liberal. For example, we determined that with $\pi = 0.01$ and $N = 200$, a 95% Jeffreys confidence bound only achieved 87% coverage. We agree with Casella [24] that confidence intervals (and confidence bounds) should perform as advertised; they should never provide substantially less than $1 - \alpha$ coverage.

A popular "common-sense" prior for the analysis of binary data has long been the Bayes-Laplace prior, which is simply the uniform distribution on 0-1 assigned to $\pi$ and is equivalent to the Beta(1,1) distribution. Tuyl, Gerlac and Mengersen [26] argue strongly for the desirability of this prior based on its predictive properties. The Bayes-Laplace prior leads to what we call the Bayes-Laplace confidence bound, which is easily shown to be $Beta_{1-\alpha}(1, N+1)$ and is equivalent to the Clopper-Pearson confidence bound based on $N + 1$ observations (see Appendix S1; Prior Matching). There is essentially no practical difference between the Clopper-Pearson and Bayes-Laplace confidence bounds coverages for moderate sample sizes; in our example above where Jeffreys bounds achieve 87% coverage, Clopper-Pearson and Bayes-Laplace both achieve 100%. While the Bayes-Laplace confidence bound will be slightly more liberal than the Clopper-Pearson, it still tends to be conservative. In a surveillance context, this conservatism is preferable to the liberal error associated with use of Jeffreys prior. We prefer Bayes-Laplace over the "Clopper-Pearson prior" $Beta(1, b \to 0)$, since the latter lacks intuitive motivation and can elicit computational difficulties in the Bayesian MCMC sampling framework (e.g., WinBUGS seems to have problems if $b$ is much less than 0.01).

In the Bayesian context, Bayes-Laplace credible bounds inherit the desirable frequentist characteristics of Bayes-Laplace confidence bounds obtained by prior matching. The problem is that confidence bounds for the $C = 0$ situation seem difficult to generalize beyond the SRS setting, whereas credible bounds seem naturally generalizable, as we will demonstrate. The Bayes-Laplace credible bound is found by solving $\alpha = (1 - \pi_t)^N + 1$, which is easily done by hand calculator. We show how this can also be done in WinBUGS (Software Code S1; Program 1) because it provides a useful stepping stone for later development. If we set $N = 297$, we find the $1 - \alpha$ 95% percentile of the posterior distribution to be $\pi = 0.01$, which although practically the same as the Clopper-Pearson confidence bound has a very different interpretation.

## The Two Meanings of Statistical Assurance

Given the importance of confidence and credible bounds to our approach, some background on both is useful. Both impart information about the statistical assurance of parameter values, but the nature of this assurance is very different and worth understanding in the disease surveillance context. It is not uncommon for practitioners to have an unclear understanding of how to interpret a frequentist confidence bound. (Anyone who feels they really understand confidence intervals should read BCD and see if the feeling remains!) A confidence bound is a random variable. A $1 - \alpha$ upper confidence bound computed from data as $\pi_U$ means that in an infinite number of future sets of samples from the same population with true prevalence $\pi$, if $\pi_U$ is always computed in the same way in these future samples, in at least $(1 - \alpha) * 100\%$ of the infinite future cases $\pi < \pi_U$ would be true. Thus a confidence bound is a statement about the behavior of a random bound in a series of hypothetical sample sets generated from the same underlying process. The confidence bound generated from a given sample of data can be considered one realization from these sample sets. As such, the frequentist confidence bound provides an indirect, yet intuitive (some would claim), measure of assurance regarding $\pi < \pi_U$ in the sample at hand. Many practitioners erroneously conclude that confidence is simply the probability that $\pi < \pi_U$, but this is the definition of a Bayesian credible bound [19]. This difference in interpretation reflects the frequentist versus Bayesian interpretation of probability – "the probabilities of things and the probabilities of our beliefs about things" [27].

Confidence bounds can be criticized for the convoluted interpretation that they require when used as a data interpretation tool (e.g., [19]). On the other hand, there seems to be agreement, even among most Bayesians, that the frequentist notion of coverage probability inherent in confidence bounds is a desirable performance metric for assurance measures. The usual criticism of credible bounds is that it requires the subjective specification of prior belief. It could be argued that the ideal assurance measure shares the strong points of both confidence and credible bounds: credible bounds that enjoy the clear Bayesian interpretation yet achieve good coverage behavior when viewed as frequentist confidence bounds. This justifies our use of the Bayes-Laplace confidence/credible bound (see Appendix S1; Prior Matching). However, it is not the clarity of the Bayesian interpretation that primarily motivates our Bayesian approach. With auxiliary data (a learning set), there appears to be no way forward with respect to

extending frequentist confidence bounds, while the way is clear with Bayesian credible bounds. We consider this in more detail next.

## Model Implementation

### Changing Scales – Binary Regression Models for Surveillance Data

It is traditional to analyze binary event data, such as disease test data, with logistic regression. In essence, the logistic function remaps prevalence $\pi$ from 0 to 1 to a new scale, the logistic scale, which covers the entire real line. Most software programs allow fitting a regression model without any covariates, that is, an intercept-only, or grand mean model. On the logistic scale, this can be represented as $\text{logit}(\pi) = \mu$, where logit() refers to the logistic transformation of prevalence. If one attempts to fit this model using traditional frequentist logistic regression software for the case where no events ($C = 0$) were observed, it will fail because the traditional large sample approximations methods used by popular software break down.

However, the no event case presents no particular challenge in the Bayesian context. This is because Bayesian computations are essentially exact and not based on large sample approximations (WinBUGS uses numerical methods to obtain exact results – the longer it is allowed to run, the smaller the numerical error becomes in general. In contrast, traditional generalized linear model software uses numerical methods to obtain approximate results; numerical errors can be reduced by more iterations but approximation error cannot.)

We illustrate how this is done in WinBUGS (Software Code S1; Program 2) for the surveillance situation where 297 animals were sampled with no positives. We use the complementary log-log (cloglog) link instead of the logistic link, but the basic principle remains the same. We used the logistic link above because readers are much more likely to be familiar with it than the cloglog link, but we develop in the Appendix (Appendix S1; Weight Models) why the cloglog link is better suited to our goals. At this point, it may appear the cloglog transform is simply adding an additional, apparently pointless, step beyond our previous Bayes-Laplace approach. Our reason for presenting this stepping stone becomes clear in the next two sections when we consider auxiliary data from outside the surveillance area.

### Modeling Auxiliary Information

Suppose we have sampled an area known to have CWD; we refer to this as auxiliary information or the learning data set ($L$). Sex is known to be a risk factor for CWD; we will use it for illustration. We will use $x$ to indicate sex, with $x = 0$ for females and $x = 1$ for males. Let $N_x$ be the sex-specific sample size, and let $C_x$ be the respective number of positives found. For illustration, assume $N_0 = N_1 = 200, C_0 = 10$, and $C_1 = 20$; the observed (empirical or apparent) prevalence in males is twice that of females. We could fit the model $\text{cloglog}(C_i / N_i) = \mu_L + \beta x_i$, where $i$ refers to the $i$-th category of samples. Because $x$ is the male indicator, the intercept $\mu_L$ is the cloglog-transformed female prevalence in the learning data set. In this model, $\beta$ is referred to as the log hazard ratio, and $w = \exp(\beta)$ is the hazard ratio (Appendix S1). We will refer to $w$ and estimates of it as "nominal weights".

This model can be readily fitted to the auxiliary data using traditional generalized linear model software. This model is also easily fitted with WinBUGS (Software Code S1; Program 3). (The large-variance normal prior on $\beta$ is a traditional approach to establishing an essentially vague yet proper prior; see for example

Appendix C of [28].) For our hypothetical example the posterior mean (and standard deviation) for the male log hazard ratio $\beta$ is 0.656 (0.379). The posterior mean for the hazard ratio $w = \exp(\beta)$, or nominal weight, is 2.07; very close to the observed 2:1 prevalence ratio observed in the data. As noted, the analyses up to this point could be done with either traditional frequentist or Bayesian software. The problem with the frequentist approach would arise when one then attempts to integrate surveillance data in which no positives were observed.

When we obtain a point estimate of the nominal weight $w$ our certainty in it will depend on the strength of the learning set, just as for any regression coefficient in general. If our data set is small and we obtain an estimate of $w$ of 2, we may be reluctant to conclude that a male is actually worth 2 females, but our certainty in this should increase as the sample size increases. We later describe how to calculate modified weights (which we refer to as real weights) that adjust for such uncertainty due to sample size.

### Augmented Surveillance

We now combine our hypothetical surveillance sample of 297 animals and our learning sample from before. Will the learning data set change our conclusions about surveillance? As we will see, the answer is that it depends. Let $\delta_i$ be an indicator variable for whether the $i$-th sample is from the surveillance ($\delta_i = 1$) or learning data set ($\delta_i = 0$). The model for the augmented analysis then becomes $\text{cloglog}(C_i / N_i) = (1 - \delta_i)\mu_L + \delta_i \mu_S + \beta x_i$, where $\mu_L$ and $\mu_S$ are data-set specific female intercept terms for the learning and surveillance data sets respectively. Note that we can back-transform $\mu_S$ to $\pi_S$, the prevalence in the surveillance sample. Given how the model is parameterized, this is the female prevalence, which we have established as the baseline.

Suppose all 297 surveillance subjects are females. If we run this analysis (Software Code S1; Program 4) and establish a 95% credible bound for $\pi_S$, we find it is $\pi_S = 0.01$. This is exactly as it was before in the absence of any auxiliary learning data. This is exactly as it should be. In the auxiliary analysis, the baseline was established as the females. As the reference group, the observation of a female provides a unit amount of information in the surveillance sample.

Now suppose all 297 surveillance subjects are males (Software Code S1; Program 5). We now find the 95% credible bound for $\pi_S$ to be 0.0058. Recall that $\pi_S$ is the prevalence for the baseline female group; we can now be 95% certain that female prevalence $\pi_S$ is less than 0.0058 with 297 male samples in contrast to 0.01 with 297 female samples. Because the auxiliary sample showed males have a higher risk of infection than the female reference class, they contain more information regarding freedom-from-disease, and hence the smaller bound.

If these models were attempted with traditional maximum likelihood software, they would fail because the MLE for $\mu_S$ in the absence of any positive surveillance events is negative infinity, on the boundary of parameter space. Even if this is "patched" by assigning some small number, usual methods for estimating the standard error of the estimate of $\mu_S$ will fail. (Technically speaking, this failure results from a violation of what are called the "usual regularity conditions" on which traditional standard error approximations are based – in particular the parameter estimate is not in the interior of the parameter space as required.).

Returning to our augmented analysis, the nominal weight of 2.07 suggests that 1 male is worth a little more than 2 females. But this assessment ignores statistical uncertainty in the nominal weight estimate. We can account for this uncertainty by progressively decreasing the surveillance sample of males until the 95% credible bound matches the target $\pi_S = 0.01$, which

occurs at about $N_1 = 173$ males. We call this approach "target bound-matching". Thus, a male surveillance sample is worth about $(297/173) = 1.7$ females, given the information, albeit imperfect, from our learning data set. We will refer to weights obtained in this manner, by target bound-matching, as real weights.

## Model Results

### Weights in General

WM proposed the idea of weights or "points" that could be assigned to an animal to reflect its value for detecting disease, relative to some reference class of animals for which the point value was 1. Under WM's derivation, the parametric expression of their weight was $w_{WM} = \pi_1 / \pi_0$ (considering just two classes, with class 0 being the reference class). Under our derivation (Appendix S1) the parametric expression for our (nominal) weight is $w = \log(1 - \pi_1) / \log(1 - \pi_0)$. Generally speaking, our derivation of $w$ reflects how sample sizes and prevalences influence the probability of detecting at least 1 positive subject in a sample. The different derivations of $w$ versus $w_{WM}$ lead to different behaviors. Because $w$ is based on the probability of detecting at least one positive, $\pi_1 = 1$ has special significance because it means if even one class 1 animal is sampled, a positive will be detected with certainty. When $\pi_1 = 1$, we say that class 1 constitutes a "perfect sentinel" (only one sample is needed), and in which case $w = +\infty$ which is arguably desirable behavior (regardless of the prevalence of the reference class, only one perfect sentinel needs to be sampled). Figure 1 displays the parametric relationship between $w$ and $w_{WM}$, and in particular it shows how they depart as $\pi_1 \to 1$.

These are parametric expressions; in reality one uses estimates of these quantities. As these parametric expressions suggest, the quality of the weight estimates rest largely on the quality of the prevalence estimates. If the prevalence estimates are of low quality with substantial uncertainty, estimates of $w$ and $w_{WM}$ should not be taken at face value but should be discounted in some way for estimation uncertainty, which is considered next.

### Nominal Weights versus Real Weights

As illustrated previously, we propose a method to obtain weights that are adjusted for uncertainty through a process we call "target bound-matching", we refer to these uncertainty adjusted weights as "real weights". For large data sets with many positive cases, real weights and nominal weights should correspond. Here we are primarily interested in the factors that cause them to not correspond, that is, what aspects of an auxiliary data set gives rise to uncertainty when it comes to estimating nominal weights? Considering just two classes, there are 4 statistics involved in estimating weights, which are $N_0$, $N_1$, $C_0$, and $C_1$: the sample sizes in the two classes, and the number of positives in the two classes, respectively. In this 4-dimensional statistics space, what factors result in large departures between real and nominal weights? This requires exploring this sample space in a systematic manner; we were interested in exploring regions of the space that correspond with potential real world scenarios. One factor we wanted to examine was the role of the empirical prevalence ratio, $\hat{\phi} = \hat{\pi}_1 / \hat{\pi}_0$, where $\hat{\pi}_i = C_i / N_i$. Thus we did two sets of analyses, one for $\hat{\phi} = 2$ and one for $\hat{\phi} = 10$. Within each observed prevalence ratio we looked at the effect of total sample size for sample sizes of $N_0 = N_1 = 100$ and $N_0 = N_1 = 200$. With $\hat{\phi}$ and $N_i$ fixed, it was an easy matter to compute all values of $C_i$ consistent with the fixed $\hat{\phi}$ and $N_i$, which we did. We then compute the corresponding estimated nominal weights $\hat{w}$ and real weights $R$ which we

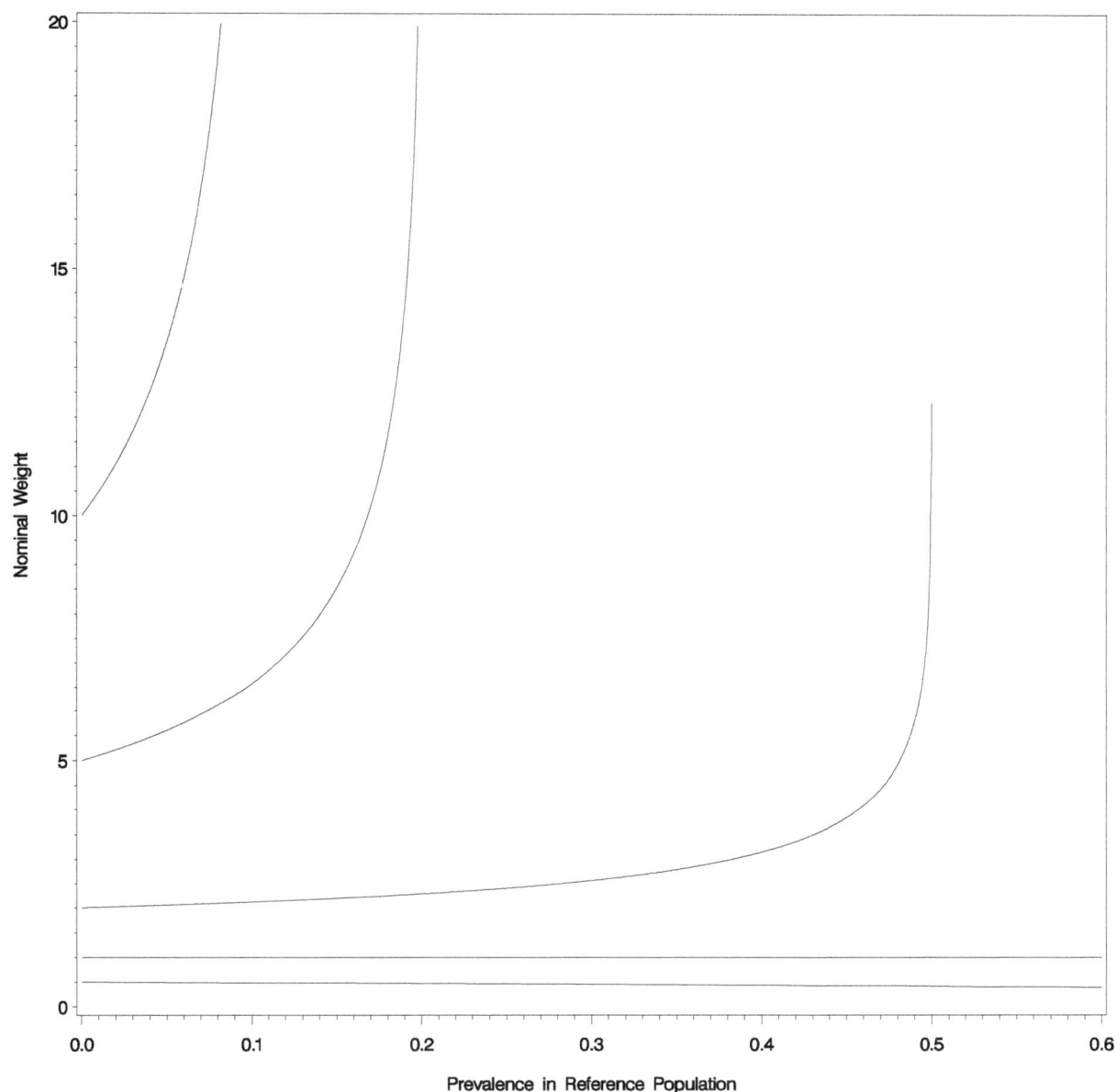

**Figure 1. Nominal weights as a function of the prevalence ratio** $\pi_1 / \pi_0$ **and prevalence** $\pi_0$. Nominal weights are shown for 5 fixed prevalence ratios: 10, 5, 2, 1, and 0.5, which are in ascending order in the figure. The x-axis is the denominator prevalence $\pi_0$. Nominal weights increase rapidly as the numerator prevalence $\pi_1$ approaches 1; as the numerator class becomes more like a "perfect sentinel".

expressed as the ratio $\hat{w}/R$ for standardization; the results surprised us somewhat (Figure 2).

The observed prevalence ratio and total sample size has relatively little influence over the estimated nominal weight/real weight ratio. The primary determinate seemed to the number of events (positives) $C_i$, while the number of trials $N_i$ needed to observe these events seem to have little influence. Figure 2 also clearly illustrates that there is a point of diminishing returns, where the real weights get very close to the nominal weights, and relatively little is learned with additional sampling. The practical implication for the learning set appears to be that one should seek a happy medium; if few positives are observed, the real weights will be low, but beyond a certain number of positives the additional gain in real weight is negligible.

## Real Data Application

Using the auxiliary data from WM's Table 1 of Colorado mule deer/CWD data[15], we first compute point estimates for weights that are not adjusted for uncertainty. We do this in three ways. We used SAS PROC GENMOD (Software Code S1; Program 8) under WM's Poisson assumption to obtain MLEs of their weights $w_{WM}$. As we note above, we need to use a Bayesian approach for augmented (surveillance and auxiliary combined) analyses, but the auxiliary data alone can be equally well analyzed by either Bayesian or frequentist methods, and it is interesting to do so for comparative purposes. We computed Bayesian nominal weights for our binomial model (Software Code S1; Program 6) and their maximum likelihood equivalents using SAS PROC GENMOD (Software Code S1; Program 8). As expected, our estimated

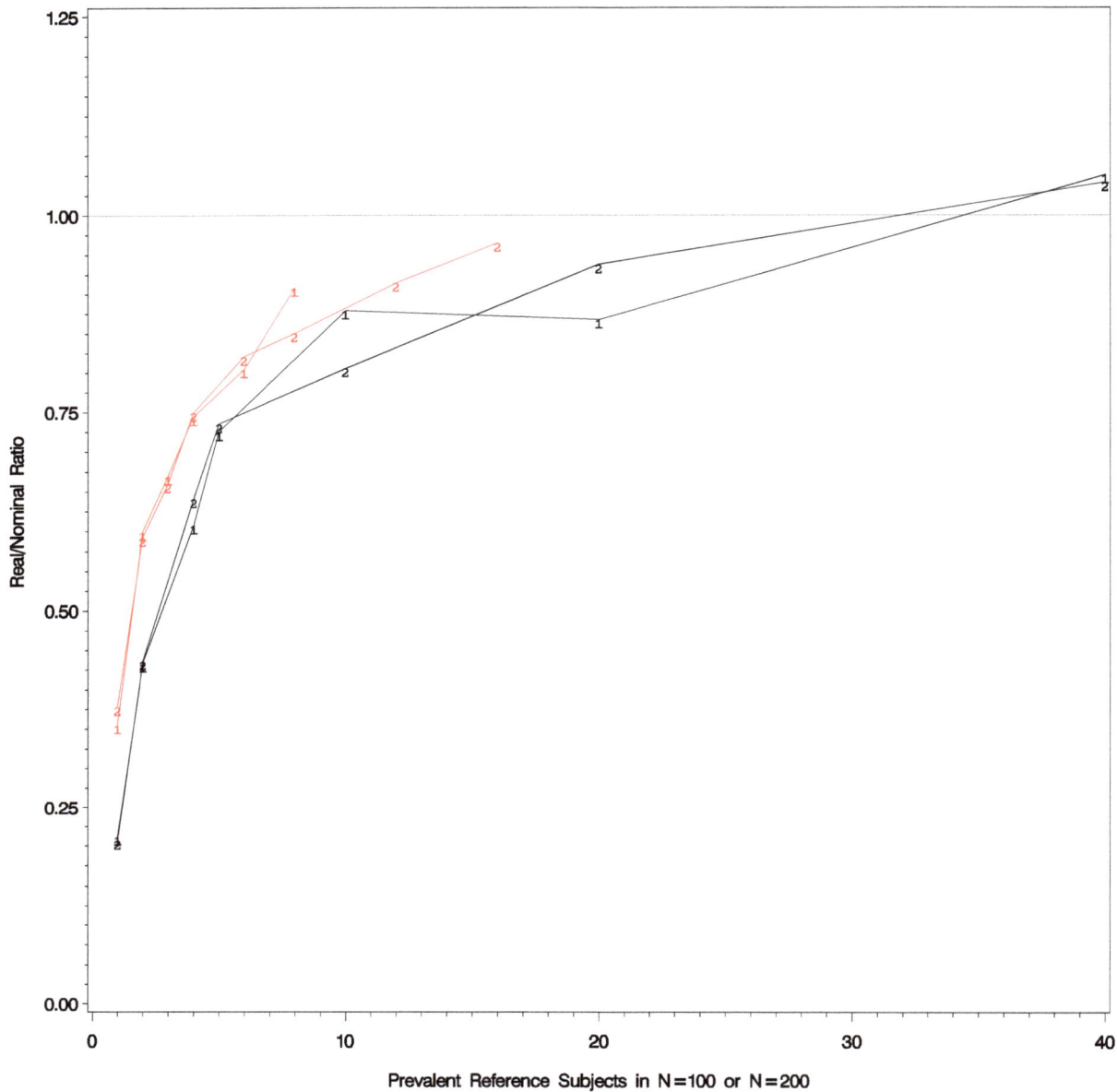

**Figure 2. Factors controlling the departure of real and nominal weights.** The red curves correspond to a prevalence ratio of 10, and the black curves correspond to a prevalence ratio of 2. For each fixed prevalence ratio, two sample sizes $N_0 = N_1 = 100$(plotting symbol = 1) and $N_0 = N_1 = 200$(plotting symbol = 2) are shown. For a fixed prevalence ratio and sample size, one can vary the number of positives in class 0 ($C_0$), and compute the corresponding number of positives in class 1 ($C_1$). The x-axis is $C_0$. One can then compute the nominal and real weights from $C_0, C_1, N_0,$ and $N_1$. The primary determinate for departures between the real and nominal weights appears to be the number of positives in the sample (x-axis), and not the total sample size (1 versus 2 plotting symbol). The apparent prevalence ratio (red versus black) appears to play a minor secondary role.

nominal weights are higher than estimated WM's weights in high prevalence situations (Table 1) because of the sort of behavior demonstrated in Figure 1. The Bayesian and frequentist estimates of our nominal weights are the same for practical purposes.

We then used credible bound matching in our Bayesian model to obtain real weights for the Colorado data set (Table 2). The real weights closely matched the estimated nominal weights obtained from the learning data for all but the three lowest weighted classes. This stability reflects the relatively large number of positives in most of the learning set categories.

## Discussion

We think real weights are useful to motivate the notion that targeted surveillance schemes should accommodate uncertainty. We also think they are a useful design tool for researchers tasked with conducting surveillance – if testing resources are limited, real weights can be used as a rule-of-thumb to prioritize samples during the design and implementation phases. For example, using the Colorado data for illustration, if$\Pr(\pi < 0.01) \geq 0.95$ is the goal, and harvested-adult-males are deemed a reasonable reference category for$\pi$, this goal can be achieved with a surveillance sample of 297 harvested-adult-males. But this goal could also be achieved

**Table 1.** Estimates of nominal CWD surveillance weights for 8 classes of mule deer from Colorado (data from WM[15]) using a binomial complementary log-log regression model with Bayesian and maximum likelihood approaches, as well as a Poisson regression model.

| Mortality Source | Binomial | | Poisson | C/N |
| | Bayesian (SD) | MLE (SD) | MLE (SD) | |
|---|---|---|---|---|
| Suspect-F | 14.1 (2.40) | 14.1 (2.4) | 11.6 (1.6) | 40/111 |
| Suspect-M | 12.2 (2.05) | 12.2 (2.06) | 10.3 (1.46) | 40/125 |
| Other | 1.9 (0.24) | 1.9 (0.25) | 1.9 (0.24) | 77/1,300 |
| Harvest-adult-M | 1 (NA) | 1 (NA) | 1 (NA) | 313/10,046 |
| Harvest-adult-F | 0.57 (0.06) | 0.57 (0.06) | 0.58 (0.06) | 104/5,782 |
| Harvest-juv-F | 0.44 (0.15) | 0.44 (0.15) | 0.45 (0.15) | 9/645 |
| Harvest-juv-M | 0.25 (0.08) | 0.25 (0.08) | 0.25 (0.08) | 11/1,329 |
| Harvest-fawn | 0.03 (0.03) | 0. 03 (0.03) | 0.03 (0.03) | 1/999 |

Notes: The *Harvest-adult-M* category is used as the reference class in these analyses, as in WM [15]. We provide both the count of CWD positive animals (*C*) and the total number sampled (*N*) from WM [15].

with as few as 22 suspect-females (297/13.5). In many cases, it may not be possible to simply sample the highest weight subjects, but one could still focus on generally high weight subjects. For example, if one summed up the real weights for 10 suspect-females, 10 suspect-males, and 23 others, the summed real weight is 297.7. When we calculate the exact posterior credible bound for such an observation (Software Code S1; Program 7), we observe $Pr(\pi < 0.0096) \geq 0.95$, so we have slightly overshot our goal (which is usually not a bad thing).

As this illustrates, we have noticed that in general real weights do not exhibit perfect additivity, in particular when the discrepancy between real and nominal weights is large (not illustrated). Thus, although we feel that real weights are a useful design tool for planning and prioritizing samples and "getting in the ballpark" with respect to the effective sample size, we advocate exact posterior bounds as we just illustrated to evaluate the specific performance of a surveillance sample.

Typically, logistics constrain the number of surveillance samples that a monitoring agency can obtain. Real weights allow the agency to realistically prioritize high-value animals. By summing weights, they can also keep track of how well a surveillance program is progressing by summarizing the "effective" sample size

in terms of a synthetic sample of all reference animals; however we recommend some caution in this respect. As we note, real weights are not purely additive, and we advocate that exact posterior bounds be used to rigorously determine whether the surveillance goal of $Pr(\pi < \pi_t) \geq 1 - \alpha$ has been achieved. Summed real weights should be viewed as rules-of-thumb, and should be useful in designing and monitoring a surveillance effort.

The choice of reference class is mainly a matter of common sense; it should be some class of animals in which one would be interested in statements about disease presence, typically a common class. This notion is sometimes criticized for its apparent arbitrariness; but this completely misses the point – such criticism is akin a saying the Celsius scale measures temperature better than Fahrenheit. Indeed, without such standardization, it seems essentially impossible to make meaningful comparative statements about how well surveillance has been performed in various units. Clearly, a surveillance sample of 297 harvest-fawns is not equivalent to a sample of 297 harvest-adult-males; only an approach such as ours allows an "apples-to-apples" comparison of certainty of "freedom-from-disease" from different areas.

For CWD, the standard USDA certified tests are regarded as being essentially 100% specific. However, for an animal that has

**Table 2.** Nominal and real surveillance weights calculated using data from WM[15].

| Mortality Source | Nominal Weight (SD) | Real Weight (*R_i*) | C/N |
|---|---|---|---|
| Suspect-female | 14.1 (2.40) | 13.5 | 40/111 |
| Suspect-male | 12.2 (2.05) | 11.9 | 40/125 |
| Other | 1.9 (0.24) | 1.9 | 77/1,300 |
| Harvest-adult male | 1 (NA) | 1 | 313/10,046 |
| Harvest-adult female | 0.57 (0.06) | 0.57 | 104/5,782 |
| Harvest-yearling female | 0.44 (0.15) | 0.39 | 9/645 |
| Harvest-yearling male | 0.25 (0.07) | 0.23 | 11/1,392 |
| Harvest-fawn | 0.03 (0.03) | 0.006 | 1/999 |

For real weights, a sample equivalent to $N_{Harvest-adult-males} = 297$ reference class animals was needed to obtain the target goal, which is for the posterior probability $Pr(\pi_t \leq 0.01) \geq 0.95$.
Notes: Values for nominal weights are the Bayesian posterior means of the hazard ratios. Real weights were obtained by posterior credible bound matching, described in the text.

just recently experienced an infection event, it may not test positive, so in this sense the test may not be 100% sensitive, but it is very difficult to quantify this. The most straightforward approach would be to recognize the possibility that apparent prevalence might be lower than true prevalence, and set an appropriately conservative (small) threshold for $\pi_t$. If sensitivity and specificity can be quantified, extensions similar to Cameron and Baldock [21] could be explored. Another potential modification would be to include a finite population correction factor if the population size is known [21]; our approach is conservative for small populations, that is, the actual assurance level will probably be higher than the nominal $1 - \alpha$ level, which is appropriate for disease surveillance.

Ideally, we recommend agencies collect learning data from their unique disease systems for subsequent calculation of real weights in their surveillance efforts. If relatively local data are available, the desirability of including spatial structure as a risk factor, similar to that employed for disease risk mapping [29], could be explored. If relatively local data are not available, caution should be exercised when generalizing information from other systems. As we presented our approach, we always included the data from the learning set directly into the augmented analysis of the surveillance data. However, we could have partitioned our analyses into two steps – first obtain the posterior distributions for the log hazards from the learning set, and then use these posteriors as priors in the evaluation of the surveillance set, perhaps using normal approximations. If we have doubts about the generalizability of the learning set to our surveillance set, we could manipulate the priors going into the surveillance analysis from the learning set to reflect this added uncertainty, for example increasing their variance to evaluate the sensitivity of the results to this added uncertainty. This is a natural application of the Bayesian concept of uncertainty.

## Supporting Information

**Appendix S1 Prior Matching and Weight Models.** The technical details behind prior matching and our derivation of sample weight models is given here.

**Software Code S1 Software Code for Examples.** The WinBUGS and SAS code is given here for all of our examples.

## Acknowledgments

We thank Glen Sargeant, Mike Samuel and several anonymous reviewers for comments on earlier drafts. The use of trade names or products does not constitute endorsement by the U.S. Government.

## Author Contributions

Conceived and designed the experiments: DMH CSJ RER DPW. Analyzed the data: DMH CSJ DPW. Contributed reagents/materials/analysis tools: DMH CSJ RER DPW. Wrote the paper: DMH CSJ RER DPW.

## References

1. Anonymous (1995) Ordonnance sur les épizooties du 27 Juin 1995. Swiss Federal Veterinary Office, 89 pages.
2. Dufour B, Pouillot R, Toma B (2001) Proposed criteria to determine whether a territory is free of a given animal disease. Vet Res 32: 545–563.
3. Doherr MG, Audigé L, Salman MD, Gardner IA (2003) Use of animal monitoring and surveillance systems when the frequency of health-related events is near zero. Pages 135–147 in Salman MD, editor. Animal disease surveillance and survey systems – methods and applications, Iowa State Press, Ames, Iowa, USA.
4. Salman M (2003) Animal Disease surveillance and survey systems: Methods and applications, Iowa State Press, Ames, Iowa, USA.
5. Daszak P, Cunningham AA, Hyatt AD (2000) Emerging infectious diseases of wildlife – threats to biodiversity and human health. Science 287: 443–449.
6. Wobeser G (2002) Disease management strategies for wildlife. Rev Sci Tech 21: 159–178.
7. Ziller M, Selhorst T, Teuffert J, Kramer M, Schlüter H (2002) Analysis of sampling strategies to substantiate freedom from disease in large areas. Prev Vet Med 52: 333–343.
8. Cameron A, Gardner I, Doherr MG, Wagner B (2003) Sampling considerations in surveys and monitoring and surveillance systems. Pages 47–66 in M. D. Salman, editor. Animal disease surveillance and survey systems – methods and applications. Iowa State Press, Ames, Iowa, USA.
9. Office International des Epizooties (OIE) (2010) Terrestrial Animal Health Code. Available: http://www.oie.int/. Accessed 2014 Mar 7.
10. Centers for Disease Control and Prevention - Chronic Wasting Disease - Available: http://www.cdc.gov/ncidod/dvrd/cwd/. Accessed 2014 Mar 7.
11. Samuel MD, Joly DO, Wild MA, Wright SD, Otis DL, et al. (2003) Surveillance strategies for detecting chronic wasting disease in free-ranging deer and elk: results of a CWD surveillance workshop, 10–12 December 2002, United States Geological Survey National Wildlife Health Center, Madison, Wisconsin, USA. Available: http://www.nwhc.usgs.gov/publications/fact_sheets/pdfs/cwd/CWD_Surveillance_Strategies.pdf. Accessed 2014 Mar 7.
12. Joly DO, Samuel MD, Langenberg JA, Rolley RE, Keane DP (2009) Surveillance to detect chronic wasting disease in Wisconsin white-tailed deer. J Wildl Dis 45: 989–997.
13. Nusser SM, Clark WR, Otis DL, Huang L (2008) Sampling considerations for disease surveillance in wildlife populations. J Wildl Manage 72: 52–60.
14. Diefenbach DR, Rosenberry CS, Boyd RC (2004) Efficacy of detecting chronic wasting disease via sampling hunter-killed white-tailed deer. Wildl Soc Bull 32: 267–272.
15. Walsh DP, Miller MW 2010. A weighted surveillance approach for detecting chronic wasting disease foci. J Wildl Dis 46: 118–135.
16. Cannon RM (2002) Demonstrating disease freedom – combining confidence intervals. Prev Vet Med 52: 227–249.
17. Reid N, Mukerjee R, Fraser DAS (2003) Aspects of matching priors. Pages 31–43 in Moore M, Froda S, Léger C, editors. Mathematical Statistics and Applications: Festschrift for Constance van Eeden, Institute of Mathematical Statistics, Beachwood, Ohio, USA .
18. Lunn D, Thomas A, Best N, Spiegelhalter DJ (2000) WinBUGS – A Bayesian modeling framework: concepts, structure, and extensibility. Stat Comput 10: 325–337.
19. Hoenig JM, Heisey DM (2001) The abuse of power: The pervasive fallacy of power calculations for data analysis. Am Stat 55: 19–24.
20. Dayton PK (1998) Reversal of the burden of proof in fisheries management. Science 279: 821–822.
21. Cameron AR, Baldock FC (1998) A new probability formula for surveys to substantiate freedom from disease. Prev Vet Med 34: 1–17.
22. Brown LD, Cai TT, DasGupta A (2001) Interval estimation for a binomial proportion. Stat Sci 16: 101–133.
23. Cai TT (2005) One-sided confidence intervals in discrete distributions. J Stat Plan Inference 131: 63–88.
24. Casella G (2001) Comment - Interval estimation for a binomial proportion. Stat Sci 16: 121–122.
25. Ghosh M (2001) Comment - Interval estimation for a binomial proportion. Stat Sci 16: 124–125.
26. Tuyl F, Gerlac R, Mengersen K (2009) Posterior predictive arguments in favor of the Bayes-Laplace prior as the consensus prior for binomial and multinomial parameters. Bayesian Anal 4: 151–158.
27. Fienberg SE (2006) When did Bayesian inference become "Bayesian"? Bayesian Anal 1: 1–40.
28. Gelman A, Carlin JB, Stern HS, Rubin DB (2004) Bayesian Data Analysis, Chapman and Hall, New York, New York, USA.
29. Osnas EE, Heisey DM, Rolley RE, Samuel MD (2009) Spatial and temporal patterns of chronic wasting disease: fine-scale mapping of a wildlife epidemic in Wisconsin. Ecol Appl 19: 1311–1322.

# 10

# A Pilot Study Exploring the Use of Breath Analysis to Differentiate Healthy Cattle from Cattle Experimentally Infected with *Mycobacterium bovis*

**Christine K. Ellis[1,2], Randal S. Stahl[3], Pauline Nol[4], W. Ray Waters[5], Mitchell V. Palmer[5], Jack C. Rhyan[4], Kurt C. VerCauteren[2], Matthew McCollum[4], M. D. Salman[1]***

**1** Animal Population Health Institute, College of Veterinary Medicine and Biomedical Sciences, Colorado State University, Fort Collins, Colorado, United States of America, **2** United States Department of Agriculture, Animal Plant and Health Inspection Service, Wildlife Services, National Wildlife Research Center, Fort Collins, Colorado, United States of America, **3** United States Department of Agriculture, Animal Plant and Health Inspection Service, Wildlife Services, National Wildlife Research Center, Fort Collins, Colorado, United States of America, **4** United States Department of Agriculture, Animal Plant and Health Inspection Service, Veterinary Services, Wildlife Livestock Disease Investigations Team, Fort Collins, Colorado, United States of America, **5** United States Department of Agriculture, Agricultural Research Service, National Animal Disease Center, Ames, Iowa, United States of America

## Abstract

Bovine tuberculosis, caused by *Mycobacterium bovis*, is a zoonotic disease of international public health importance. Ante-mortem surveillance is essential for control; however, current surveillance tests are hampered by limitations affecting ease of use or quality of results. There is an emerging interest in human and veterinary medicine in diagnosing disease via identification of volatile organic compounds produced by pathogens and host-pathogen interactions. The objective of this pilot study was to explore application of existing human breath collection and analysis methodologies to cattle as a means to identify *M. bovis* infection through detection of unique volatile organic compounds or changes in the volatile organic compound profiles present in breath. Breath samples from 23 male Holstein calves (7 non-infected and 16 *M. bovis*-infected) were collected onto commercially available sorbent cartridges using a mask system at 90 days post-inoculation with *M. bovis*. Samples were analyzed using gas chromatography-mass spectrometry, and chromatographic data were analyzed using standard analytical chemical and metabolomic analyses, principle components analysis, and a linear discriminant algorithm. The findings provide proof of concept that breath-derived volatile organic compound analysis can be used to differentiate between healthy and *M. bovis*-infected cattle.

**Editor:** Mónica V. Cunha, INIAV, I.P.- National Institute of Agriculture and Veterinary Research, Portugal

**Funding:** USDA-APHIS (United States Department of Agriculture's Animal and Plant Health Inspection Service) funded the study. The funders had no role in study design, data collection and analysis, decision to publish, or preparation of the manuscript.

**Competing Interests:** The authors have declared that no competing interests exist.

\* E-mail: m.d.salman@colostate.edu

## Introduction

Bovine tuberculosis (bTB) is caused by *Mycobacterium bovis*, a zoonotic pathogen of importance to public health and international trade [1,2]. Globally approximately 8.8 million incident cases of human tuberculosis occurred in 2010 [3], and while *M. tuberculosis* was responsible for the majority of those cases, an unknown proportion were likely attributable to *M. bovis* [4,5]. Eradication programs and milk pasteurization have decreased the incidence of bTB in developed countries [6]; however, in developing countries, disease prevalence in cattle may approach 10–14% [7,8]. Presently, in the United States of America (USA), ante-mortem surveillance tests for cattle include the caudal fold skin test (CFT), the comparative cervical skin test (CCT), and the interferon gamma assay (IFN-γ, IGRA; Bovigam, Prionics Ag, Schlieren-Zurich, Switzerland). While these tests have reasonable sensitivities and specificities [1,6,9], all take 48–72 hours to produce results, and require multiple animal handlings (CFT, CCT) or specialized laboratory procedures (IFN-γ). In addition, performance of these tests can be compromised by factors affecting the immune response or confounding test interpretation [10]. Other *in vitro* assays (i.e., serologic assays, lymphocyte proliferation assay, polymerase chain reaction) have limitations associated with their accuracy and execution relative to ante mortem surveillance [6].

There is emerging interest in diagnosing disease via identification of volatile organic compounds (VOCs) produced by pathogens, host-pathogen interactions, and biochemical pathways. Volatile organic compounds may be found in the blood, breath, feces, sweat, skin, urine, and vaginal fluids of humans and animals [11–13]. The suite of VOCs found in these samples is influenced by host biological variables such as age, breed, gender, genetics, metabolic function, and physiological status; environmental factors including diet, climate, husbandry, and seasonal variation; symbiotic and infectious microbe-host interactions; and patho-physiological responses to infections, toxins, or endogenous metabolic pathway perturbations [11,14]. Volatile organic compound analysis has been used in human and veterinary medicine to explore suites of VOCs associated with infectious diseases [14–21], metabolic disorders and diseases [22–25], neoplasia

[11,26,27], and organ transplant rejection [28]. Additionally, analysis of VOCs may prove useful for investigating metabolic and biosynthetic pathway processes associated with homeostasis and pathophysiological responses to disease. In cattle VOC analysis has been explored as a method for diagnosis of bovine respiratory disease [20], brucellosis [14], bovine tuberculosis [29], Johne's disease [14,30], ketoacidosis [31,32], and normal rumen physiology.

Studies searching for host-derived biomarkers of disease have classically been conducted using biofluids, cells, or tissues. Such biomarkers are likely present as well in expired air, since breath contains hundreds of endogenous and exogenous VOCs [33,34]. To date, VOC analysis has been used to search for unique biomarkers associated with *M. bovis* and *M. tuberculosis* in serum samples [14,35,36], cell cultures [36–41], tissues [42], and breath [18,29,36]. Most research has attempted to isolate unique VOC biomarkers that would indicate presence of mycobacterial infection, with little work done to investigate potential changes within host VOC profiles that represent host-pathogen interactions or host responses to disease presence. Development of a highly sensitive and specific diagnostic tool capable of identifying such changes in VOC profiles would be of value in that sample collection would be non-invasive, easily repeatable, cost and labor efficient, and could be used in a point-of-care or "cow-side" setting. In this paper, we present the results of a pilot study exploring the concept of using VOC biomarkers in breath as a means to differentiate between non-infected cattle and cattle experimentally infected with *M. bovis*.

## Materials and Methods

### Ethics Statement

Strict biosafety level-3 (BSL-3) safety protocols were followed during all challenge and animal handling procedures to protect personnel from exposure to *M. bovis*. All animal work was reviewed and approved by the Institutional Biosafety and Animal Care and Use Committees (IACUC) of the United States Department of Agriculture (USDA), Agricultural Research Service (ARS), National Animal Disease Center (NADC), Ames, Iowa, USA; and the USDA, Animal and Plant Health Inspection Service (APHIS), National Wildlife Research Center (NWRC), Fort Collins, Colorado, USA prior to initiation of studies.

### Mycobacterium bovis challenge strains

Two strains of *M. bovis* were used for challenge inoculum: (1) *M. bovis* strain 95-1315 (USDA, APHIS designation) originally isolated from a white-tailed deer in Michigan, USA [43]; (2) *M. bovis* strain 10-7428_CO_Dairy_10-A (*M. bovis* strain 10-7428; USDA, APHIS designation) a recent isolate from Colorado, USA. Strains were prepared using standard procedures in Middlebrook 7H9 liquid media (Becton Dickinson, Franklin Lakes, NJ) [44].

### Animals and Mycobacterium bovis challenge

Male Holstein calves (n = 23, approximately 1 year of age) were obtained from a *M. bovis* and *M. avium paratuberculosis*-free herd in Wisconsin, USA, transported to NADC, and housed outdoors for approximately 2 months prior to placement into a BSL-3 agricultural facility at NADC. Animals were randomized to three treatment groups: non-infected controls (n = 7); animals receiving $10^4$ colony forming units (cfu) *M. bovis* strain 95-1315 (n = 8); animals receiving $10^4$ cfu *M. bovis* strain 10-7428 (n = 8) by aerosol as described by Palmer et al 2002 [45]. Each treatment group was housed according to IACUC guidelines in separate biocontainment rooms with no exchange of air, feed or water occurring between rooms. All animals were housed under the same environmental conditions, fed the same diet, and were allowed to acclimate to the new environment for approximately 3 months prior to initiation of *M. bovis* challenge studies.

### Diagnostic Tests Performed

Blood was collected from all calves at 2 weeks pre-challenge and at 2, 3, 4, 6, 8, and 12 weeks post-challenge for *in vitro* evaluation of cellular immune responses (CMI) to mycobacterial antigens including recombinant Early Secretory Antigenic Target -6kDa: Culture Filtrate Protein 10 fusion protein (rESAT-6:CFP10), overlapping (14 mer) peptide cocktail of ESAT-6:CFP10, *M. bovis* purified protein derivative (PPD), and *M. avium* PPD using the Bovigam assay [46]. Comparative cervical tuberculin (CCT) skin tests were performed at 12 weeks post-challenge as specified for the eradication of bovine tuberculosis in the United States [47]. All animals were humanely euthanized approximately 3.5 months after challenge by intravenous administration of sodium pentobarbital and necropsied. Tissues collected for bacteriologic isolation of *M. bovis* and histopathologic analysis included: parotid, medial retropharyngeal, mediastinal, and tracheobronchial lymph nodes; lung; and liver. Tissues were processed for isolation of *M. bovis*, and gross and microscopic lesions present were staged I–IV as previously described [45,48].

### Collection of VOC samples

Breath sample collection was conducted 90 days post inoculation (DPI) and took place over three days, with one day dedicated to each treatment group (Day 1: control treatment group; Day 2: *M. bovis* strain 95-1315; Day 3: *M. bovis* strain 10-7428). Sampling commenced and concluded at the same time each day. Collection intervals per calf were approximately consistent for every animal in the study. A modified equine nebulization mask (Aeromask, Trudell Medical International, London, Ontario, Canada) was used for breath sample collection. Modifications included installment of three one-way valves to which charcoal filters were affixed to remove environmental VOCs from inspired air, installment of a one-way valve to allow excess expired air to escape, modification of the silicon gasket to allow proper fitting to the muzzle of the test subjects, and placement of a port at the apex of the mask to allow attachment of the breath sample kit. Breath sample kits consisted of: a 5 cm section of Tygon tubing (3/8 inch OD, ¼ inch ID) (Thermo Fisher Scientific, Inc., Waltham, MA, USA), a 3-piece bioaerosol cassette (SKC Inc., Eighty Four, PA, USA) containing a 37 mm 0.22 um PTFE filter (Tisch Scientific, North Bend, OH, USA) and a 37 mm cellulose pad (SKC Inc. Eighty Four, PA, USA); a 20 cm section of Tygon tubing; a Tenax sorbent cartridge (SKC Inc. Eighty Four, PA, USA); and a 20 cm section of Tygon tubing attached to a vacuum pump (AirChek XR5000, SKC Inc., Eighty Four, PA, USA). Each calf was restrained unhaltered in a standard cattle stanchion. The mask was held over the animal's muzzle and breath samples were collected at a rate of 1 L/min for 2 minutes (min). For background control, room air samples were collected three times during the duration of animal sampling each day using the same apparatus without the mask attached. Immediately post-collection, each Tenax cartridge was capped, placed in a Whirl-Pack (Nasco, Fort Atkinson, WI, USA) and stored at −80°C. Samples were transported on dry ice to NWRC, and stored at −80°C until analysis.

### Method Validation

To establish the working range of the gas chromatography/ mass spectrometry (GC/MS) analysis method, 50 mg Tenax samples were spiked with 0.01 ml of a low (~5 µg/mL) or high

(~250 µg/mL) alkane stock solution containing each of the following alkanes: decane (C10); undecane (C11); dodecane (C12); tridecane (C13); and tetradecane (C14). Samples were allowed to equilibrate following vortexing, at room temperature for 45 minutes. Samples were extracted in 0.5 mL hexane and analyzed by GC/MS using the same method for the breath samples to establish repeatability and limits of detection for the method. Linearity for the method was established across the range of 0.24–10.0 µg/mL for each of the alkanes. Spiked samples were replicated at n = 5 and the process was repeated on three separate occasions to allow for inter- and intra-day comparisons for method performance. Method limits of detection for each of the alkanes were calculated as a concentration that would produce a peak height three times the base line noise, measured peak to peak, based on the total ion current (TIC) chromatograms from the low fortified samples. Inter-day recoveries were evaluated based on the magnitude of the standard deviation as a percent of the target concentration (+/−20%), while intra-day recoveries were compared using ANOVA at $\alpha = 0.05$.

## Sample Preparation for GC/MS Analysis and GC/MS Conditions

One Tenax sorbent cartridge from each animal was used for GC/MS analysis. A 50 mg sample of Tenax was extracted from each cartridge, and mixed with 0.5 mL hexane solvent. Each sample was sonicated for 10 minutes and the solvent then decanted into a GC vial. Analysis was performed using an Agilent 6890 GC coupled with an Agilent 5973 MS. Five microliters of sample solvent were injected into the GC in pulsed spitless mode. The inlet port temperature was 235°C, and the pulse pressure was 206.8 kPa (30 psi) for 0.5 minutes. The carrier gas was helium delivered with an average velocity of 59.0 cm/s. The column used was a DB-5 ms 30 m×250 µm column with a film thickness of 0.25 µm (J&W Scientific, Agilent Technologies, Santa Clara, CA, USA). Analytes were eluted from this column using a thermal gradient starting at 30°C and ramping at a rate of 5°C/1.0 min to a final temperature of 150°C. The total GC run time was 26.5 min. The temperature of the transfer line was 280°C. The MS was operated in positive ion mode, performing a total ion scan ranging from 10 to 550 m/z with a threshold of 150 m/z at a scan rate of 20 Hz. The MS source was operated at 230°C with the quad set to 150°C. Data were generated as raw Agilent.dat files.

## Data Processing

Data were analyzed qualitatively to identify VOCs present in the chromatograms, and quantitatively to determine if treatment group effects could be detected based on the ion abundances in the observed peaks. Chromatograms were baseline corrected using the region from 23–25 min, allowing for greater feature distinction in the chromatograms. Significant peak features in the chromatograms were identified using two different approaches. Initially features were identified using the Agilent Enhanced Chemstation MSD Data Analysis Tool software (Agilent Technologies, Santa Clara, CA, USA) and tentative peak compound identification was determined using the National Institute of Science and Technology (NIST) W8N08 database (www.nist.gov). Peaks were identified as significant if the total peak area exceeded 5000 across all ions in the peak. Compounds identified in the chromatograms using this approach were evaluated as possible metabolites using the Kyoto Encyclopedia of Genes and Genomes Database (KEGG) (www.genome.jp/kegg/) [49].

Chromatograms were also processed using XCMS Online (www.xcmsonline.scripps.edu) [49,50] [51]. Briefly, this software identifies single ion (m/z) features that are significantly different

across chromatograms grouped by treatment. Peaks identified in the chromatograms are aligned by a mean retention time calculated across all chromatograms evaluated in the data set. Peak features with relative intensity variance between sample groups are identified and a cross-sample peak-matching is performed in the METLIN Metabolite Database, identifying peaks that may represent metabolites [50,52]. The ions identified in this analysis as significantly different across treatment groups were then used in the chemometric analysis described below.

## Statistical Analysis

Mass spectral data from the XCMS Online analyses were used to construct two sets of principle components analysis (PCA) and linear discriminant analysis (LDA) classification models using the chemometrics statistical package in "R" [53]. Initial PCAs were calculated using the data from the control and one *M. bovis* treatment group. The individual ions were median centered and scaled to a variance of 1.0 using the median absolute deviation. Outliers were identified as exceeding regular observations by the 97.5% quantile of a standard normal distribution of either distance value, and by visually plotting the score distance and the orthogonal distance against the sample number. Identified outliers were removed from subsequent analyses. Principle component analysis scores from *M. bovis* treatment groups were compared to the same control treatment group, and then used to parameterize LDA classification models using 2, 3, or 4 PCA scores [51].

The LDA classification models were written as two class models; classifying a sample as either a control or one of the *M. bovis* strains. A training dataset was constructed by randomly distributing two-thirds of the data, and a classification dataset was constructed from the remaining one-third of the data. The LDA classification was performed for 100 iterations and the resulting predicted classification of each test animal in a given iteration was compared to the actual treatment group assignment. Misclassification rates were calculated as a percentage of the total number of test animals misclassified per iteration of the model.

We compared the ability of our LDA classification models to correctly identify control *vs.* infected cattle to currently used surveillance tests by calculating diagnostic sensitivity and specificity using the PCA scores generated from the XCMS Online analysis. The best LDA classification model was used for each calculation (four PCA scores *M. bovis* strain 95-1315; three PCA scores *M. bovis* strain 10-7428). For both *M. bovis* strains, the numbers of true positive (*M. bovis*-infected) and true negative (control) samples classified across 100 iterations of the classification simulation were summed. Samples that were misclassified as falsely positive (negative sample incorrectly classified as positive) or falsely negative (positive sample incorrectly classified as negative) were also summed. Diagnostic sensitivity was calculated as the total number of true positives divided by the sum of the true positives plus false negatives. Diagnostic specificity was calculated as the sum of all true negative samples divided by sum of the true negative plus false positive samples [54]. These values are reported as percentages.

## Results

### Diagnostic Tests

Specific CMI responses of all calves prior to and during the study are reported elsewhere [46]. Briefly, prior to initiation of the study, in some calves, Bovigam assay results demonstrated responses to *M. avium* PPD that exceeded respective responses to *M. bovis* PPD indicating environmental exposure to ubiquitous non-tuberculous *Mycobacteria* spp. (NTM). During the study, the

CMI responses of all *M. bovis*-inoculated calves to mycobacterial antigens were robust, with no significant differences noted between animals infected with *M. bovis* strain 95-1315 *vs. M. bovis* strain 10-7428. As early as three weeks post-challenge, CMI responses by all *M. bovis*-inoculated calves exceeded the pre- and post-challenge responses by the uninoculated controls. All calves inoculated with *M. bovis*, regardless of strain, were classified as reactors based upon standard interpretation of the CCT skin test 12 weeks after challenge. Calves in the non-infected control group were classified as negative on CCT skin test. During the study, no significant differences in clinical disease severity were observed between calves infected with *M. bovis* strain 95-1315 *vs. M. bovis* strain 10-7428. The severity of disease present grossly and microscopically was mild in both *M. bovis*-inoculated treatment groups. Similar gross and microscopic lesions were observed in the mediastinal and tracheobronchial lymph nodes and lungs of all *M. bovis*-inoculated calves examined (*M. V. Palmer, unpublished data*). *M. bovis* was isolated by culture from all calves inoculated with *M. bovis* strain 95-1315 or *M. bovis* strain 10-7428. *Mycobacterium bovis* was not isolated from the non-infected control group.

## Method validation

Method validation recoveries of low and high target concentrations for the alkanes were as follows: decane 0.55, and 5.5 µg/mL; undecane 0.52 and 5.2 µg/mL, dodecane 0.52 and 5.2 µg/mL, and for both tridecane and tetradecane 0.53 and 5.3 µg/mL. The retention times observed for each of the compounds were 8.9 minutes for decane; 12 minutes for undecane; 15.1 minutes for dodecane; 18 minutes for tridecane; and 20.8 minutes for tetradecane. The observed mean (mean +/- 1 standard deviation) concentrations determined for each of the alkanes in the extracting solutions across the three repetitions of the procedure are presented in Table 1. All observed concentrations fell within 20% of the target. Standard deviations for the means fell within 10% of the mean. Limits of detection for each of the compounds across three repetitions of the extraction procedure consistently fell below 0.1 µg/mL. The concentrations of each of the alkanes observed across the three intraday repetitions of the procedure at

the high and low fortification levels were not significantly different at the $\alpha = 0.05$ significance level.

## Compound identification

The peaks identified by the Agilent analysis were quantified and peak areas could be tentatively determined for 14 compounds (Table 2) using the NIST W8NO8 mass spectral library. The volatile compounds tentatively identified included acetals; alcohols; aldehydes; amines; hydrocarbons; ketones; an amino acid; a piperidine compound; and a pyrrolidine compound. Five compounds (4-hydroxy-4-methyl-2-pentanone, benzaldehyde, 1-ethyl-2-pyrrolidinone, $\alpha$, $\alpha$ - dimethyl-benzenemethanol, and nonanal) were present in significantly greater concentration ($p<0.05$) in the *M. bovis*-infected treatment groups.

## Cloud Plots

The two aligned between-groups comparisons generated by XCMS Online are presented as cloud plots (Figure 1 A and B) [49,55]. XCMS Online identified 137 peak features in the *M. bovis* strain 95-1315 *vs.* control group comparison, with 17 up-regulated features of statistical significance ($p<0.05$, $>1.5$ fold intensity change between treatment groups) present in the infected treatment group chromatograms (Figure 1A). There were 171 peak features identified in the *M. bovis* strain 10-7428 *vs.* control groups comparison with 51 features identified as significantly different between groups ($p<0.01$, $>1.5$ fold intensity change between treatment groups) (Figure 1B).

## Principle Components Analysis

Principle components analysis plots were constructed using the first two principle components scores based on all the features identified in the XCMS Online analysis of the chromatograms. The ability to distinguish between *M. bovis*-infected and control group samples based on the spatial distribution of the treatment group scores is illustrated in Figure 2A and B. In both comparisons there is distinct clustering of treatment group samples and a well-defined separation between the infected group and control group

**Table 1.** Solvent extraction method development mean alkane concentrations observed across replicates.

| Replicate/Alkane (ppm) | C10 (decane) | C11 (undecane) | C12 (dodecane) | C13 (tridecane) | C14 (tetradecane) |
|---|---|---|---|---|---|
| **Day 1** | | | | | |
| Low Mean | 0.52+0.01 | 0.48+0.00 | 0.49+0.02 | 0.50+0.01 | 0.48+0.01 |
| High Mean | 5.70+0.33 | 5.55+0.35 | 5.67+0.37 | 5.82+0.38 | 5.89+0.44 |
| MLOD | 0.056 | 0.068 | 0.079 | 0.067 | 0.068 |
| **Day 2** | | | | | |
| Low Mean | 0.47+0.05 | 0.42+0.05 | 0.43+0.04 | 0.45 + 0.05 | 0.47+0.06 |
| High Mean | 5.06+0.59 | 4.75+0.60 | 4.87+0.62 | 4.87 + 0.63 | 4.93+0.65 |
| MLOD | 0.051 | 0.060 | 0.048 | 0.059 | 0.056 |
| **Day 3** | | | | | |
| Low Mean | 0.53+0.05 | 0.50+0.06 | 0.51+0.05 | 0.51 + 0.05 | 0.51+0.05 |
| High Mean | 5.70+0.33 | 5.55+0.35 | 5.67+0.37 | 5.82 + 0.38 | 5.89+0.44 |
| MLOD | 0.070 | 0.093 | 0.087 | 0.075 | 0.092 |
| **ANOVA Results** | | | | | |
| **Low Fortification** | Df = 2,12 | Df = 2,12 | Df = 2,12 | Df = 2,12 | Df = 2,12 |
| **Comparison** | F = 0.78 | F = 1.99 | F = 3.24 | F = 1.22 | F = 0.004 |
| **F$_{critical}$ =3.89** | P = 0.49 | P = 0.18 | P = 0.07 | P = 0.33 | P = 0.995 |
| **High** | Df = 2,12 | Df = 2,12 | Df = 2,12 | Df = 2,12 | Df = 2,12 |
| **Fortification** | F = 1.36 | F = 2.38 | F = 1.88 | F = 3.00 | F = 2.42 |
| **Comparison** | P = 0.29 | P = 0.13 | P = 0.20 | P = 0.088 | P = 0.13 |

**Table 2.** Total Ion Chromatogram (TIC) peak area summary results of VOC profiles across treatment groups.

| Compound | Major m/z | Retention Time (min) | Control Mean | Control Standard Deviation | bTB strain 10-7428 Mean | bTB strain 10-7428 Standard Deviation | bTB strain 95-1315 Mean | bTB strain 95-1315 Standard Deviation | ANOVA (df 2, 19) F statistic | p-value |
|---|---|---|---|---|---|---|---|---|---|---|
| 1,1-diethoxyethane | 45, 73,103 | 3.28 | 5013 | 3964 | 92881 | 148133 | 75599 | 179478 | 0.863 | 0.438 |
| Toluene | 91, 65, 39 | 3.78 | 15729 | 3106 | 11740 | 3284 | 13232 | 3190 | 2.930 | 0.078 |
| Diethylamine | 41, 56, 44 | 4.37 | 8363 | 5154 | 11084 | 4265 | 8756 | 7168 | 0.527 | 0.599 |
| 4-hydroxy-4-methyl-2-pentanone | 43, 57, 58 | 5.46 | 8540 | 1491 | 23982 | 9902 | 18286 | 6603 | 8.905 | 1.87E-03 |
| Styrene | 104, 78, 51 | 6.37 | 21439 | 21783 | 17429 | 3627 | 15621 | 4002 | 0.390 | 0.682 |
| Benzaldehyde | 77, 106, 105, | 8.31 | 13449 | 5213 | 15314 | 2932 | 9442 | 3312 | 3.606 | 0.047 |
| 1-ethenyl-2-pyrrolidinone | 56, 111, 55 | 9.65 | 3838 | 4841 | 12382 | 5837 | 9649 | 7045 | 3.930 | 0.031 |
| 1-methyl-3-piperidinone | 43, 84, 113 | 9.77 | 4294 | 4439 | 10136 | 7923 | 8690 | 5222 | 1.780 | 0.950 |
| 2-ethyl-1-hexanol | 57, 43, 42, | 10.44 | 54162 | 25339 | 52353 | 41487 | 47641 | 34600 | 0.066 | 1.937 |
| α-acetophenone | 105, 77, 51 | 11.50 | 18646 | 10814 | 15665 | 4136 | 12354 | 8959 | 1.011 | 0.383 |
| α,α-dimethyl-benzenemethonol | 43, 121, 77 | 12.18 | 13372 | 11406 | 33399 | 13490 | 23657 | 12264 | 4.813 | 0.020 |
| 3-heptanone | 43, 57, 71 | 12.72 | 5820 | 13272 | 3361 | 3655 | 3366 | 3668 | 0.237 | 0.792 |
| Nonanal | 57, 41, 56 | 12.87 | 29126 | 11982 | 72466 | 20903 | 51064 | 23526 | 9.210 | 0.002 |
| 1-1-dimethyl-2-(1-methylethyl) cyclopropane | 151, 69, 41 | 21.78 | 49884 | 23201 | 54879 | 24983 | 57668 | 52478 | 0.038 | 0.963 |

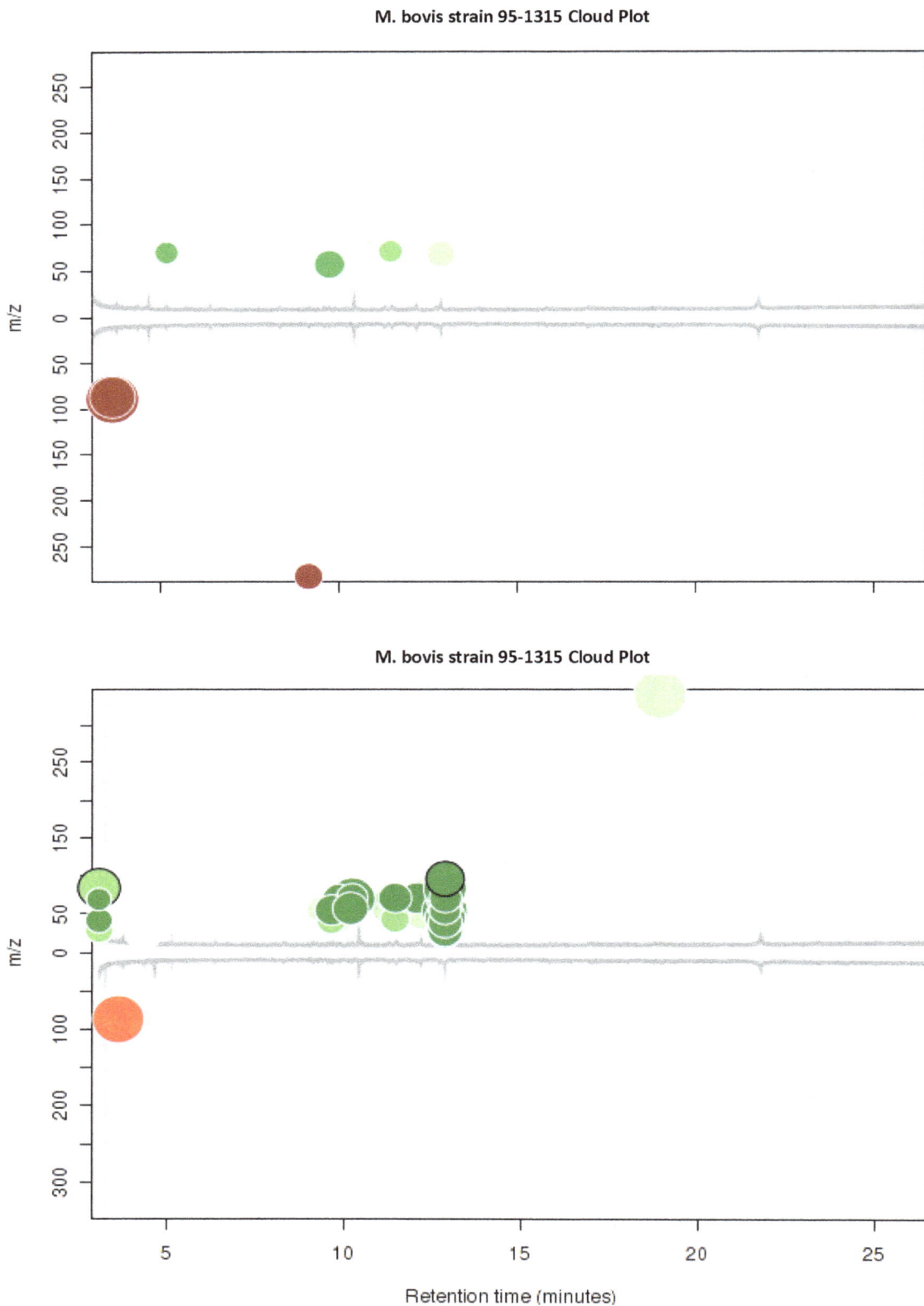

**Figure 1. Cloud plots of aligned GC/MS chromatograms generated with XCMS Online.** (**A**) Control vs. *M. bovis* strain 95-1315 analysis. (**B**) Control vs. *M. bovis* strain 10-7428 analysis. Control treatment group chromatograms are depicted below the X-axis, and *M. bovis*-infected chromatograms are positioned above. Up-regulated features of statistical significance are identified with green-colored circles located at the top of the plot, and down-regulated features are identified by red-colored circles located at the bottom of the plot. The color intensity of each circle represents the statistical significance of the feature difference, with brighter circles having lower p-values. The diameter of each circle represents a log-fold increase or decrease in abundance (i.e., larger circles correspond to peaks with greater fold differences).

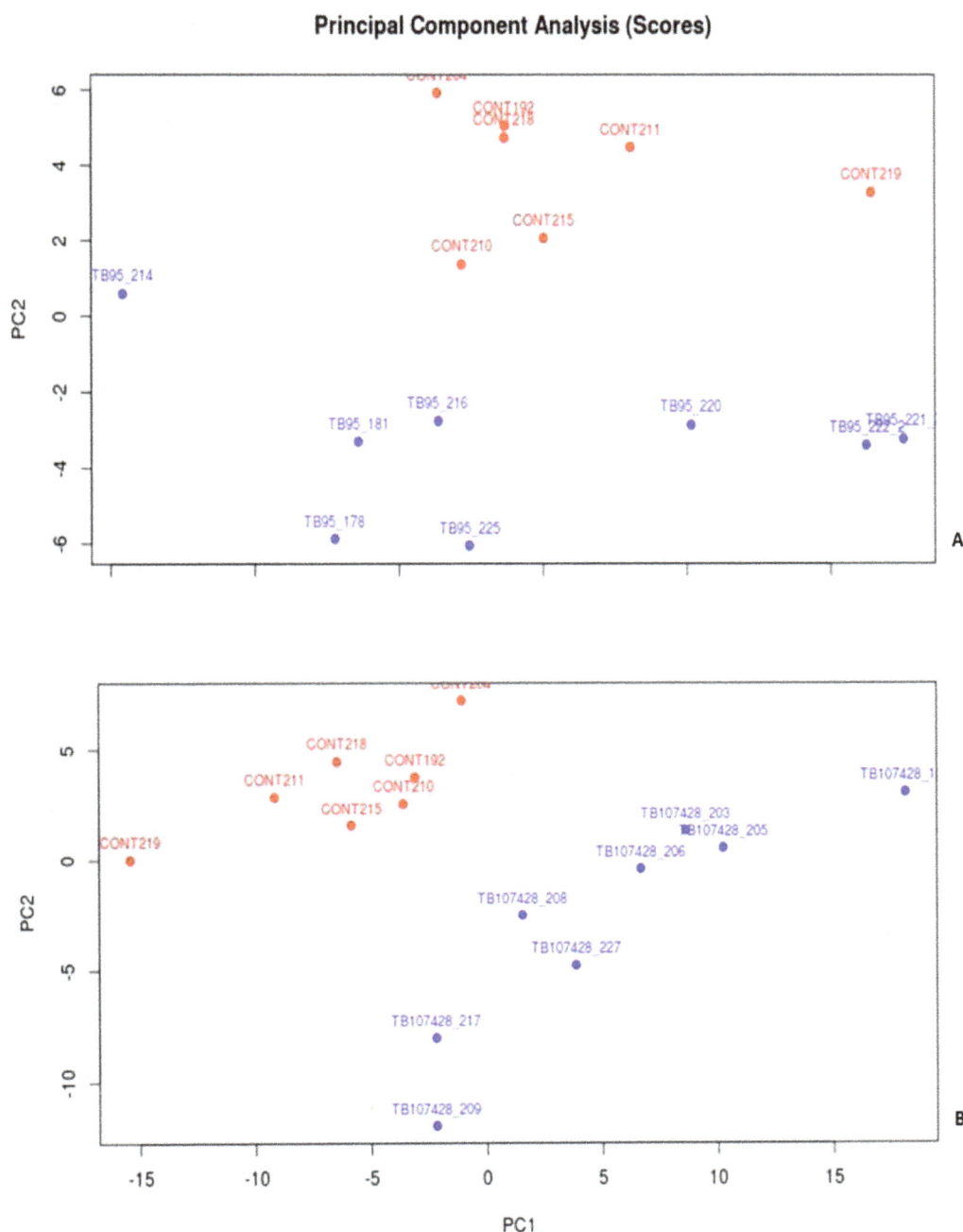

**Figure 2. Principle Components Analysis results. (A)** Control vs. *M. bovis* strain 95-1315. **(B)** Control vs. *M. bovis* strain 10-7428.

sample clusters, indicating that the VOC profiles of the *M. bovis*-infected cattle are distinctly different from those of the control cattle. It is interesting to note that while the chromatograms of *M. bovis* strain 95-1315-infected cattle did not contain many statistically significant peaks (n = 17; p<0.05, >1.5 fold intensity change between treatment groups) (Figure 1A), the magnitude of peaks present did allow for differentiation, particularly after relaxing the 1.5 fold increase criteria and including ion fragments that met only the p<0.05 criteria.

## Linear Discriminant Analysis and Sensitivity and Specificity

Linear discriminant analysis models based on ions identified by XCMS Online as significantly different across treatment groups (p<0.01, *M. bovis* strain 10-7428; p<0.05, *M. bovis* strain 95-1315) did allow for classification (Table 3). The misclassification probabilities (combined false positive and false negative) for the control vs. *M. bovis* strain 10-7428 model were 11.25%, 8.75%, and 12.00%; and the misclassification probabilities for the control vs. *M. bovis* strain 95-1315 model were 22.09%, 17.50% and 2.25% (based on 2, 3, or 4 principle component scores, respectively). Based on the LDA model classifications, the

**Table 3.** Misclassification rates for Least Discriminant Analysis (LDA) models based on Principle Components Analysis (PCA) scores for XCMS Online data.

| Number of PCA Scores Used in the Model | bTB strain 95-1315 *vs.* Control | bTB strain 10-7428 *vs.* Control |
|---|---|---|
| 2 | 22.09% | 11.25% |
| 3 | 17.50% | 8.75% |
| 4 | 2.25% | 12.00% |
| bTB (+) samples | n = 7 | n = 7 |
| Control samples | n = 8 | n = 7 |
| Number of variables | 16 | 51 |
| Training Data Set | n = 10 | n = 10 |
| Classification Data Set | n = 5 | n = 4 |

sensitivity and specificity for the control vs. *M. bovis* strain 10-7428 and control vs. *M. bovis* strain 95-1315 were 83.8% and 96.4% (based on the three score model) and 97.4% and 99.2% (based on the 4 score model), respectively.

## Discussion

In this pilot study we demonstrate that it is possible to discriminate between healthy cattle and cattle experimentally infected with *M. bovis* at 90 DPI, using GC/MS analysis of breath samples. The analytical and statistical approaches we describe provide a means of identifying compounds from breath analysis that may be diagnostically significant in identifying the presence of bovine tuberculosis infection. The cloud plots generated in the XCMS Online analysis demonstrate it is possible to differentiate between infected and healthy calves based on changes in ion intensities associated with VOCs common across the treatment groups. The results of our PCA further demonstrate this capability based on the distinct clustering of within group samples and the clear separation of between groups samples. The robustness of our models is supported by the low misclassification rates present in the LDA and by the calculated sensitivity and specificity values of our classification models, as those values observed compare favorably with the standard ante-mortem surveillance tests used in the United States [6,9,56,57]. Our results were unexpected in that the intent of our work was to identify unique VOCs in the breath of *M. bovis*-infected cattle, based on the results of other studies exploring VOC analysis as a means of diagnosing tubercular disease in cattle [29] and other animal species [42,58], with potential applications to humans [18,36,38,39,55]. However, our findings lead us to consider that the VOCs identified in our study represent up- or down-regulation of metabolic pathways, physiological or immune responses, or homeostatic perturbations caused by *M. bovis* infection.

The calves in our study were procured from a herd in which bovine tuberculosis- and *M. avium paratuberculosis*-infections were not reported or observed, were held in a controlled environment under observation for months prior to the start of and throughout the duration of the study, and were screened for exposure to *M. bovis*, *M. avium*, and *M. avium paratuberculosis* prior to challenge. In some animals, responses to *M. avium* PPD did exceed respective responses to *M. bovis* PPD prior to experimental infection with *M. bovis* indicating environmental exposure to ubiquitous NTM [46]. In general, NTM are rapidly cleared by cattle; thus, it was not anticipated that transient exposure and sensitization of the cattle to NTM would result in significant interference with detection and

interpretation of *M. bovis* specific VOCs. The robust immune responses, gross pathologic and histopathologic observations, and bacteriological results in all *M. bovis* infected animals *vs.* controls lead us to state with confidence that the changes noted in the VOC profiles of the *M. bovis*-infected calves in our study were likely caused by *M. bovis* infection. We cannot, however, state that the changes noted in the breath VOC profiles are exclusive to *M. bovis* infection. Our findings do demonstrate that it is possible to differentiate between healthy and diseased calves, when *M. bovis* is present as the infectious agent. These results illustrate the need for further research exploring the breath VOC profiles of healthy cattle and those experiencing disease caused by *M. bovis* and other etiological agents in order to more thoroughly evaluate the robustness of VOC analysis as a disease detection method. To date, limited research has been conducted exploring the use of VOC analysis as a means to differentiate between healthy cattle and cattle infected with any etiological agent [19,20,29,31,32,59–61]. This is likely due partly to the practical difficulties in adapting human breath sampling and analysis strategies to cattle, and in interpreting VOC profiles produced by animals that have a microbial fermentation-driven digestive system.

Tenax is widely used to concentrate nonpolar VOCs in air samples and is typically thermally desorbed before being analyzed by GC/MS [62]. However, Tenax has also been solvent extracted when used in air or aqueous phase sampling, particularly in environmental applications where large molecular weight compounds are being monitored [63–66]. The decision to use a solvent extraction method in this study was driven by the possibility that large organic molecules entrained in breath water vapor might be retained on the Tenax and would not be thermally labile. This is presently the subject of ongoing work.

We were able to provide tentative identification of 14 compounds using the Agilent Enhanced Chemstation MSD Data Analysis Tool/NIST W8N08 (Table 1). Seven of the compounds have been previously described in association with cattle [19,29,31,32,67–71], or as potential biomarkers for *M. bovis* [29,40] or *M. tuberculosis* [41,72] (Table 4). Tentative identification and change in peak intensity of nonanal is interesting as this compound is a lipid peroxidation by-product present in the breath of healthy humans and detected in greater concentrations in the breath of humans with respiratory tract disease [73,74]. Potential metabolic pathway associations were identified for 6 compounds (toluene; styrene; benzaldehyde; 2-ethyl-1-hexanol; α-acetophenone; 1, 1-dimethyl 2-(1-methylethyl) cyclopropane)(Table 4). Review of the literature identified one other study exploring the VOC profiles of cattle infected with *M. bovis*. In that study 16

**Table 4.** Comparison of compounds identified in cattle and humans.

| Compound | Cattle | Humans | Culture | Potential metabolic pathway [78] | Other [71,79] |
|---|---|---|---|---|---|
| 1,1-Diethoxyethane | | | | | Found in onions, grapes. Used as a flavoring ingredient in fruit and alcohols. Endogenous metabolite. Food metabolite. |
| Toluene | Ketosis [31,32] BRD [19] M. bovis [29] | | | M. tuberculosis M. bovis BCG Bos tarus | Found in allspice, lime oil and some foods. Food metabolite. Toxin and pollutant metabolite. Found in some plants. |
| Diethylamine | Healthy [70] | | | | Occurs naturally in some foods and plants. Endogenous metabolite. |
| 4-Hydroxy-4-methyl-2-pentanone | | | M. tuberculosis [41] | | Also known as diacetone alcohol. Found in fruits. Endogenous metabolite. Food metabolite. |
| Styrene | Healthy [67] | Tuberculosis [72] | | M. tuberculosis M. bovis BCG Bos tarus | Found naturally in some plants and a variety of foods including fruits, vegtables, nuts, beverages, meats and dairy products. Exhibits signaling and catabolic functions. Food metabolite. Biofunctions include catabolism and signaling. |
| Benzaldehyde | | | | M. tuberculosis M. bovis BCG Bos tarus | Occasionally found as a volatile compound in urine. Food additive. By-product in phenylalanine metabolism. |
| 1-Ethenyl-2-pyrrolidinone | | | | | Also known as polyvidone. Used as a food additive. 2-pyrrolidinone is a lactam cyclization product of gamma-aminobutyric acid (GABA). Food metabolite. |
| 1-Methyl-3-piperidinone | | | | | |
| 2-Ethyl-1-hexanol | Healthy [69] | | | M. tuberculosis M. bovis BCG Bos tarus | May occur naturally in some fruits and grains, olive oil, tobacco, and teas. Endogenous metabolite. Food metabolite. Biofunctions include cell signaling, energy source, and membrane integrity. |
| α-Acetophenone | Healthy [69] BRD [19] M. bovis [29] | | | M. tuberculosis M. bovis BCG Bos tarus | Found in some plants. Used as a food flavoring ingredient. Additive in cigarettes. Has anti-fungal properties. Drug metabolite. Food metabolite. |
| α,α-Dimethyl-benzenemethanol | | | | | |
| 3-Heptanone | | | | | Found naturally in spearmint. Used as a flavoring ingredient. Endogenous metabolite. Food metabolite. |
| Nonanal | BRD [19] M. bovis [29] | Tuberculosis [72] Asthma, COPD [73,74] | | M. tuberculosi M. bovis BCG Bos tarus | Lipid peroxidation by-product |
| 1-1-Dimethyl-2-(1-methylethyl) cyclopropane | | | | | Cyclopropane fatty acids are produced by some microorganisms and plants. American Oil Chemists Society (AOCS) Lipid Library www.lipidlibrary.aocs.org |

VOCs were tentatively identified, with 10 VOCs present in the breath of all the cattle sampled, four VOCs apparently exclusive to healthy cattle, and two VOCs apparently exclusive to cattle infected with *M. bovis*. Only two VOCs were consistent between that study and our study. Acetophenone was found in the breath of all cattle in both studies. Nonanal was present in the breath of all cattle in our study, but was absent from the breath VOC profiles of *M. bovis*-infected cattle and present only in a subset of healthy cattle in the other study [29].

While it is conceivable that some VOCs produced by monogastric animals, humans, cattle, and bacteria may be similar, there is limited continuity in the suites of VOCs identified when comparing studies performed on healthy cattle *vs.* cattle with BRD or *M. bovis* infection, studies of healthy humans *vs.* humans with tuberculosis, and between *M. tuberculosis* cultures grown *in vitro* in different types of solid and liquid media [18–20,29,31,32,41,59,61,67,68,72,75]. Volatile compounds identified as biomarkers for specific pathogens in culture or preliminary human or animal testing have been found in the breath of normal subjects and subjects with diseases of different etiology, or associated with specific foods or other materials [41,73,76]. Likely explanations for these inconsistencies include individual variability; similarities in host response to pathogen presence; pathobiological similarities between pathogens; endogenous and exogenous factors; and, relative to cattle, the dynamic nature of rumen gases. Identifying endogenous and exogenous factors that may affect VOC suite composition and concentrations of VOCs present in breath is important. Endogenous VOCs are comprised of bloodborne compounds produced by metabolic, hemostatic, or pathologic processes that passively diffuse across the blood-alveolar interface or are produced within the respiratory tract. Exogenous VOCs present in the environment that are passively inspired then expired, or are present in food and water may be inadvertent contaminants [76].

The diverse methods of VOC collection and analytical methods that have been used are likely to have contributed to the variability in results as well. For example, methods of sample collection have included Tedlar bags, Tenax sorbent cartridges, and SPME fibers of various types [19,20,29,35,60,61,67,75], and sample analysis methods have included, but have not been limited to, thermal desorption-GC/MS [19,61,67], proton-transfer-reaction mass spectrometry (PTR-MS)[75], electronic nose technology coupled with GC/MS [35,60], nanotechnology based artificial nose (NANOSE) in combination with GC/MS [29], in addition to our solvent sample extraction-GC/MS method. The methods of VOC identification when performed have been variable as well.

Our study demonstrates the importance of analysis method and database selection for purposes of compound identification. The Agilent Enhanced Chemstation MSD Data Analysis Tool/NIST W8N08 search emphasized identification of unique chromatographic features, whereas the XCMS Online/METLIN search focused upon identification of feature differences between groups, with emphasis on minor peaks within chromatograms. Standard chemical databases such as NIST W8N08 contain many classes of compounds including industrial solvents, toxicants, and biohazardous materials. Metabolomic database searches appear more likely sources for identification of compounds produced by living organisms or cell-based structures; however, the number of compounds and species represented in metabolomics databases are often limited [49,77]. Utilizing a combined chemometric-bioinformatics approach may provide the best method for identification of unique or dysregulated peaks within chromatograms until such time that metabolomic databases are capable of functioning as standalone references.

The potential influence of endogenous and exogenous VOCs, the variability in collection strategy, analysis methodology, and VOC identification underscores the difficulty of identification of VOCs as biomarkers for specific pathogens or diseases, and the need for cross-validation and standardization of breath analysis methods. It will be especially important to consider the potential

confounding influences of endogenous and exogenous VOC sources when performing breath analysis on animals under field conditions. In principle, breath analysis could be applicable to all animal species, although modification of systems used in human breath analysis is required. In many animal species sample collection is not voluntary and collection of an alveolar breath sample is not possible. This necessitates capture of breath samples via mask or nasal collection systems [61], and expectations that samples will likely contain VOCs derived from the upper respiratory or gastrointestinal tracts.

The strengths of this study include the ability to control for many endogenous and exogenous factors that might affect breath VOC profiles. The test subjects were all male Holstein calves of the same approximate age housed under the controlled environmental and dietary conditions. Inoculum preparation and the nebulization method used were consistent. Sample collection was conducted over the same time period on consecutive days, and sample handling was consistent across all treatment groups. Limitations of this study include the low number of study animals, immunological evidence of prior exposure to NTM in some of the test subjects, and lack of comparative breath analysis research in healthy cattle, tuberculous cattle, or cattle infected with BRD or other etiological agents.

Continued investigation and refinement of our breath collection system and our methods may lead to development of diagnostic strategies and disease surveillance monitoring systems that could preclude individual animal handling. Advantages to such systems would include decreased stress on individual animals, decreased cost and labor, ability to screen groups of animals, and potential surveillance of wildlife reservoirs of zoonoses and diseases of agricultural importance. Future work should include continued research using experimentally infected cattle and naturally infected cattle, multiple time point sample collections, collection of biofluid and tissue samples, increased sample sizes, comparative studies examining the VOC profiles produced by cattle with other infectious diseases and by cattle housed in different environments and fed different diets, and compound confirmation using reference standards. The eventual transfer of developed laboratory methods to portable GC-MS or Electric Nose systems would be beneficial and future work will ideally incorporate such tools.

## Acknowledgments

USDA is an equal opportunity provider and employer. Mention of trade names or commercial products in this publication is solely for the purpose of providing specific information and does not imply recommendation or endorsement by the U.S. Department of Agriculture.

## Author Contributions

Conceived and designed the experiments: CKE RSS PN WRW MVP JCR MM KCV MDS. Performed the experiments: CKE RSS PN WRW MVP. Analyzed the data: CKE RSS. Contributed reagents/materials/analysis tools: RSS PN WRW MVP JCR MM KCV MDS. Wrote the paper: CKE RSS PN. Editing and final manuscript approval: WRW MVP JCR MM KCV MDS.

## References

1. Biet F, Boschiroli ML, Thorel MF, Guilloteau LA (2005) Zoonotic aspects of Mycobacterium bovis and Mycobacterium avium-intracellulare complex (MAC). Vet Res 36: 411–436.

2. Schiller I, Oesch B, Vordermeier HM, Palmer MV, Harris BN, et al. (2010) Bovine Tuberculosis: A Review of Current and Emerging Diagnostic Techniques in View of their Relevance for Disease Control and Eradication. Transbound Emerg Dis 57: 205–220.

3. World Health Organization (2011) Global Tuberculosis Control 2011. WHO report 2011. Geneva: WHO.

4. Cosivi O, Grange JM, Daborn CJ, Raviglione MC, Fujikura T, et al. (1998) Zoonotic tuberculosis due to Mycobacterium bovis in developing countries. Emerg Infect Dis 4: 59–70.

5. Cleaveland S, Shaw DJ, Mfinanga SG, Shirima G, Kazwala RR, et al. (2007) Mycobacterium bovis in rural Tanzania: Risk factors for infection in human and cattle populations. Tuberculosis 87: 30–43.

6. de la Rua-Domenech R, Goodchild AT, Vordermeier HM, Hewinson RG, Christiansen KH, et al. (2006) Ante mortem diagnosis of tuberculosis in cattle: A review of the tuberculin tests, γ-interferon assay and other ancillary diagnostic techniques. Res Vet Sci 81: 190–210.

7. Ameni G, Amenu K, Tibbo M (2003) Bovine tuberculosis: prevalence and risk factor assessment in cattle and cattle owners in Wuchale-Jida district, Central Ethiopia. Int J Appl Res Vet Med 1: 17–26.

8. Abubakar U, Ameh J, Abdulkadir I, Salisu I, Okaiyeto S, et al. (2011) Bovine Tuberculosis in Nigeria: A Review. Vet Res 4: 24–27.

9. Waters W, Palmer M, Whipple D, Slaughter R, Jones S (2004) Immune responses of white-tailed deer (Odocoileus virginianus) to Mycobacterium bovis BCG vaccination. J Wildl Dis 40: 66–78.

10. Kaneen JB, Pfeiffer D (2006) Epidemiology of Mycobacterium bovis. In: Thoen C. O SJH, Gilsdorf M J., editor. Mycobacterium bovis Infection in Animals and Humans. Ames, IA: Blackwell Publishing.pp. 2602–2608.

11. Shirasu M, Touhara K (2011) The scent of disease: volatile organic compounds of the human body related to disease and disorder. J Biochem 150: 257–266.

12. Ma W, Clement B, Klemm W (1995) Cyclic changes in volatile constituents of bovine vaginal secretions. J Chem Ecol 21: 1895–1906.

13. Klemm WR, Hawkins GN, Santos EDL (1987) Identification of compounds in bovine cervico-vaginal mucus extracts that evoke male sexual behavior. Chem Senses 12: 77–87.

14. Knobloch H, Köhler H, Nicola C, Reinhold P, Turner C, et al. (2009) Volatile Organic Compound (VOC) Analysis For Disease Detection: Proof Of Principle For Field Studies Detecting Paratuberculosis And Brucellosis. AIP Conf Proc 1137: pp. 195–197.

15. Garner CE, Smith S, Baridhan PK, Ratcliffe NM, Probert CSJ (2009) A pilot study of faecal volatile organic compounds in faeces from cholera patients in Bangladesh to determine their utility in disease diagnosis. Trans R Soc Trop Med Hyg 103: 1171–1173.

16. Probert C, Ahmed I, Khalid T, Johnson E, Smith S, et al. (2009) Volatile organic compounds as diagnostic biomarkers in gastrointestinal and liver diseases. J Gastrointestin Liver Dis 18: 337–343.

17. Liddell K (1976) Smell as a diagnostic marker. Postgrad Med J 52: 136–138.

18. Phillips M, Basa-Dalay V, Bothamley G, Cataneo RN, Lam PK, et al. (2010) Breath biomarkers of active pulmonary tuberculosis. Tuberculosis 90: 145–151.

19. Spinhirne JP, Koziel JA, Chirase NK (2004) Sampling and analysis of volatile organic compounds in bovine breath by solid-phase microextraction and gas chromatography–mass spectrometry. J Chromatogr A 1025: 63–69.

20. Burciaga-Robles LO, Holland BP, Step DL, Krehbiel CR, McMillen GL, et al. (2009) Evaluation of breath biomarkers and serum haptoglobin concentration for diagnosis of bovine respiratory disease in heifers newly arrived at a feedlot. Am J Vet Res 70: 1291–1298.

21. Guamán AV, Carreras A, Calvo D, Agudo I, Navajas D, et al. (2012) Rapid detection of sepsis in rats through volatile organic compounds in breath. J Chromatogr B 881–882: 76–82.

22. Chen S, Zieve L, Mahadevan V (1970) Mercaptans and dimethyl sulfide in the breath of patients with cirrhosis of the liver. Effect of feeding methionine. J Lab Clin Med 75: 628.

23. Kaji H, Hisamura M, Saito N, Murao M (1978) Gas chromatographic determination of volatile sulfur compounds in the expired alveolar air in hepatopathic subjects. J Chromatogr 145: 464.

24. Leopold DA, Preli G, Moxell MM, Youngenlob SL, Wright HN (1990) FIsh-odor syndrome presenting as dysosmia. Arch Otolaryngol Head Neck Surg 116: 354–355.

25. Moorhead KT, Hill JV, Chase JG, Hann CE, Scotter JM, et al. (2011) Modelling acute renal failure using blood and breath biomarkers in rats. Comput Methods Programs in Biomed 101: 173–182.

26. Phillips M, Cataneo RN, Ditkoff BA, Fisher P, Greenberg J, et al. (2006) Prediction of breast cancer using volatile biomarkers in the breath. Breast Cancer Res Treat 99: 19–21.

27. Phillips M, Gleeson K, Hughes JMB, Greenberg J, Cataneo RN, et al. (1999) Volatile organic compounds in breath as markers of lung cancer: a cross-sectional study. The Lancet 353: 1930–1933.

28. Phillips M, Boehmer JP, Cataneo RN, Cheema T, Eisen HJ, et al. (2004) Heart allograft rejection: detection with breath alkanes in low levels (the HARDBALL study). Journal Heart Lung Transplant 23: 701–708.

29. Peled N, Ionescu R, Nol P, Barash O, McCollum M, et al. (2012) Detection of volatile organic compounds in cattle naturally infected with Mycobacterium bovis. Sens Actuators B Chem 171–172: 588–594.

30. Purkhart R, Köhler H, Liebler-Tenorio E, Meyer M, Becher G, et al. (2011) Chronic intestinal Mycobacteria infection: discrimination via VOC analysis in exhaled breath and headspace of feces using differential ion mobility spectrometry. J Breath Res 5: 027103.

31. Elliott-Martin R, Mottram T, Gardner J, Hobbs P, Bartlett P (1997) Preliminary investigation of breath sampling as a monitor of health in dairy cattle. J Ag Eng Res 67: 267–275.

32. Mottram TT, Dobbelaar P, Schukken YH, Hobbs PJ, Bartlett PN (1999) An experiment to determine the feasibility of automatically detecting hyperketo-naemia in dairy cows. Livest Prod Sci 61: 7–11.

33. Manolis A (1983) The diagnostic potential of breath analysis. Clinical chemistry 29: 5–15.

34. Phillips M, Herrera J, Krishnan S, Zain M, Greenberg J, et al. (1999) Variation in volatile organic compounds in the breath of normal humans. J Chromatogr B: Biomed Sci Appl 729: 75–88.

35. Fend R, Kolk AHJ, Bessant C, Buijtels P, Klatser PR, et al. (2006) Prospects for clinical application of electronic-nose technology to early detection of Mycobacterium tuberculosis in culture and sputum. J Clin Microbiol 44: 2039–2045.

36. Weiner J, Parida SK, Maertzdorf J, Black GF, Repsilber D, et al. (2012) Biomarkers of inflammation, immunosuppression and stress with active disease are revealed by metabolomic profiling of tuberculosis patients. PloS one 7: e40221.

37. Pavlou AK, Magan N, Jones JM, Brown J, Klatser P, et al. (2004) Detection of Mycobacterium tuberculosis (TB) in vitro and in situ using an electronic nose in combination with a neural network system. Biosen Bioelect 20: 538–544.

38. Syhre M, Chambers ST (2008) The scent of Mycobacterium tuberculosis. Tuberculosis 88: 317–323.

39. Syhre M, Manning L, Phuanukoonnon S, Harino P, Chambers ST (2009) The scent of Mycobacterium tuberculosis – Part II breath. Tuberculosis 89: 263–266.

40. McNerney R, Mallard K, Okolo PI, Turner C (2012) Production of volatile organic compounds by mycobacteria. FEMS Microbiol Lett 328: 150–156.

41. Nawrath T, Mgode GF, Weetjens B, Kaufmann SHE, Schulz S (2012) The volatiles of pathogenic and nonpathogenic mycobacteria and related bacteria. Beilstein J Org Chem 8: 290.

42. Somashekar BS, Amin AG, Rithner CD, Troudt J, Basaraba R, et al. (2011) Metabolic Profiling of Lung Granuloma in Mycobacterium tuberculosis Infected Guinea Pigs: Ex vivo 1H Magic Angle Spinning NMR Studies. J Proteome Res 10: 4186–4195.

43. Schmitt S, Fitzgerald S, Cooley T, Bruning-Fann C, Sullivan L, et al. (1997) Bovine tuberculosis in free-ranging white-tailed deer from Michigan. J Wildl Dis 33: 749–758.

44. Larsen MH, Biermann K, Jacobs WR (2005) Laboratory Maintenance of Mycobacterium tuberculosis. Current Protocols in Microbiology: John Wiley & Sons, Inc.

45. Palmer MV, Waters WR, Whipple DL (2002) Aerosol delivery of virulent Mycobacterium bovis to cattle. Tuberculosis 82: 275–282.

46. Bass KE, Nonnecke BJ, Palmer MV, Thacker TC, Hardegger R, et al. (2013) Clinical and Diagnostic Developments of a Gamma Interferon Release Assay (Bovigam^TM) for Use in Bovine Tuberculosis Control Programs. Clin Vaccine Immunol

47. USDA, APHIS(2005) Bovine Tuberculosis Eradication Uniform Methods and Rules 602 (APHIS 91-45-011). U. S. Government Printing Office, Washington, DC: 1–20.

48. Waters WR, Palmer MV, Nonnecke BJ, Thacker TC, Scherer CFC, et al. (2007) Failure of a Mycobacterium tuberculosis δRD1 δpanCD double deletion mutant in a neonatal calf aerosol M. bovis challenge model: Comparisons to responses elicited by M. bovis bacille Calmette Guerin. Vaccine 25: 7832–7840.

49. Smith CA, Maille GO, Want EJ, Qin C, Trauger SA, et al. (2005) METLIN: A Metabolite Mass Spectral Database. Ther Drug Monit 27: 747–751.

50. Smith CA, Want EJ, O'Maille G, Abagyan R, Siuzdak G (2006) XCMS: Processing Mass Spectrometry Data for Metabolite Profiling Using Nonlinear Peak Alignment, Matching, and Identification. Anal Chem 78: 779–787.

51. Team R (2005) R Foundation for Statistical Computing. Vienna, Austria.

52. Tautenhahn R, Patti GJ, Rinehart D, Siuzdak G (2012) XCMS Online: A Web-Based Platform to Process Untargeted Metabolomic Data. Anal Chem 84: 5035–5039.

53. Varmusa K, Filzmoser P (2009). Introduction to Multivariate Statistical Analysis in Chemometrics. Boca Raton, FL: CRC Press, Taylor & Francis Group.

54. Gerstman (2003) Epidemiology Kept Simple: an Introduction to Traditional and Modern Epidemiology. Hoboken, New Jersey: Wiley-Liss, Inc.

55. Kwiatkowska S, Szkudlarek U, Łuczyńska M, Nowak D, Zięba M (2007) Elevated exhalation of hydrogen peroxide and circulating IL-18 in patients with pulmonary tuberculosis. Respir Med101: 574–580.

56. Aranaz A, De Juan L, Montero N, Sánchez C, Galka M, et al. (2004) Bovine tuberculosis (Mycobacterium bovis) in wildlife in Spain. J Clin Microbiol 42: 2602–2608.

57. Pollock JM, Girvin RM, Lightbody KA, Neill SD, Clements RA, et al. (2000) Assessment of defined antigens for the diagnosis of bovine tuberculosis in skin test-reactor cattle. Vet Rec 146: 659–665.

58. Spooner AD, Bessant C, Turner C, Knobloch H, Chambers M (2009) Evaluation of a combination of SIFT-MS and multivariate data analysis for the diagnosis of Mycobacterium bovis in wild badgers. Analyst 134: 1922–1927.

59. Dobbelaar P, Mottram T, Nyabadza C, Hobbs P, Elliott-Martin RJ, et al. (1996) Detection of ketosis in dairy cows by analysis of exhaled breath. Vet Q 18: 151–152.

60. Fend R, Geddes R, Lesellier S, Vordermeier H-M, Corner L, et al. (2005) Use of an electronic nose to diagnose Mycobacterium bovis infection in badgers and cattle. Journal of clinical microbiology 43: 1745–1751.

61. Turner C, Knobloch H, Richards J, Richards P, Mottram TTF, et al. (2012) Development of a device for sampling cattle breath. Biosyst Eng 112: 75–81.

62. Spinhirne JP, Koziel JA, Chirase NK (2003) A Device for Non-invasive On-site Sampling of Cattle Breath with Solid-Phase Microextraction. Biosyst Eng 84: 239–246.

63. Cai L, Koziel J, Davis J, Lo Y-C, Xin H (2006) Characterization of volatile organic compounds and odors by in-vivo sampling of beef cattle rumen gas, by solid-phase microextraction, and gas chromatography–mass spectrometry–olfactometry. Anal Bioanal Chem 386: 1791–1802.

64. Jeanbourquin P, Guerin PM (2007) Sensory and behavioural responses of the stable fly Stomoxys calcitrans to rumen volatiles. Med Vet Entomol 21: 217–224.

65. Sorooshian A, Murphy S, Hersey S, Gates H, Padro L, et al. (2008) Comprehensive airborne characterization of aerosol from a major bovine source. Atmos Chem Phys Discuss 8: 10415–10479.

66. Bolton EE, Wang Y, Thiessen PA, Bryant SH (2008) Chapter 12 PubChem: Integrated Platform of Small Molecules and Biological Activities. In: Ralph AW, David CS, editors. Annual Reports in Computational Chemistry: Elsevier.pp. 217–241.

67. Phillips M, Cataneo RN, Condos R, Ring Erickson GA, Greenberg J, et al. (2007) Volatile biomarkers of pulmonary tuberculosis in the breath. Tuberculosis 87: 44–52.

68. Corradi M, Rubinstein I, Andreoli R, Manini P, Caglieri A, et al. (2003) Aldehydes in Exhaled Breath Condensate of Patients with Chronic Obstructive Pulmonary Disease. Am J Respir Crit Care Med 167: 1380–1386.

69. Westhoff M, Litterst P, Maddula S, Bödeker B, Rahmann S, et al. (2010) Differentiation of chronic obstructive pulmonary disease (COPD) including lung cancer from healthy control group by breath analysis using ion mobility spectrometry. Int J Ion Mobil Spectrom 13: 131–139.

70. Shaw SL, Mitloehner FM, Jackson W, DePeters EJ, Fadel JG, et al. (2007) Volatile Organic Compound Emissions from Dairy Cows and Their Waste as Measured by Proton-Transfer-Reaction Mass Spectrometry. Environ Sci Tech 41: 1310–1316.

71. Uhde E (1999) Application of solid sorbents for the sampling of volatile organic compounds in indoor air. Organic Indoor Air Pollutants: Occurrence-Measurement-Evaluation.

72. Nunez AJ, González LF, Janák J (1984) Pre-concentration of headspace volatiles for trace organic analysis by gas chromatography. J Chromatogr 300: 127–162.

73. Leuenberger C, Pankow JF (1984) Tenax GC cartridges in adsorption/solvent extraction of aqueous organic compounds. Anal Chem 56: 2518–2522.

74. Hawthorne SB, Miller DJ (1986) Extraction and recovery of organic pollutants from environmental solids and Tenax-GC using supercritical CO2. J Chromatogr Sci 24: 258–264.

75. Middleditch B (1989) Analytical Artifacts-GC, MS, HPLC, TLC and PC. J Chromatogr Library 44, Elsevier, Amsterdam.

76. Patti GJ, Yanes O, Siuzdak G (2012) Innovation: Metabolomics: the apogee of the omics trilogy. Nat Rev Mol Cell Biol 13: 263–269.

77. Scott-Thomas A, Syhre M, Epton M, Murdoch DR, Chambers ST Assessment of potential causes of falsely positive Mycobacterium tuberculosis breath test. Tuberculosis.

78. The Kyoto Encylopedia of Genes and Genomes (KEGG) Database. Available: http://www.genome.jp/kegg/kegg1.html. Accessed: 10 Jun 2013.

79. Wishart DS, Knox C, Guo AC, Eisner R, Young N, et al. (2009) HMDB: a knowledge base for the human metabolome. Nucleic Acids Res 37: D603–D610.

# 11

# Disease and Predation: Sorting out Causes of a Bighorn Sheep (*Ovis canadensis*) Decline

**Joshua B. Smith[1]\*, Jonathan A. Jenks[1], Troy W. Grovenburg[1], Robert W. Klaver[2]**

**1** Department of Natural Resource Management, South Dakota State University, Brookings, South Dakota, United States of America, **2** Iowa Cooperative Fish and Wildlife Research Unit and Department of Natural Resource Ecology and Management, Iowa State University, Ames, Iowa, United States of America

## Abstract

Estimating survival and documenting causes and timing of mortality events in neonate bighorn sheep (*Ovis canadensis*) improves understanding of population ecology and factors influencing recruitment. During 2010–2012, we captured and radiocollared 74 neonates in the Black Hills, South Dakota, of which 95% (70) died before 52 weeks of age. Pneumonia (36%) was the leading cause of mortality followed by predation (30%). We used known fate analysis in Program MARK to estimate weekly survival rates and investigate the influence of intrinsic variables on 52-week survival. Model $\{S_{1\ wk,\ 2-8\ wks,\ >8\ wks}\}$ had the lowest $AIC_c$ (Akaike's Information Criterion corrected for small sample size) value, indicating that age (3-stage age-interval: 1 week, 2–8 weeks, and >8 weeks) best explained survival. Weekly survival estimates for 1 week, 2–8 weeks, and > 8 weeks were 0.81 (95% CI = 0.70–0.88), 0.86 (95% CI = 0.81–0.90), and 0.94 (95% CI = 0.91–0.96), respectively. Overall probability of surviving 52 weeks was 0.02 (95% CI = 0.01–0.07). Of 70 documented mortalities, 21% occurred during the first week, 55% during weeks 2–8, and 23% occurred >8 weeks of age. We found pneumonia and predation were temporally heterogeneous with lambs most susceptible to predation during the first 2–3 weeks of life, while the greatest risk from pneumonia occurred from weeks 4–8. Our results indicated pneumonia was the major factor limiting recruitment followed by predation. Mortality from predation may have been partly compensatory to pneumonia and its effects were less pronounced as alternative prey became available. Given the high rates of pneumonia-caused mortality we observed, and the apparent lack of pneumonia-causing pathogens in bighorn populations in the western Black Hills, management activities should be geared towards eliminating contact between diseased and healthy populations.

**Editor:** Axel Janke, BiK-F Biodiversity and Climate Research Center, Germany

**Funding:** Funding for this study was provided by Federal Aid to Wildlife Restoration administered by South Dakota Department of Game, Fish, and Parks (Study No. 7537), and the Wild Sheep Foundation (http://www.wildsheepfoundation.org/). The funders had no role in study design, data analysis, decision to publish, or preparation of the manuscript. The authors acknowledge that members of the funding agency participated in capture of study animals.

**Competing Interests:** The authors have declared that no competing interests exist.

\* E-mail: joshua.smith@sdstate.edu

## Introduction

Bighorn sheep (*Ovis canadensis*) populations in North America have declined dramatically since European settlement [1]. These declines have been attributed to an array of environmental and demographic factors including: unregulated hunting, predation, habitat loss, and diseases [2,3]. While transplant efforts have proved effective in increasing overall bighorn numbers, many herds remain genetically and geographically isolated and often fail to recover to historical levels [4]. One of the major challenges currently facing managers attempting to restore these populations is low lamb recruitment.

In ungulates, juvenile survival is typically more variable than adult survival; thus, juvenile survival often has the greatest impact on population trajectories [5,6]. While numerous studies have used vaginal implant transmitters (VITs) or intensely-monitored females to radiocollar and examine neonate survival of elk (*Cervus elaphus*, [7]) and deer (*Odocoileus* sp., [8,9]), the steep and rugged terrain often used for lambing and rearing young [10] has precluded or severely limited this technique for neonate bighorn sheep [11]. Instead, most researchers have relied on visual observations of marked ewes for lambs at-heel, or lamb:ewe ratios in the herd [12–16]. Reliance on such metrics potentially allows reasonable assessments of overall recruitment into the population; however, it may obscure timing, causes of mortality, and may not reflect total mortality as such things as stillborn and early-age mortalities may be misconstrued as non-lambing events. Furthermore, it precludes the use of intrinsic variables (e.g., sex, weight) in survival analyses.

Documenting cause of mortality of juveniles is particularly important for bighorn sheep as many populations commonly experience pneumonia outbreaks that result in partial or complete die-offs [17,18]. These die-offs are typically followed by years of depressed lamb recruitment that hinder population recovery. Additionally, cougar (*Puma concolor*) predation on adults has been shown to contribute to some bighorn sheep population declines [19–22] with higher rates of predation occurring during declines in primary prey [23]. Predation by cougars also was the suspected cause of reduced lamb survival in the eastern Black Hills [24].

As in many other regions of the United States [25], native bighorn sheep were extirpated from the Black Hills, South Dakota, around the early 1900 s [24] and western South Dakota around 1925 [26]. Reintroductions and transplants beginning in 1965 resulted in the establishment of 5 subherds in the Black Hills region. Beginning in 2006, surveys conducted annually by South Dakota Department of Game, Fish and Parks (SDGF&P) indicated significant declines in bighorn lamb recruitment in 3 subherds (i.e., Rapid Creek, Hill City, and Spring Creek) in the east-central Black Hills (SDGF&P, Rapid City, SD, unpublished data). Our objectives were to radiocollar neonate bighorn sheep to: 1) estimate survival and document cause-specific mortality of bighorn lambs in the eastern Black Hills, South Dakota and 2) determine the influence of intrinsic variables on neonate survival.

## Materials and Methods

### Study Area

The Black Hills are located in southwestern South Dakota and eastern Wyoming, USA. Topography of the area varied from steep ridges, rock outcrops, canyonlands, and gulches to upland prairie, rolling hills, and tablelands. Elevations ranged from 973 to 2,202 m above mean sea level (msl; [27]). Ponderosa pine (*Pinus ponderosa*) forest comprised 83% of the landscape [28]. Mixed grass prairie (5%), riparian (4%), aspen (*Populus tremuloides*)-mixed conifer forest (3%), and developed open space (2%) were other major land cover types present in our study area [28]. During our study, average annual precipitation in the project area was 53 cm. Mean temperatures ranged from a maximum of 28°C in July to a minimum of −10°C in January. Climate values were based on data collected at the Hill City, South Dakota weather station from 1981–2010 [29].

The study area for this project was located in the east-central portion of the Black Hills with bighorn sheep habitat encompassing an area of approximately 26,000 ha. Each herd maintained distinct wintering areas; however, we did observe some range overlap between Spring Creek and Rapid Creek ewes during the lambing season (Figure 1). Over the course of our study, no range overlap was observed between our study herds and that of other herds in the Black Hills. In 2010, breeding-age ewe population estimates were: Rapid Creek = 56, Spring Creek = 50, and Hill City = 10 (SDGF&P, Rapid City, SD, unpublished data). Estimated proportion of ewes collared by herd across years ranged from: Rapid Creek 25%–29% (2010–2012), Spring Creek 30%–42% (2010–2012), and Hill City 90%–100% (2011–2012). Previously, no all-age pneumonia outbreaks had been detected in these herds, although several lambs had tested positive for pneumonia prior to 2010 (S. Griffin, SDGF&P, Rapid City, SD, personal communication). There were no domestic sheep grazing allotments within the Black Hills National Forest; however, several small domestic sheep and goat flocks were kept on private lands within bighorn sheep use areas. Other ungulates in the study area included mule deer (*Odocoileus hemionus*), white-tailed deer (*O. virginianus*), mountain goats (*Oreamnos americanus*), and elk. In addition to cougars, other potential predators of bighorn sheep included coyotes (*Canis latrans*) and bobcats (*Lynx rufus*).

### Ewe Capture

We captured adult ewes using a drop-net baited with weed-free alfalfa hay or sheep were chemically immobilized (BAM; 0.43 mg/kg butorphanol, 0.29 mg/kg azaperone, 0.17 mg/kg medetomidine) via dart rifle (Dan-Inject, Børkop, Denmark, EU). We estimated ewe age class (1 year, 2 years, 3 years, or ≥4 years) based on tooth replacement [30]. We evaluated pregnancy status of ewes via ultrasonography (Universal Ultrasound, Bedford Hills, NY, USA) at time of capture. We fitted pregnant ewes with M3930 VITs manufactured by Advanced Telemetry Systems (ATS; Isanti, MN) with a redesigned wing system and antenna length of 6 cm [31]. Ewes that were not pregnant or not checked for pregnancy at the time of capture were not fitted with VITs. Methods of VIT deployment followed Bishop et al. [31]. In addition to receiving VITs, all ewes were fitted with very high frequency (VHF) collars (M252OB or G2110D; ATS) that were uniquely marked to facilitate individual identification.

### Lamb Capture Using Ewes with VITs

Prior to the lambing season, radiocollared ewes were monitored 1–3 times per week from the ground using hand-held directional antennas (Telonics, Inc., Mesa, AZ), or from a Cessna 182 airplane. We listened for possible VIT expulsion each time we located ewes. When we detected an expelled VIT prior to the lambing season, we retrieved it using ground telemetry, ascertained if the ewe had aborted the fetus on-site, and estimated date of expulsion as the mean date between the first mortality signal and the last active signal received.

During the lambing season in May and June, ewes with VITs were checked once daily to determine if the VIT had been expelled. If the radio signal indicated a VIT had been expelled and terrain permitted, personnel would use telemetry to locate the expelled VIT on foot and retrieve it. If the VIT was located at a birth site and the lamb was present, we attempted to hand-capture it. If the dam had moved away from the VIT or if a lamb was not located in the vicinity of the ewe, we searched the area surrounding the ewe's location and the VIT location, and if a lamb was located we attempted capture. In the event the VIT was prematurely expelled based on a lack of evidence of birthing activities at the VIT site and observation of the ewe without a lamb, we intensively monitored the individual ewe's behavior. If we subsequently established the ewe had lambed, we attempted to capture the lamb once it was observed.

### Lamb Capture Using Ewes without VITs

We monitored radiocollared ewes without VITs on a near daily basis for movement patterns indicative of parturition and presence of newborn lambs via radio-telemetry and visual observation from a distance. When we detected a newborn lamb, we assessed its degree of mobility using observations of ambulatory movements. We attempted hand-capture from the ground if the lamb seemed sufficiently immobile and the terrain was accessible. We waited until animals bedded down before attempting capture. Solitary ewe-lamb pairs were preferred; however, we also attempted captures of lambs associated with small groups of ewes. Once animals bedded down, we noted location of the animals in relation to topography and notable landmarks. Ideally, while attempting to avoid detection (e.g., by climbing up the opposite side of a ridge), two people approached the animals from above. When detection by the animals was imminent, we rapidly approached the animals' location causing the ewe to flee, and the lamb would hide or attempt to flee at which time we attempted to capture the lamb.

### Lamb Handling and Marking

We physically restrained each captured lamb, blindfolded, and fitted the lamb with an expandable, 62 g VHF collar equipped with a 4-hr or 8-hr mortality switch (Model M4210; ATS). Additionally, we determined sex, age, and weight of captured lambs. We monitored lamb survival after capture using telemetry to determine if lambs had died or were abandoned as a result of our capture activities. We attempted to keep handling time to <5 minutes. All capture and handling procedures were approved by the South Dakota State University Animal Care and Use Committee (Approval number 09–019A) and followed recommendations of the American Society of Mammalogists [32].

We monitored lambs and ewes daily for 60 days post-capture and 3–4 times/week thereafter from the ground using a receiver and hand-held directional antenna (Telonics, Inc.) or from a

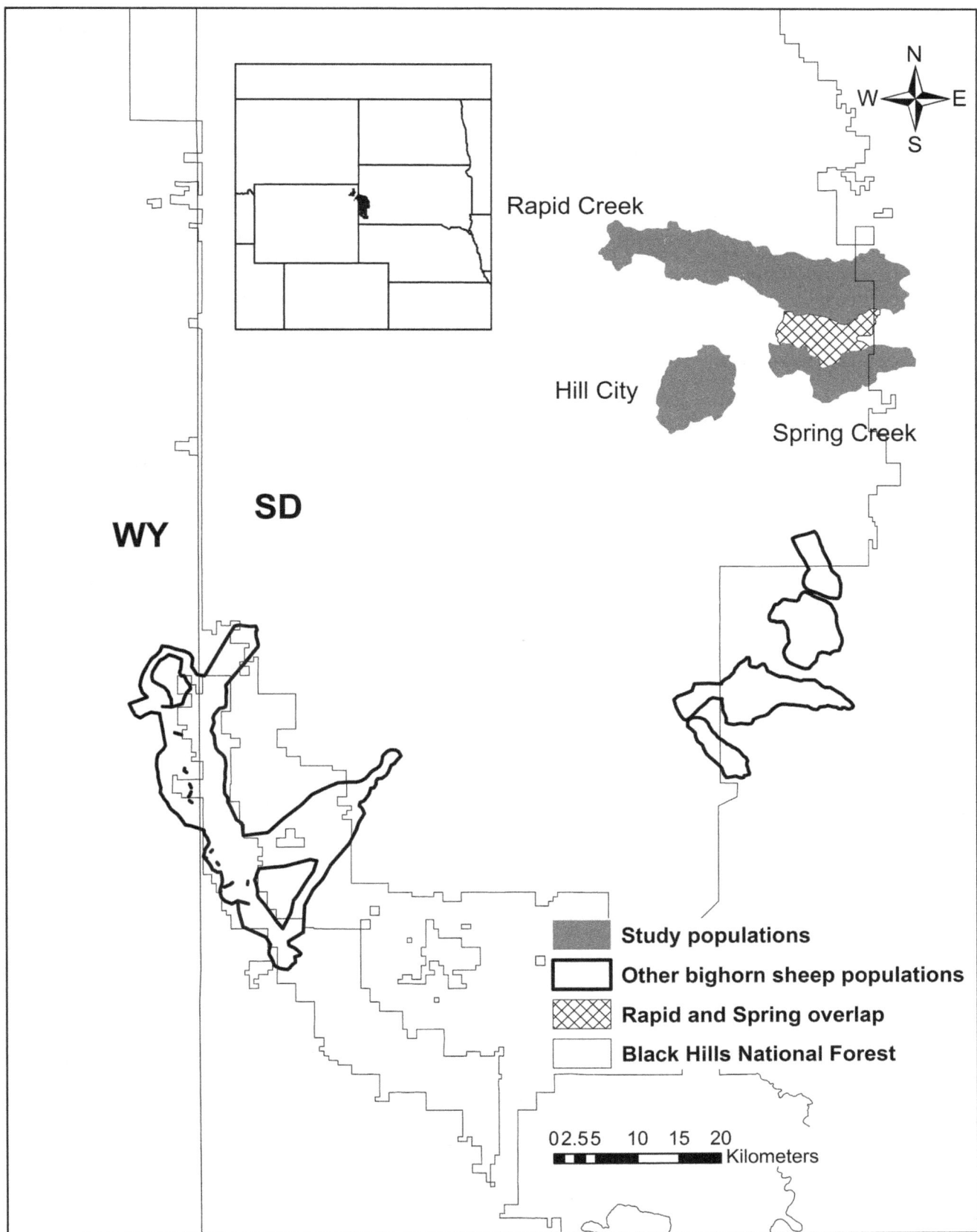

**Figure 1.** Bighorn sheep populations and locations of study populations in the Black Hills, South Dakota, USA, 2010–2012.

Cessna 182 airplane. When we detected a mortality signal, we immediately located the collar, and recorded evidence at the site of mortality to determine cause of death. If we could not determine cause of death in the field, we transported animals to the Washington Animal Disease Diagnostic Laboratory (WADDL) at Washington State University for further examination. We classified mortalities as predation based on observations at the mortality site including, bite marks, caching, plucking, blood, and consumption of carcass. To estimate survival and determine factors influencing lamb survival, we used the known fate model with the logit-link function in Program MARK [33]. We estimated weekly survival for 52 weeks post capture. Intrinsic variables included capture year, sex, herd, mass at capture, age at capture, winter severity, cougar population estimate for the Black Hills, birth timing (early, peak, and late), and 4 age-intervals (Table 1).

## Survival Analysis

We determined age of the lamb at capture on the basis of new hoof growth measurements and texture, umbilicus condition, behavioral characteristics such as mobility, the presence of afterbirth, and wet fur. We calculated winter severity by summing days with measurable snow accumulation with days that were $\leq -7°C$ based on data obtained from Hill City (for Spring Creek and Hill City herds) and Rapid City (for Rapid Creek herd), South Dakota weather stations from 2009–2012 [29]. Cougar population estimates were based on mark/recapture and modeling of the Black Hills cougar population (J. A. Jenks, South Dakota State University, Brookings, SD, unpublished data). Stage-interval models were constructed to test hypotheses regarding lamb susceptibility to various sources of mortality (e.g., predation vs. pneumonia). For birth timing, we grouped neonates into 3 periods: peak born (date when 50% of known lambs were born ±3 days), early (born >3 days before peak parturition date), and late (born >3 days after peak parturition date). We also considered 4 age-intervals: 1) a 2-stage model ($S_{1wk, >1 wk}$) in which neonate survival varied from <1 week versus >1 week post birth, 2) a 3-stage model ($S_{1 wk, 2–4 wks, >4 wks}$) in which neonate survival varied

among 1 week, 2–4 weeks, and >4 weeks post birth, 3) a 3-stage model ($S_{1 wk, 2–8 wks, >8 wks}$) in which neonate survival varied among 1 week, 2–8 weeks, and >8 weeks post birth, and 4) a 4-stage model ($S_{1 wk, 2–4 wks, 5–8 wks, >8 wks}$) in which neonate survival varied among 1 week, 2–4 weeks, 5–8 weeks, and >8 weeks post birth (Table 1).

We based a priori model construction on variables we considered biologically meaningful to neonate ecology and used Akaike's Information Criterion corrected for small sample size ($AIC_c$) to select models that best described the data. We compared $AIC_c$ values to select the most parsimonious model and considered models differing by $\leq 2$ $\Delta AIC_c$ from the selected model as potential alternatives [34]. We used Akaike weights ($w_i$) as an indication of support for each model. Because there is no current goodness-of-fit test statistic available for known fate models, we investigated model robustness by artificially inflating $\hat{c}$ (i.e., a model term representing overdispersion) from 1.0 to 3.0 (i.e., no dispersion to extreme dispersion) to simulate various levels of dispersion reflected in Quasi-$AIC_c$ ($QAIC_c$; [7,35]). Additionally, as some lambs were collared from the same ewe over multiple years, we performed a data-bootstrap analysis [36] in Program MARK to estimate overdispersion as a function of lamb maternity. Our bootstrap analysis was performed on our top ranked survival model and comprised 10,000 replicate datasets generated by resampling our data with replacement after removing lambs associated with each ewe across years.

We calculated a cumulative incidence function (CIF) to estimate cause-specific mortality related to pneumonia and predation to measure the contribution of each to survival rates [37]. We used the *wild 1* package [38] in Program R to calculate CIF for all individuals that survived $\geq 1$ day. We used a log-rank test to evaluate whether observed differences between cumulative mortality curves differed between the 2 mortality factors using the *survival* package [39] in Program R. The test computes a $\chi^2$ statistic for observed and expected mortality events during each time step and tests the null hypothesis of no difference between mortality curves.

**Table 1.** A priori models constucted to determine the influence of intrinsic variables on bighorn sheep neonate survival in the Black Hills, South Dakota, USA, 2010–2012.

| Model | K[a] | Description |
|---|---|---|
| $S_{constant}$ | 1 | Survival was constant |
| $S_{vit status}$ | 2 | Survival varied by whether ewe was vitted or non-vitted |
| $S_{age at capt}$ | 2 | Survival varied by age at capture of neonates |
| $S_{weight}$ | 2 | Survival varied by birth weight of neonates |
| $S_{birth timing}$ [b] | 3 | Survival varied by birth timing (early, late, and peak) |
| $S_{year}$ | 3 | Survival varied by year |
| $S_{winter severity}$ | 2 | Survival varied by previous winter severity |
| $S_{cougar pop}$ | 2 | Survival varied by estimated cougar population |
| $S_{herd}$ | 3 | Survival varied by herd |
| $S_{sex}$ | 2 | Survival varied by gender |
| $S_{1 wk, >1 wk}$ | 2 | Survival varied by age in 2 stages |
| $S_{1 wk, 2–4 wks, >4 wks}$ | 3 | Survival varied by age in 3 stages |
| $S_{1 wk, 2–8 wks, >8 wks}$ | 3 | Survival varied by age in 3 stages |
| $S_{1 wk, 2–4 wks, 5–8 wks, > 8 wks}$ | 4 | Survival varied by age in 4 stages |

[a]Number of parameters.
[b]Peak = date when 50% of known lambs were born +/−3 days, early = born >3 days before peak parturition date, and late = born >3 days after peak parturition date.

## Results

From February 2010 to April 2012, we captured and radio-collared 55 adult ewes (3 at 3 years of age; 52 at ≥4 years of age) and deployed 62 VITs [11]. From May 2010 to June 2012, we captured and radiocollared 77 neonates (25 in 2010, 25 in 2011, and 27 in 2012), 2 of which were from unmarked ewes (lamb capture by ewe VIT status summarized in Smith et al. [11]). Peak parturition occurred on 13 May 2010 (range = 2–31 May), 16 May 2011 (range = 4–26 May), and 16 May 2012 (range = 30 April–6 June). Of the 77 neonates radiocollared, 14 (18.2%) were born early, 40 (51.9%) were born during the peak period, and 23 (29.9%) were born late. Estimated age at capture ranged from < 0.01 to 2 days and 54% of lambs were <1 day old at capture; mean age and weight at capture was 0.8 days (SE = 0.1, $n = 70$) and 4.7 kg (SE = 0.1, $n = 75$), respectively. We documented 72 mortalities from capture to 52 weeks post capture; 24 in 2010, 23 in 2011, and 25 in 2012. However, in 2012, 2 lambs died from possible capture-related activity and 1 lamb was transported to a captive facility following possible capture-related abandonment; thus, we censored them from survival analyses. Additionally, 1 lamb in 2010 was right-censored 163 days post capture after we determined the collar was no longer on the animal. In addition to the 70 mortalities of radiocollared lambs, we documented 5 mortalities of lambs <24 hrs old; 3 stillborn, 1 predation, and 1 hypothermia. Because they were not collared, these animals also were excluded from survival analyses. Mean age at death was 42 days (SE = 5, $n = 70$).

From model results on survival analysis, we considered {$S_{1 \text{ wk}, 2–8 \text{ wks}, >8 \text{ wks}}$} as the best approximating model ($w_i = 0.59$). Remaining models were ≥2.00 $\Delta AIC_c$ units from this model, and the weight of evidence supporting this model was 1.4 times greater than all other models combined (Table 3). While 2 models, {$S_{1 \text{ wk}, 2–4 \text{ wks}, 5–8 \text{ wks}, >8 \text{ wks}}$} and {$S_{\text{birth timing}}$}, were within ≤2.73 $\Delta AIC_c$ units from our top model, we excluded them for the following reasons; 1) survival estimates for weeks 2–4 (0.86, SE = 0.03) vs weeks 5–8 (0.86, SE = 0.03) from model {$S_{1 \text{ wk}, 2–4 \text{ wks}, 5–8 \text{ wks}, >8 \text{ wks}}$} were not significantly different and were virtually identical to the 2–8 week survival estimate (0.86, SE = 0.02) obtained from model {$S_{1 \text{ wk}, 2–8 \text{ wks}, >8 \text{ wks}}$}, 2) given the lack of discrepancy between these 2 models, removal of model {$S_{1 \text{ wk}, 2–8 \text{ wks}, >8 \text{ wks}}$} resulted in weight of evidence supporting our top ranked model ($w_i = 0.73$) 2.7 times greater than all other models combined, and 3) the model {$S_{\text{birth timing}}$} 95% CI for the β estimate for early born lambs incorporated 0. Furthermore, model {$S_{1 \text{ wk}, 2–8 \text{ wks}, >8 \text{ wks}}$} had the lowest $QAIC_c$ when $\hat{c} = 2.0$ (moderate dispersion; $QAIC_c$ wt = 0.34) and through $\hat{c} = 3.0$ (extreme dispersion; $QAIC_c$ wt = 0.20). The β estimate and 95% confidence intervals for the intercept (default >8 weeks survival period; 2.78, 95% CI = 2.28 to 3.29), 1 week (−1.36, 95% CI = −2.11−−0.60), and 2–8 weeks age intervals (−0.96, 95% CI = −1.57−−0.36), indicated β ≠ 0; thus, we considered survival was best explained by 3-stage age-intervals. Weekly survival estimates for 1 week, 2–8 weeks, and >8 weeks were 0.81 (95% CI = 0.70–0.88), 0.86 (95% CI = 0.81–0.90), and 0.94 (95% CI = 0.91–0.96), respectively; overall probability of surviving 52 weeks was 0.02 (95% CI = 0.01–0.07). Of 70 mortalities used in covariate models, 15 (21.4%) occurred during the first week, 39 (55.7%) during weeks 2–8, and 16 (22.9%) occurred >8 weeks of age. Results of data bootstrapping analyses provided limited evidence for over-dispersion (i.e., limited sibling dependence) due to lambs being collared from the same female over multiple years ($\hat{c} = 1.23$). Our estimate of $\hat{c}$ indicates sample variance was slightly underestimated; however, as we observed no change in our top ranked survival

model after inflating $\hat{c}$ to 3.0, we believe multiple births from some ewes had little impact on our overall estimate of survival.

Pneumonia was the leading cause of mortality (35.7%, $n = 25$) followed by predation (30.0%, $n = 21$); we were unable to determine ultimate cause of death for 7 (10%) mortalities (Table 2). We verified cougar predation in 15 (71%) predation events, and suspected felid (cougar or bobcat) on 5 (24%) other occasions; canid (coyote or domestic dog [*C. lupus familiaris*]) was suspected in 1 (5%) instance. Additionally, we suspected pneumonia as the ultimate (6 unknowns) or proximate cause of death (1 predation event) in 7 other instances. In 6 cases, carcasses were too degraded for definitive diagnosis; however, carcasses were intact (i.e., no evidence of predation) and the mortalities occurred during peak times when lambs were most susceptible to the disease (Figure 2). Additionally, in one cougar-killed lamb we obtained sufficient tissue for analysis and pneumonia was detected.

The mortality curve from pneumonia was significantly different from predation ($X^2 = 4.56$, $df = 1$, $P = 0.04$), with average age of lambs succumbing to predation (35.5 days, SE = 8.9 days; median = 17.5 days) younger in age than those succumbing to pneumonia (60.3 days, SE = 9.8 days; median = 48.0 days). Risk of predation peaked around 21 days of age while pneumonia exhibited 2 peak periods, 28 and 49 days, before tapering off around day 84 (Figure 2). The CIF indicated the risk of mortality from predation (0.45, 95% CI = 0.30–0.58) was higher than for pneumonia (0.14, 95% CI = 0.02–0.25) during the first 21 days of life, while pneumonia (0.54, 95% CI = 0.39–0.68) was higher than predation (0.20, 95% CI = 0.05–0.34) for lambs surviving >21 days. Overall CIF for pneumonia and predation were 0.37 (95% CI = 0.25–0.48) and 0.30 (95% CI = 0.17–0.42), respectively.

## Discussion

Nearly all lambs in the herds we studied died in their first year, and all but one died by the age of 2. Of 82 documented birthing events only 3 (4%) lambs survived to 1 year of age (2 in 2011 and 1 in 2012). However, both surviving lambs from 2011 ultimately died the following year; one was struck by a vehicle while migrating back to the lambing grounds at just over 1 year of age and the other was found dead of unknown causes at approximately 16 months of age. Based on our sample of 74 collared animals, recruitment averaged 0.04 (SD = 0.04) across years (2010 = 0.00, 2011 = 0.08, 2012 = 0.04) and was lower than previous regional estimates (range = 0.10–0.28; 2007–2009; SDGF&P, Rapid City, SD, unpublished data) but was within the range of recruitment observed in 9 populations of bighorn sheep in the Hells Canyon area of Idaho, Oregon, and Washington that displayed evidence of pneumonia epizootics ($\bar{x} = 0.17$, SD = 0.11, range 0.39–0.00; [15]).

Similar to our study, Cassirer and Sinclair [15] determined that pneumonia (86%) was the leading known cause of lamb mortality. However, they relied on visual observations and documented only 1 (4%) predation event. Based on our observations, ewes that lost lambs as a result of predation were more likely to leave the area where the predation event occurred, while ewes that lost lambs as a result of other mortality events (e.g., pneumonia, starvation) were more likely to remain in the general vicinity. When attempting to retrieve lambs that died from causes other than predation, we routinely observed ewes in the same area as the recently deceased lamb; however, on only one occasion did we observe a ewe within sight of a lamb that was killed by a predator. As a consequence of observed ewe behavior, relying on visual observations would have led to an underestimate of mortality from predation.

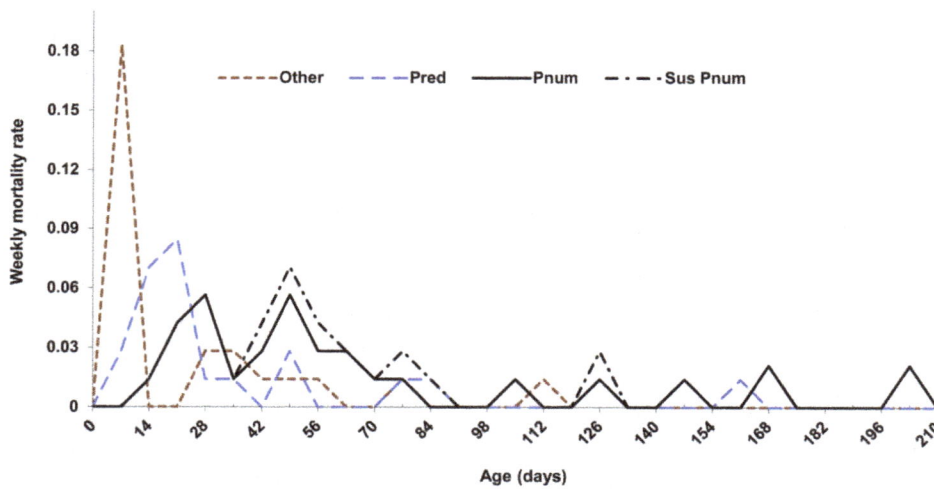

**Figure 2. Average weekly mortality rate comparison of bighorn lamb mortality events.** Average weekly mortality rate comparison for other[a], predation, pneumonia, and suspected pneumonia[b] mortality events of bighorn lambs in the Black Hills, South Dakota, USA, 2010–2012. [a] Other includes all causes of mortality other than predation and pneumonia. [b] Suspected pneumonia includes mortalities in which we assumed pneumonia was the ultimate or proximate cause of death in addition to confirmed pneumonia mortality events.

Furthermore, we documented 5 lamb mortalities prior to capture (e.g., they died ≤24 hrs old), and had we been relying solely on visual observations these events would most likely have been misconstrued as non-lambing events resulting in a lower assessment of overall lamb mortality. It is worth noting that despite having numerous ewes instrumented with VITs and attempting to obtain visual observations on ewes not instrumented with VITs on a near daily basis, we observed several instances where ewes had apparently given birth (e.g., presence of afterbirth on the animal) yet we were unable to find the lamb. Although of minimal importance in our study, with higher survival, these mortalities could contribute significantly to total estimates of survival.

Model selection results indicated that neonate survival was best explained by 3-stage age-intervals. Previous research examining neonate survival in deer [9] and elk [7] have identified similar 3-phase models as best explaining survival. However, their results were mainly attributed to different predator avoidance strategies

(e.g., hiding vs. fleeing; [40]) typically exhibited in these species. Rather than a difference in life-history phases, we believe our results were more a reflection of the different mortality sources acting at distinct time periods on these populations. For instance, during the first week of life lambs were most likely to die of causes other than predation or pneumonia (e.g., handling, starvation, infection), while during the second and third weeks of life lambs experienced the greatest risk of mortality from predation, and at > 3 weeks pneumonia was the leading cause of mortality (Figure 2). Gaillard et al. [5] noted that preweaning juvenile mortality typically occurs within 1 month of birth, yet, due to the presence of pneumonia, we observed no difference in survival from 2–8 weeks of life.

Summer pneumonia epizootics resulting in high rates of lamb mortality followed a similar pattern to those documented in other populations [15,41], with relatively few deaths occurring in the first few weeks. Lambs as young as 11 days died from pneumonia although the majority occurred ≥4 weeks of age (Figure 2).

**Table 2.** Cause-specific mortality of neonate bighorn sheep in the Black Hills, South Dakota, 2010–2012.

| Cause-specific mortality | n | % |
|---|---|---|
| Pneumonia | 25 | 35.7% |
| Predation | 21 | 30.0% |
| Starved | 8 | 11.4% |
| Unknown | 7 | 10.1% |
| Ewe died | 3 | 4.3% |
| Abandoned | 1 | 1.4% |
| Contagious eczema (CE) | 1 | 1.4% |
| Hypothermia | 1 | 1.4% |
| Infection | 1 | 1.4% |
| Underweight | 1 | 1.4% |
| Vehicle | 1 | 1.4% |

**Table 3.** Top-ranked survival models of neonate bighorn sheep from birth to 52 weeks post capture in the Black Hills, South Dakota, USA, 2010–2012 when ĉ (a model term representing overdispersion) was 1.0 (i.e., assumed no dispersion).

| Model[a] | $AIC_c$[b] | $\Delta AIC_c$[c] | $w_i$[d] | $K$[e] | Deviance |
|---|---|---|---|---|---|
| {$S_{1\ wk,\ 2-8\ wks,\ >8\ wks}$} | 429.67 | 0.00 | 0.59 | 3 | 423.64 |
| {$S_{1\ wk,2-4\ wks,\ 5-8\ wks,\ >8\ wks}$} | 431.70 | 2.02 | 0.36 | 4 | 423.63 |
| {$S_{birth\ timing}$} | 432.40 | 2.73 | 0.26 | 3 | 426.36 |
| {$S_{1\ wk,2-4\ wks,\ >4\ wks}$} | 436.25 | 6.58 | 0.02 | 3 | 430.22 |

[a]Composition and description of models are listed in Table 1.
[b]Akaike's Information Criterion corrected for small sample size (Burnham and Anderson 2002).
[c]Difference in $AIC_c$ relative to min. AIC.
[d]Akaike wt (Burnham and Anderson 2002).
[e]Number of parameters.

Cassirer and Sinclair [15] found that highest rates of pneumonia-related mortality occurred between 6–8 weeks post birth and suggested that morbidity may have coincided with the waning of passive immunity acquired from colostrum [42]. We found pneumonia-related mortality occurred slightly earlier, peaking from 4–7 weeks; however, we observed a definitive lull in mortality around week 5 (Figure 2). Lack of mortality at that time may simply be a result of sample size, or perhaps a function of the vigor in which the epizootic operated within each of the 3 herds. We did, however, find that birth weights of lambs that died of pneumonia ≤35 days old, were on average lighter (4.23 kg, SE = 0.14; $n = 9$) than lambs that died of pneumonia >35 days old (4.97 kg, SE = 0.10; $n = 14$) suggesting that heavier lambs lived longer.

Predation was our second leading cause of mortality with the greatest risk occurring primarily around 2–3 weeks of age. It is likely that decreased mobility during this time predisposed lambs to predation, although we suspect that changes in prey density also may explain some of the decreased risk at >3 weeks. For instance, birth peak for bighorn sheep was approximately 15 May across years, while the birth peak in the Black Hills for mule deer was 7–14 June [43], for white-tailed deer it was 7–17 June [44], and for elk it was 28 May–4 June (Schmitz 2010, SDGF&P, unpublished data). If risk of predation was strictly a function of lamb mobility we would expect no difference in predation based on birth timing (e.g., early, peak, or late). However, if predation was a function of prey density we would expect a decrease in risk from early to late born lambs as other prey became available. Early, peak, and late born lambs represented 18% ($n = 14$), 52% ($n = 40$), and 30% ($n = 23$), respectively, of all documented mortality events; yet, they made up 29% ($n = 6$), 62% ($n = 13$), and 10% ($n = 2$), respectively, of predation events. The decreasing trend in relative predation risk we observed between birth periods, and the decreased susceptibility to predation after 3 weeks of life, indicates that prey density could influence neonate lamb risk of predation, and supports others (e.g., [45]) who have hypothesized cougar predation on bighorn sheep is reduced when primary prey (deer; *Odocoileus spp.*) are more abundant.

Cassirer and Sinclair [15] noted a lack of lesions in predator-killed animals, no interaction between predation and disease-related mortality, and suggested that disease did not increase adult sheep vulnerability to predation. We, however, had evidence to the contrary in lambs. Although most predation events resulted in nearly the entire carcass being consumed, we were able to test one lamb that died at 81 days of age, and a second uncollared lamb that was found in the same cache pile. Both lambs were killed by a cougar the night before and laboratory (WADDL) results confirmed both had lesions consistent with bronchopneumonia. This was the only time we documented 2 lambs killed on the same evening by the same predator, and the fact that both were pneumonia positive suggests that disease can increase lamb vulnerability to predation. Additionally, the one lamb that died as a result of canid predation occurred when the lamb was approximately 158 days of age which, we assume, would have been sufficiently mobile to avoid canid predators had it been healthy. Yet, this lamb was observed 3 days prior to the mortality event and appeared gaunt and lethargic. Studies of domestic calves (*Bos taurus*) have indicated animals inoculated with *Mannheimia haemolytica* (one of the pathogens hypothesized to cause pneumonia in bighorn sheep) spent less time feeding and more time resting than control animals [46]. If these same behavioral characteristics were exhibited in bighorn lambs they would likely experience greater risk to predation.

Even though we considered only one model as best approximating survival, we did glean information from other models that was noteworthy. First, model {$S_{age \, at \, capt}$} 95% CI for the β estimate incorporated 0 (−0.16, 95% CI = −0.62–0.31) and the estimate suggested no positive relationship between age at capture and survival. Based on these results, it did not seem that capturing younger lambs during the first few hours of life, a time we hypothesized may be a critical bonding period, influenced survival. Additionally, model {$S_{birth \, timing}$} indicated that peak (0.90, 95% CI = 0.86–0.92) and early (0.93, 95% CI = 0.87–0.96) born lambs exhibited higher survival than late (0.78, 95% CI = 0.66–0.86) born lambs. As noted above, late born lambs were less likely to suffer mortality from predation, however, the opposite trend was observed for late born lambs dying of pneumonia. Late born lambs were 1.5 times (11 observed vs 7.1 expected) more likely to die of pneumonia than expected by chance, which was higher than for early (1.2; 6 observed vs 5 expected) or peak (0.6; 8 observed vs 12.9 expected) born lambs. This trend may simply be a function of late born lamb availability, as they were less likely to die of predation, or it could be a result of increased horizontal disease transmission. For example, lambs born early in the season would be present when sheep densities were at their lowest as most ewes had not given birth and remained on wintering grounds. Lambs born later in the year would arrive as sheep densities on the lambing grounds were at their highest. Assuming lamb immune systems are weakest during the first few weeks of life, late born lambs would have a much greater chance of coming into contact with other diseased animals, which could increase their chance of contracting the disease.

The sustained high levels of juvenile mortality we observed indicate these 3 populations are declining, primarily as a result of chronic pneumonia epizootics. Whether these pathogens are being maintained and transmitted among populations via bighorn sheep movements or from contact with domestic sheep and goats remains unclear. Over the course of our study we observed no range overlap between the Hill City and the other 2 subherds, and limited overlap during the lambing season between Rapid Creek and Spring Creek subherds (Figure 1). However, our sample of collared adults only included females, and it could be male movements, especially during the breeding season, could account for pathogen transmission. Conversely, bighorn sheep habitat in the Black Hills is made up of a matrix of public and private lands with several domestic sheep and goats present in areas adjacent to primary habitats or along known dispersal corridors. As effective buffers between domestics and bighorns have been identified as 20–40 km [47,48], the potential exists for all 3 herds to have contact with domestic sheep and goats, precipitating pneumonia-caused mortality.

## Conclusions

We provide the first evaluation of the influence of intrinsic variables on neonate bighorn sheep survival and a quantitatively robust assessment of cause-specific mortality. Pneumonia was the major factor limiting recruitment followed by predation, although mortality from predation seemed to be partly compensatory to pneumonia and its effects were less pronounced as alternative prey became available. Given the politically untenable prospect of culling herds (J. Kanta, SDGF&P, personal communication), and the current lack of effective vaccines for wild bighorn sheep [16,49], it seems current declines in these 3 populations will likely go unabated. Future research assessing the role of male dispersal in perpetuating disease among populations, experimenting with vaccines that have shown promise in captive bighorns at reducing pneumonia-caused mortality [50], and quantifying the relationship between disease and predation at limiting bighorn sheep populations is warranted. Furthermore, given the high rates of pneumonia-caused mortality we observed, and the apparent lack of pneumonia-causing pathogens in bighorn populations in the western Black Hills (B. Parr, South Dakota State University, Brookings, SD, unpublished data), management activities should be geared towards eliminating contact between diseased and healthy populations.

## Acknowledgments

We thank S. Griffin, J. Broecher, B. Juarez, B. Tycz, L. Meduna., L. Dahl, J. Kanta, A. Lindbloom, T. Berdan, J. Schmit, and J. Felio for capture and monitoring assistance and F. Cassirer for helpful comments on our manuscript. Thanks also to the Civil Air Patrol and pilots L. Becht and G. Kirk for assistance with flight time. Any use of trade, firm, or product names is for descriptive purposes only and does not imply endorsement by the U.S. Government.

## Author Contributions

Conceived and designed the experiments: JBS JAJ. Performed the experiments: JBS JAJ. Analyzed the data: JBS JAJ TWG RWK. Contributed reagents/materials/analysis tools: JBS JAJ TWG RWK. Wrote the paper: JBS JAJ TWG RWK. Collected field data: JBS.

## References

1. Buechner HK (1960) The bighorn sheep in the United States, its past, present, and future. Wildl Monogr 4: 1–174.

2. Singer FJ, Zeigenfuss LC, Spicer L (2001) Role of patch size, disease, and movement in rapid extinction of bighorn sheep. Conserv Biol 15: 1347–1354.

3. Wehausen JD, Kelley ST, Ramey RR (2011) Domestic sheep, bighorn sheep, and respiratory disease: a review of the experimental evidence. California Fish and Game 97: 7–24.

4. Fitzsimmons NN, Buskirk SW, Smith MH (1995) Population history, genetic variability, and horn growth in bighorn sheep. Conserv Biol 9: 314–323.

5. Gaillard JM, Festa-Bianchet M, Yoccoz NG, Loison A, Toigo C (2000) Temporal variation in fitness components and population dynamics of large herbivores. Annu Rev Ecol Syst 31: 367–393.

6. Raithel JD, Kauffman M, Pletscher DH (2007) Impact of spatial and temporal variation in calf survival on the growth of elk populations. J Wildl Manage 71: 795–803.

7. Barber-Meyer SM, Mech LD, White PJ (2008) Elk calf survival and mortality following wolf restoration to Yellowstone National Park. Wildl Monogr 169: 1–30.

8. Bishop CJ, Freddy DJ, White GC, Watkins BE, Stephenson T, et al. (2007) Using vaginal implant transmitters to aid in capture of mule deer neonates. J Wildl Manage 71: 945–954.

9. Grovenburg TW, Swanson CC, Jacques CN, Klaver RW, Brinkman TJ, et al. (2011) Survival of white-tailed deer neonates in Minnesota and South Dakota. J Wildl Manage 75: 213–220.

10. Shackleton DM, Shank CC, Wikeem BM (1999) Natural history of Rocky Mountain and California bighorn sheep. In: Valdez R, Krausman PR, editors. Mountain sheep of North America. Tucson: The University of Arizona Press. 78–138.

11. Smith JB, Walsh DP, Goldstein EJ, Parsons ZD, Karsch RC, et al. (2013) Techniques for capturing bighorn sheep lambs. Wildl Soc Bull: In Press.

12. Woodard TN, Gutierrez RJ, Rutherford WH (1974) Bighorn lamb production, survival, and mortality in South-Central Colorado. J Wildl Manage 38: 771–774.

13. Wehausen JD, Bleich VC, Blong B, Russi TL (1987) Recruitment dynamics in a Southern-California mountain sheep population. J Wildl Manage 51: 86–98.

14. Cook JG, Arnett E, Irwin LL, Lindzey FG (1990) Population dynamics of two transplanted bighorn sheep herds in southcentral Wyoming. Proceedings of the Biennial Symposium of the Northern Wild Sheep and Goat Council 7: 19–30.

15. Cassirer EF, Sinclair AE (2007) Dynamics of pneumonia in a bighorn sheep metapopulation. J Wildl Manage 71: 1080–1088.

16. Sirochman MA, Woodruff KJ, Grigg JL, Walsh DP, Huyvaert KP, et al. (2012) Evaluation of management treatments intended to increase lamb recruitment in a bighorn sheep herd. J Wildl Dis 48: 781–784.

17. Onderka DK, Wishart WD (1984) A major bighorn sheep die-off from pneumonia in southern Alberta. Proceedings of the Biennial Symposium of the Northern Wild Sheep and Goat Council 4: 356–363.

18. Festa-Bianchet M (1988) A pneumonia epizootic in bighorn sheep, with comments on preventive management. Proceedings of the Biennial Symposium of the Northern Wild Sheep and Goat Council 6: 66–76.

19. Ross PI, Jalkotzy M, Festa-Bianchet M (1997) Cougar predation on bighorn sheep in southwestern Alberta during winter. Can J Zool 75: 771–775.

20. Wehausen JD (1996) Effects of mountain lion predation on bighorn sheep in the Sierra Nevada and Granite Mountains of California. Wildl Soc Bull 24: 471–479.

21. Rominger EM, Whitlaw HA, Weybright DL, Dunn WC, Ballard WB (2004) The influence of mountain lion predation on bighorn sheep translocations. J Wildl Manage 68: 993–999.

22. Festa-Bianchet M, Coulson T, Gaillard JM, Hogg J, Pelletier F (2006) Stochastic predation events and population persistence in bighorn sheep. Proc R Soc B Biol Sci 273: 1537–1543.

23. Kamler JF, Lee RM, deVos JC, Ballard WB, Whitlaw HA (2002) Survival and cougar predation of translocated bighorn sheep in Arizona. J Wildl Manage 66: 1267–1272.

24. South Dakota Department of Game, Fish and Parks (2007). Rocky mountain bighorn sheep management plan South Dakota. Available: http://gfp.sd.gov/wildlife/management/plans/. Accessed 7 June 2013.

25. Valdez R, Krausman PR (1999) Description, distribution, and abundance of mountain sheep in North America. In: Valdez R, Krausman PR, editors. Mountain Sheep of North America. Tucson: University of Arizona Press. 3–22.

26. Zimmerman TJ (2008) Evaluation of an augmentation of Rocky Mountain bighorn sheep at Badlands National Park, South Dakota. Disseration. Brookings: South Dakota State University.

27. Froiland SG (1990) Natural History of the Black Hills and Badlands. Sioux Falls: The Center for Western Studies. 225 p.

28. USGS Gap Analysis Program. 2013. National GAP analysis landcover data portal. Available: http://gapanalysis.usgs.gov/gaplandcover/data/download/. Accessed 13 March 2013.

29. National Oceanic and Atmospheric Administration (2013) Summary of monthly normals 1981–2010. Available: http://www.ncdc.noaa.gov/cdo-web/search. Accessed 13 March 2013.

30. Krausman PR, Bowyer RT (2003) Mountain Sheep. In: Feldhamer GA, Thompson BC, Chapman JA, editors. Wild mammals of North America: biology, management, and conservation. Baltimore: Johns Hopkins University Press. 1095–1115.

31. Bishop CJ, Anderson CR, Walsh DP, Bergman EJ, Kuechle P, et al. (2011) Effectiveness of a redefined vaginal implant transmitter in mule deer. J Wildl Manage 75: 1797–1806.

32. Sikes RS, Gannon WL, Animal Care and Use Committee of the American Society of Mammalogists (2011) Guidelines of the American Society of Mammalogists for the use of wild animals in research. J Mammal 92: 235–253.

33. White GC, Burnham KP (1999) Program MARK: survival estimation from populations of marked animals. Bird Study 46: 120–138.

34. Burnham KP, Anderson DR (2002) Model selection and inference: a practical information-theoretic approach. New York: Springer-Verlag. 488 p.

35. Devrie JH, Citta JJ, Lindberg MS, Howerter DW, Anderson MG (2003) Breeding-season survival of mallard females in the prairie pothole region of Canada. J Wildl Manage 67: 551–563.

36. Bishop CJ, White GC, Lukacs PM (2008) Evaluating dependence among mule deer siblings in fetal and neonatal survival analyses. J Wildl Manage 72: 1085–1093.

37. Heisey DM, Patterson BR (2006) A review of methods to estimate cause-specific mortality in presence of competing risks. J Wildl Manage 70: 1544–1555.

38. Sargeant GA (2011) wildl: R Tools for Wildlife Research and Management. R package version 1.09.

39. Therneau T (2013) A Package for Survival Analysis in S. R package version 2.37–4, <http://CRAN.R-project.org/package = survival.> Accessed 9 June 2013.

40. Lent PC (1974) Mother-infant relationships in ungulates. In: Geist V, and Walther F, editors. The behaviour of ungulates and its relation to management. Morges: IUCN Publication 24. 14–55.

41. Enk TA, Picton HD, Williams JS (2001) Factors limiting a bighorn sheep population in Montana following a dieoff. Northwest Sci 75: 280–291.

42. Miller MW, Conlon JA, McNeil HJ, Bulgin JM, Ward ACS (1997) Evaluation of a multivalent Pasteurella haemolytica vaccine in bighorn sheep: safety and serologic responses. J Wildl Dis 33: 738–748.

43. Schmitz LE (2010) Mortality and habitat use of mule deer fawns in the southern Black Hills, South Dakota, 2003–2007. Pierre: South Dakota Game, Fish, and Parks Report No.2010–05. 1–64.

44. Schmitz LE (2006) Ecology of white-tailed deer in South Dakota: growth, survival, and winter nutrition. Dissertation. Brookings: South Dakota State University.

45. Logan KA, Sweanor LL (2001) Desert puma: evolutionary ecology and conservation of an enduring carnivore. Washington: Island Press. 1–463.

46. Theurer ME, Anderson DE, White BJ, Miesner MD, Mosier DA, et al. (2013) Effect of Mannheimia haemolytica pneumonia on behavior and physiologic responses of calves during high ambient environmental temperatures. J Anim Sci 8: 3917–3929.

47. Singer FJ, Williams ES, Miller MW, Zeigenfuss LC (2000) Population growth, fecundity, and survivorship in recovering populations of bighorn sheep. Restor Ecol 8: 75–84.

48. Monello RJ, Murray DL, Cassirer EF (2001) Ecological correlates of pneumonia epizootics in bighorn sheep herds. Can J Zool 79: 1423–1432.

49. Cassirer EF, Rudolph KM, Fowler P, Coggins VL, Hunter DL, et al. (2001) Evaluation of ewe vaccination as a tool for increasing bighorn lamb survival following pasteurellosis epizootics. J Wildl Dis 37: 49–57.

50. Subramaniam R, Shanthalingam S, Bavananthasivam J, Kugadas A, Potter KA, et al. (2011) A multivalent *Mannheimia-Bibersteinia* vaccine protects bighorn sheep against *Mannheimia haemolytica* challenge. Clin Vaccine Immunol 18: 1689–1694.

# 12

# Incidence of Infection in *Prnp* ARR/ARR Sheep following Experimental Inoculation with or Natural Exposure to Classical Scrapie

**Martin Jeffrey[1]\*, Stuart Martin[1], Francesca Chianini[2], Samantha Eaton[2¤], Mark P. Dagleish[2], Lorenzo González[1]**

**1** Animal Health and Veterinary Laboratories Agency (AHVLA-Lasswade), Pentlands Science Park, Bush Loan, Penicuik, Midlothian, Scotland, United Kingdom, **2** Moredun Research Institute, Pentlands Science Park, Bush Loan, Penicuik, Midlothian, Scotland, United Kingdom

## Abstract

The prion protein gene (*Prnp*) is highly influential in determining risk and susceptibility of sheep exposed to classical scrapie. Sheep homozygous for alanine at codon 136 and arginine at codons 154 and 171 (ARR/ARR) of the *Prnp* gene are historically considered to be highly resistant to classical scrapie, although they form a significant fraction of cases of atypical scrapie. To date, experimental transmission of prions to ARR/ARR sheep has only been achieved with the BSE agent and mostly by the intracerebral route. We summarise here the results of six separate studies, in which 95 sheep of the ARR/ARR genotype were naturally exposed to (n = 18) or experimentally challenged with (n = 77) natural or experimental sources of classical scrapie by the oral, intra-intestinal, subcutaneous or intracerebral routes and allowed to survive for periods of up to 94 months post-infection. Only the intracerebral route resulted in disease and/or amplification of disease associated PrP (PrP$^d$), and only in two of 19 sheep that survived for longer than 36 months. Discriminatory immunohistochemistry and Western blot confirmed the scrapie, non-BSE signature of PrP$^d$ in those two sheep. However, the neuropathological phenotype was different from any other scrapie (classical or atypical) or BSE source previously reported in sheep of any *Prnp* genotype. These studies confirm the widely held view that ARR/ARR sheep are highly resistant to classical scrapie infection, at least within their commercial lifespan. Moreover, within the constraints of the present studies (only two infected sheep), these results do not support the suggestion that atypical scrapie or BSE are generated by adaptation or mutation of classical scrapie in sheep of resistant ARR/ARR genotype.

**Editor:** Andrew C. Gill, University of Edinburgh, United Kingdom

**Funding:** The UK government supported these projects through the following Defra approved grants: SE1851, SE1948, SE1949, SE1951/1955, SE1952 and SE1953. The funders had no role in study design, data collection and analysis, decision to publish, or preparation of the manuscript.

**Competing Interests:** The authors have declared that no competing interests exist.

\* E-mail: martin.jeffrey@ahvla.gsi.gov.uk

¤ Current address: Division of Neurobiology, The Roslin Institute and Royal (Dick) School of Veterinary Studies, University of Edinburgh, Easter Bush, Midlothian, Scotland, United Kingdom

## Introduction

The transmissible spongiform encephalopathies (TSEs) are characterised by the accumulation of abnormal forms of a host-coded, cell membrane sialoglycoprotein called prion protein (PrP). Scrapie, or classical scrapie, of sheep and goats is the archetypal TSE and has been recognised as contagious outbreaks of disease for several centuries. More recently, a novel, apparently non-contagious or sporadic form of sheep TSE, originally called Nor 98 [1] and now more commonly referred to as atypical scrapie, has been recognised in Europe and elsewhere.

The prion protein gene (*Prnp*) controls susceptibility to both atypical and classical scrapie [2]. Sheep bearing alanine (A) or valine (V) at codon 136 and glutamine (Q) at codon 171 of PrP are susceptible to classical scrapie. In contrast, classical scrapie is rarely reported in sheep homo- or hetero-zygous for the allele that bears A at codon 136 and arginine (R) at codons 154 and 171. In separate UK studies, sheep scrapie was not identified in aged ARR/ARR or ARQ/ARR sheep in flocks or geographical regions with endemic scrapie [3,4,5,6]. Other epidemiological studies also show that scrapie is very rare in ARQ/ARR sheep and absent from ARR/ARR sheep in the UK [7]. However, single cases of natural scrapie infection in ARR/ARR sheep have been reported from Germany, France [8] and possibly also Japan [9].

In contrast, atypical scrapie is relatively common in sheep that are homozygous or heterozygous for ARR alleles but is rare in genotypes considered highly susceptible to classical scrapie such as the VRQ/VRQ genotype [10]. In addition, ARR/ARR sheep succumb to cattle and sheep BSE infection following intracerebral challenge, albeit with extended incubation periods relative to homozygous ARQ sheep [11,12]. ARR/ARR sheep orally [13] or intra-splenically [14] dosed with BSE may also sustain infection though development of clinical disease was not achieved by these routes.

Over the last two decades, we have performed several experiments in which ARR/ARR sheep have been exposed to natural scrapie or have been experimentally challenged by different routes. The purpose of this report is to draw together the data from those studies and report the susceptibility of ARR/ARR sheep to classical scrapie.

## Materials and Methods

All studies, including experimental inoculations, care of animals and euthanasia, were carried out in accordance with the UK Animal (Scientific Procedures) Act 1986. Studies 1 and 3–6 were performed at the Moredun Research Institute under licenses from the UK Government Home Office number 60/2656 (renewed in 2005 with number 60/3646). Study 2 was carried out at the Agricultural Development and Advisory Service facilities at High Mowthorpe under project license number 70/5155. Animals were monitored daily for the presence of neurological signs compatible with scrapie and were euthanized once those signs reached a standard, pre-determined end point (for details refer to [15]), when showing signs of intercurrent disease unresponsive to treatment, or for welfare reasons. In most cases, however, sheep were killed at the scheduled termination of the different studies. In all cases, euthanasia was performed by intravenous injection of barbiturate overdose followed by exsanguination.

### ARR/ARR sheep included in the different studies

Ninety-five ARR/ARR sheep were included in the following six studies (Table 1 and Fig. 1):

**Study 1 (Natural infection).** In a closed flock of Suffolk sheep, in which the average incidence of scrapie in ARQ/ARQ sheep over a nine-year period was 84% [15], 18 ARR/ARR sheep were allowed to survive for over 48 months (Table 1 and Fig. 1). These ARR/ARR sheep were reared from birth in continuous contact with scrapie infected individuals.

**Study 2 (Oral infection with sheep scrapie).** 26 ARR/ARR Cheviot lambs were orally dosed at 2–3 weeks of age on five consecutive days with 1 g of a brain pool homogenate (total dose 5 g) and were allowed to survive for 14 to 92 months post-infection (mpi; Table 1 and Fig. 1). The brain pool homogenate (RBP1) was made from whole brains taken from 17 scrapie affected sheep of five different breeds and four Prnp genotypes (VRQ/VRQ, VRQ/ARQ, ARQ/ARQ and VRQ/ARR), which originated from six different farms. After challenge with the same 5 g oral dose, this inoculum produced attack rates of 100% in VRQ homozygous sheep [16,17] and of 64% in ARQ/ARR sheep [18]. A 1 g dose of the same inoculum administered also by the oral route gave rise to

100% attack rates in VRQ/VRQ, VRQ/ARQ, VRQ/ARR and ARQ/ARQ sheep [17,18].

**Study 3 (Oral infection with experimental murine-adapted scrapie).** A total of 12 Suffolk or Cheviot ARR/ARR sheep between the ages of 3–5 months were orally dosed with 25 ml of a 20% suspension of brain from scrapie affected mice (5 g tissue equivalent). Three sheep each were infected with the murine adapted strains ME7, 22 A, 79 A, or 87 V, all of which were originally derived from scrapie affected sheep, and killed between 35–47 mpi (Table 1 and Fig. 1). The rationale for this experiment and the results of challenging sheep of other genotypes with the same murine strains were reported by Sisó et al., [19]. Briefly, oral challenge of VRQ/VRQ sheep with the same 5 g dose induced 100% attack rate with ME7, 50% with 22 A, 33% with 79 A and 0% with 87 V. Attacks rates for the same dose and route in ARQ/ARQ sheep (some of which were polymorphic at codons 112, 141, or 168) were 86% with ME7, 83% with 22 A, 17% with 79 A and 0% with 87 V. All four murine scrapie strains produced 100% attack rates in VRQ/VRQ and ARQ/ARQ sheep when administered by a combined oral, subcutaneous and intracerebral route.

**Study 4 (Inoculation of intestinal loops with sheep scrapie).** Single isolated gut loops were created as described previously [20] in six two month-old, scrapie-free ARR/ARR Suffolk lambs. Loops were created to include the distal ileum with its continuous Peyer's patch and inoculated with 5 ml of a Suffolk scrapie brain 20% homogenate (1 g tissue equivalent). Two sheep were killed at 16 and 47 mpi because of intercurrent health problems; the remaining 4 sheep were healthy when killed at the end of the experiment at 70–72 mpi (Table 1). The inoculum was sourced from scrapie confirmed clinical cases (pool of 10 ARQ/ARQ sheep) from the naturally infected Suffolk flock described above (study 1, see Fig. 1). In a different experiment, the same inoculum was used to infect sheep of the VRQ/VRQ, VRQ/ARQ and ARQ/ARQ genotypes either by the oral or subcutaneous routes with 100% attack rates in all cases [21].

**Study 5 (Sub-cutaneous inoculation with sheep scrapie).** 13 New Zealand-derived ARR/ARR Suffolk lambs were subcutaneously inoculated at 6 months of age with 1 ml of a 10% clarified homogenate of the same inoculum as used in study 4 (0.1 g tissue equivalent; Fig.1). The injection was done in the drainage area of the right prefemoral lymph node, as described in detail previously [22]. Seven ARR/ARR sheep were killed at

**Table 1.** Design of the different studies.

| Study No. | Exposure | Source | Dose | Months post-infection or age at post-mortem examination | | | | | | | | Total |
|---|---|---|---|---|---|---|---|---|---|---|---|---|
| | | | | 0–12 | 13–24 | 25–36 | 37–48 | 49–60 | 61–72 | 73–84 | 85–96 | |
| 1 | Natural | ARQ/ARQ | n/a | | | | | 9 | 5 | 1 | 3 | 18 |
| 2 | Oral | Sheep pool | 5 | | 3 | 3 | 3 | 3 | 3 | | 11 | 26 |
| 3 | Oral | Murine strains | 5 | | | 6 | 6 | | | | | 12 |
| 4 | Intraintestinal | ARQ/ARQ | 1 | | 1 | | 1 | | 4 | | | 6 |
| 5 | Subcutaneous | ARQ/ARQ | 0.1 (+2*) | 7 | 2 | | | | | | 4* | 13 |
| 6a | Intracerebral | ARQ/ARQ | 0.1 | | | | 2 | | 4 | 4 | | 10 |
| 6b | Intracerebral | VRQ/VRQ | 0.1 | 1 | | | | | 1 | 8 | | 10 |
| Total | | | | 1 | 11 | 11 | 12 | 12 | 17 | 13 | 18 | 95 |

Age in months for naturally exposed sheep of study 1; months post-infection for all other studies. Sheep pool, pool of 17 scrapie brains (VRQ/VRQ = 6, VRQ/ARQ = 6, ARQ/ARQ = 4, VRQ/ARR = 1).
Murine strains, sheep dosed with 22 A or 87 V killed at 35 mpi; sheep dosed with ME7 or 79 A killed at 47 mpi. Dose in grams: n/a, not applicable;
*, four sheep were boosted with 2 g of inoculum by the subcutaneous route (months post-inoculation correspond to those of original challenge).

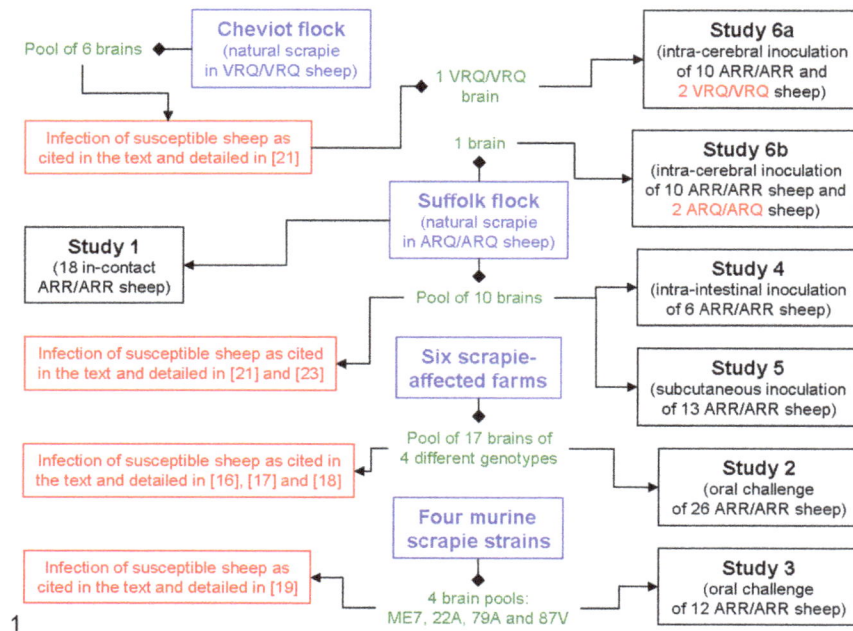

**Figure 1. Design of the different studies with reference to the source of the inocula used.** In green, inocula used; in blue, source of the inocula; in black use of the inocula for the six different studies on ARR/ARR sheep; in red, use of the same inocula to challenge sheep of susceptible genotypes.

22 mpi and two at 29 and 32 mpi; the remaining four were re-challenged subcutaneously at 32 mpi with 10 ml (5 ml in each flank) of a 20% dilution of the same inoculum (2 g tissue equivalent) and killed 58 to 62 months after the second inoculation (90 to 94 months after the original challenge; Table 1). The inoculum used induced infection in 100% ARQ/ARQ Suffolk sheep without threonine polymorphism at codon 112 when injected by the same subcutaneous route [23].

**Study 6 (Intracerebral inoculation with sheep scrapie).** In study 6a, 10 ARR/ARR Suffolk sheep were intracerebrally challenged at four months of age with 0.5 ml of a 20% sheep scrapie brain homogenate (0.1 g tissue equivalent) using a scrapie brain homogenate derived from an ARQ/ARQ sheep from the naturally infected Suffolk flock described above (Fig. 1). Two sheep were found dead at 39 and 43 mpi, another four were culled at 61 to 72 mpi due to welfare issues and the remaining four were killed at the end of the experiment (79 mpi; Table 1). Two age-matched ARQ/ARQ sheep were also inoculated (same inoculum, route and dose) and died at ~17 mpi with a pathological and biochemical scrapie phenotype indistinguishable from that of the inoculum donor and other ARQ/ARQ sheep in their flock.

In study 6b, 10 ARR/ARR Cheviot sheep were also intracerebrally challenged at the same age and with the same dose as the Suffolk sheep but with an inoculum derived from a VRQ/VRQ Cheviot sheep that succumbed to confirmed scrapie after oral infection with a brain pool homogenate of six natural scrapie cases in sheep of the same breed and genotype all derived from the same flock (Fig. 1; for details of this source see [21]). Two sheep were found dead at 11 and 72 mpi, one was killed with terminal neurological signs at 74 mpi and the remaining seven were culled at the end of the experiment (79 mpi; Table 1). Two age-matched VRQ/VRQ sheep were also inoculated (same inoculum, route and dose) and died at ~5 mpi with a pathological

and biochemical scrapie phenotype that was indistinguishable from that of the donor sheep.

## Laboratory examinations

From each of the above studies, a detailed necropsy was performed and samples of lymphoid tissues, digestive tract, brain and spinal cord, peripheral and autonomic nervous system tissues, striated muscles and other organs were taken for immunohistochemical (IHC) examinations, as detailed in table 2. Tissues were processed to paraffin wax and stained with haematoxylin and eosin (brain only) or subjected to IHC labelling for disease associated PrP (PrP$^d$) using R145 monoclonal antibody (binding to ovine PrP amino acid [aa] sequence 222–226 [24]) as described previously [11]. Two additional PrP antibodies, F99 (aa sequence 220–225 [25]) and 3F10 (aa sequence 137–151 [26]) were used in serial sections to help confirming low levels of PrP$^d$ accumulation found with R145. In addition, 2A11 (aa sequence 163–171 [27], and SAF 84 (aa sequence 166–172 [28]), monoclonal antibodies that do not recognize R at codon 171 were also used on tissue sections where positive PrP$^d$ labelling was detected with R145.

Western blotting (WB) was carried out in samples of medulla oblongata and/or cerebellum of all sheep using P4 (aa sequence 93–99 [29]) and SAF84 PrP antibodies as described previously [21] to detect protease resistant PrP (PrP$^{res}$). In addition, samples of five different brain areas from the only sheep that developed clinical scrapie were examined with L42 (aa sequence 148–153 [28]) and F99 PrP monoclonal antibodies.

The Bio- Rad TeSeE ELISA is the screening test used in the current statutory UK small ruminant TSE surveillance programme, and was used to test cerebellum samples from all 20 intracerebrally challenged ARR/ARR sheep and the four controls of that experiment (study 6).

**Table 2.** Details of tissues examined routinely by IHC in ARR/ARR sheep of the different studies.

| Tissue | Study number | | | | | |
|---|---|---|---|---|---|---|
| | 1 | 2 | 3 | 4 | 5 | 6 |
| **Lymphoid tissues** | | | | | | |
| Pharyngeal tonsil | | X | | | | |
| Palatine tonsil | X | X | X | X | X | X |
| Nictitating membrane | | X | | | X | X |
| Medial retropharyngeal LN | X | X | X | X | | X |
| Lateral retropharyngeal LN | | X | | | | |
| Submandibular LN | | X | | | X | X |
| Parotid LN | | X | | | | |
| Prescapular LN | | X | | | X | X |
| Tracheobronchial LN | | X | | | | |
| Mediastinal LN | | X | | | | |
| Mesenteric LN | | X | X | | X | X |
| Ileocecal LN | | X | | | | |
| Inguinal LN | | X | | | X | |
| Popliteal LN | | X | | | X | |
| Spleen | | X | X | | X | X |
| **Digestive tract** | | | | | | |
| Oesophagus | | X | | | | |
| Rumen | | X | | | | |
| Reticulum | | X | | | | |
| Omasum | | X | | | | |
| Abomasum | | X | | | | |
| Duodenum | | X | | | | |
| Jejunum | | X | | X | X | |
| Ileum | X | X | X | | X | X |
| Caecum | | X | | | | |
| Colon | | X | | | X | |
| Rectum | X | X | | | X | X |
| **Central nervous system** | | X | X | X | X | |
| Frontal cortex | | X | X | X | X | |
| Corpus striatum | X | X | X | X | X | |
| Thalamus/hypothalamus | | | | X | | |
| Hippocampus | | X | X | | X | X |
| Midbrain | | X | X | X | X | X |
| Cerebellum | X | X | X | X | X | |
| Medulla oblongata | | X | X | X | X | X |
| Obex | X | X | X | X | X | X |
| Cervical spinal cord | | X | | | X | X |
| Thoracic spinal cord | | X | | | X | X |
| Lumbar spinal cord | | X | | | X | X |
| Retina | | | | | X | X |
| **Peripheral nervous system** | | | | | | |
| Trigeminal G | | X | | | X | X |
| Nodose G | | X | | | X | X |
| Cranial cervical G | | X | | | | |
| Stellate G | | X | | | | X |
| Sympathetic chain | | X | | | X | X |

**Table 2.** Cont.

| Tissue | Study number | | | | | |
|---|---|---|---|---|---|---|
| | 1 | 2 | 3 | 4 | 5 | 6 |
| Vago-sympathetic trunk | | X | | | | |
| Vagus nerve | | X | | | X | X |
| Cranial mesenteric G | | X | | | X | X |
| Radial nerve | | X | | | | |
| Sciatic nerve | | | | | X | X |
| **Muscles and other organs** | | | | | | |
| Semitendinous muscle | | | | | X | X |
| Intercostal muscle | | | | | X | X |
| Occular muscles | | | | | X | X |
| Tongue | | | | | | X |
| Heart | X | X | | | X | |
| Lung | | X | | | | |
| Liver | | X | | | | |
| Kidney | | X | | | | |
| Adrenal gland | | X | | | X | X |

LN, lymph node; G, ganglion.
Most digestive tract tissues provided opportunity to examine both nervous and lymphoid components.
Tissues examined in each study (for description of each study refer to text) are marked with an X.

## Results

### Attack rates

None of the 64 sheep surviving for less than 72 months after scrapie challenge showed any post-mortem indication of PrP$^d$ accumulation. These included 14 naturally exposed sheep, 27 orally dosed (including the 12 dosed with murine scrapie), all six receiving intra-intestinal inoculation, nine injected subcutaneously and six infected intracerebrally. Among the remaining 33 sheep, which were aged or survived for 72 or more mpi, none of the four naturally exposed, the 11 orally dosed with sheep scrapie or the four inoculated subcutaneously were positive for PrP$^d$/PrP$^{res}$, either by IHC or WB, in any of the tissues examined. Of the 14 sheep challenged by the intracerebral route only two, one Cheviot and one Suffolk sheep, showed PrP$^d$ accumulation, as described below. In summary, these results indicate attack rates of 0% in sheep naturally exposed or experimentally infected by routes other than the intracerebral, regardless of their survival time. For intracerebrally challenged sheep, attack rates would vary between 10% (2/20), if all inoculated sheep are considered, and 14.3% (2/14), if only those coeval or older than the first indication of infection (72 mpi) are accounted for.

### PrP$^d$ positive ARR/ARR Suffolk sheep

One neurologically unremarkable ARR/ARR Suffolk sheep intracerebrally challenged with ARQ/ARQ Suffolk scrapie was culled at 72 mpi because of persistent lameness and problems related to its hooves. On histological examination of the brain this sheep showed neuropil vacuolation in the thalamus. Immunohistochemistry confirmed PrP$^d$ accumulation in the thalamus (Fig. 2a), the midbrain, the parietal cerebral cortex and the obex. PrP$^d$ was almost exclusively present in the form of particulate accumulation within the neuropil. In the obex, sparse particulate deposits of PrP$^d$

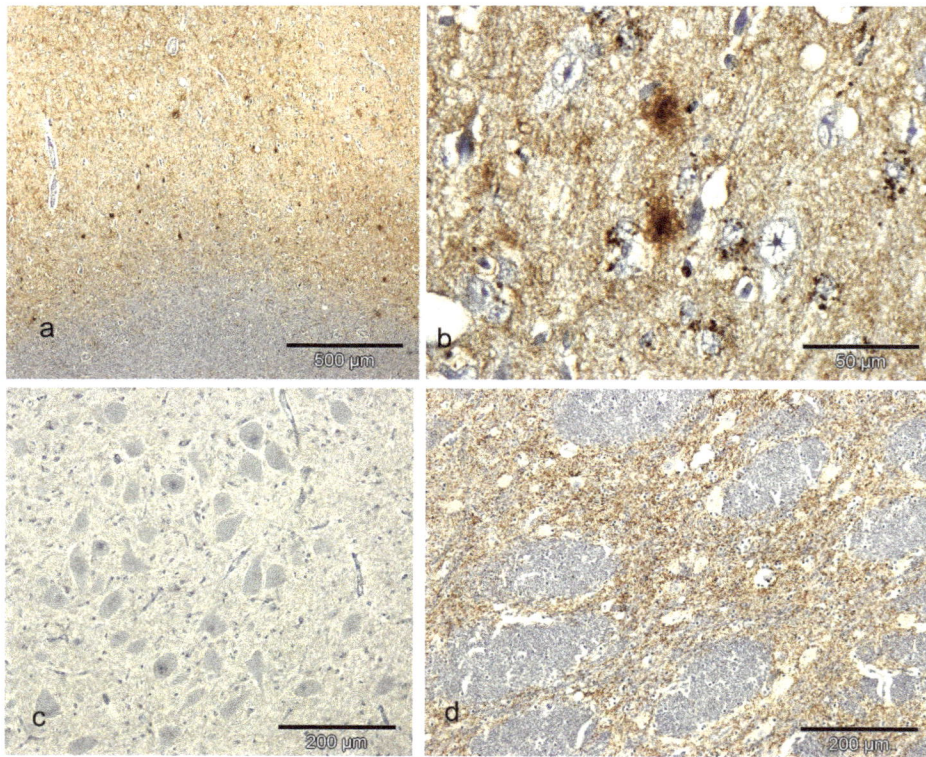

**Figure 2. PrP^d accumulation in CNS tissues of clinically affected and pre-clinical ARR/ARR sheep.** a) Cerebral cortex of an ARR/ARR Cheviot sheep challenged with a VRQ/VRQ scrapie source showing marked diffuse particulate PrP^d accumulation in grey matter with multifocal mini-plaque like accumulations. Bar = 500 μm. IHC with R145 PrP antibody and haematoxylin counterstaining. b) Detail of the cerebral cortex of the ARR/ARR scrapie affected Cheviot sheep showing diffuse, marked intra-astrocytic PrPd and multifocal intense mini-plaque–like PrP^d accumulations. Bar = 50 μm. IHC with R145 PrP antibody and haematoxylin counterstaining. c) Pre-clinical ARR/ARR Suffolk sheep challenged with ARQ/ARQ scrapie sources. Note absence of detectable PrP^d accumulation in the dorsal motor nucleus of the vagal nerve. Bar = 200 μm. IHC with R145 PrP antibody and haematoxylin counterstaining. d) Pre-clinical ARR/ARR Suffolk sheep showing diffuse grey matter PrP^d accumulation in the thalamus. Bar 200 μm. IHC with R145 PrP antibody and haematoxylin counterstaining.

were present in the spinal tract of the trigeminal nerve but not in the dorsal motor nucleus of the vagus nerve (Fig. 2b). Immuno-reactivity to R145 antibody was confirmed by positive immuno-labelling with F99 and 3F10 but no PrP^d was detected with either SAF 84 or 2A11, confirming the ARR variant of the protein.

PrP^res was not detected by WB or ELISA done on brain samples and all other tissues examined by IHC were also negative.

## PrP^d positive ARR/ARR Cheviot sheep

One ARR/ARR Cheviot sheep intracerebrally challenged with VRQ/VRQ Cheviot scrapie collapsed after a short clinical course of 3 weeks, in which the animal displayed vague neurological signs, and was killed at 75 mpi. The brain showed severe vacuolation throughout all grey matter regions and PrP^d was also present throughout all neuroanatomical areas of the brain and spinal cord. A wide range of PrP^d types [30] were present including types consistent with intra-neuronal and intra-glial and several extra-cellular types. Most of the latter were in the form of coarse or fine diffuse particulate PrP^d in the grey matter neuropil, while glial associated perivascular aggregates were infrequent. In the thalamus and cerebral cortex, distinctive, multifocal, intensely-labelled mini plaque-like deposits and marked intra-astrocytic PrP^d accumulations were observed (Fig. 2c,d). Labelling was absent when R145 positive areas were incubated with antibodies 2A11 or SAF 84. Neither the pattern of vacuolation nor the pattern and distribution of PrP^d accumulation was consistent with that of the

VRQ/VRQ Cheviot donor or the two positive control sheep. These showed less intense and less widespread vacuolation (Fig. 3a,b), predominant stellate type of PrP^d and absence of mini plaques, although the intra-glial, intra-neuronal and diffuse particulate PrP^d types were in common with ARR/ARR sheep (Fig. 3c,d).

PrP^d accumulation was not detected in the lymphoid system, digestive tract or in most of the peripheral nervous system and other tissues examined. In the retina, diffuse PrP^d labelling was found in the outer plexiform layer and coarse particulate deposits in the inner plexiform layer and in the soma of retinal ganglion cells (Fig 4a). Low levels of PrP^d accumulation were found in the trigeminal ganglion's satellite cells (Fig 4b) and in intrafusal fibres of the infra-orbital muscles (Fig 4c). In trigeminal ganglion peri-axonal PrP^d accumulation was detected in myelinated axons. Incubation of serial sections with F99 (Fig 4d) and 3F10 confirmed the specificity of labelling in these tissues.

Western blotting of brain samples incubated with P4, L42 or F99 (Fig. 5a) confirmed the presence of PrP^res in the obex, frontal cortex, thalamus, midbrain and cerebellum. The highest signal was detected in cerebellum. In almost all brain areas tested the strongest PrP^res signal was obtained from the monoglycosylated fraction, which contrasted with the strongest signal of the diglycosylated fraction in the VRQ/VRQ donor and control recipients (Figs. 5a and 5b). The mobility of the unglycosylated fraction corresponded to a molecular weight of ~20 to 21 kDa,

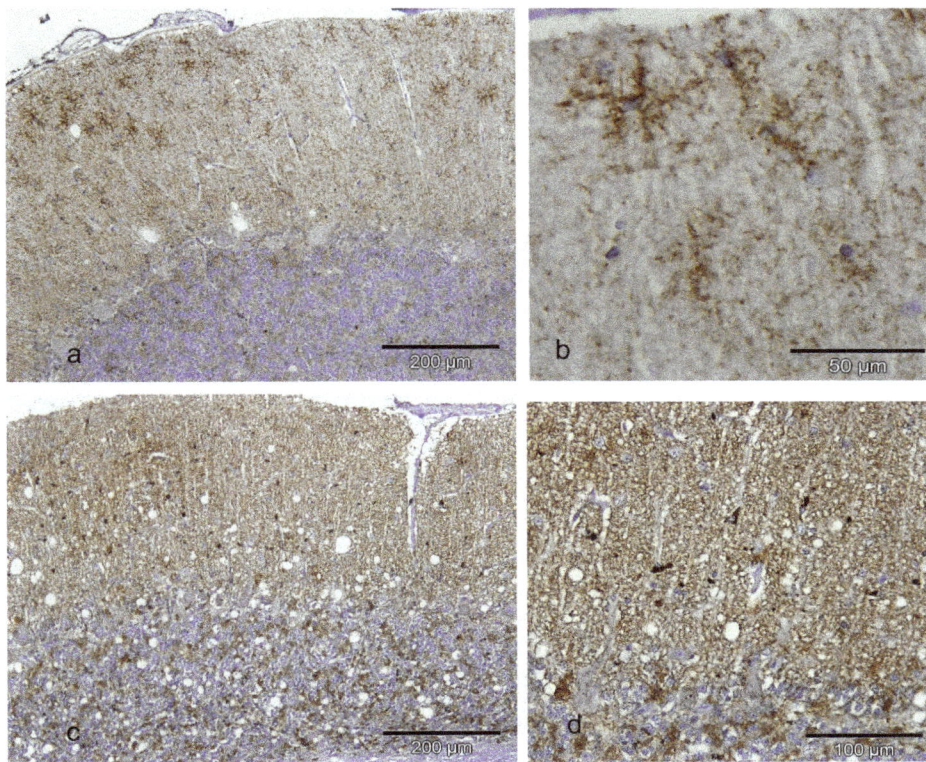

**Figure 3. PrP$^d$ labelling and vacuolation in the cerebellar cortex of VRQ/VRQ and ARR/ARR sheep.** a) VRQ/VRQ sheep showing diffuse particulate and stellate types of PrP$^d$ accumulation in the cerebellar molecular layer. Vacuolation is relatively subtle. Bar 200 μm. IHC with R145 PrP antibody and haematoxylin counterstaining. b) VRQ/VRQ sheep showing detail of the stellate type of PrP$^d$ accumulation centred on glial cell nuclei in the molecular layer of the cerebellum. Bar 50 μm. IHC with R145 PrP antibody and haematoxylin counterstaining. c) ARR/ARR sheep showing diffuse particulate but not stellate PrP$^d$ accumulation in both molecular and internal granule cell layers and prominent intra-glial types of PrP$^d$ accumulation in the cerebellar molecular layer. Vacuolation is abundant. Bar 200 μm. IHC with R145 PrP antibody and haematoxylin counterstaining. d) ARR/ARR sheep showing detail of the intensity of particulate type of PrP$^d$ accumulation and intense granular PrP$^d$ accumulation associated with glial cell nuclei (intra-microglial type) in the cerebellar molecular layer. Bar 100 μm. IHC with R145 PrP antibody and haematoxylin counterstaining.

similar to that of the VRQ/VRQ and ARQ/ARQ controls and consistent with classical scrapie. When the same brain samples were incubated with SAF84 (Fig. 5a), no signal or only trace signals were obtained for any of the bands. These observations are in agreement with the 2A11 and SAF84 IHC results, and indicate that PrP$^{res}$ was of the ARR variant.

The Bio-Rad TeSeE ELISA gave positive test values in brain samples from VRQ/VRQ and ARQ/ARQ positive scrapie controls and from the clinically affected ARR/ARR Cheviot sheep.

## Discussion

In agreement with previously published studies, the above experiments show that ARR/ARR sheep are extremely resistant to classical scrapie when naturally exposed to a highly contaminated environment or when infected by experimental protocols that approximate natural exposure. However, experimental intra-cerebral challenge shows that it is possible to induce disease in sheep of this genotype, albeit with low attack rates and incubation periods that are years longer than those in sheep of susceptible genotypes. Therefore, these data provide proof of principle that ARR/ARR sheep are susceptible to UK classical sheep scrapie sources albeit only by a highly artificial and efficient route of challenge.

The experimental gut loop protocol circumvents transit of orally dosed infectivity through the upper part of the alimentary system, avoiding enzymatic degradation of PrP$^d$. It thus maximises the opportunity of transport of infectivity across the intestinal barrier to permit amplification of infectivity in gut associated lymphoid tissues of susceptible sheep [20]. Despite this and a relatively large dose, this route did not result in generalised or even localised amplification of PrP$^d$ in ARR/ARR sheep. Equally, oral and subcutaneous infection did not result in transmission of infection. Failure to induce classical scrapie using these routes of inoculation is more relevant to natural disease than the intra-cerebral route, particularly when considering that the volumes of inocula used were in excess of those likely to be found under environmental conditions of even the highest infectivity pressure. The lack of transmission in these experiments is consistent with the absence of infection in ARR/ARR sheep exposed for prolonged periods to a highly contaminated environment (the "natural infection" group) and with many other epidemiological studies of natural scrapie in the UK [3,4,5,6,7] and elsewhere [31] which do not report classical scrapie in ARR/ARR sheep.

However, single cases of classical scrapie have been reported in ARR/ARR sheep from Japan [9], Germany and France [8], and in all instances by the detection of PrP$^{res}$ in Western blot analyses of brain samples. The Japanese case, a Suffolk sheep, appeared to be clinically affected but no data are available about the clinical or pathological phenotype of the disease. The German case, a black-

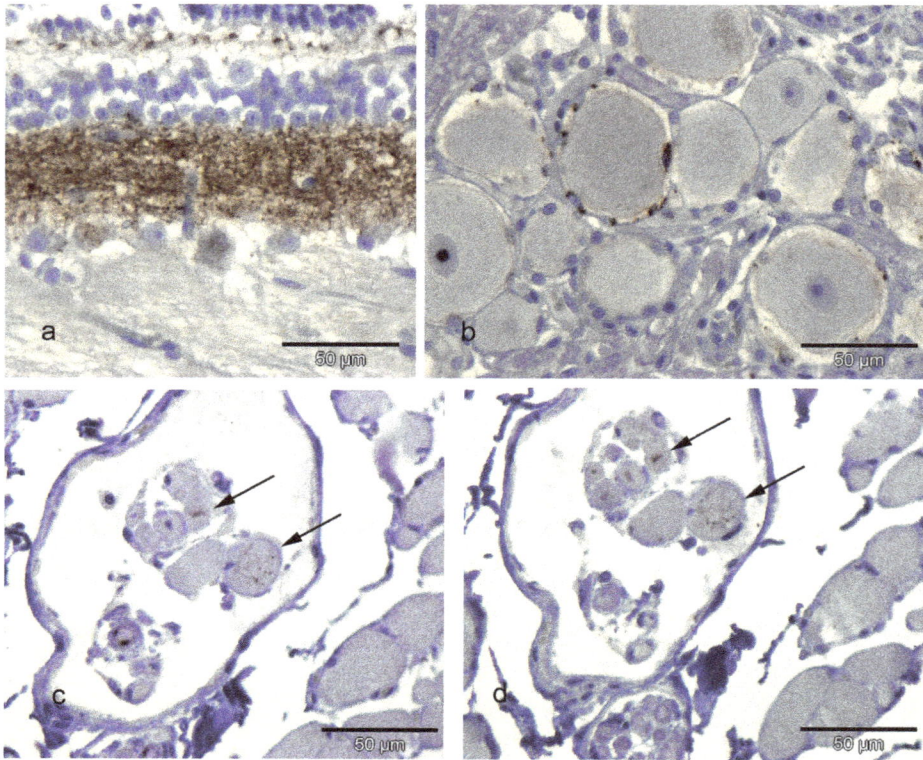

**Figure 4. Additional tissues of ARR/ARR clinically affected Cheviot sheep showing PrP$^d$ accumulation.** a) Retina showing diffuse PrP$^d$ accumulation in outer plexiform layer and granular accumulations in inner plexiform layer and retinal ganglion cells. Bar = 50 μm. IHC with R145 PrP antibody and haematoxylin counterstaining. b) Trigeminal ganglion showing granular PrP$^d$ accumulation in satellite cells Bar = 50 μm. IHC with R145 PrP antibody and haematoxylin counterstaining. c) Muscle spindle from ocular muscle showing weak granular PrP$^d$ accumulation in intrafusal muscle fibres (arrows). Bar = 50 μm. IHC with R145 PrP antibody and haematoxylin counterstaining. d) The same muscle spindle as in c) labelled with anti- PrP antibody F99. The same intrafusal muscle fibres as with R145 are labelled (arrows). Bar = 50 μm. IHC with F99 PrP antibody and haematoxylin counterstaining.

headed German mutton sheep, was apparently healthy and the French case, a 5 year-old sheep, showed neurological signs of histopathologically confirmed listeriosis. Detailed data on clinico-pathological phenotypes are not available for either case, although the French case was successfully transmitted to Tg338 mice [8]. These reports suggest that cases of classical scrapie may occur naturally in ARR/ARR sheep, although all epidemiological and experimental evidence indicate that such occurrences would be sporadic or exceptional. However, more frequent detection of such cases may be hampered by current sampling strategies which focus on the hind brain, as shown by the failure of statutory ELISA testing to detect the single pre-clinically affected intra-cerebrally challenged Suffolk sheep in the present study.

ARR/ARR sheep also appear to be much more resistant to infection with classical scrapie than with experimental sheep BSE. Thus, ARR/ARR sheep intra-cerebrally challenged with 0.5 mg tissue equivalent of sheep BSE (i.e., allowing for potential differences in infectious titre, a 500 times smaller dose than in the scrapie experiment reported here) developed clinical disease with a 100% attack rate and a survival time of $49 \pm 5$ months [12]. Similarly, ARR/ARR sheep intra-cerebrally challenged with cattle BSE showed figures of 56% attack rate and $49 \pm 13$ months survival time (Houston et al., unpublished observations). More-over, susceptibility of ARR/ARR sheep to sheep BSE by the oral route [13] and to cattle BSE by the intra-splenic route [14] has been documented, while oral, intra-intestinal and sub-cutaneous

challenge with sheep scrapie and murine adapted sheep scrapie failed to transmit infection, at least as judged by PrP$^d$ or PrP$^{res}$ detection. The difference in pathogenicity of BSE and scrapie agents for ARR/ARR sheep does not appear to be a property of the agents *per se* as this difference in pathogenicity is not observed in sheep of other genotypes. For example, oral infection of ARQ/ARQ sheep (without polymorphisms at codons 112 or 141) with ARQ/ARQ sheep scrapie results in complete attack rates and short survival times of $23 \pm 2$ months [21], while sheep of the same genotype inoculated by the same route and with the same 5 g dose of ARQ/ARQ sheep BSE also showed a 100% attack rate and survival times of $23 \pm 2$ months (first passage) or $25 \pm 2$ months (second passage) [32]. Similarly, oral infection of VRQ/VRQ sheep with ARQ/ARQ sheep scrapie produces a 100% attack rate with survival times of $47 \pm 7$ months [21] and infection of sheep of the same genotype with cattle BSE by the same route and dose also results in complete attack rate figures and survival times of ~59 months (Jeffrey et al., unpublished observations). It is worth pointing out that despite the studies reported here using a variety of natural and experimental scrapie sources, all of which proved to be infectious for sheep of susceptible *Prnp* genotypes [15,16,17,18,19,21,23], the number of such sources was limited. We cannot therefore rule out the possibility that other sources or strains of classical scrapie could result in higher attack rates or different disease phenotypes in ARR/ARR sheep, as is found with the BSE agent.

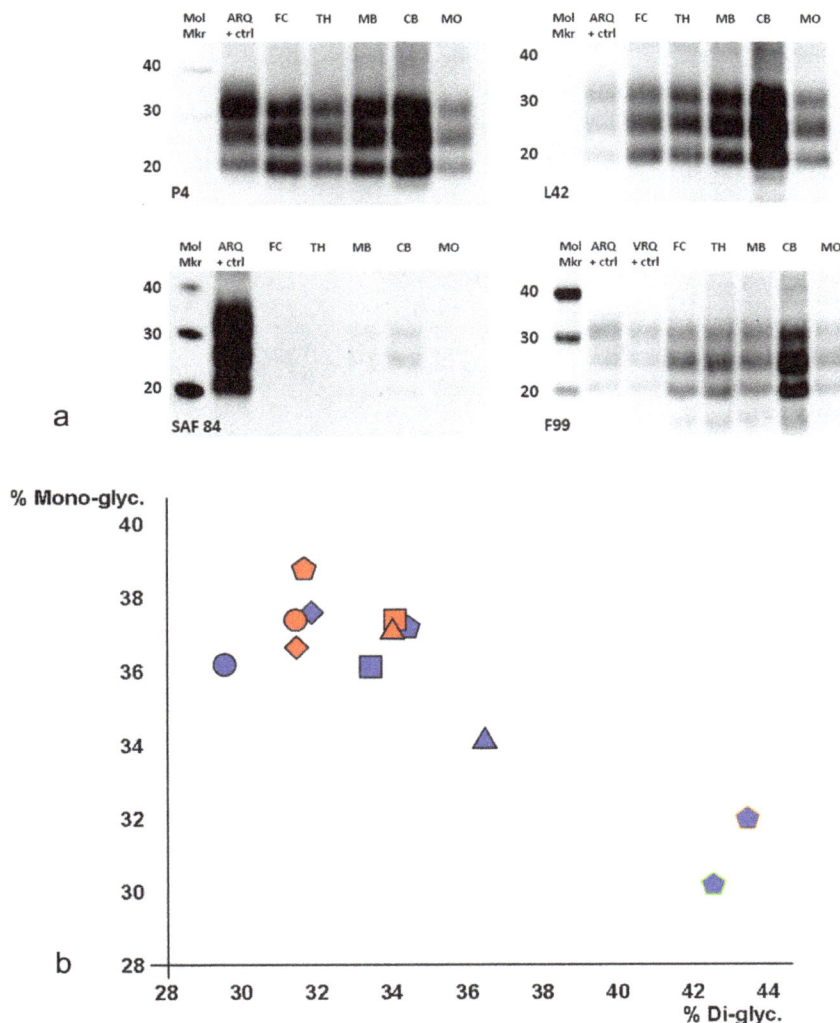

**Figure 5. Western blotting of different brain areas of ARR/ARR clinically affected Cheviot sheep.** a) Western blots of brain tissue with 4 different PrP antibodiesImmunoblots of frontal cortex (FC) thalamus (TH) midbrain (MB) cerebellum (CB) and medulla at the level of the obex (MO) each showed significant accumulation of PrP[res] with antibodies P4, L42, and F99. With each of these antibodies the cerebellum showed the greatest concentration of PrP[res]. Compared with ARQ/ARQ and VRQ/VRQ scrapie positive control obex samples, the mono-glycosylated band predominates in most of the ARR/ARR samples. The unglycosylated band from all ARR/ARR and positive control samples has a molecular weight of ~20 to 21 kDa. No labelling or only trace labelling was found when the antibody SAF84 was used. Mol mkr: molecular weight marker (Note: the molecular weight marker produced a very faint signal with L42. To position the weight reference values the blot was digitally overexposed but it is the original, non-saturated blot that is reproduced). b) Graph showing the proportion of di-glycosylated and mono-glycosylated PrP[res] for brain from the clinically affected ARR/ARR sheep in comparison with ARQ/ARQ and VRQ/VRQ controls. For each of the brain sites the mono-glycosylated fraction of PrP[res] was present in a relatively greater amount than the di-glycosylated fraction when labelled with either P4 or L42 antibodies. In contrast both VRQ/VRQ control and ARQ/ARQ positive controls had a relatively greater amount of di-glycosylated PrP[res]. Values for P4 antibody are shown in blue and for L42 in red; frontal cortex, diamonds; thalamus, squares; midbrain, triangles; cerebellum, circles; obex, pentagons; the Suffolk sheep ARQ/ARQ positive control (obex) is outlined in orange and the Cheviot sheep VRQ/VRQ positive control (obex) is outlined in green.

Although the pathological and biochemical features of the single clinical scrapie case in an ARR/ARR genotype in our studies was consistent with classical rather than atypical scrapie or BSE, the disease phenotype was dissimilar to the VRQ/VRQ case that provided the inoculum and to the two VRQ/VRQ positive control sheep challenged with the same inoculum. The pathological phenotype of this single ARR/ARR scrapie case has little resemblance to any other classical scrapie source the authors have examined in any sheep breed or *Prnp* genotype. This suggests that although some sort of modification occurs on passage of classical scrapie into ARR/ARR sheep, such change does not result in the emergence of atypical scrapie or BSE and also reinforces the notion that the interaction between the infecting source and the *Prnp* genotype of the host has significant impact on the susceptibility to scrapie and on the disease phenotype [21].

## Acknowledgments

This study describes the outcome of six large experiments carried out over almost two decades. Thanks are due to numerous individuals within the former VLA (now AHVLA) and Moredun Research Institute for performing some of the experimental procedures, the husbandry and necropsies of sheep.

## Author Contributions

Conceived and designed the experiments: MJ LG MD. Performed the experiments: MJ LG SM SE MD FC. Analyzed the data: MJ SM LG MP

SE FC. Contributed reagents/materials/analysis tools: MJ FC MP LG SM SE. Wrote the paper: MJ LG.

## References

1. Benestad SL, Sarradin P, Thu B, Schonheit J, Tranulis MA, et al. (2003) Cases of scrapie with unusual features in Norway and designation of a new type, Nor98. Vet Rec 153: 202–208.

2. Goldmann W (2008) PrP genetics in ruminant transmissible spongiform encephalopathies. Vet Res 39: 30–41.

3. González L, Dagleish MP, Bellworthy SJ, Siso S, Stack MJ et al. (2006) Post-mortem diagnosis of preclinical and clinical scrapie in sheep by the detection of disease associated PrP in their rectal mucosa. Vet Rec 158: 325–331.

4. Jeffrey M, Martin S, Thomson JR, Dingwall WS, Begara-McGorum I, et al.(2001) Onset and distribution of tissue PrP accumulation in scrapie-affected Suffolk sheep as demonstrated by sequential necropsies and tonsillar biopsies. J Comp Pathol 125: 48–57.

5. Jeffrey M, Begara-McGorum I, Clark S, Martin S, Clark J, et al. (2002) Occurrence and distribution of infection-specific PrP in tissues of clinical scrapie cases and cull sheep from scrapie-affected farms in Shetland. J Comp Pathol 127: 264–273.

6. McIntyre KM, Gubbins S, Goldmann W, Hunter N, Baylis M (2008) Epidemiological characteristics of classical scrapie outbreaks in 30 sheep flocks in the United Kingdom. PLoS One 3(12): e3994.

7. Tongue SC, Pfeiffer DU, Warner R, Elliot H, del Río Vilas V (2006) Estimation of the relative risk of developing clinical scrapie: the role of prion protein (PrP) genotype and selection bias. Vet Rec 158: 43–50.

8. Groschup MH, Lacroux C, Buschmann A, Luhken G, Mathey J, et al. (2007) Classic scrapie in sheep with the ARR/ARR prion genotype in Germany and France. Emerg Infect Dis 13: 1201–1207.

9. Ikeda T, Horiuchi M, Ishiguro N, Muramatsu Y, Kaiuwe CD, et al. (1995) Amino acid polymorphisms of PrP with reference to onset of scrapie in Suffolk and Corriedale sheep in Japan. J Gen Virol 76: 2577–2581.

10. Benestad SL, Arsac JN, Goldmann W, Noremark M (2008) Atypical/Nor98 scrapie: properties of the agent, genetics, and epidemiology. Vet Res 39: 19–26.

11. González L, Martin S, Houston FE, Hunter N, Reid HW, et al. (2005) Phenotype of disease associated PrP accumulation in the brain of bovine spongiform encephalopathy experimentally infected sheep. J Gen Virol 86: 827–838.

12. González L, Chianini F, Martin S, Sisó S, Gibbard L, et al. (2007) Comparative titration of experimental ovine BSE infectivity in sheep and mice. J Gen Virol 88: 714–717.

13. Andreoletti O, Morel N, Lacroux C, Rouillon V, Barc C, et al. (2006) Bovine spongiform encephalopathy agent in spleen from an ARR/ARR orally exposed sheep. J Gen Virol 87: 1043–1046.

14. Bencsik A, Baron T (2007) Bovine spongiform encephalopathy agent in a prion protein (PrP) ARR/ARR genotype sheep after peripheral challenge: Complete immunochemical analysis of disease-associated PrP and transmission studies to ovine-transgenic mice. J Infect Dis 195: 989–996.

15. González L, Dagleish MP, Martin S, Finlayson J, Sisó S, et al. (2012) Factors influencing temporal variation of scrapie incidence within a closed Suffolk sheep flock. J Gen Virol 93: 203–211.

16. Ryder SJ, Dexter GE, Heasman L, Warner R, Moore SJ (2009) Accumulation and dissemination of prion protein in experimental sheep scrapie in the natural host. BMC Vet Res 5: 9–14.

17. González L, Pitarch JL, Martin S, Thurston L, Moore J, et al. (In press) Identical pathogenesis and neuropathological phenotype of scrapie in valine, arginine, glutamine/valine, arginine, glutamine sheep infected experimentally by the oral and conjunctival routes. J Comp Pathol (In press: http://dx.doi.org/10.1016/j.jcpa.2013.06.006).

18. González L, Pitarch JL, Martin S, Thurston L, Simmons H, et al. (In press) Influence of polymorphisms in the prion protein gene on the pathogenesis and neiropathological phenotype of sheep scrapie after oral infection. J Comp Pathol (In press: http://dx.doi.org/10.1016/j.jcpa.2013.10.00).

19. Sisó S, Chianini F, Eaton S, Witz J, Hamilton S, et al. (2012) Disease phenotype in sheep after infection with cloned murine scrapie strains. Prion 2: 1–10.

20. Jeffrey M, González L, Espenes A, Press C, Martin S, et al. (2006) Transportation of prion protein across the intestinal mucosa of scrapie-susceptible and scrapie-resistant sheep. J Pathol 209: 4–14.

21. González L, Jeffrey M, Dagleish MP, Goldmann W, Sisó S, et al. (2012) Susceptibility to scrapie and disease phenotype in sheep: cross-PRNP genotype experimental transmissions with natural sources. Vet Res 43: 55.

22. Eaton SL, Rocchi M, González L, Hamilton S, Finlayson J, et al. (2007) Immunological differences between susceptible and resistant sheep during the preclinical phase of scrapie infection. J Gen Virol 88: 1384–1391.

23. Chianini F, Sisó S, Ricci E, Eaton SL, Finlayson J, et al. (2013) Pathogenesis of scrapie in ARQ/ARQ sheep after subcutaneous infection: Effect of lymphad-enectomy and immune cell subset changes in relation to prion protein Vet immunol immunopath 152: 348–358.

24. Jeffrey M, González L, Chong A, Foster J, Goldmann W, et al. (2006) Ovine infection with the agents of scrapie (CH1641 isolate) and bovine spongiform encephalopathy: Immunochemical similarities can be resolved by immunohis-tochemistry. J Comp Pathol 134: 17–29.

25. Spraker TR, ORourke KI, Balachandran A, Zink RR, Cummings BA, et al. (2002) Validation of monoclonal antibody F99/97.6.1 for immunohistochemical staining ofbrain and tonsil in mule deer (Odocoileus hemionus) with chronic wasting disease. J Vet Diag Invest 14: 3–7.

26. Choi JK, Park SJ, Jun YC, Oh JM, Jeong BH, et al. (2006) Generation of monoclonal antibody recognized by the GXXXG motif (glycine zipper) of prion protein. Hybrid (Larchmt.) 25: 271–277.

27. Brun A, Castilla J, Ramirez MA, Prager K, Parra B, et al. (2004) Proteinase K enhanced immunoreactivity of the prion protein-specific monoclonal antibody 2A11. Neurosci Res 48: 75–83.

28. Jacobs JG, Bossers A, Rezaei H, van Keulen LJ, McCutcheon S, et al. (2011) Proteinase K-resistant material in ARR/VRQ sheep brain affected with classical scrapie is composed mainly of VRQ prion protein. J Virol 85: 12537–12546.

29. Thuring CMA, van Keulen LJM, Langeveld JPM, Vromans MEW, van Zijderveld FG, et al. (2005) Immunohistochemical distinction between preclinical bovine spongiform encephalopathy and scrap[ie infection in sheep. J Comp Pathol 132: 59–69.

30. Jeffrey M, González L (2004) Pathology and pathogenesis of bovine spongiform encephalopathy and scrapie. In Mad cow disease and related spongiform encephalopathies Ed. DA . Harris, Pub Springer –Verlag Berlin, Heidelberg. pp 65–98.

31. Elsen JM, Amigues Y, Schelcher F, Ducrocq V, Andreoletti O, et al. (1999) Genetic susceptibility and transmission factors in scrapie: detailed analysis of an epidemic in a closed flock of Romanov. Arch Virol 144: 431–445.

32. Stack M, González L, Jeffrey M, Martin S, Macaldowie C, et al. (2009) Three serial passages of bovine spongiform encephalopathy in sheep do not significantly affect discriminatory test results. J Gen Virol, 90, 764–768.

# 13

# Healthy Animals, Healthy People: Zoonosis Risk from Animal Contact in Pet Shops, a Systematic Review of the Literature

**Kate D. Halsby[1]\*, Amanda L. Walsh[1], Colin Campbell[2], Kirsty Hewitt[1,3], Dilys Morgan[1]**

1 Gastrointestinal, Emerging and Zoonotic Infections Department, Public Health England, London, United Kingdom,, 2 Centre for the Epidemiological Study of Sexually Transmitted Infections and AIDS of Catalonia (CEEISCAT) – ICO, Hospital Universitari Germans Trias i Pujol, Badalona, Spain, 3 London/KSS Specialty School of Public Health, London Deanery, London, United Kingdom

## Abstract

*Background:* Around 67 million pets are owned by households in the United Kingdom, and an increasing number of these are exotic animals. Approximately a third of pets are purchased through retail outlets or direct from breeders. A wide range of infections can be associated with companion animals.

*Objectives:* This study uses a systematic literature review to describe the transmission of zoonotic disease in humans associated with a pet shop or other location selling pets (incidents of rabies tracebacks and zoonoses from pet food were excluded).

*Data sources:* PubMed and EMBASE.

*Results:* Fifty seven separate case reports or incidents were described in the 82 papers that were identified by the systematic review. Summary information on each incident is included in this manuscript. The infections include bacterial, viral and fungal diseases and range in severity from mild to life threatening. Infections associated with birds and rodents were the most commonly reported. Over half of the reports describe incidents in the Americas, and three of these were outbreaks involving more than 50 cases. Many of the incidents identified relate to infections in pet shop employees.

*Limitations:* This review may have been subject to publication bias, where unusual and unexpected zoonotic infections may be over-represented in peer-reviewed publications. It was also restricted to English-language articles so that pathogens that are more common in non-Western countries, or in more exotic animals not common in Europe and the Americas, may have been under-represented.

*Conclusions/implications:* A wide spectrum of zoonotic infections are acquired from pet shops. Salmonellosis and psittacosis were the most commonly documented diseases, however more unusual infections such as tularemia also appeared in the review. Given their potential to spread zoonotic infection, it is important that pet shops act to minimise the risk as far as possible.

**Editor:** Martyn Kirk, The Australian National University, Australia

**Funding:** The authors have no support or funding to report.

\* E-mail: kate.halsby@phe.gov.uk

## Introduction

Rising numbers of household pets, in particular exotic species, means that an increasing number of people are exposed to the risk of acquiring zoonotic disease from companion animals. Around 67 million pets are now owned by UK households, with 13 million households in the UK (48%) owning at least one pet in 2012 [1]. Traditional pets such as dogs and cats remain the most popular (23% of UK households own a dog and 19% of UK households own a cat) [1], however there has been an increased ownership of exotic pets in recent years, though accurate figures are difficult to obtain. This increase is due in part to the 2007 modification to The Dangerous Wild Animals Act 1976 [2]. This act lists animals for which licenses are required in the UK in order to keep the animal as a pet, whilst the modification to the act removed some exotic animals from the list.

A wide range of infections can be associated with companion animals, including parasitic, bacterial, fungal and viral diseases [3–5]. Of those transmitted by bites and scratches, pasteurellosis, cat-scratch disease, and various aerobic and anaerobic infections are predominant. Other common infections are gastrointestinal (e.g. campylobacter, salmonella), dermatologic (e.g. dermatophytoses, scabies), respiratory (e.g. psittacosis) and multisystemic (e.g. toxoplasmosis, leishmaniasis) [3].

The top five sources for acquiring a pet are: friend/acquaintance, rescue centre, pet shop, recommended breeder, and private advertisement [6]. There are studies in the literature examining animal infections in pet shops and other retail outlets [7–10], but little exploration of human infections arising from these facilities. Whilst owning a pet will always result in a small risk of zoonotic illness to the owners and those that the pet comes into contact with, a sick animal in a pet shop can potentially spread the illness to other animals within the shop, and to a large number of geographically distributed owners as newly purchased pets are taken home. Pet shops can therefore act as a nexus point for zoonotic disease.

## Methods

In September 2012, a systematic literature review was performed in order to identify any reports of human infection acquired (or where the report's authors inferred that it had been acquired) from a pet shop or other location selling pets, or an animal reported to have been acquired from such a premises.

### Search Strategy and Selection Criteria

Data for this review were identified by searches of PubMed and EMBASE, and through the references of papers identified by the review (references at all stages of publication were considered). We used the following Boolean search statement: ("pet shop" OR "pet store" OR "pet" OR "companion animal") AND ("zoonoses" OR "zoonosis" OR "Human infection" OR "Human case"). Articles in English were selected (although foreign language publications were accepted where an English abstract was available and contained sufficient information to fulfill the inclusion criteria), and no date restrictions were applied to the searches. (The main PubMed database contains manuscripts dating back to 1966, whilst EMBASE covers manuscripts from 1974 onwards.).

The abstracts of the articles were examined and retained if they referred to: i) human cases of zoonotic infection, with ii) a link to a pet or companion animal. The full text was then examined and retained if reference was made to: i) human cases of zoonotic infection, ii) which came from a pet (or a potential pet), and iii) where the animal had a link to a pet shop or other location that sells or distributes companion animals. The following information was extracted from the articles: zoonosis/agent, country (of infection or report if not known), year of infection (or report if not known), type of animal, setting (e.g. pet store, pet distributor), number of human cases associated with pet shop (or other location selling/distributing companion animals), age of human cases, method of transmission (e.g. bite or scratch), and type of contact (e.g. domestic or occupational). The information was extracted by the principal investigator and reviewed by a co-author.

A number of articles considered during the systematic review described rabid animals which had been sold in pet shops, and the extensive contact tracing for postexposure prophylaxis (PEP) which had to be conducted as a result. These were not included in this review since none of the articles documented a human case of rabies that had arisen from such animals. Further articles considered by the systematic review described cases of zoonotic infection associated with pet food and treats, purchased in pet shops. These were also not included in the review since the inclusion criteria required the pet itself to have a link to the pet shop.

## Results

One thousand and eighty seven papers were identified by the initial systematic literature review. Nine hundred and forty five of these were English-language articles, of which 265 were retained based on abstracts, and 66 met the full text inclusion criteria. The original search also identified 142 foreign language papers, of which five had sufficient information in the English abstract to include the paper in the final review. In addition, twelve potential articles were identified through the references of included papers, of which eleven met the inclusion criteria themselves.

A total of 82 papers fulfilled the criteria of the systematic review.

The results of the literature review are presented in Table 1 (where a particular incident was described by more than one paper in the review, only primary paper(s) are included in the table; articles which discussed the incident only by reference to the primary paper(s) were not included). If the country of the incident was not stated, it was assumed to be the authors' country. If a year of incident was not given, the year of publication of the paper was used as a proxy. The number of infections refers to the human cases linked to pet shops in each article, not the total number of human cases discussed.

Table 1 therefore summarises the cases of disease associated with a pet shop that were identified by the literature review. Fifty seven cases of disease or incidents associated with pet shops or other facilities distributing companion animals were included. Bacterial, viral and fungal diseases were all identified, and ranged in severity from mild to life threatening. For example, infection with ringworm (Dermatophytosis) was noted in several articles, with four separate examples in Japanese pet shop employees and customers [11–14]. Zoophilic dermatophyte infections are rarely serious, generally self-limiting and respond well to treatment [15]. In contrast, two articles describing infection with rat bite fever (*Streptobacillus moniliformis* or *Spirillum minus*) were identified by the review [16,17], one of which occurred in a pet shop employee and resulted in his death. Rat bite fever has a mortality rate of up to 13% in untreated cases [18].

The infection described most often was psittacosis (n = 18), followed by salmonellosis (n = 12) (Table 2). All of the psittacosis infections were associated with birds (where the putative animal source was identified), and no other avian infection was recorded in the review. The next group of animals most commonly referenced were rodents (n = 11), including rats, mice and prairie dogs. Four papers reported that the infections occurred through scratches or bites, two through oral transmission, one through a wound from a rat cage, and seven through other direct contact (including one paper with cases infected by a mixture of bites and direct contact). The review also included one paper (detailing a salmonellosis infection) which specified that the case had had no direct contact with the pet. In the remaining papers the method of transmission was not specified for some or all of the cases (n = 42). This includes 17 of the 18 papers reporting psittacosis incidents; it is likely that many of these infections occurred via airborne transmission.

Thirty of the papers referenced incidents in the Americas, nineteen referenced incidents in Europe, and eight referenced incidents in South East Asia. The majority of the papers described individual case reports or outbreaks of fewer than ten cases associated with pet shops (or other locations selling/distributing companion animals) (n = 42), with only three describing outbreaks with 50 cases or more (an outbreak of lymphocytic choriomeningitis virus in hamsters, an outbreak of monkeypox in prairie dogs, and an outbreak of salmonellosis in African dwarf frogs). Twenty-two of the incidents involved adults only, three involved children only, 11 involved both adults and children, and 21 did not specify the age of some or all of the cases.

Thirty-five papers described an incident associated with a pet shop, eight were associated with a breeder or distributor, five with

**Table 1.** Cases of zoonoses associated with pet shops identified by the systematic literature review.

| Zoonosis/agent | Country | Year | Animal | Setting | Human cases associated with pet shops | Age: child (≤16 years)/adult | Transmission | Probable type of contact: Occ/dom/visitor* | Comment | Main ref |
|---|---|---|---|---|---|---|---|---|---|---|
| Bartonellosis | USA | 1994 | Cats | Animal shelter | 1 case | Adult | Multiple scratches | >1 category | Case adopted kittens from animal shelter. Case had high antibody titres to Bartonella henselae. The kittens were blood culture positive. | [30] |
| Blastomycosis | USA | 2009 | Kinkajou | Educational organisation | 1 case | Adult | Bitten on finger | Dom | Case was bitten by a wild-born pet kinkajou (a rainforest mammal related to a raccoon) from an educational organisation. The animal died shortly afterwards. Blastomycosis DNA sequences from the patient isolate and kinkajou tissues were indistinguishable. | [31] |
| Cowpox | France | 2011 | Rats | Pet store | 1 case | Adult | Direct contact | Dom | Case fell ill after buying two rats from a pet store. Other rats from the store had died but were not investigated. | [32] |
| Cowpox | Germany | 2009 | Rats | Pet shop | 5 cases | 2 × child, 3 × adult | Direct contact | Dom | Five cases occurred in two families that had purchased rats from the same pet shop. Some of the rats developed skin lesions after purchase. | [33] |
| Cowpox | France | 2009 | Rats | Pet store; pet breeder | 4 cases | 1× child, 3× adult | Scratches | Dom | Four cases of infection from sick pet rats from the same pet store. The human cases were shown to be infected by a unique cowpox virus strain. All four pet rats died. | [34] |
| Cowpox | Germany | 2008 | Rats | Pet shops; wholesaler | 6 cases | 2× child, 4× adult | 3 × direct contact, 3 × not specified | Dom | Five cases of cowpox, and one putative case, among pet rat owners. All had contact with rats recently purchased from pet shops that had sourced from same wholesaler. | [35] |
| Cryptosporidiosis | USA | 2007 | Unknown | Pet shop | 1 case | Adult | Direct contact | >1 category | A pet shop employee was infected with Cryptosporidium horse genotype. Case reported no contact with horses although did have contact with numerous other animals. | [36] |
| Edwardsiella tarda | USA | 1981 | Turtle | Pet shop | 1 case | Adult | Oral | Dom | The patient was infected with Edwardsiella tarda, an organism associated with cold blooded animals. Patient's son had recently purchased a turtle from a pet shop. Patient drank from a glass containing tank water. No specimens were available from turtle or tank. | [37] |
| Lymphocytic choriomeningitis virus (LCMV) | Romania | 2008 | Unknown | Pet shop | 2 cases | Adults | Not specified | Occ | A case of LCMV infection in a pet store worker, and evidence of a previous infection in one other employee. No samples were taken from rodents at the store. | [38] |

**Table 1.** Cont.

| Zoonosis/agent | Country | Year | Animal | Setting | Human cases associated with pet shops | Age: child (≤16 years)/adult | Transmission | Probable type of contact: Occ/dom/visitor* | Comment | Main ref |
|---|---|---|---|---|---|---|---|---|---|---|
| LCMV | USA | 2005 | Hamsters | Pet store; pet distributor | 1 case (plus 4 secondary cases via a common organ donor) | Not specified | Not specified | Dom | Organ donor exposed to LCMV by hamster recently purchased from a pet store (although there was no evidence of LCMV infection in the donor). Illness occurred in four organ transplant recipients, 3 of whom died. More LCMV-infected hamsters were found in both the pet store and the distribution centre. Phylogenetic analysis linked the human and animal infections, including the donor hamster. | [39] |
| LCMV | USA | 1974 | Hamster | Pet distributor | 181 cases | Not specified: ages ranged from 2 to 74 years | Not specified | Dom | 181 symptomatic laboratory confirmed cases in persons with hamsters sourced from a single distributor. Breeder was an employee of a biological products firm that had previously been associated with outbreaks of LCMV from hamsters used for tumor research. | [40] |
| LCMV | USA | 1974 | Hamster | Pet shop | 6 cases | 2 × child, 4 × adult | All direct contact, incl 2 × bite | Dom | Two individuals living in same household contracted severe infection from a hamster (proven to have LCMV) recently purchased from a local pet shop. Three additional members of the family and a neighbor had a mild illness with raised antibody titres to LCMV (all handled the hamster and its bedding). | [41] |
| Leptospirosis | UK | 2006 | Rats | Pet shop | 1 case | Adult | Not specified | Dom | Case purchased two pet rats from a pet shop three months prior to falling ill. Leptospiral DNA was detected in both rats, and other rats from same litter. | [42] |
| Leptospirosis | Austria | 2001 | Unknown | Pet shop | 1 case | Adult | Not specified | Occ | Case worked in a pet shop. No discussion of possible exposures. | [43] |
| Leptospirosis | USA | 1971 | Mice | Pet shop | 1 case | Adult | Oral | Dom | Case of leptospirosis acquired from pet mice recently purchased from a pet shop. Infection may have been acquired when the case's daughter used his toothbrush to clean the mouse-cage. | [44] |

**Table 1.** Cont.

| Zoonosis/agent | Country | Year | Animal | Setting | Human cases associated with pet shops | Age: child (≤16 years)/adult | Transmission | Probable type of contact: Occ/dom/visitor* | Comment | Main ref |
|---|---|---|---|---|---|---|---|---|---|---|
| Monkeypox | USA | 2003 | Prairie dogs | Pet store; distributor | 20 cases (part of an outbreak involving 72 cases) | i) 11 cases: 3–43y, ii) 9 cases: 5× child, 4× adult | i) 11 cases: All direct contact, incl 2× scratch/bite, 3× open wounds, ii) 9 cases: not specified | i) 11 cases: >1 category, ii) 9 cases: >1 category | Outbreak of monkeypox, including two pet store employees and two animal distributors. Acquired from prairie dogs which entered the community through pet shops and pet swap meets. Papers detail two clusters within the outbreak: i) 11 cases and ii) nine cases. | [45,46] |
| MRSA | Canada | 2006 | Cats | Rescue centre | 4 cases | Not specified | 1× direct contact, 3× not specified | >1 category | Two kittens from a rescue centre were infected with *Staphyloccocus aureus*. Some of their littermates had previously died of an unknown disease. Indistinguishable strains were isolated from both owners, one veterinary employee (out of 24 people tested) and the operator of the rescue centre, as well as another cat in the household. | [47] |
| Psittacosis | Brazil | 2012 | Unknown | Pet shop | 1 case | Adult | Not specified | Occ | Case contracted *Chlamydophila psittaci* after starting work at a pet shop. | [48] |
| Psittacosis | Japan | 2004 | Birds | Pet shop | 2 cases | Adults | Not specified | Occ | An elderly couple who ran a pet shop (selling psittacine birds) contracted psittacosis. No bird sampling was conducted. | [49] |
| Psittacosis | Belgium | 1988–2003 | Birds | Breeding facilities | 7 cases | Adults | Not specified | >1 category | *C. psittaci* DNA detected in 6/46 owners of pet birds obtained from six different breeding facilities. All of these had birds that tested positive for *C. psittaci* by PCR or culture. A veterinary student working at the facilities was also culture positive and had mild illness. | [50] |
| Psittacosis | Japan | 2001 | Birds | Pet shop | 2 cases | Adults | Not specified | Occ | Cases worked in a pet shop where some parakeets had recently died. [Article in Japanese] | [51] |
| Psittacosis | Slovenia | Unclear: 1991–2001 | Birds | Pet shops; breeders | 9 cases | Not specified | Not specified | Occ | Nine pet shop keepers/breeders (out of 86 pet shop keepers/breeders [10.5%]) were seropositive for *C. psittaci*. Second study from 1997 of pet store salesmen, breeders, veterinary employees and employees in the animal slaughter industry showed highest seropositivity (18.2%) was found in salesmen from pet stores. | [52] |
| Psittacosis | USA | 1980s | Birds | Pet shops | Unknown | Not specified | Not specified | Occ | 10% of psittacosis cases reported to CDC during the 1980s (where the source of infection was known) occurred in pet shop employees. | [53] |

**Table 1.** Cont.

| Zoonosis/agent | Country | Year | Animal | Setting | Human cases associated with pet shops | Age: child (≤16 years)/adult | Transmission | Probable type of contact: Occ/dom/visitor* | Comment | Main ref |
|---|---|---|---|---|---|---|---|---|---|---|
| Psittacosis | USA | 1997 | Birds | Pet stores | i) 1 case, ii) Unknown | Not specified | Not specified | i) Dom, ii) >1 category | i) One individual with a positive antibody titre was found amongst a group of pet bird owners who were tested after the bird lot from which their pets came was confirmed to have chlamydiosis, ii) Birds from pet stores were tested for *C. psittaci* following illness in pet store employees and bird owners. Persons with high antibody levels had been exposed to PCR positive birds. | [54] |
| Psittacosis | USA | 1997 | Unknown | Pet shop | 1 case (also 7 secondary nosocomial cases) | Not specified | Not specified | Occ | A pet shop worker was hospitalised with psittacosis. | [55] |
| Psittacosis | USA | 1997 | Bird | Pet distributor | 1 case | Adult | Direct contact | Occ | A dealer in exotic animals became ill after handling a dead cockatiel. | [56] |
| Psittacosis | USA | 1995 | Birds | Pet stores; distributor | Unknown (35 households) | Not specified | Not specified | Dom | Avian chlamydiosis detected in a shipment of >700 pet birds to a particular distributor. Among people who purchased birds sourced from this distributor, evidence of transmission of psittacosis was found in 35 (30.7%) households when clinical and serological case definitions were combined. | [57] |
| Psittacosis | Spain | 1993 | Birds | Pet shop | 4 cases | Not specified | 2 × direct contact, 2 × not specified | Dom | Two cases each bought a parakeet at the same pet shop. Additional serological evidence of infection in two of the cases' relatives. [Article in Spanish] | [58] |
| Psittacosis | UK | 1991 | Birds | Pet shop | 7 cases | 1 × child, 6 × adult | Not specified | >1 category | An outbreak of seven cases of *C. psittaci* originating from a local pet shop. All cases had links to the shop, and three were employees. The shop had recently taken delivery of four love-birds, two of which had been unwell and died. None of the birds were tested. | [59] |
| Psittacosis | Sweden | 1977 | Unknown | Pet shop | 1 case (also 11 secondary cases, of which 9 nosocomial) | Adult | Not specified | Visit | Case visited two pet shops prior to his (fatal) illness. Two parrots in the shops had been bought from a wholesaler connected with a previous outbreak [60], but attempts to isolate chlamydiae failed. Eleven secondary cases occurred. | [61] |
| Psittacosis | Japan | 1976 | Birds | Pet shop | 1 case | Adult | Not specified | Visit | Case visited a pet shop 11 days prior to falling ill with psittacosis. [Article in Japanese] | [62] |

**Table 1.** Cont.

| Zoonosis/agent | Country | Year | Animal | Setting | Human cases associated with pet shops | Age: child (≤16 years)/adult | Transmission | Probable type of contact: Occ/dom/visitor* | Comment | Main ref |
|---|---|---|---|---|---|---|---|---|---|---|
| Psittacosis | UK | 1974 | Birds | Pet shop | 3 cases | 1× adult, 2× not specified | 2× direct contact, 1× not specified | Occ | The owner of a pet shop became ill after acquiring parrots from a dealer connected with a previous outbreak [63]. A second shipment of parrots was kept in the same cage. One parrot died; two people who had cared for it fell ill with compatible symptoms. | [64] |
| Psittacosis | UK | 1973 | Birds | Private pet distributor | 3 cases | Not specified | Not specified | >1 category | A pet distributor and a husband-wife couple fell ill after being in proximity to a sick parrot. | [63] |
| Psittacosis | Sweden | 1967–1969 | Birds | Pet shop | 18 cases | Not specified | Not specified | >1 category | 13/24 cases of ornithosis were probably infected from the same pet shop and five more got their birds from a wholesale dealer who provided birds to the pet shop. Attempts to culture from the birds were not successful. | [60] |
| Psittacosis | Sweden | 1963 | Birds | Pet shop | 13 cases | 1× child, 12× adult | Not specified | >1 category | 13 cases of ornithosis were associated with a pet shop. Birds at the shop were culture positive for *C. psittaci*. | [65] |
| Rat bite fever | USA | 2004 | Rat | Pet shop | 1 case | Adult | Finger wound from cage | Occ | Pet shop employee sustained a minor finger wound from a rat cage and died from sepsis and multi-organ failure 59 days later. | [16] |
| Rat bite fever | UK | 2001 | Rat | Pet shop | 1 case | Child | Bitten on finger | Visit | A case of septic arthritis of the hip in a teenager following a bite on the finger from a rat in a pet shop. *Streptobacillus moniliformis* was cultured from joint fluid. | [17] |
| Ringworm | Japan | 2006 | Unknown | Pet shop | 1 case | Adult | Direct contact | Occ | A case of tinea corporis (*Arthroderma benhamiae*) in a pet store employee. Likely that patient was infected through contact with an animal in the pet shop where she handled small animals. | [11] |
| Ringworm | Japan | 2002 | Unknown | Pet shop | 1 case | Not specified | Not specified | Occ | Pet shop worker with *Arthroderma benhamiae* lesions on face and hand, unknown exposure. [Article in Japanese.] | [12] |
| Ringworm | Japan | 2002 | Hedgehog | Pet shop | 1 case | Adult | Not specified | Dom | Case had a lesion on her palm. Had bought a hedgehog from a pet shop four years prior. Isolates from the patient and hedgehog were identified as *Trichophyton mentagrophytes* var. *erinacei*. | [13] |
| Ringworm | Slovakia | 2002 | Guinea pig | Zoo | 2 cases | 1× adult, 1× child | Not specified | Dom | Two cases of infection in a family which kept a guinea pig obtained from a zoo. Samples from cases and guinea pig were identified as *T. mentagrophytes* var. *quinckeanum*. | [66] |

**Table 1.** Cont.

| Zoonosis/agent | Country | Year | Animal | Setting | Human cases associated with pet shops | Age: child (≤16 years)/adult | Transmission | Probable type of contact: Occ/dom/visitor* | Comment | Main ref |
|---|---|---|---|---|---|---|---|---|---|---|
| Ringworm | USA | 2000 | Hedgehogs | Pet store | 3 cases | Adults | 1× direct contact, 2× not specified | >1 category | Three patients developed culture positive ringworm after handling or purchasing African pygmy hedgehogs from pet stores. Two isolates were atypical *Trichophyton mentagrophytes* and one was *T. mentagrophytes var erinacei*. | [67] |
| Ringworm | Japan | 1991 | Dog | Pet shop | 1 case | Adult | Not specified | Dom | Case purchased a puppy from a pet shop four weeks before presenting with symptoms. The puppy was asymptomatic, but *Microsporum canis* was isolated from both case and puppy. | [14] |
| Salmonellosis | USA | 2009–2011 | African dwarf frogs | Breeder; pet distributor | 56 cases | Not specified | Not specified | >1 category | 56/86 patients with *Salmonella* Typhimurium who were interviewed had recent contact with African dwarf frogs sourced through two distributors from the same breeder. These cases were amongst 224 reported with a unique strain. | [68] |
| Salmonellosis | USA | 2007 | Turtles | Pet store | 16 cases | Not specified (for the 16 linked to pet stores) | Not specified (for the 16 linked to pet stores) | Dom (possibly with additional exposures) | 16/78 cases with S. Java who were interviewed had recent exposure to turtles purchased in retail pet stores. Samples collected from six turtles (or their habitats) yielded the outbreak strain. These cases were amongst 107 infected with the same strain of S. Java. | [69] |
| Salmonellosis | USA | 2004 | Rodents | Pet distributors | 13 cases | Not specified | Not specified | Dom | 13/22 cases of S. Typhimurium who were interviewed had exposure to rodents purchased from pet stores. Seven distributors were identified but no single source was found. These cases were amongst 28 reported with matching isolates. | [70] |
| Salmonellosis | Canada | 2000–2003 | Fish | Pet shops | 33 cases | Not specified | Not specified | Dom | S. Java was detected in 8/34 pet shops from which 33 individuals with S. Java infection had purchased tropical fish. | [71] |
| Salmonellosis | USA | 1999–2000 | Cats | Rescue shelter | 4 cases (and two secondary cases) | Not specified | Not specified | Dom | Four people with S. Typhimurium infection adopted kittens from an animal shelter. Isolates from nine adopted cats from the shelter were indistinguishable from the human isolates by PFGE. Two secondary cases occurred. (One further human isolate was found to have the same PFGE pattern, but no connection to the shelter.) | [72] |
| Salmonellosis | Ireland | 1999 | Terrapins | Pet shop | 8 cases | 7× child, 1× adult | Not specified | Not specified (either dom or "close contact") | Eight cases of S. Tel-el-kebir had contact with pet terrapins purchased from the same pet shop. | [73] |

**Table 1.** Cont.

| Zoonosis/agent | Country | Year | Animal | Setting | Human cases associated with pet shops | Age: child (≤16 years)/adult | Transmission | Probable type of contact: Occ/dom/visitor* | Comment | Main ref |
|---|---|---|---|---|---|---|---|---|---|---|
| Salmonellosis | Canada | 1995–1997 | Pygmy hedgehogs; sugar gliders | Stock farm; breeders | 10 cases | 9× child, 1× adult | 1× direct contact, 9× not specified | >1 category | Nine cases of S. Tilene had contact with families owning African Pygmy hedgehogs, and one case's family owned sugar gliders. The sugar gliders and all but one of the hedgehogs had been directly acquired from breeding herds or stock farms. In most cases, S. Tilene was isolated from the implicated animals or animals from the same breeders. | [74,75] |
| Salmonellosis | USA | 1994 | Iguana | Pet stores; pet show | Unknown (17 households) | Not specified | Not specified | Dom | 25/32 S. Marina cases had a history of exposure to an iguana in the week before illness. Of these, cases from sixteen households obtained their iguana from a pet store and one obtained theirs from a pet show. | [76] |
| Salmonellosis | USA | 1994 | Hedgehogs | Breeders | 1 case | Child | No direct contact | >1 category | A case of S. Tilene in a 10-month old baby whose family owned a breeding herd of 80 African Pygmy hedgehogs. One of three hedgehogs tested yielded S. Tilene. | [77] |
| Salmonellosis | Japan | 1985 | Turtle | Pet shops | 2 cases | 1× adult, 1× child | Not specified | Dom | Two cases of S. Paratyphi B occurred in a family who had a pet turtle positive for the same organism. Investigations also detected this pathogen in turtles or turtle tanks in 4/12 pet shops in the city. | [78]** |
| Salmonellosis | USA | 1983 | Turtles | Pet shops | 12 cases | 11× child, 1× adult | 1× direct contact, 11× not specified | Dom | 12/83 cases of Salmonella had a history of exposure or probable exposure to turtles from pet shops. Turtles were collected from pet shops in Puerto Rico and pooled into 'lots' for testing; all lots included at least one animal that was culture-positive for Salmonella. Contamination is believed to have occurred at the turtle farm prior to distribution. | [79] |
| Salmonellosis | USA | 1970–1971 | Turtles | Pet shops; department store | i) 2 cases, ii) 36 cases (possibly more, but not stated) | i) 2× child, ii) not specified | Not specified | Dom | i) Case study of two siblings with S. Hartford infection from a pet turtle (also positive for S. Hartford) purchased at a department store, ii) Also report of six surveys of laboratory-confirmed cases of salmonellosis, where 193/1239 patients with salmonellosis owned pet turtles (it was noted that all the turtles from one survey (36 patients) came from pet shops or department stores). | [80] |

**Table 1. Cont.**

| Zoonosis/agent | Country | Year | Animal | Setting | Human cases associated with pet shops | Age: child (≤16 years)/adult | Transmission | Probable type of contact: Occ/dom/visitor* | Comment | Main ref |
|---|---|---|---|---|---|---|---|---|---|---|
| Toxocariosis | USA | 1989 | Dog | Pet store | 1 case | Child | Not specified | Dom | Young girl suffered permanent loss of vision due to ocular toxocariasis after her parents purchased a puppy from a pet store. | [81] |
| Tularemia | USA | 2002 | Prairie dogs | Pet distributor | 1 case | Adult | Direct contact | Occ | 61 prairie dogs at a pet distributor tested positive for *Francisella tularensis*. An animal handler at the facility showed serological evidence of recent infection. | [82] |

*Occ = occupational (exposure associated with case's place of work); dom = domestic (pet owned by case or relative/friend of case), visitor = case visited place of likely exposure, outside of domestic setting).
**The original source paper for this incident (Murao T et al (1985) Ann Rep Fukuoka City Inst Hyg Environ, 10, 70–71) is only available in Japanese. The paper by Nagano contains sufficient information to include the incident in this review.

some other facility (an animal shelter, an educational organization, two rescue centres, and a zoo; all of which sold or distributed animals to members of the public), and the remaining nine incidents involved more than one type of facility (most commonly involving both a distributor and pet shop). Twenty-five of the papers involved infections occurring in a domestic setting, fourteen in an occupational setting and three described infections occurring after a visit to a pet shop. Fifteen papers covered outbreaks where the cases fell into more than one category or where the setting was unspecified.

## Discussion

Pet shops can play an important role in the control of zoonotic infections from companion animals. They are the initial point at which members of the public can access information and advice on the risks associated with their newly purchased pets. Unfortunately, there is evidence to suggest that pet shop employees do not adequately understand or control the risks. A 2003 poll (commissioned by The Royal Society for the Prevention of Cruelty to Animals) of 300 pet shops which reported trading in exotic pets, asked pet shops whether any illnesses contracted by a client's prospective pet could be passed onto humans; 36% answered "No, not at all" [19]. It is important that zoonotic risks are recognized and addressed because the consequences of these infections can be very serious.

The systematic literature review described in this manuscript identified 82 papers covering 57 separate human infections, outbreaks or incidents believed to have been associated with pet shops. Although the review was conducted in a systematic manner, the authors acknowledge that this list is not comprehensive; in order to be comprehensive, individual searches would have to be conducted for each potential zoonotic disease, and zoonotic incidents are often not written up in peer-reviewed journals. However, the review does present a representative sample of papers derived from a well-defined set of search criteria.

A wide spectrum of infections acquired from pet shops was identified by the review. Salmonellosis and psittacosis were the most commonly documented diseases, however more unusual infections such as tularemia were also identified. Many of the references relate to infections in pet shop employees, where often the precise source of infection was undetermined but the pet shop was assumed to be involved. The animals involved in the transmission of these infections were varied, including birds, mammals and rodents, and cover both common household pets, such as dogs and cats, and more exotic creatures, such as iguanas and prairie dogs. Some zoonotic infections were associated with a variety of different companion animals (e.g. salmonellosis), whereas others were associated with only a narrow range of species (e.g. psittacosis). Whilst some of the pathogens identified in Table 1 are commonly foodborne (e.g. *Salmonella*), or transmitted by other established routes of zoonotic infection, e.g. bites and scratches, this review demonstrates that more unexpected routes exist, and that transmission through animal contact should be considered when defining strategies to prevent disease in the population.

There are other organisms which have been identified in pet shop animals, and which have the potential to cause human infection, but which were not identified in this literature review. For example, infections caused by *Yersinia pseudotuberculosis* and *Y. enterocolitica* may be contracted from pet rodents, however this is uncommon because the usual serotypes found in rodents do not affect humans. The lack of clinical signs in animals affected by these infections may increase the likelihood of transmission of the

**Table 2.** Incidents/outbreaks identified by the review, by zoonotic agent and animal category.

| Zoonosis/agent | Birds | Cats/dogs | Hamsters/ guinea pigs | Hedgehogs | Rodents | Turtles | Other | Not known | Total |
|---|---|---|---|---|---|---|---|---|---|
| LCMV | 0 | 0 | 3 | 0 | 0 | 0 | 0 | 1 | 4 |
| Leptospirosis | 0 | 0 | 0 | 0 | 2 | 0 | 0 | 1 | 3 |
| Pox virus | 0 | 0 | 0 | 0 | 5 | 0 | 0 | 0 | 5 |
| Psittacosis | 15 | 0 | 0 | 0 | 0 | 0 | 0 | 3 | 18 |
| Ringworm | 0 | 1 | 1 | 2 | 0 | 0 | 0 | 2 | 6 |
| Salmonellosis | 0 | 1 | 0 | 1 | 1 | 4 | 5 | 0 | 12 |
| Other | 0 | 3 | 0 | 0 | 3 | 1 | 1 | 1 | 9 |
| Total | 15 | 5 | 4 | 3 | 11 | 5 | 6 | 8 | 57 |

organism from pet to human; guinea pigs are commonly infected with *Y. pseudotuberculosis* and clinical signs are usually subacute, similarly *Y. enterocolitica* is usually asymptomatic in rodents [20]. It is also likely that other zoonotic organisms may have passed from pet shop animals to humans and caused disease, but have not been documented because of under-diagnosis and under-reporting, and a lack of follow-up of sporadic infections, e.g. cryptosporidium, giardia.

There are some diseases which were unexpected omissions in this review, e.g. pasteurellosis. A number of articles concerning pasteurella infections were initially accepted into the review on the basis of their abstracts, however they were not included in the final results because they did not specifically refer to pet shops. This might reflect a publication bias; because infections with *Pasteurella* spp. are commonly associated with animal exposures, case studies might not be written up in the literature. In addition, the association of pasteurellosis with cat and dog bites is very well established, so where articles on pasteurella infections do occur, links to pets and pet shops may not be deemed to be of sufficient interest to warrant inclusion in the final publication. Similarly, this may explain why the literature review included only one article on cat scratch disease. It is therefore important to note that unusual and unexpected zoonotic infections may be over-represented in peer-reviewed publications, and in this review.

A further limitation of this review was its restriction to English-language papers. Although a small number of foreign-language manuscripts were included where a translated abstract was available and provided sufficient information to fulfill the inclusion criteria, 137 out of 142 foreign-language papers were nonetheless excluded. The countries associated with incidents in this review (predominantly the Americas and Europe), reflect this bias. This may imply that pathogens that are more common in non-Western countries, or in more exotic animals not common in Europe and the Americas, were under-represented.

Incidents of rabies tracebacks and zoonoses from pet food were excluded from this review. They are nonetheless important public health considerations and can require a large amount of resource to deal with appropriately. For example, in the US in 1994, significant numbers of people were exposed to a rabid kitten in a pet shop and, although no human cases resulted, the final cost of the investigation and prophylaxis was estimated to be over $1 million with 665 people receiving prophylaxis [21,22]. Such incidents are not necessarily unusual, and Rotz *et al.* summarise 22 large-scale incidents of exposure to rabid or presumed rabid animals (defined as administration of PEP to 25 or more people after an exposure) that occurred in the US between 1990 and 1996 [23]. The increase in *Salmonella* Typhimurium, designated definitive type 191a (DT191a), was an example of an outbreak from pet food detected in the UK in December 2008. The increase was found to be associated with raw frozen mice used as reptile feed and sold through wholesalers and distributors [24]. Revised infection control guidance for reptile owners and handlers has been published on the Health Protection Agency (HPA) website [25]. It is therefore important to note that there will be further significant events associated with pet shops beyond those summarized in this manuscript, which must be kept in mind when considering the importance of such facilities in the zoonotic transmission of disease.

While many zoonotic infections associated with pet shops are likely to result in single cases or familial incidents, e.g. rat bite fever, such premises also have the potential to amplify the risk of spread. A sick animal in a pet shop can potentially transmit the illness to other animals within the shop, and therefore to a large number of new pet owners, who may be geographically dispersed. Pet shops (and other locations that sell animals) can additionally act as a type of leisure activity, with families visiting to see and handle the animals, and potentially becoming exposed to zoonotic diseases even though they do not own a pet of their own. As such, pet shops can be the focus of very large outbreaks of disease, such as the 2003 incident in the USA where prairie dogs infected with monkeypox were widely disseminated through pet shops and pet swap meets, and resulted in over 50 cases of human disease. Such disease outbreaks can have a significant public health burden in the direct morbidity and mortality to cases, in financial and logistical impacts on laboratories and healthcare providers, and in the time and expertise required to investigate exposures and follow up potentially infected animals and human cases and contacts. The precise public health impacts will vary according to the zoonosis and the size of incident.

Given their potential to spread zoonotic infections, it is important that pet shops act to minimise the risk as far as possible. The current legislative framework is biased towards animal welfare in the UK, with few recommendations seeking explicitly to protect human health. However, those exposures that fall within occupational health and safety are an exception: employee safety is covered by health and safety at work legislation, and the Control Of Substances Hazardous to Health (COSHH) regulations additionally cover the health of other people who may be exposed to hazards in the workplace, including customers.[26–28] Local Authorities have powers to impose conditions on the licensing of pet shops, and most adopt model standards published by the Local Government Association which includes taking all reasonable precautions to prevent the outbreak and spread of disease [29].

Whilst proposing specific recommendations to improve control measures associated with companion animals in pet shops is beyond the scope of this paper, legislative authorities might consider more stringent oversight of pet breeders and distributors before animals enter the market. Alternatively, practical hygiene measures similar to those implemented on farms open to the public could be made mandatory in pet shops, and information leaflets on zoonotic risks and prevention measures for prospective pet owners could be provided to help to reduce the risk of infection.

## Acknowledgments

The authors would like to thank the reviewers of this manuscript for their valuable contributions.

## Author Contributions

Conceived and designed the experiments: DM CC K. Hewitt. Analyzed the data: K. Halsby AW CC. Wrote the paper: K. Halsby CC. Prepared Table 1: K. Halsby AW. Read and commented on draft manuscript: K. Halsby CC K. Hewitt AW DM. Initiated and supervised the development of the paper: DM. Suggested and developed the public health proposals put forward at the end of the discussion section: DM.

## References

1. Pet Food Manufacturers association (2012) Pet population 2008 to 2012. Available: http://www.pfma.org.uk/pet-population-2008-2012. Accessed 28 January 2014.
2. [Anonymous] (2007) The Dangerous Wild Animals Act 1976 (Modification) (No. 2) Order 2007. Available: www.legislation.gov.uk/uksi/2007/2465/introduction/made. Accessed 28 January 2014.
3. Geffray L (1999) Infections associated with pets. Rev Med Interne 20: 888–901.
4. Plaut M, Zimmerman EM, Goldstein RA (1996) Health hazards to humans associated with domestic pets. Annu Rev Public Health 17: 221–245.
5. Day MJ, Breitschwerdt E, Cleaveland S, Karkare U, Khanna C, et al. (2012) Surveillance of zoonotic infectious disease transmitted by small companion animals. Emerg Infect Dis [Internet] Available: http://dx.doi.org/10.3201/eid1812.120664. Accessed 28 January 2014.
6. Pet Food Manufacturers association (2014) Pet statistics FAQ's. Available: http://www.pfma.org.uk/faqs/pet-statistics. Accessed 28 January 2014.
7. Stehr-Green JK, Murray G, Schantz PM, Wahlquist SP (1987) Intestinal parasites in pet store puppies in Atlanta. Am J Public Health 77: 345–346.
8. Oxberry SL, Hampson DJ (2003) Colonisation of pet shop puppies with *Brachyspira pilosicoli*. Vet Microbiol 93: 167–174.
9. Bugg RJ, Robertson ID, Elliot AD, Thompson RC (1999) Gastrointestinal parasites of urban dogs in Perth, Western Australia. Vet J 157: 295–301.
10. Itoh N, Itagaki T, Kawabata T, Konaka T, Muraoka N, et al. (2011) Prevalence of intestinal parasites and genotyping of *Giardia intestinalis* in pet shop puppies in east Japan. Vet Parasitol 176: 74–78.
11. Shiraki Y, Hiruma M, Matsuba Y, Kano R, Makimura K, et al. (2006) A case of tinea corporis caused by *Arthroderma benhamiae* (teleomorph of *Tinea mentagrophytes*) in a pet shop employee. J Am Acad Dermatol 55: 153–154.
12. Mochizuki T (2002) Molecular epidemiology of Japanese isolates of *Arthroderma benhamiae* by polymorphisms of non-transcribed spacer region of the ribosomal DNA. [Article in Japanese]. Nihon Ishinkin Gakkai Zasshi 43: 1–4.
13. Mochizuki T, Takeda K, Nakagawa M, Kawasaki M, Tanabe H, et al. (2005) The first isolation in Japan of *Trichophyton mentagrophytes* var. *erinacei* causing tinea manuum. Int J Dermatol 44: 765–768.
14. Katoh T, Maruyama R, Nishioka K, Sano T (1991) Tinea corporis due to *Microsporum canis* from an asymptomatic dog. J Dermatol 18: 356–359.
15. Palmer SR, Soulsby L, Simpson DIH (Editors) (1998) Zoonoses: Biology, clinical practice, and public health control. New York: Oxford University Press.
16. Shvartsblat S, Kochie M, Harber P, Howard J (2004) Fatal rat bite fever in a pet shop employee. Am J Ind Med 45: 357–360.
17. Downing ND, Dewnany GD, Radford PJ (2001) A rare and serious consequence of a rat bite. Ann R Coll Surg Engl 83: 279–280.
18. Elliott SP (2007) Rat bite fever and *Streptobacillus moniliformis*. Clin Microbiol Rev 20: 13–22.
19. Ipsos MORI (2004) Exotic pets. Available: http://www.ipsos-mori.com/researchpublications/researcharchive/912/Exotic-Pets.aspx. Accessed 28 January 2014.
20. Chomel BB (1992) Zoonoses of house pets other than dogs, cats and birds. Pediatr Infect Dis J 11: 479–487.
21. CDC (1995) Mass treatment of humans exposed to rabies - New Hampshire, 1994. MMWR Morb Mortal Wkly Rep 44: 484–486.
22. Noah DL, Smith MG, Gotthardt JC, Krebs JW, Green D, et al. (1996) Mass human exposure to rabies in New Hampshire: exposures, treatment, and cost. Am J Public Health 86: 1149–1151.
23. Rotz LD, Hensley JA, Rupprecht CE, Childs JE (1998) Large-scale human exposures to rabid or presumed rabid animals in the United States: 22 cases (1990–1996). J Am Vet Med Assoc 212: 1198–1200.
24. HPA (2009) Reptile-associated salmonella infections (*S.* Typhimurium DT 191a)- an update. HPR 3: Online report. Available: http://www.hpa.org.uk/hpr/archives/2009/news3109.htm#dt191a. Accessed 28 January 2014.
25. HPA (2009) Reducing the risks of salmonella infection from reptiles. Available: http://www.hpa.org.uk/Topics/InfectiousDiseases/InfectionsAZ/Salmonella/GeneralInformation/salmReptiles. Accessed 28 January 2014.
26. [Anonymous] (2002) The Control of Substances Hazardous to Health Regulations 2002. Available: http://www.legislation.gov.uk/uksi/2002/2677/made. Accessed 28 January 2014.
27. [Anonymous] (2003) The Control of Substances Hazardous to Health (Amendment) Regulations 2003. Available: http://www.legislation.gov.uk/uksi/2003/978/made. Accessed 28 January 2014.
28. [Anonymous] (2004) The Control of Substances Hazardous to Health (Amendment) Regulations 2004. Available: http://www.legislation.gov.uk/uksi/2004/3386/made. Accessed 28 January 2014.
29. Local Government Association (2006) Pet Animals Act 1951: model standards for pet shop licence conditions. Available: http://www.local.gov.uk/web/guest/publications/-/journal_content/56/10171/3378153/PUBLICATION-TEMPLATE. Accessed 28 January 2014.
30. Breitschwerdt EB, Kordick DL (1995) Bartonellosis. J Am Vet Med Assoc 206: 1928–1931.
31. Harris JR, Blaney DD, Lindsley MD, Zaki SR, Paddock CD, et al. (2011) Blastomycosis in man after kinkajou bite. Emerg Infect Dis 17: 268–270.
32. Elsendoorn A, Agius G, Le Moal G, Aajaji F, Favier AL, et al. (2011) Severe ear chondritis due to cowpox virus transmitted by a pet rat. J Infect 63: 391–393.
33. Campe H, Zimmermann P, Glos K, Bayer M, Bergemann H, et al. (2009) Cowpox virus transmission from pet rats to humans, Germany. Emerg Infect Dis 15: 777–780.
34. Ninove L, Domart Y, Vervel C, Voinot C, Salez N, et al. (2009) Cowpox virus transmission from pet rats to humans, France. Emerg Infect Dis 15: 781–784.
35. Becker C, Kurth A, Hessler F, Kramp H, Gokel M, et al. (2009) Cowpox virus infection in pet rat owners. Dtsch Arztebl Int 106: 329–334.
36. Xiao L, Hlavsa MC, Yoder J, Ewers C, Dearen T, et al. (2009) Subtype analysis of Cryptosporidium specimens from sporadic cases in Colorado, Idaho, New Mexico, and Iowa in 2007: widespread occurrence of one *Cryptosporidium hominis* subtype and case history of an infection with the Cryptosporidium horse genotype. J Clin Microbiol 47: 3017–3020.
37. Nagel P, Serritella A, Layden TJ (1982) *Edwardsiella tarda* gastroenteritis associated with a pet turtle. Gastroenterology 82: 1436–1437.
38. Ceianu C, Tatulescu D, Muntean M, Molnar GB, Emmerich P, et al. (2008) Lymphocytic choriomeningitis in a pet store worker in Romania. Clin Vaccine Immunol 15: 1749.
39. Amman BR, Pavlin BI, Albarino CG, Comer JA, Erickson BR, et al. (2007) Pet rodents and fatal lymphocytic choriomeningitis in transplant patients. Emerg Infect Dis 13: 719–725.
40. Gregg MB (1975) Recent outbreaks of lymphocytic choriomeningitis in the United States of America. Bull World Health Organ 52: 549–553.
41. Hirsch MS, Moellering RC Jr, Pope HG, Poskanzer DC (1974) Lymphocytic-choriomeningitis virus infection traced to a pet hamster. N Engl J Med 291: 610–612.
42. Gaudie CM, Featherstone CA, Phillips WS, McNaught R, Rhodes PM, et al. (2008) Human *Leptospira interrogans* serogroup Icterohaemorrhagiae infection (Weil's disease) acquired from pet rats. Vet Rec 163: 599–601.
43. Finsterer J, Stollberger C, Sehnal E, Stanek G (2005) Mild leptospirosis with three-year persistence of IgG- and IgM-antibodies, initially manifesting as carpal tunnel syndrome. J Infect 51: E67–E70.
44. Friedmann CT, Spiegel EL, Aaron E, McIntyre R (1973) Leptospirosis ballum contracted from pet mice. Calif Med 118: 51–52.
45. Reed KD, Melski JW, Graham MB, Regnery RL, Sotir MJ, et al. (2004) The detection of monkeypox in humans in the Western Hemisphere. N Engl J Med 350: 342–350.
46. Kile JC, Fleischauer AT, Beard B, Kuehnert MJ, Kanwal RS, et al. (2005) Transmission of monkeypox among persons exposed to infected prairie dogs in Indiana in 2003. Arch Pediatr Adolesc Med 159: 1022–1025.
47. Weese JS, Dick H, Willey BM, McGeer A, Kreiswirth BN, et al. (2006) Suspected transmission of methicillin-resistant *Staphylococcus aureus* between domestic pets and humans in veterinary clinics and in the household. Vet Microbiol 115: 148–155.

48. Budoia J, Tagliari C, Villa R, Gatto S, Bedin V (2012) Dermatologic manifestation of psittacosis. J Am Acad Dermatol 66: 108.

49. Saito T, Ohnishi J, Mori Y, Iinuma Y, Ichiyama S, et al. (2005) Infection by *Chlamydophila avium* in an elderly couple working in a pet shop. J Clin Microbiol 43: 3011–3013.

50. Vanrompay D, Harkinezhad T, van de Walle M, Beeckman D, van Droogenbroeck C, et al. (2007) *Chlamydophila psittaci* transmission from pet birds to humans. Emerg Infect Dis 13: 1108–1110.

51. Maegawa N, Emoto T, Mori H, Yamaguchi D, Fujinaga T, et al. (2001) Two cases of *Chlamydia psittaci* infection occurring in employees of the same pet shop [Article in Japanese]. Nihon Kokyuki Gakkai Zasshi 39: 753–757.

52. Dovc A, Dovc P, Kese D, Vlahovic K, Pavlak M, et al. (2005) Long-term study of Chlamydophilosis in Slovenia. Vet Res Commun 29: 23–36.

53. [Anonymous] (2000) Compendium of measures to control *Chlamydia psittaci* infection among humans (psittacosis) and pet birds (avian chlamydiosis), 2000. MMWR Recomm Rep 49: 1–17.

54. Messmer TO, Skelton SK, Moroney JF, Daugharty H, Fields BS (1997) Application of a nested, multiplex PCR to psittacosis outbreaks. J Clin Microbiol 35: 2043–2046.

55. Hughes C, Maharg P, Rosario P, Herrell M, Bratt D, et al. (1997) Possible nosocomial transmission of psittacosis. Infect Control Hosp Epidemiol 18: 165–168.

56. Gregory DW, Schaffner W (1997) Psittacosis. Semin Respir Infect 12: 7–11.

57. Moroney JF, Guevara R, Iverson C, Chen FM, Skelton SK, et al. (1998) Detection of chlamydiosis in a shipment of pet birds, leading to recognition of an outbreak of clinically mild psittacosis in humans. Clin Infect Dis 26: 1425–1429.

58. Viciana P, Bozada JM, Martin-Sanz V, Martinez-Marcos F, Martin A, et al. (1993) Psittacosis of avian origin as etiology of community-acquired pneumonia with severe onset. [Article in Spanish]. Rev Clin Esp 192: 28–30.

59. Morrison WM, Hutchison RB, Thomason J, Harrington JH, Herd GW (1991) An outbreak of psittacosis. J Infect 22: 71–75.

60. Jernelius H, Pettersson B, Schvarcz J, Vahlne A (1975) An outbreak of ornithosis. Scand J Infect Dis 7: 91–95.

61. Broholm KA, Bottiger M, Jernelius H, Johansson M, Grandien M, et al. (1977) Ornithosis as a nosocomial infection. Scand J Infect Dis 9: 263–267.

62. Kanazawa Y, Suga S, Niwayama S (1976) A case of psittacosis treated with rifampicin (author's transl). [Article in Japanese]. Jpn J Antibiot 29: 601–606.

63. [Anonymous] (1973) An outbreak of psittacosis. Br Med J 4: 58.

64. [Anonymous] (1975) Psittacosis in a pet shop. Br Med J 1: 283.

65. Alestig K, Bakos K, Barr J, Heller L (1963) An Ornithosis epidemic in Orebro. Acta Med Scand 174: 441–449.

66. Bilek J, Baranova Z, Kozak M, Fialkovicova M, Weissova T, et al. (2005) *Trichophyton mentagrophytes* var. *quinckeanum* as a cause of zoophilic dermatomycosis in a human family. Bratisl Lek Listy 106: 383–385.

67. Rosen T (2000) Hazardous hedgehogs. South Med J 93: 936–938.

68. CDC (2011) Notes from the field: Update on human *Salmonella* Typhimurium infections associated with aquatic frogs – United States, 2009–2011. MMWR Morb Mortal Wkly Rep 60: 628.

69. Harris JR, Bergmire-Sweat D, Schlegel JH, Winpisinger KA, Klos RF, et al. (2009) Multistate outbreak of *Salmonella* infections associated with small turtle exposure, 2007–2008. Pediatrics 124: 1388–1394.

70. Swanson SJ, Snider C, Braden CR, Boxrud D, Wunschmann A, et al. (2007) Multidrug-resistant *Salmonella enterica* serotype Typhimurium associated with pet rodents. N Engl J Med 356: 21–28.

71. Gaulin C, Vincent C, Ismail J (2005) Sporadic infections of *Salmonella* Paratyphi B, Var. Java associated with fish tanks. Can J Public Health 96: 471–474.

72. Wright JG, Tengelsen LA, Smith KE, Bender JB, Frank RK, et al. (2005) Multidrug-resistant *Salmonella* Typhimurium in four animal facilities. Emerg Infect Dis 11: 1235–1241.

73. Lynch M, Daly M, O'Brien B, Morrison F, Cryan B, et al. (1999) *Salmonella tel-el-kebir* and terrapins. J Infect 38: 182–184.

74. Anand CM, Fonseca K, Longmore K, Rennie R, Chui L, et al. (1997) Epidemiological investigation of *Salmonella tilene* by pulsed-field gel electrophoresis and polymerase chain reaction. Can J Infect Dis 8: 318–322.

75. Craig C, Styliadis S, Woodward D, Werker D (1997) African pygmy hedgehog-associated *Salmonella tilene* in Canada. Can Commun Dis Rep 23: 129–131.

76. Mermin J, Hoar B, Angulo FJ (1997) Iguanas and *Salmonella marina* infection in children: a reflection of the increasing incidence of reptile-associated salmonellosis in the United States. Pediatrics 99: 399–402.

77. CDC (1995) African pygmy hedgehog-associated Salmonellosis - Washington, 1994. MMWR Morb Mortal Wkly Rep 44: 462–463.

78. Nagano N, Oana S, Nagano Y, Arakawa Y (2006) A severe *Salmonella enterica* Serotype Paratyphi B infection in a child related to a pet turtle, *Trachemys scripta elegans*. Jpn J Infect Dis 59: 132–134.

79. Tauxe RV, Rigau-Perez JG, Wells JG, Blake PA (1985) Turtle-associated salmonellosis in Puerto Rico. Hazards of the global turtle trade. JAMA 254: 237–239.

80. Lamm SH, Taylor A Jr, Gangarosa EJ, Anderson HW, Young W, et al. (1972) Turtle-associated salmonellosis. I. An estimation of the magnitude of the problem in the United States, 1970–1971. Am J Epidemiol 95: 511–517.

81. Jack DC (1997) The legal implications of the veterinarian's role as a private practitioner and health professional, with particular reference to the human-animal bond: Part 2, The veterinarian's role in society. Can Vet J 38: 653–659.

82. Avashia SB, Petersen JM, Lindley CM, Schriefer ME, Gage KL, et al. (2004) First reported prairie dog-to-human tularemia transmission, Texas, 2002. Emerg Infect Dis 10: 483–486.

# 14

# Prevalence of Disorders Recorded in Dogs Attending Primary-Care Veterinary Practices in England

**Dan G. O'Neill[1]\*, David B. Church[2], Paul D. McGreevy[3], Peter C. Thomson[3], Dave C. Brodbelt[1]**

1 Veterinary Epidemiology, Economics and Public Health, Royal Veterinary College, London, United Kingdom, 2 Small Animal Medicine and Surgery Group, Royal Veterinary College, London, United Kingdom, 3 Faculty of Veterinary Science, University of Sydney, Sydney, New South Wales, Australia

## Abstract

Purebred dog health is thought to be compromised by an increasing occurence of inherited diseases but inadequate prevalence data on common disorders have hampered efforts to prioritise health reforms. Analysis of primary veterinary practice clinical data has been proposed for reliable estimation of disorder prevalence in dogs. Electronic patient record (EPR) data were collected on 148,741 dogs attending 93 clinics across central and south-eastern England. Analysis in detail of a random sample of EPRs relating to 3,884 dogs from 89 clinics identified the most frequently recorded disorders as otitis externa (prevalence 10.2%, 95% CI: 9.1–11.3), periodontal disease (9.3%, 95% CI: 8.3–10.3) and anal sac impaction (7.1%, 95% CI: 6.1–8.1). Using syndromic classification, the most prevalent body location affected was the head-and-neck (32.8%, 95% CI: 30.7–34.9), the most prevalent organ system affected was the integument (36.3%, 95% CI: 33.9–38.6) and the most prevalent pathophysiologic process diagnosed was inflammation (32.1%, 95% CI: 29.8–34.3). Among the twenty most-frequently recorded disorders, purebred dogs had a significantly higher prevalence compared with crossbreds for three: otitis externa (P = 0.001), obesity (P = 0.006) and skin mass lesion (P = 0.033), and popular breeds differed significantly from each other in their prevalence for five: periodontal disease (P = 0.002), overgrown nails (P = 0.004), degenerative joint disease (P = 0.005), obesity (P = 0.001) and lipoma (P = 0.003). These results fill a crucial data gap in disorder prevalence information and assist with disorder prioritisation. The results suggest that, for maximal impact, breeding reforms should target commonly-diagnosed complex disorders that are amenable to genetic improvement and should place special focus on at-risk breeds. Future studies evaluating disorder severity and duration will augment the usefulness of the disorder prevalence information reported herein.

**Editor:** Cheryl S. Rosenfeld, University of Missouri, United States of America

**Funding:** This study was part of a Ph.D. study that was financially supported by the RSPCA (http://www.rspca.org.uk/sciencegroup/companionanimals). The funders had no role in study design, data collection and analysis, decision to publish, or preparation of the manuscript.

**Competing Interests:** The authors have declared that no competing interests exist.

\* E-mail: doneill@rvc.ac.uk

## Introduction

The domestic dog (*Canis lupus familiaris*) has become integral to modern human family life, with the UK dog population estimated to be 8–10 million [1,2,3] and 24–31% of UK households estimated to own at least one dog [1,2]. Although humans benefit from dog ownership both physically [4,5] and mentally [6,7], it is increasingly questioned whether modern breeding practices have allowed dog health and welfare to derive comparable benefits [8,9]. Although the dog is now the most phenotypically diverse mammal at a species level [10], genetic diversity has been greatly reduced within modern breeds [11] because of breeding practices that include closed stud books [12], structured inbreeding [11] and reproductive dominance of popular sires [13]. Additionally, selection pressure within breeds towards phenotypic exaggeration driven by breed standards [8], have increased the potential for conformation-associated disease [14]. Each of the 50 most popular breeds in the UK has at least one reported conformational predisposition to disease [15] and almost 400 non-conformational inherited disorders have been identified [16]. Conversely, implicit acceptance of the statement that purebred dogs are plagued with many inherited diseases [17] has contributed to a widespread belief that crossbred dogs are substantially healthier than purebreds [18].

Following claims in the BBC documentary *Pedigree Dogs Exposed* that purebred dog health was deteriorating because of inbreeding and ill-advised breed standards [19], three major reports concurred that pedigree breeding practices did impose welfare costs on dogs but, more crucially, concluded that a critical data gap on disorder prevalence information in UK dogs constrained effective reforms [20,21,22]. Prevalence data have been published on only 1% of inherited disorders affecting popular UK dog breeds [23]. Effective welfare reform of pedigree dog-breeding must be underpinned by scientifically valid prioritisation of disorders based on reliable and comparable prevalence data [12,24]. However, differing case definitions, study populations, geographical locations, data quality and data collection periods between published studies, combined with substantial data gaps, have constrained efforts to prioritise disorders in domestic dogs [9]. Application of health data collected via a single national surveillance system has been proposed for effective disorder prioritisation, with the critical first step being the generation of reliable disorder prevalence values [12].

Systematised collection, mergence and analysis of electronic patient record (EPR) data from primary-care veterinary practices has been proposed for generation of reliable prevalence data relating to the overall dog population [12,20]. Contemporaneous recording of clinical information by veterinary health professionals during episodes of care for every patient treated minimises selection and recall biases in primary-care practice EPR data [20]. By contrast, referral caseloads may show selection bias towards more complicated disorders [25], questionnaire surveys may incur selection, recall and misclassification biases [26], and pet insurance data are limited by selection bias emerging from age restrictions, financial excesses and owner attributes [27].

This study aimed to use a database of merged primary-care practice EPRs to estimate the prevalence of the most frequently recorded disorders and syndromes in dogs attending primary-care veterinary practices in England. The study further aimed to evaluate associations between the occurrence of common disorders with purebred/crossbred status and with popular breeds. It was hypothesised that purebred dogs have a higher prevalence of common disorders compared with crossbred dogs.

## Materials and Methods

Ethics statement: Ethics approval was granted by the RVC Ethics and Welfare Committee (reference number 2010 1076).

The VetCompass Animal Surveillance project collates de-identified EPR data from primary-care veterinary practices in the UK for epidemiological research [28]. The current study included data collected from all clinics within the Medivet Veterinary Group, a large network of integrated veterinary practices covering central and south-eastern England [29]. Practitioners recorded summary diagnosis terms from an embedded standard nomenclature, the VeNom codes [30], at episodes of clinical care. EPR data were extracted from practice management systems (PMSs) using integrated clinical queries [31] and uploaded to a secure structured query language (SQL) database. Information collected included patient demographic (animal identification number, species, breed, date of birth, sex, neuter status, insurance status, microchip number and weight) and clinical information (free-form text clinical notes, VeNom summary diagnosis terms and treatment, with relevant dates) data fields.

The study sampling frame included all dogs that had at least one EPR (clinical note, weight recording or treatment dispensed) recorded within the VetCompass Animal Surveillance database from September 1, 2009 to March 31, 2013. Sample size calculations estimated that, from a study population of 140,000 dogs, a sample of 3,648 animals was required to represent a disorder with 2.5% expected frequency with a precision of 0.5% at a 95% confidence level [32].

A random sample of dogs was selected from the overall sampling frame using an online random number generator (www.random.org). Clinical notes and VeNom summary diagnosis terms recorded during the study period were reviewed in detail, and the most definitive diagnostic term recorded for each disorder diagnosed within individual dogs was manually coded using the most appropriate VeNom term. Elective (e.g. neutering) or prophylactic (e.g. vaccination) clinical events were not included. Multiple counting of disorder events for ongoing cases was avoided by including recurring diagnoses of ongoing conditions only once (e.g. repeated events of otitis externa) and by including only the final diagnosis term recorded in cases with diagnosis revision over time (e.g. following clinical work-up or trial therapy), based on the assumption that diagnostic accuracy increased over time [33]. The parent term was used for disorders that encompassed multiple child terms [34] (e.g. a parent term *road traffic accident* (RTA) may have multiple child terms such as *laceration*, *fracture* and *hypovolaemic*

*shock*). Disorder events that were aetiologically independent despite sharing the same disorder term name (e.g. novel traumatic events) were included separately. No distinction was made between pre-existing and incident disorder presentations. Disorders described within the clinical notes using presenting sign terms (e.g. 'vomiting and diarrhoea'), but without a formal clinical diagnostic term being recorded, were included using the first sign listed (e.g. vomiting). Dental disorders were included only if surgical or medical intervention were recommended.

Recognisable single breeds [35] were grouped as 'purebred' while all other dogs were grouped as 'crossbred'. Purebreds were further categorised by Kennel Club (KC) breed-recognition (recognised/not recognised) and KC breed group (gundog, hound, pastoral, terrier, toy, utility, working) [36]. Neuter status was defined by the final EPR neuter value and was combined with sex to create four categories: female entire, female neutered, male entire and male neutered. Insurance and microchip values characterized the existence of a positive status at any time during the study period. The maximum bodyweight (kg) recorded for dogs aged over one year was categorised into seven groups (<10.0, 10.0–19.9, 20.0–29.9, 30.0–39.9, 40.0–49.9, ≥50.0, and 'no recorded weight'). The age (years) at the final EPR was categorised into five groups (<1.0, 1.0–2.9, 3.0–5.9, 6.0–9.9, ≥10.0). Time contributed to the study for each dog was calculated as the period from the date of the earliest EPR to the date of the latest EPR. The date and manner (euthanasia or non-assisted) [37] of deaths recorded during the study were identified.

VeNom diagnostic terms for all recorded disorders were extracted and mapped to three systems of terms for analysis: diagnosis-level precision, mid-level precision and syndromic classification. Diagnosis-level terms were one-to-one descriptors of the original extracted terms at the maximal diagnostic precision recorded within the clinical notes (e.g. *inflammatory bowel disease* would remain as *inflammatory bowel disease*). Mid-level precision terms were one-to-one descriptors of original diagnosis terms defined at a general level of diagnostic precision (e.g. *inflammatory bowel disease* would map to *enteropathy*). Syndromic classification used three taxonomic groupings: body location, organ system and pathophysiologic process. The number of syndromic terms that could be mapped from each original diagnostic term was not limited.

Study data were exported from the VetCompass database to a spreadsheet (Microsoft Office Excel 2007, Microsoft Corp.) for checking and cleaning before further export to Stata Version 11.2 (Stata Corporation) for statistical analyses. Demographic variables were described statistically for the overall study population and the sample group. Prevalence values with 95% confidence intervals (CI) were tabulated for the twenty most prevalent diagnosis-level and mid-level disorders and for all syndromic terms, and were reported across all sampled dogs, purebreds only and crossbreds only. Prevalence values for purebred and crossbred dogs were compared statistically using the chi-squared test with Holm-adjusted P-values to account for multiple testing effects [38]. Statistical significance was set at the 5% level. The CI estimates were derived from standard errors based on approximation to the normal distribution for disorders with ten or more events recorded [39], but the Wilson approximation method was used for disorders with fewer than ten events recorded [40]. Prevalence (95% CI) values for the twenty most prevalent diagnosis-level and mid-level disorders and for all syndromic terms were similarly derived, reported and compared for popular breeds and crossbreds (popular breeds had ≥100 dogs in the sample group).

## Results

The overall population comprised 148,741 dogs attending 93 clinics across central and south-eastern England. Demographic examination of dogs with information available indicated that 117,179 (78.9%) were purebred, 71,002 (48.0%) were female, 61,120 (41.1%) were neutered, 43,435 (29.2%) were insured and 41,071 (27.6%) were microchipped. The median weight was 18.2 kg (interquartile range (IQR): 9.4–29.0, range: 0.68–105.0) and the median age was 4.5 years (IQR: 1.6–8.7, range: 0.0–27.4) (Table 1).

The study sample comprised 3,884 dogs attending 89 clinics. Of dogs with information available, 3,079 (79.4%) were purebred, 1,817 (47.0%) were female, 1,735 (44.7%) were neutered, 1,226 (31.6%) were insured and 1,151 (29.6%) were microchipped. The median weight was 17.3 kg (IQR: 9.1–28.4, range: 1.3–100.6) and the median age was 4.8 years (IQR: 1.8–9.1, range: 0.0–21.24). The most popular seven breeds accounted for 1,431 (36.8%) of the study sample dogs (Table 1). Of the sampled dogs, 373 (9.7%) died during the study period, with a median (IQR, range) age at death of 12.3 years (9.2–14.4, 0.0–21.0) and 336 (88.9%) deaths involving euthanasia. Overall, 2,945 (75.8%) dogs had at least one disorder diagnosed, with the remainder having no disorders diagnosed during the study period. The median (IQR, range) number of disorders diagnosed per dog was 1.0 (1.0–3.0, 0.0–21.0). The median (IQR, range) time contributed to the study per dog was 0.7 years (0.0–3.5, 0.0–1.9). The sample and study populations were similar across all measures assessed.

Among the sampled dogs, 8,025 unique disorder events were recorded encompassing 430 distinct diagnosis-level disorder terms. The most prevalent diagnosis-level disorders recorded were otitis externa (number of events: 396, prevalence: 10.2%, 95% CI: 9.1–11.3), periodontal disease (361, 9.3%, 95% CI: 8.3–10.3), anal sac impaction (277, 7.1%, 95% CI: 6.1–8.1) and overgrown nails (276, 7.1%, 95% CI: 6.1–8.2). Purebred dogs had a significantly higher prevalence compared with crossbreds for three of the twenty most-prevalent diagnosis-level disorders: otitis externa (P = 0.001), obesity (P = 0.006) and skin mass lesion (P = 0.033) (Table 2). The prevalence of five of the twenty most-prevalent diagnosis-level disorders differed statistically significantly between popular breeds: periodontal disease (P = 0.002), overgrown nails (P = 0.004), degenerative joint disease (P = 0.005), obesity (P = 0.001) and lipoma (P = 0.003) (Table 3).

Within 54 mid-level diagnosis terms, the most prevalent disorders were enteropathic (n = 692, prevalence: 17.8%, 95% CI: 16.0–19.6), dermatological (602, 15.5%, 95% CI: 13.9–17.1), musculoskeletal (457, 11.8%, 95% CI: 10.6–12.9) and aural (426, 11.0%, 95% CI: 9.8–12.2). Purebred dogs showed a significantly higher prevalence than crossbreds for four of the twenty most-prevalent mid-level disorders: dermatological (P = 0.004), aural (P = 0.001), ophthalmological (P = 0.032) and obesity (P = 0.009) (Table 4). Statistically significant differences in prevalence values were shown between the most popular breeds in eight of the twenty most-frequent mid-level disorders: musculoskeletal (P = 0.002), claw/nail (P = 0.008), dental (P = 0.007), neoplastic (P = 0.001), anal sac (P = 0.006), obesity (P = 0.004), cardiac (P = 0.005) and brain (P = 0.003) (Table 5).

Syndromic classification analysis indicated that the most prevalent body locations affected in dogs were the head-and-neck (n = 1,273, prevalence = 32.8%, 95% CI: 30.7–34.9), abdomen (993, 25.6%, 95% CI: 23.6–27.5) and limb (679, 17.5%, 95% C: 15.9–19.1). Purebreds had significantly higher prevalence values compared with crossbreds for two of the eight body locations: head-and-neck (P = 0.003) and tail (P = 0.038) disorders. The most

prevalent organ systems affected were the integument (1,408, 36.3%, 95% CI: 33.9–38.6), digestive (1,144, 29.5%, 95% CI: 27.5–31.5) and musculoskeletal (573, 14.8%, 95% CI: 13.8–16.0) (Table 6). Purebreds had significantly higher prevalence values than crossbreds for two of fifteen organ systems, namely integument (P = 0.001) and auditory (P = 0.002) (Table 6). The most prevalent pathophysiologic processes recorded were inflammation (1,246, 32.1%, 95% CI: 29.8–34.3), mass/swelling (625, 16.1%, 95% CI: 14.6–17.6) and traumatic (557, 14.3%, 95% CI: 12.8–15.9). Purebreds had significantly higher prevalence values than crossbreds for two of twenty-one pathophysiological processes: inflammatory (P = 0.006) and nutritional (P = 0.0014) disorders (Table 7). Statistically significant differences in prevalence values between the most popular breeds were shown for 5/8 body location terms, 5/15 organ system terms and 5/21 pathophysiologic processes (Tables 8, 9 &10).

## Discussion

This study reported the most prevalent disorders recorded in dogs attending primary-care veterinary practices in England as otitis externa, periodontal disease and anal sac impaction, while the most prevalent disorder groups were enteropathic, dermatological and musculoskeletal. The head-and-neck was the most prevalent body location affected, the integument was the most prevalent organ system affected, and inflammation was the most prevalent pathophysiologic process. Some evidence was shown to support higher disorder prevalence in purebred dogs compared with crossbred dogs and for important differences in disorder prevalence between breeds.

The current study was designed to fill a critical data gap relating to disorder prevalence information that has been identified as a constraint to improving dog welfare by effective reform of purebred dog-breeding [20,21,22]. Unacceptably high occurrence of inherited disorders in purebred dogs has been discussed since over half a century ago [41,42,43,44], leading to implementation of disease control measures such as defined health schemes [45,46,47,48] and revised KC recommendations and rules for registration and showing [44,49]. However, the current state and predicted trajectory of purebred dog health remain contentious despite these and other ongoing health measures, suggesting that these earlier breeding reforms that were developed without access to prioritisation information on the overall disorder burden may at best have been sub-optimal, and potentially even counter-productive [50].

Primary-care veterinary clinical data have been proposed as a superior data resource for clinical research in dogs [12,20]. Although useful, alternative data sources including referral practice data [51,52,53], pet insurance databases [27], official health schemes [54,55,56] and large scale questionnaire surveys [26,57,58,59] are reported to suffer many limitations for the generation of prevalence values that can be generalised to the wider dog population. Analyses based on primary-care veterinary EPR data benefit from open-ended data collection allowing generation of stronger evidence from cohort compared with cross-sectional study designs [60,61,62]. Selection bias is reduced by merging data collected from a miscellany of practices [63] and recall and misclassification biases are reduced by collection of clinical notes recorded contemporaneously by veterinary clinicians during episodes of care [64]. Veterinary primary-care denominator populations are well-characterised demographically within PMSs and include all practice-attending animals, whether presenting healthy or sick, linked with comprehensive clinical documentation that facilitates internal validation [27]. Registra-

**Table 1.** Demographic information for sampled (n = 3,884) and overall study population (n = 148,741) dogs attending primary veterinary practices in England.

| Variable | Category | Sample: No. (%) | Population: No. (%) |
|---|---|---|---|
| Sex/neuter | Female entire | 981 (25.4) | 40,514 (27.4) |
| | Female neutered | 836 (21.6) | 30,488 (20.6) |
| | Male entire | 1,152 (29.8) | 46,459 (31.4) |
| | Male neutered | 899 (23.2) | 30,635 (20.7) |
| Microchip | Not microchipped | 2,733 (70.4) | 107,670 (72.4) |
| | Microchipped | 1,151 (29.6) | 41,071 (27.6) |
| Purebred status | Crossbred | 797 (20.6) | 31,354 (21.1) |
| | Purebred | 3,079 (79.4) | 117,179 (78.9) |
| Popular breeds | Crossbreed | 797 (20.5) | 31,354 (21.1) |
| | Labrador Retriever | 339 (8.7) | 13,328 (9.0) |
| | Staffordshire Bull Terrier | 334 (8.6) | 12,212 (8.2) |
| | Jack Russell Terrier | 262 (6.8) | 10,006 (6.7) |
| | Cocker Spaniel | 133 (3.4) | 5,579 (3.8) |
| | German Shepherd Dog | 132 (3.4) | 5,314 (3.6) |
| | Yorkshire Terrier | 127 (3.3) | 4,880 (3.3) |
| | Border Collie | 104 (2.7) | 3,997 (2.7) |
| | Other named breeds | 1,656 (42.6) | 62,071 (41.7) |
| KC[a]- breed[b] | Not KC-recognised | 306 (9.9) | 11,717 (10.0) |
| | KC-recognised | 2,773 (90.1) | 105,462 (90.0) |
| KC[a] group[c] | Gundog | 737 (26.6) | 28,832 (27.3) |
| | Hound | 178 (6.4) | 6,505 (6.2) |
| | Pastoral | 284 (10.2) | 11,530 (10.9) |
| | Terrier | 561 (20.2) | 21,481 (20.4) |
| | Toy | 474 (17.1) | 17,215 (16.3) |
| | Utility | 330 (11.9) | 11,573 (11.0) |
| | Working | 209 (7.5) | 8,326 (7.9) |
| Weight (kg) | No recorded weight | 1,260 (32.4) | 52,308 (35.2) |
| | <10.0 | 769 (19.8) | 26,786 (18.0) |
| | 10.0–19.9 | 695 (17.9) | 25,278 (17.0) |
| | 20.0–20.99 | 579 (14.9) | 21,869 (14.7) |
| | 30.0–30.9 | 390 (10.0) | 15,255 (10.3) |
| | 40.0–40.9 | 130 (3.4) | 5,118 (3.4) |
| | ≥50.0 | 61 (1.6) | 2,127 (1.4) |
| Age (years) | <1.0 | 588 (15.2) | 24,915 (16.8) |
| | 1.0–2.9 | 791 (20.4) | 30,747 (20.7) |
| | 3.0–5.9 | 877 (22.6) | 33,500 (22.5) |
| | 6.0–9.9 | 811 (20.9) | 30,811 (20.7) |
| | ≥10.0 | 814 (21.0) | 28,664 (19.3) |
| Insurance | Non-insured | 2,658 (68.4) | 105,306 (70.8) |
| | Insured | 1,226 (31.6) | 43,435 (29.2) |

[a]KC The Kennel Club.
[b]Percentage values based on purebred only.
[c]Percentage values based on KC-recognised dogs only.

tion databases from primary-care practices are more representative of the national dog population than other databases available for research purposes; 77% of UK dogs are registered with a veterinary practice compared with just 42% of UK dogs that are insured and 31% of UK dogs that are registered with the KC [2].

Previous large-scale studies using primary-care practice clinical data have been variably successful and have encountered problems with sustainability. A cross-sectional study of paper-based clinical records for 7,146 dogs from eight UK practices described demographic and morbidity results but concluded that direct electronic extraction of clinical data and implementation of

Table 2. Prevalence results for the most frequent disorders recorded in dogs, purebreds only and crossbreds only that attended primary veterinary practices in England.

| Disorder | Overall | | | Purebred | | Crossbred | | |
|---|---|---|---|---|---|---|---|---|
| | No. | Prev[a]% | 95% CI[b] | Prev[a]% | 95% CI[b] | Prev[a]% | 95% CI[b] | P-value |
| Otitis externa | 396 | 10.2 | 9.1–11.3 | 11.2 | 10.0–12.4 | 6.5 | 4.7–8.3 | **0.001** |
| Periodontal disease | 361 | 9.3 | 8.3–10.3 | 9.4 | 8.2–10.5 | 9.2 | 7.4–11.0 | 1.000 |
| Anal sac impaction | 277 | 7.1 | 6.1–8.1 | 7.1 | 6.0–8.1 | 7.5 | 5.7–9.4 | 1.000 |
| Overgrown nails | 276 | 7.1 | 6.1–8.2 | 6.9 | 5.8–8.0 | 8.0 | 6.1–9.9 | 1.000 |
| Degenerative joint disease | 256 | 6.6 | 5.7–7.5 | 6.4 | 5.3–7.4 | 7.5 | 5.7–9.4 | 1.000 |
| Diarrhoea | 249 | 6.4 | 5.5–7.4 | 6.8 | 5.6–8.0 | 4.9 | 3.4–6.4 | 0.255 |
| Obesity | 238 | 6.1 | 5.2–7.1 | 6.7 | 5.6–7.9 | 3.9 | 2.3–5.5 | **0.006** |
| Traumatic injury | 214 | 5.5 | 4.7–6.4 | 5.5 | 4.4–6.5 | 5.7 | 3.6–7.7 | 1.000 |
| Conjunctivitis | 192 | 4.9 | 4.1–5.8 | 5.2 | 4.2–6.2 | 4.1 | 2.8–5.5 | 1.000 |
| Vomiting | 159 | 4.1 | 3.3–4.9 | 4.0 | 3.1–4.9 | 4.5 | 3.0–6.0 | 1.000 |
| Heart murmur | 153 | 3.9 | 3.3–4.5 | 4.1 | 3.5–4.7 | 3.4 | 2.1–4.7 | 1.000 |
| Lipoma | 137 | 3.5 | 2.8–4.2 | 3.5 | 2.7–4.2 | 3.8 | 2.7–4.9 | 1.000 |
| Dermatitis | 134 | 3.5 | 2.8–4.1 | 3.5 | 2.8–4.3 | 3.1 | 1.9–4.4 | 1.000 |
| Skin hypersensitivity | 113 | 2.9 | 2.3–3.5 | 3.2 | 2.5–3.9 | 1.8 | 0.9–2.6 | 0.116 |
| Skin mass | 110 | 2.8 | 2.3–3.4 | 3.2 | 2.6–3.8 | 1.5 | 0.6–2.4 | **0.033** |
| Claw injury | 103 | 2.7 | 2.1–3.2 | 2.6 | 2.0–3.2 | 2.6 | 1.5–3.8 | 1.000 |
| Behavioural | 99 | 2.6 | 2.1–3.0 | 2.6 | 2.1–3.1 | 2.4 | 1.4–3.4 | 1.000 |
| Gastroenteritis | 99 | 2.6 | 2.0–3.1 | 2.4 | 1.9–2.9 | 3.1 | 2.0–4.3 | 1.000 |
| Dog bite injury | 97 | 2.5 | 1.9–3.1 | 2.4 | 1.7–3.1 | 2.9 | 1.8–4.0 | 1.000 |
| Laceration | 92 | 2.4 | 1.8–2.9 | 2.5 | 1.8–3.1 | 2.0 | 1.1–2.9 | 0.446 |

P-values (Holm-adjusted) represent comparison between purebreds and crossbreds.
[a]Prev prevalence.
[b]95% CI 95% confidence interval.

standardised coding for breeds and disorders were required to sustain long-term data collection [65]. In the US, the National Companion Animal Study (NCAS) reported overall disorder prevalence values using electronic records from 86,772 dogs attending 63 private practices. However, prevalence estimation was based only on the 36% of animals that had at least one coded disorder term recorded and the full clinical notes were not accessible for case-finding and internal validation exercises [66]. The National Companion Animal Surveillance System (NCASP) was established using EPR data from over 500 Banfield Pet Hospitals, but this system focused on the threat of emerging infection, terrorist attack or natural disaster rather than disorder prevalence [67] and has since been discontinued [68].

A standardised veterinary lexicon is critical for large-scale epidemiological application of secondary clinical data [52,65,69,70]. The VeNom codes [30] offers an open-access veterinary nomenclature that has been developed collaboratively between university and primary-care practice groups and facilitates both direct coding by attending clinicians at the point of clinical care and also retrospective coding by researchers during analysis. The VeNom coding ontology that is made available for point-of-care coding defines multiple clinical fields including species (45 terms), dog breeds (767), cat breeds (101), presenting complaints (201), diagnostic tests (39), diagnoses (2,291) and procedures (780).

The current study indicated that otitis externa (10.2%), periodontal disease (9.3%), anal sac impaction (7.1%) and overgrown nails (7.1%) were the most prevalent disorders recorded

in dogs attending veterinary practices in England. A US primary-care study similarly identified dental calculus (20.5%), gingivitis (19.5) and otitis externa (13.0%) as the most prevalent diagnoses in dogs, but reported the prevalence of anal sac disease at only 2.5%, and did not even include nail disorders within the common disorders diagnosed [70]. An under-developed coding system, inconsistent case definitions and selection bias from inclusion of only the one-third of animals that had at least one coded diagnosis term within the US study may explain these differing prevalence trends and underscores the importance of standardised coding systems for reliable comparisons between studies. The high frequency of dental disease reported in the US study may have resulted from inclusion of animals with any recorded dental abnormality, regardless of severity. By contrast, the current study aimed to report the occurrence of dental disorders that currently warranted treatment in the opinion of the attending clinician. Study-inclusion of dental abnormalities of any nature provides information on the summative effects from both current and potential future clinically-significant dental disease whereas including just current clinically-significant cases provides evidence on the current welfare implications of dental disease. Both approaches have merit and add to our understanding of the substantial clinical relevance of dental disorders to the health and welfare of dogs. A UK primary-care study using paper-based clinical records identified the most prevalent disorders of dogs as overgrown nails (2.7%), ascarid worm problems (2.3%), anal sac impaction (2.1%), dental calculus (1.8%), fleas (1.8%), bacterial otitis externa (1.7%), waxy otitis externa (1.2%), diarrhoea/

**Table 3.** Prevalence results for frequent disorders recorded in popular breeds (number of dogs) from 3,884 randomly sampled dogs attending primary veterinary practices in England.

| Disorder | Prevalence percentage (95% confidence interval) | | | | | | | | |
| | Crossbred (797) | Labrador Retriever (339) | Staffordshire Bull Terrier (334) | Jack Russell Terrier (262) | Cocker Spaniel (133) | German Shepherd Dog (132) | Yorkshire Terrier (127) | Border Collie (104) | P-Value |
|---|---|---|---|---|---|---|---|---|---|
| Otitis externa | 6.5 (4.7–8.3) | 11.8 (8.8–15.7) | 9.9 (7.1–13.6) | 6.9 (4.4–10.6) | 8.3 (4.7–14.2) | 11.4 (7.0–17.9) | 7.9 (4.3–13.9) | 1.9 (0.5–6.7) | 0.084 |
| Periodontal disease | 9.2 (7.4–11.0) | 3.2 (1.8–5.7) | 2.4 (1.2–4.7) | 9.5 (6.6–13.7) | 12.8 (8.1–19.5) | 4.5 (2.1–9.6) | 25.2 (18.6–33.4) | 6.7 (3.3–13.3) | **0.002** |
| Anal sac impaction | 7.5 (5.7–9.4) | 4.7 (2.9–7.5) | 3.3 (1.9–5.8) | 6.9 (4.4–10.6) | 12.0 (7.5–18.6) | 6.1 (3.1–11.5) | 6.3 (3.2–11.9) | 2.9 (1.0–8.1) | 0.066 |
| Overgrown nails | 8.0 (6.1–9.9) | 6.5 (4.3–9.6) | 3.9 (2.3–6.5) | 13.7 (10.1–18.4) | 2.3 (0.8–6.4) | 1.5 (0.4–5.4) | 15.0 (9.8–22.2) | 1.0 (0.2–5.3) | **0.004** |
| Degenerative joint disease | 7.5 (5.9–9.6) | 11.5 (8.5–15.3) | 5.4 (3.4–8.4) | 4.2 (2.4–7.4) | 1.5 (0.4–5.3) | 6.8 (3.6–12.5) | 1.6 (0.4–5.6) | 11.5 (6.7–19.1) | **0.005** |
| Diarrhoea | 4.9 (3.4–6.4) | 8.3 (5.8–11.7) | 4.8 (3.0–7.6) | 4.6 (2.6–7.8) | 9.8 (5.8–16.0) | 8.3 (4.7–14.3) | 5.5 (2.7–10.9) | 7.7 (4.0–14.5) | 1.000 |
| Obesity | 3.9 (2.3–5.5) | 13.0 (9.8–17.0) | 6.0 (3.9–9.1) | 5.3 (3.2–8.8) | 8.3 (4.7–14.2) | 2.3 (0.8–6.5) | 0.8 (0.1–4.3) | 6.7 (3.3–13.3) | **0.001** |
| Traumatic injury | 5.7 (3.6–7.7) | 5.3 (3.4–8.2) | 4.5 (2.7–7.3) | 6.1 (3.8–9.7) | 5.3 (2.6–10.5) | 4.6 (2.1–9.6) | 3.2 (1.2–7.8) | 4.8 (2.1–10.8) | 1.000 |
| Conjunctivitis | 4.1 (2.8–5.5) | 4.1 (2.5–6.8) | 5.1 (3.2–8.0) | 4.2 (2.4–7.4) | 6.8 (3.6–12.4) | 0.0 (0.0–2.8) | 7.1 (3.8–12.9) | 4.8 (2.1–10.8) | 1.000 |
| Vomiting | 4.5 (3.0–6.0) | 3.8 (2.3–6.5) | 3.9 (2.3–6.5) | 5.7 (3.5–9.2) | 2.3 (0.8–6.4) | 4.6 (2.1–9.6) | 3.2 (1.2–7.8) | 1.9 (0.5–6.7) | 1.000 |
| Heart murmur | 3.4 (2.1–4.7) | 1.5 (0.6–3.4) | 2.7 (1.4–5.0) | 3.8 (2.1–6.9) | 3.8 (1.6–8.5) | 1.5 (0.4–5.4) | 7.1 (3.8–12.9) | 4.8 (2.1–10.8) | 0.837 |
| Lipoma | 3.8 (2.7–4.9) | 9.1 (6.5–12.7) | 2.1 (1.0–4.3) | 2.7 (1.3–5.4) | 6.0 (3.1–11.4) | 1.5 (0.4–5.4) | 2.1 (0.0–2.9) | 5.8 (2.7–12.0) | **0.003** |
| Dermatitis | 3.1 (1.9–4.4) | 1.5 (0.6–3.4) | 3.6 (2.1–6.2) | 3.4 (1.8–6.4) | 3.0 (1.2–7.5) | 3.0 (1.2–7.5) | 4.7 (2.2–9.9) | 6.7 (3.3–13.3) | 1.000 |
| Skin hypersensitivity | 1.8 (0.9–2.6) | 3.8 (2.3–6.5) | 5.1 (3.2–8.0) | 3.1 (1.6–5.9) | 1.5 (0.4–5.3) | 3.0 (1.2–7.5) | 3.2 (1.2–7.8) | 2.9 (1.0–8.1) | 1.000 |
| Skin mass | 1.5 (0.6–2.4) | 3.2 (1.8–5.7) | 3.9 (2.3–6.5) | 2.3 (1.1–4.9) | 3.8 (1.6–8.5) | 3.0 (1.2–7.5) | 2.4 (0.8–6.7) | 3.0 (1.0–8.1) | 1.000 |
| Claw injury | 2.6 (1.5–3.8) | 3.8 (2.3–6.5) | 3.6 (2.1–6.2) | 2.7 (1.3–5.4) | 2.3 (0.8–6.4) | 3.0 (1.2–7.5) | 3.9 (1.7–8.9) | 2.9 (1.0–8.1) | 1.000 |
| Undesirable behaviour | 2.4 (1.4–3.4) | 3.0 (1.6–5.3) | 2.7 (1.4–5.0) | 1.5 (0.6–3.9) | 3.0 (1.2–7.5) | 7.6 (4.2–13.4) | 2.4 (0.8–6.7) | 5.8 (2.7–12.0) | 0.208 |
| Gastro–enteritis | 3.1 (2.0–4.3) | 4.4 (2.7–7.3) | 1.5 (0.6–3.5) | 1.9 (0.8–4.4) | 3.0 (1.2–7.5) | 0.8 (0.1–4.2) | 3.9 (1.7–8.9) | 3.9 (1.5–9.5) | 1.000 |
| Dog bite injury | 2.9 (1.8–4.0) | 1.5 (0.6–3.4) | 3.0 (1.6–5.4) | 3.8 (2.1–6.9) | 3.8 (1.6–8.5) | 1.5 (0.4–5.4) | 0.0 (0.0–2.9) | 1.0 (0.2–5.3) | 1.000 |
| Laceration | 2.0 (1.2–3.2) | 3.5 (2.0–6.1) | 2.4 (1.2–4.7) | 2.7 (1.3–5.4) | 3.0 (1.2–7.5) | 0.8 (0.1–4.2) | 1.6 (0.4–5.6) | 2.9 (1.0–8.1) | 1.000 |

P-values (Holm-adjusted) represent comparison between breeds.

**Table 4.** Prevalence results for the most frequent mid-level disorders recorded in dogs, purebreds only and crossbreds only that attended primary veterinary practices in England.

| Mid-level disorder | Overall | | | Purebred | | Crossbred | | P-value |
|---|---|---|---|---|---|---|---|---|
| | No. | Prev[a]% | 95% CI[b] | Prev[a]% | 95% CI[b] | Prev[a]% | 95% CI[b] | |
| Enteropathic | 692 | 17.8 | 16.0–19.6 | 17.7 | 15.8–19.7 | 18.3 | 15.4–21.2 | 1.000 |
| Dermatological | 602 | 15.5 | 13.9–17.1 | 16.5 | 14.6–18.4 | 11.9 | 10.0–13.9 | **0.004** |
| Musculoskeletal | 457 | 11.8 | 10.6–12.9 | 11.2 | 9.8–12.6 | 14.1 | 11.8–16.3 | 0.130 |
| Aural | 426 | 11.0 | 9.8–12.2 | 12.0 | 10.7–13.3 | 7.2 | 5.3–9.0 | **0.001** |
| Ophthalmological | 406 | 10.5 | 9.1–11.8 | 11.1 | 9.7–12.6 | 7.9 | 6.1–9.7 | **0.032** |
| Claw/nail | 400 | 10.3 | 9.1–11.5 | 10.1 | 8.8–11.5 | 10.9 | 9.0–12.9 | 1.000 |
| Dental | 386 | 9.9 | 8.8–11.1 | 10.0 | 8.8–11.2 | 9.8 | 7.9–11.7 | 1.000 |
| Neoplastic | 367 | 9.5 | 8.2–10.7 | 9.6 | 8.2–10.9 | 9.2 | 7.2–11.1 | 1.000 |
| Traumatic injury (not incl. bites) | 351 | 9.0 | 8.0–10.1 | 9.1 | 7.8–10.3 | 8.9 | 6.6–11.2 | 1.000 |
| Anal sac | 337 | 8.7 | 7.5–9.8 | 8.6 | 7.3–9.9 | 9.0 | 7.1–11.0 | 1.000 |
| Obesity | 238 | 6.1 | 5.2–7.1 | 6.7 | 5.6–7.9 | 3.9 | 2.3–5.5 | **0.009** |
| Mass lesion | 235 | 6.1 | 5.2–6.9 | 6.4 | 5.3–7.4 | 4.9 | 3.4–6.4 | 0.726 |
| Behavioural | 233 | 6.0 | 5.3–6.85 | 5.8 | 4.9–6.7 | 6.9 | 5.1–8.7 | 1.000 |
| Upper respiratory tract | 223 | 5.7 | 4.9–6.5 | 5.6 | 4.6–6.6 | 6.4 | 4.6–8.2 | 1.000 |
| Cardiac | 219 | 5.6 | 4.8–6.5 | 5.9 | 5.0–6.7 | 4.9 | 3.1–6.7 | 1.000 |
| Parasitic | 172 | 4.4 | 3.8–5.1 | 4.2 | 3.5–5.0 | 5.3 | 3.7–6.8 | 1.000 |
| Congenital | 171 | 4.4 | 3.7–5.1 | 4.6 | 3.7–5.4 | 3.9 | 2.6–5.2 | 1.000 |
| Bite injury | 148 | 3.8 | 3.0–4.6 | 3.7 | 2.9–4.6 | 4.1 | 2.8–5.5 | 1.000 |
| Urinary | 126 | 3.2 | 2.7–3.8 | 3.4 | 2.7–4.1 | 2.8 | 1.6–3.9 | 1.000 |
| Brain | 122 | 3.1 | 2.5–3.7 | 3.2 | 2.6–3.8 | 3.1 | 1.9–4.4 | 1.000 |

P-values (Holm-adjusted) represent comparison between purebreds and crossbreds.
[a]Prev prevalence.
[b]95% CI 95% confidence interval.

vomiting (1.0%) and *Otodectes* otitis externa (0.9%) [65]. Although the predominance of aural, nail, anal sac and dental disorders identified was consistent with the current study, the older study reported *prevalence per consultation* values, leading to apparently lower prevalence values than the current study that reported *period prevalence per dog*. The substantially lower prevalence of parasitic disorders reported in the current study may also reflect increasing adoption and effectiveness of prophylactic parasiticides in the intervening fifteen years since the previous study [71,72].

Although diagnosis-level disorder terms are useful to describe disorders at their precision of clinical diagnosis, sole reliance on these terms for research may mask important underlying disorder concepts because of fragmentation into multiple terms along diagnostic pathways. The current study grouped clinically-related diagnosis-level terms (430 unique terms) into appropriate, composite mid-level disorder terms (54 unique terms) for further analysis. Selection of cut-off points for amalgamation along diagnostic precision pathways aimed to optimise interpretability whilst still retaining adequate precision [73]. The predominant mid-level disorders (enteropathic, dermatological, musculoskeletal and aural) differed from the predominant diagnosis-level disorders (otitis externa, periodontal disease, anal sac impaction, overgrown nails), suggesting that such hierarchical analysis can offer useful insights that may otherwise be missed.

Syndromic surveillance is based on clinical features that are discernible even from early presentation and are not dependent on complete or even correct diagnosis for elucidation of diagnostic patterns [74]. Although veterinary clinical diagnostic accuracy

may have improved over recent years, diagnostic discrepancies have been identified in 15% of cases undergoing necropsy [75]. Syndromic surveillance has been applied within human bioterrorism surveillance [76] and for analysis of canine insurance data [77,78]. The three syndromic classification systems used in the current study (body location, organ system and pathophysiology) were selected for their potential welfare importance via breed conformation and genetic effects [15]. The syndromic coding system used in the current study was adapted from VeNom codes and other published veterinary lexicons in line with the disorder types recorded within the study [25,79]. Progression towards a standardised syndromic terminology would facilitate future inter-study comparisons and meta-analyses [80].

The results from syndromic analyses in the current study identified the most prevalent body locations affected by disorders in dogs as the head-and-neck (32.8%), abdomen (25.6%) and limb (17.5%). Morphologic diversity between breeds resulting from artificial selection towards the extremes of breed standard morphometrics [81] has been associated with conformational predisposition for disorders [15,20]. The predominance of disorders identified affecting the head-and-neck reaffirm the importance of this body area to dog health [82].

The most affected organ systems identified by the current study were the integument (36.3%), digestive (29.5%) and musculoskeletal (14.8%). Swedish insurance data analysis similarly identified the most prevalently affected organs systems as the integument (3.2%), gastrointestinal (2.7%) and genital (2.5%) [83]. A consistently high prevalence reported by these studies for disorders

**Table 5.** Prevalence results for frequent mid-level disorders recorded in popular breeds (number of dogs) attending primary veterinary practices in England.

| Mid-level disorder | Prevalence percentage (95% confidence interval) | | | | | | | | P-value |
| | Crossbred (797) | Labrador Retriever (339) | Staffordshire Bull Terrier (334) | Jack Russell Terrier (262) | Cocker Spaniel (133) | German Shepherd Dog (132) | Yorkshire Terrier (127) | Border Collie (104) | |
| --- | --- | --- | --- | --- | --- | --- | --- | --- | --- |
| Enteropathic | 18.3 (15.4-21.2) | 22.7 (18.6-27.5) | 13.2 (10.0-17.2) | 15.3 (11.4-20.1) | 18.8 (13.1-26.3) | 20.5 (14.5-28.1) | 16.5 (11.1-24.0) | 17.3 (11.2-25.7) | 1.000 |
| Dermatological | 11.9 (10.0-13.9) | 16.8 (13.2-21.2) | 14.7 (11.38-18.9) | 13.0 (9.4-17.6) | 9.8 (5.8-16.0) | 18.9 (13.2-26.5) | 18.1 (12.4-25.7) | 18.3 (12.0-26.8) | 0.715 |
| Musculoskeletal | 14.1 (11.8-16.3) | 16.2 (12.7-20.5) | 8.4 (5.9-11.9) | 7.3 (4.7-11.1) | 3.0 (1.2-7.5) | 16.7 (11.3-24.0) | 6.3 (3.2-11.9) | 16.4 (10.5-24.6) | **0.002** |
| Aural | 7.2 (5.3-9.0) | 12.1 (9.0-16.0) | 11.1 (8.1-14.9) | 7.6 (5.0-11.5) | 9.0 (5.2-15.1) | 11.4 (7.0-17.9) | 7.9 (4.3-13.9) | 4.8 (2.1-10.8) | 0.828 |
| Ophthalmological | 7.9 (6.1-9.7) | 6.8 (4.6-10.0) | 8.1 (5.6-11.5) | 8.0 (5.3-11.9) | 12.0 (7.5-18.7) | 2.3 (0.8-6.5) | 12.6 (7.9-19.5) | 12.5 (7.5-20.2) | 0.261 |
| Claw/nail | 10.9 (9.0-12.9) | 10.9 (8.0-14.7) | 7.5 (5.1-10.8) | 14.9 (11.1-19.7) | 5.3 (2.6-10.5) | 5.3 (2.6-10.5) | 19.7 (13.7-27.5) | 5.8 (2.7-12.0) | **0.008** |
| Dental | 9.8 (7.9-11.7) | 3.8 (2.3-6.5) | 3.0 (1.6-5.4) | 11.5 (8.1-15.9) | 12.8 (8.1-19.5) | 5.3 (2.6-10.5) | 25.2 (18.5-33.4) | 7.7 (4.0-14.5) | **0.007** |
| Neoplastic | 9.2 (7.2-11.1) | 14.8 (11.4-18.9) | 6.6 (4.4-9.8) | 4.6 (2.6-7.8) | 13.5 (8.7-20.4) | 4.6 (2.1-9.6) | 6.3 (3.2-11.9) | 8.7 (4.6-15.6) | **0.001** |
| Traumatic injury (not bites or claw) | 8.9 (6.6-11.2) | 11.2 (8.3-15.0) | 7.88 (5.4-11.2) | 9.2 (6.2-13.3) | 10.5 (6.4-16.9) | 6.1 (3.1-11.5) | 3.9 (1.7-8.9) | 9.6 (5.3-16.8) | 1.000 |
| Anal sac | 9.0 (7.1-11.0) | 5.9 (3.9-8.9) | 3.6 (2.1-6.2) | 9.9 (6.9-14.1) | 13.5 (8.7-20.4) | 6.8 (3.6-12.5) | 6.3 (3.2-11.9) | 2.9 (1.0-8.1) | **0.006** |
| Obesity | 3.9 (2.3-5.5) | 12.98 (9.81-16.98) | 6.0 (3.9-9.1) | 5.3 (3.2-8.8) | 8.3 (4.7-14.2) | 2.3 (0.8-6.5) | 0.8 (0.1-4.3) | 6.7 (3.3-13.3) | **0.004** |
| Mass lesion | 4.9 (3.4-6.4) | 8.26 (5.78-11.68) | 6.6 (4.4-9.8) | 5.0 (2.9-8.3) | 6.8 (3.6-12.4) | 6.1 (3.1-11.5) | 7.9 (4.3-13.9) | 8.7 (4.6-15.6) | 1.000 |
| Behavioural | 6.9 (5.1-8.7) | 4.7 (2.9-7.5) | 5.1 (3.2-8.0) | 7.6 (5.0-11.5) | 6.8 (3.6-12.4) | 12.9 (8.2-19.7) | 3.9 (1.7-8.9) | 8.7 (4.6-15.6) | 0.460 |
| Upper respiratory tract | 6.4 (4.6-8.2) | 6.2 (4.1-9.3) | 6.3 (4.2-9.4) | 5.7 (3.5-9.2) | 2.3 (0.8-6.4) | 3.0 (1.2-7.5) | 7.1 (3.8-12.9) | 2.9 (1.0-8.1) | 1.000 |
| Cardiac disorder | 4.9 (3.1-6.7) | 1.5 (0.6-3.4) | 3.0 (1.6-5.4) | 6.5 (4.1-10.1) | 4.5 (2.1-9.5) | 1.5 (0.4-5.4) | 10.2 (6.1-16.7) | 5.8 (2.7-12.0) | **0.005** |
| Parasitic | 5.3 (3.7-6.8) | 3.5 (2.0-6.1) | 4.8 (3.0-7.6) | 3.4 (1.8-6.4) | 8.3 (4.7-14.2) | 2.3 (0.8-6.5) | 4.7 (2.2-9.9) | 1.9 (0.5-6.7) | 1.000 |
| Congenital | 3.9 (2.6-5.2) | 2.4 (1.2-4.6) | 2.1 (1.0-4.3) | 3.8 (2.2-6.9) | 3.8 (1.6-8.5) | 0.8 (0.1-4.2) | 6.3 (3.2-11.9) | 1.9 (0.5-6.7) | 1.000 |
| Bite injury | 4.1 (2.8-5.5) | 3.8 (2.3-6.5) | 4.29 (2.5-6.9) | 5.0 (2.9-8.3) | 4.5 (2.1-9.5) | 2.3 (0.8-6.5) | 1.6 (0.4-5.6) | 1.9 (0.5-6.7) | 1.000 |
| Urinary | 2.8 (1.6-3.9) | 4.7 (2.9-7.5) | 2.4 (1.2-4.6) | 1.9 (0.8-4.4) | 3.0 (1.2-7.5) | 3.0 (1.2-7.5) | 2.4 (0.8-6.7) | 3.9 (1.5-9.5) | 1.000 |
| Brain | 3.1 (1.9-4.4) | 3.2 (1.8-5.7) | 0.6 (0.2-2.2) | 2.3 (1.1-4.9) | 3.0 (1.2-7.5) | 4.6 (2.1-9.6) | 1.6 (0.4-5.6) | 9.6 (5.3-16.8) | **0.003** |

P-values (Holm-adjusted) represent comparison between breeds. ($n = 3,884$).

**Table 6.** Prevalence of syndromic disorders affecting body location and organ system recorded in overall dogs, purebreds only and crossbreds only that attended primary veterinary practices in England.

| | Overall | | | Purebred | | Crossbred | | P-value |
|---|---|---|---|---|---|---|---|---|
| | No. | Prev[a]% | 95% CI[b] | Prev[a]% | 95% CI[b] | Prev[a]% | 95% CI[b] | |
| **Body Location** | | | | | | | | |
| Head/neck | 1,273 | 32.8 | 30.7–34.9 | 34.0 | 31.7–36.2 | 28.5 | 24.9–32.0 | **0.003** |
| Abdomen | 993 | 25.6 | 23.6–27.5 | 25.9 | 23.7–28.0 | 24.6 | 21.5–27.7 | 1.000 |
| Limb | 679 | 17.5 | 15.9–19.1 | 17.3 | 15.5–19.1 | 18.3 | 15.7–20.9 | 1.000 |
| Anus/perineum | 359 | 9.2 | 8.1–10.4 | 9.1 | 7.8–10.5 | 9.8 | 7.6–12.0 | 1.000 |
| Thorax | 353 | 9.1 | 8.1–10.1 | 9.2 | 8.1–10.4 | 8.7 | 6.5–10.8 | 1.000 |
| Vertebral column | 78 | 2.0 | 1.5–2.5 | 2.0 | 1.5–2.6 | 2.0 | 1.0–3.0 | 1.000 |
| Pelvis | 33 | 0.9 | 0.6–1.2 | 0.9 | 0.7–1.4 | 0.5 | 0.2–1.3 | 0.684 |
| Tail | 21 | 0.5 | 0.4–0.8 | 0.7 | 0.5–1.0 | 0.0 | 0.0–0.5 | **0.038** |
| **Organ system** | | | | | | | | |
| Integument | 1,408 | 36.3 | 33.9–38.6 | 37.6 | 35.0–40.2 | 31.4 | 28.0–34.7 | **0.001** |
| Digestive | 1,144 | 29.5 | 27.5–31.5 | 29.4 | 27.2–31.6 | 30.0 | 26.6–33.3 | 1.000 |
| Musculoskeletal | 573 | 14.8 | 13.5–16.0 | 14.1 | 12.6–15.6 | 17.3 | 14.8–19.8 | 0.110 |
| Connective/Soft tissue | 503 | 13.0 | 11.6–14.3 | 13.2 | 11.6–14.7 | 12.3 | 10.2–14.4 | 1.000 |
| Ocular | 447 | 11.5 | 10.2–12.8 | 12.2 | 10.6–13.7 | 9.2 | 7.2–11.1 | 0.057 |
| Auditory | 437 | 11.3 | 10.0–12.5 | 12.3 | 11.0–13.6 | 7.4 | 5.5–9.3 | **0.002** |
| Nervous | 301 | 7.8 | 6.8–8.7 | 7.7 | 6.7–8.7 | 7.9 | 6.2–9.6 | 1.000 |
| Respiratory | 273 | 7.0 | 6.2–7.9 | 7.0 | 6.0–8.1 | 7.2 | 5.2–9.1 | 1.000 |
| Cardiovascular | 241 | 6.2 | 5.3–7.1 | 6.5 | 5.5–7.4 | 5.3 | 3.5–7.1 | 1.000 |
| Urinary | 227 | 5.8 | 5.1–6.6 | 5.9 | 4.9–6.8 | 5.8 | 4.1–7.5 | 1.000 |
| Reproductive | 184 | 4.7 | 4.1–5.4 | 4.7 | 4.0–5.5 | 4.9 | 3.5–6.3 | 1.000 |
| Endocrine | 72 | 1.9 | 1.5–2.3 | 1.8 | 1.3–2.3 | 2.1 | 1.2–3.1 | 1.000 |
| Haematopoietic | 53 | 1.4 | 1.0–1.7 | 1.4 | 1.0–1.8 | 1.3 | 0.5–2.1 | 1.000 |
| Hepatobiliary | 29 | 0.8 | 0.5–1.1 | 0.9 | 0.6–1.3 | 0.1 | 0.0–0.7 | 0.088 |
| Lymphatic | 26 | 0.7 | 0.5–1.0 | 0.6 | 0.4–1.0 | 0.9 | 0.4–1.8 | 1.000 |

P-values (Holm-adjusted) represent comparison between purebreds and crossbreds.
[a]Prev prevalence.
[b]95% CI 95% confidence interval.

**Table 7.** Prevalence of syndromic disorders related to pathophysiologic processes recorded in overall dogs, purebreds only and crossbreds only that attended primary veterinary practices in England.

| Pathophysiologic process | Overall | | | Purebred | | Crossbred | | |
|---|---|---|---|---|---|---|---|---|
| | No. | Prev^a% | 95% CI^b | Prev^a% | 95% CI^b | Prev^a% | 95% CI^b | P-value |
| Inflammation | 1,246 | 32.1 | 29.8–34.3 | 33.2 | 30.7–35.7 | 28.1 | 25.1–31.2 | **0.006** |
| Mass/swelling | 625 | 16.1 | 14.6–17.6 | 16.7 | 15.0–18.4 | 14.1 | 11.8–16.3 | 0.222 |
| Traumatic | 557 | 14.3 | 12.8–15.9 | 14.3 | 12.7–16.0 | 14.3 | 11.6–17.0 | 1.000 |
| Degenerative | 411 | 10.6 | 9.4–11.8 | 10.4 | 9.0–11.7 | 11.4 | 9.1–13.8 | 1.000 |
| Infectious | 388 | 10.0 | 9.0–11.0 | 10.3 | 9.1–11.4 | 9.0 | 6.9–11.2 | 1.000 |
| Neoplastic | 336 | 8.7 | 7.6–9.8 | 8.6 | 7.3–9.8 | 9.0 | 7.2–10.9 | 1.000 |
| Congenital/developmental | 332 | 8.6 | 7.4–9.7 | 8.9 | 7.6–10.2 | 7.3 | 5.6–9.2 | 0.870 |
| Nutritional | 320 | 8.2 | 7.1–9.4 | 8.9 | 7.5–10.2 | 5.9 | 4.3–7.5 | **0.014** |
| Behavioural | 262 | 6.8 | 5.9–7.6 | 6.5 | 5.5–7.4 | 7.9 | 6.0–9.8 | 1.000 |
| Hereditary | 232 | 6.0 | 5.1–6.9 | 6.2 | 5.1–7.3 | 5.3 | 3.5–7.0 | 1.000 |
| Parasitic | 221 | 5.7 | 5.0–6.4 | 5.5 | 4.6–6.3 | 6.7 | 5.0–8.4 | 1.000 |
| Iatrogenic | 150 | 3.9 | 3.3–4.5 | 3.7 | 3.1–4.4 | 4.4 | 2.9–5.9 | 1.000 |
| Foreign body | 109 | 2.8 | 2.3–3.3 | 2.8 | 2.3–3.4 | 2.8 | 1.6–3.9 | 1.000 |
| Death | 65 | 1.7 | 1.2–2.2 | 1.6 | 1.1–2.1 | 2.1 | 1.2–3.1 | 1.000 |
| Intoxicative | 49 | 1.3 | 1.0–1.7 | 1.3 | 1.0–1.8 | 1.1 | 0.6–2.1 | 1.000 |
| Haemostatic | 38 | 1.0 | 0.7–1.3 | 1.1 | 0.8–1.5 | 0.5 | 0.2–1.3 | 0.496 |
| Immune-mediated | 38 | 1.0 | 0.7–1.3 | 1.1 | 0.8–1.5 | 0.5 | 0.2–1.3 | 0.620 |
| Allergic | 35 | 0.9 | 0.7–1.3 | 0.9 | 0.6–1.3 | 0.9 | 0.4–1.8 | 1.000 |
| Thermoregulatory | 17 | 0.4 | 0.3–0.7 | 0.4 | 0.2–0.7 | 0.6 | 0.3–1.5 | 1.000 |
| Metabolic | 8 | 0.2 | 0.1–0.4 | 0.2 | 0.1–0.4 | 0.3 | 0.1–0.9 | 1.000 |
| Effusion | 1 | 0.0 | 0.0–0.2 | 0.0 | 0.0–0.2 | 0.0 | 0.0–0.5 | 1.000 |

P-values (Holm-adjusted) represent comparison between purebreds and crossbreds.
^aPrev prevalence.
^b95% CI 95% confidence interval.

affecting the integument and digestive systems suggests the importance of clinical emphasis on maintaining the health of these systems.

The current study identified inflammation (32.1%), mass/swelling (16.1%) and trauma (14.3%) as the most prevalent pathophysiologic processes affecting dogs. Similarly, a Swedish insurance study identified inflammation (5.4%), symptomatic (3.0%), trauma (2.7%) and neoplasia (2.1%) as the pathological processes with the highest risk of morbidity [83]. Although an essential adaptive response to injury, inflammation can behave both physiologically (restoring homeostasis) and pathologically (contributing to ongoing disease) [84]. The preponderance of inflammatory disorders affecting dogs identified by the current study suggests welfare gains from increased awareness by owners of judicious use of anti-inflammatory medications and also the value from ongoing research to better harness the healing aspects of inflammation while limiting detrimental effects [85].

The current study hypothesised that purebred dogs have higher prevalence of common disorders compared with crossbreds. This hypothesis was founded on reports and studies that concluded substantial detriment to purebred dog welfare from increasing inherited health problems induced by inbreeding and selection for extreme morphologies [15,16,20,21,22]. The study hypothesis was tested by comparing prevalence values between purebreds and crossbreds for each of the twenty most prevalent diagnosis-level and mid-level disorders and for all syndromic presentations. Purebreds showed significantly higher prevalence values for 13 of

the 84 (15.5%) disorders and syndromes evaluated. No instances were identified in which prevalence values were significantly higher in crossbred than in purebred dogs. These results provided moderate evidence for higher disorder prevalence in purebreds compared with crossbreds. However, additional analyses of severity and duration data for these disorders would enable a more comprehensive understanding of health disparities between the groups [23].

Failure to show overwhelming evidence for disorder disparity between purebred and crossbred dogs appears initially at odds with the large body of literature apparently to the contrary [20,21,22,86,87]. There are a number of possibilities for this dissonance. Breed-specific conformational disorders within purebreds may be under-reported or under-recognised by both veterinarians and owners because 'normal for breed' may have become confused with 'normal' [88]. A study of dogs clinically diagnosed with brachycephalic obstructive airway syndrome (BOAS) identified that 58% of owners reported these dogs not to have 'breathing problems' [82]. Purebred and crossbred dog categories comprise heterogeneous mosaics of size, shape and genetics. Merging this variation into single categories may have masked important effects related to specific conformational, physiological or behavioural features. Analyses of purebred or crossbred subgroups based on breed, behaviour or body attributes may better elucidate important health hazards, benefits and associations.

**Table 8.** Prevalence of syndromic diagnoses affecting body location recorded in crossbred dogs and popular breeds (number of dogs) from 3,884 randomly sampled dogs attending primary veterinary practices in England.

| Body Location | Prevalence percentage (95% confidence interval) | | | | | | | | P-Value |
|---|---|---|---|---|---|---|---|---|---|
| | Crossbred (797) | Labrador Retriever (339) | Staffordshire Bull Terrier (334) | Jack Russell Terrier (262) | Cocker Spaniel (133) | German Shepherd Dog (132) | Yorkshire Terrier (127) | Border Collie (104) | |
| Head/neck | 28.5 (24.9-32.0) | 28.6 (24.1-33.6) | 24.0 (19.7-28.8) | 30.5 (25.3-36.4) | 33.1 (25.7-41.5) | 22.7 (16.4-30.6) | 43.3 (35.0-52.0) | 35.6 (27.0-45.1) | **0.006** |
| Abdomen | 24.6 (21.5-27.7) | 32.4 (27.7-37.6) | 21.0 (16.9-25.6) | 21.0 (16.5-26.3) | 27.1 (20.2-35.2) | 25.8 (19.1-33.8) | 20.5 (14.4-28.3) | 30.8 (22.7-40.2) | **0.045** |
| Limb | 18.3 (15.7-20.9) | 20.4 (16.4-25.0) | 14.1 (10.7-18.2) | 20.2 (15.8-25.5) | 7.5 (4.1-13.3) | 13.6 (8.8-20.5) | 22.0 (15.7-30.0) | 16.3 (10.5-24.6) | **0.036** |
| Anus/perineum | 9.8 (7.6-12.0) | 6.2 (4.1-9.3) | 3.9 (2.3-6.5) | 9.9 (6.9-14.1) | 15.0 (10.0-22.1) | 9.1 (5.3-15.2) | 7.1 (3.8-12.9) | 3.8 (1.5-9.5) | **0.001** |
| Thorax | 8.7 (6.5-10.8) | 6.5 (4.3-9.6) | 6.0 (3.9-9.1) | 8.8 (5.9-12.8) | 6.0 (3.1-11.4) | 3.0 (1.2-7.5) | 13.4 (8.5-20.4) | 6.7 (3.3-13.2) | 0.294 |
| Vertebral column | 2.0 (1.0-3.0) | 1.5 (0.6-3.4) | 0.3 (0.1-1.7) | 1.1 (0.4-3.3) | 3.8 (1.6-8.5) | 1.5 (0.4-5.4) | 0.8 (0.1-4.3) | 2.9 (1.0-8.1) | 1.000 |
| Pelvis | 0.5 (0.2-1.3) | 0.6 (0.2-2.1) | 0.6 (0.2-2.2) | 0.0 (0.0-1.4) | 0.0 (0.0-2.8) | 0.0 (0.0-2.8) | 1.6 (0.4-5.6) | 1.0 (0.2-5.2) | 1.000 |
| Tail | 0.0 (0.0-0.5) | 2.4 (1.2-4.6) | 0.3 (0.1-1.7) | 0.0 (0.0-1.4) | 1.5 (0.4-5.3) | 0.0 (0.0-2.8) | 0.0 (0.0-2.9) | 1.0 (0.2-5.2) | **0.002** |

P-values (Holm-adjusted) represent comparison between breeds.

Purebred dogs comprise 75-80% of the overall UK dog population [3,28], suggesting that a high proportion of crossbreds are likely to be first or second filial offspring from purebred progenitors and could be reasonably expected to show conformational and polygenic disorder occurrence at the midpoint between the values for their parent breeds, with any additional health benefits in crossbreds resulting from hybrid vigour effects [89]. From this perspective, the less-than-overwhelming evidence provided by the current study for substantially lower prevalence values in crossbred compared with purebred dogs does not refute claims in the literature of rising prevalence values for inherited disorders within purebred dogs. Instead, this suggests that the overall disorder burden within crossbred dogs may reflect the overall disorder burden in purebreds at any point in time. For optimal understanding, disorder prevalence in purebreds should be quantified by analysing cohort health data to identify trends over time.

The most prevalent disorders identified in dogs within the current study were complex disorders that have multiple interacting environmental and genetic casual factors [90]: otitis externa [91], periodontal disease [92], anal sac disorders [93], nail disorders [94,95], degenerative joint disease [96], diarrhoea [97,98], obesity [99], traumatic injury [100], conjunctivitis [101], vomiting [101,102] and heart murmur [103,104]. It may be useful for canine health research to move away from viewing individual disorders as necessarily either inherited or non-inherited [105] and towards an acknowledgement of relevant roles for both genetic and environmental components in the majority of canine disorders [106,107,108]. This acceptance will improve decision-making on effective disease-control and breeding programs [109]. Application of estimated breeding values (EBVs) developed from summative health information derived from a range of sources, including health schemes and veterinary primary-care data, could contribute integrally to novel disorder-control programs [14,110,111].

A large body of literature supports the existence of disorder predispositions affecting most dog breeds [15,16,112]. Despite inclusion of just seven breeds in the current analysis, breed associations were identified for 33.3% (28/84) of the disorders and syndromes evaluated (diagnosis-level disorders 20% (5/20), mid-level disorders 40% (8/20) and syndromic terms 34% (15/44)). The high-risk breeds differed considerably between the disorders in the current study, suggesting that rational health control measures should focus on highly-predisposed disorders within at-risk breeds. Future breed-specific studies are recommended to report more precise prevalence estimates and for a wider range of breeds. Early studies could focus on the fourteen high-profile breeds identified by the KC as having higher health risks, mainly due to conformational problems [113].

There were some limitations to the current study. The practices participating in the study formed a single veterinary group that extended across central and south-east England and may not be representative of the overall veterinary practice structure in England. Case definitions and diagnosis recording relied heavily on the clinical acumen and note-making of attending practitioners. The researchers made no attempts to second-guess underlying disorders in cases with presenting signs (e.g. vomiting) recorded *in lieu* of formal diagnoses. Inclusion of umbrella terms such as *road traffic accident* without additional inclusion of the individual specific injuries sustained within the primary event may have reduced the apparent prevalence of fractures and lacerations but avoided multiple counting of disorder events along axes of diagnostic precision. The analyses based on popular breeds were exploratory in nature and should be validated within larger confirmatory

**Table 9.** Prevalence of syndromic diagnoses affecting organ system recorded in crossbred dogs and popular breeds (number of dogs) from 3,884 randomly sampled dogs attending primary veterinary practices in England.

| Organ system | Prevalence percentage (95% confidence interval) | | | | | | | | P-Value |
|---|---|---|---|---|---|---|---|---|---|
| | Crossbred (797) | Labrador Retriever (339) | Staffordshire Bull Terrier (334) | Jack Russell Terrier (262) | Cocker Spaniel (133) | German Shepherd Dog (132) | Yorkshire Terrier (127) | Border Collie (104) | |
| Integument | 31.4 (28.0–34.7) | 39.2 (34.2–44.5) | 36.2 (31.3–41.5) | 34.0 (28.5–39.9) | 33.8 (26.3–42.2) | 34.8 (27.3–43.3) | 42.5 (34.3–51.2) | 29.8 (21.9–39.2) | 0.816 |
| Digestive | 30.0 (26.6–33.3) | 29.8 (25.2–34.9) | 19.2 (15.3–23.7) | 28.6 (23.5–34.4) | 36.1 (28.4–44.5) | 27.3 (20.4–35.4) | 44.1 (35.8–52.8) | 26.9 (19.3–36.2) | **0.002** |
| Musculoskeletal | 17.3 (14.8–19.8) | 19.2 (15.3–23.7) | 9.6 (6.9–13.2) | 9.5 (6.5–13.7) | 6.8 (3.6–12.4) | 18.9 (13.2–26.5) | 8.7 (4.9–14.8) | 22.1 (15.2–31.0) | **0.005** |
| Connective/Soft tissue | 12.3 (10.2–14.4) | 16.2 (12.7–20.5) | 9.9 (7.1–13.6) | 9.5 (6.5–13.7) | 14.3 (9.3–21.2) | 5.3 (2.6–10.5) | 9.4 (5.5–15.8) | 17.3 (11.2–25.7) | 0.060 |
| Ocular | 9.2 (7.2–11.1) | 9.1 (6.5–12.7) | 8.7 (6.1–12.2) | 8.8 (5.9–12.8) | 12.8 (8.1–19.5) | 2.3 (0.8–6.5) | 13.4 (8.5–20.4) | 14.4 (8.9–22.4) | 0.203 |
| Auditory | 7.4 (5.5–9.3) | 12.4 (9.3–16.3) | 11.1 (8.1–14.9) | 8.4 (5.6–12.4) | 10.5 (6.4–16.9) | 11.4 (7.0–17.9) | 7.9 (4.3–13.9) | 5.8 (2.7–12.0) | 1.000 |
| Nervous | 7.9 (6.2–9.6) | 8.3 (5.8–11.7) | 3.0 (1.6–5.4) | 5.7 (3.5–9.2) | 9.0 (5.2–15.1) | 12.9 (8.2–19.7) | 3.1 (1.2–7.8) | 15.4 (9.7–23.5) | **0.003** |
| Respiratory | 7.2 (5.2–9.1) | 8.0 (5.5–11.3) | 6.9 (4.6–10.1) | 7.3 (4.7–11.0) | 3.0 (1.2–7.5) | 3.8 (1.6–8.6) | 8.7 (4.9–14.8) | 3.8 (1.5–9.5) | 1.000 |
| Cardiovascular | 5.3 (3.5–7.1) | 1.5 (0.6–3.4) | 3.3 (1.8–5.8) | 7.6 (5.0–11.5) | 5.3 (2.6–10.5) | 1.5 (0.4–5.4) | 11.0 (6.7–17.7) | 6.7 (3.3–13.2) | **0.001** |
| Urinary | 5.8 (4.1–7.5) | 5.3 (3.4–8.2) | 3.6 (2.1–6.2) | 4.6 (2.6–7.8) | 6.8 (3.6–12.4) | 4.5 (2.1–9.6) | 6.3 (3.2–11.9) | 6.7 (3.3–13.2) | 1.000 |
| Reproductive | 4.9 (3.5–6.3) | 2.7 (1.4–5.0) | 6.0 (3.9–9.1) | 5.0 (2.9–8.3) | 5.3 (2.6–10.5) | 2.3 (0.8–6.5) | 3.9 (1.7–8.9) | 1.0 (0.2–5.2) | 1.000 |
| Endocrine | 2.1 (1.2–3.1) | 1.5 (0.6–3.4) | 1.2 (0.5–3.0) | 2.3 (1.1–4.9) | 0.0 (0.0–2.8) | 0.8 (0.1–4.2) | 2.4 (0.8–6.7) | 1.9 (0.5–6.7) | 1.000 |
| Haematopoietic | 1.3 (0.7–2.3) | 2.1 (1.0–4.2) | 1.2 (0.5–3.0) | 0.4 (0.1–2.1) | 1.5 (0.4–5.3) | 1.5 (0.4–5.4) | 0.0 (0.0–2.9) | 0.0 (0.0–3.6) | 1.000 |
| Hepatobiliary | 0.1 (0.0–0.7) | 1.8 (0.8–3.8) | 0.0 (0.0–1.1) | 0.4 (0.1–2.1) | 0.0 (0.0–2.8) | 0.0 (0.0–2.8) | 0.0 (0.0–2.9) | 3.8 (1.5–9.5) | **0.004** |
| Lymphatic | 0.9 (0.4–1.8) | 0.6 (0.2–2.1) | 0.6 (0.2–2.2) | 0.4 (0.1–2.1) | 0.8 (0.1–4.1) | 0.0 (0.0–2.8) | 0.0 (0.0–2.9) | 1.0 (0.2–5.2) | 1.000 |

P-values (Holm-adjusted) represent comparison between breeds.

**Table 10.** Prevalence of syndromic diagnoses relating to pathophysiologic processes recorded in crossbred and popular breeds (number of dogs) attending primary veterinary practices in England.

| Pathophysiologic process | Prevalence percentage (95% confidence interval) | | | | | | | | P-Value |
|---|---|---|---|---|---|---|---|---|---|
| | Crossbred (797) | Labrador Retriever (339) | Staffordshire Bull Terrier (334) | Jack Russell Terrier (262) | Cocker Spaniel (133) | German Shepherd Dog (132) | Yorkshire Terrier (127) | Border Collie (104) | |
| Inflammation | 28.1 (25.1–31.2) | 37.8 (32.8–43.0) | 29.6 (25.0–34.7) | 25.2 (20.3–30.8) | 27.8 (20.9–36.0) | 32.6 (25.2–41.0) | 35.4 (27.7–44.1) | 27.9 (20.2–37.2) | 0.120 |
| Mass/swelling | 14.1 (11.8–16.3) | 23.3 (19.1–28.1) | 14.1 (10.7–18.2) | 11.1 (7.8–15.4) | 20.3 (14.3–27.9) | 12.1 (7.6–18.8) | 14.2 (9.2–21.3) | 24.0 (16.8–33.1) | **0.004** |
| Traumatic | 14.3 (11.6–17.0) | 18.3 (14.5–22.8) | 14.1 (10.7–18.2) | 14.5 (10.8–19.3) | 16.5 (11.2–23.8) | 11.4 (7.0–17.9) | 7.1 (3.8–12.9) | 15.4 (9.7–23.5) | 1.000 |
| Degenerative | 11.4 (9.1–13.8) | 15.6 (12.2–19.9) | 7.5 (5.1–10.8) | 7.6 (5.0–11.5) | 4.5 (2.1–9.5) | 9.8 (5.8–16.1) | 6.3 (3.2–11.9) | 18.3 (12.0–26.8) | **0.001** |
| Infectious | 9.0 (6.9–11.2) | 13.9 (10.6–17.9) | 7.8 (5.4–11.2) | 8.0 (5.3–11.9) | 9.0 (5.2–15.1) | 10.6 (6.4–17.0) | 7.9 (4.3–13.9) | 13.5 (8.2–21.3) | 0.990 |
| Neoplastic | 9.0 (7.2–10.9) | 15.3 (11.9–19.6) | 6.3 (4.1–9.4) | 4.6 (2.6–7.8) | 12.8 (8.1–19.5) | 2.3 (0.8–6.5) | 3.9 (1.7–8.9) | 9.6 (5.3–16.8) | **0.003** |
| Congenital | 7.3 (5.6–9.2) | 5.0 (3.2–7.9) | 4.8 (3.0–7.6) | 6.5 (4.1–10.1) | 7.5 (4.1–13.3) | 6.1 (3.1–11.5) | 11.0 (6.7–17.7) | 5.8 (2.7–12) | 1.000 |
| Nutritional | 5.9 (4.3–7.5) | 16.5 (12.9–20.8) | 7.5 (5.1–10.8) | 6.9 (4.4–10.6) | 9.8 (5.8–16.0) | 3.8 (1.6–8.6) | 2.4 (0.8–6.7) | 9.6 (5.3–16.8) | **0.002** |
| Behavioural | 7.9 (6.0–9.8) | 5.0 (3.2–7.9) | 6.6 (4.4–9.8) | 8.8 (5.9–12.8) | 6.8 (3.6–12.4) | 13.6 (8.8–20.5) | 3.9 (1.7–8.9) | 8.7 (4.6–15.6) | 0.000 |
| Hereditary | 3.3 (3.5–7.0) | 4.4 (2.7–7.2) | 3.3 (1.8–5.8) | 3.4 (1.8–6.4) | 3.0 (1.2–7.5) | 7.6 (4.2–13.4) | 11.8 (7.3–18.6) | 2.9 (1.0–8.1) | **0.025** |
| Parasitic | 6.7 (5.0–8.4) | 6.2 (4.1–9.3) | 5.7 (3.7–8.7) | 5.0 (2.9–8.3) | 9.8 (5.8–16.0) | 3.0 (1.2–7.5) | 5.5 (2.7–10.9) | 2.9 (1.0–8.1) | 1.000 |
| Iatrogenic | 4.4 (2.9–5.9) | 4.4 (2.7–7.2) | 3.0 (1.6–5.4) | 4.2 (2.4–7.4) | 3.8 (1.6–8.5) | 4.5 (2.1–9.6) | 4.7 (2.2–9.9) | 4.8 (2.1–10.8) | 1.000 |
| Foreign body | 2.8 (1.6–3.9) | 3.2 (1.8–5.7) | 1.2 (0.5–3.0) | 2.7 (1.3–5.4) | 2.3 (0.8–6.4) | 2.3 (0.8–6.5) | 0.0 (0.0–2.9) | 3.8 (1.5–9.5) | 1.000 |
| Death | 2.1 (1.2–3.1) | 1.8 (0.8–3.8) | 1.5 (0.6–3.5) | 0.8 (0.2–2.7) | 0.8 (0.1–4.1) | 2.3 (0.8–6.5) | 3.1 (1.2–7.8) | 4.8 (2.1–10.8) | 1.000 |
| Intoxicative | 1.1 (0.6–2.1) | 1.5 (0.6–3.4) | 0.9 (0.3–2.6) | 1.5 (0.6–3.9) | 0.8 (0.1–4.1) | 0.0 (0.0–2.8) | 1.6 (0.4–5.6) | 1.0 (0.2–5.2) | 1.000 |
| Haemostatic | 0.5 (0.2–1.3) | 1.5 (0.6–3.4) | 1.8 (0.8–3.9) | 1.1 (0.4–3.3) | 0.0 (0.0–2.8) | 0.8 (0.1–4.2) | 0.0 (0.0–2.9) | 2.9 (1.0–8.1) | 1.000 |
| Immune-mediated | 0.5 (0.2–1.3) | 0.0 (0.0–1.1) | 0.3 (0.1–1.7) | 0.8 (0.2–2.7) | 2.3 (0.8–6.4) | 0.0 (0.0–2.8) | 2.4 (0.8–6.7) | 1.0 (0.2–5.2) | 0.189 |
| Allergic | 0.9 (0.4–1.8) | 2.1 (1.0–4.2) | 0.6 (0.2–2.2) | 0.8 (0.2–2.7) | 0.8 (0.1–4.1) | 0.8 (0.1–4.2) | 1.6 (0.4–5.6) | 0.0 (0.0–3.6) | 1.000 |
| Thermoregulatory | 0.6 (0.3–1.5) | 0.0 (0.0–1.1) | 0.6 (0.2–2.2) | 0.8 (0.2–2.7) | 0.8 (0.1–4.1) | 0.0 (0.0–2.8) | 1.6 (0.4–5.6) | 1.0 (0.2–5.2) | 1.000 |
| Metabolic | 0.3 (0.1–0.9) | 0.0 (0.0–1.1) | 0.0 (0.0–1.1) | 0.0 (0.0–1.4) | 0.8 (0.1–4.1) | 0.0 (0.0–2.8) | 0.0 (0.0–2.9) | 0.0 (0.0–3.6) | 1.000 |
| Effusion | 0.0 (0.0–0.5) | 0.0 (0.0–1.1) | 0.0 (0.0–1.1) | 0.0 (0.0–1.4) | 0.0 (0.0–2.8) | 0.0 (0.0–2.8) | 0.0 (0.0–2.9) | 0.0 (0.0–3.6) | 1.000 |

P–values (Holm–adjusted) represent comparison between breeds.

studies [114,115]. Holm adjustments to P-values were used to constrain the number of false-positive findings resulting from interpretation of multiple comparisons [38,115,116]. The current study reported prevalence values but effective welfare prioritisation would additionally benefit from the generation of accurate data on disorder severity and duration [117].

## Conclusion

This study describes the most frequently recorded disorders in dogs in England and provides a prevalence baseline against which to measure progress in canine health. The most prevalent disorders recorded in dogs attending primary-care veterinary practices in England were otitis externa, periodontal disease and anal sac impaction, and the most prevalent disorder groups were enteropathic, dermatological and musculoskeletal. The head-and-neck was the body location most frequently affected by the disorders recorded, the integument was the most prevalent organ system affected and inflammation was the most prevalent pathophysiologic process. The study identified some evidence that purebred dogs had higher disorder prevalence compared with crossbred dogs. Substantial variation was shown across breeds in their prevalence of common disorders. These results suggest that breeding reforms should target commonly diagnosed complex disorders that are amenable to genetic improvement on a breed-by-breed basis for the greatest population impact. The prevalence information provided by this study fills a crucial data gap. Future studies of disorder severity and duration would augment the current results and contribute to increasingly effective strategies to improve dog welfare based on disorder prioritisation.

## Acknowledgments

We thank Peter Dron (RVC) for VetCompass database development and Noel Kennedy (RVC) for software and programming development. We are especially grateful to the Medivet Veterinary Partnership and the other UK practices and clients who are participating in VetCompass.

## Author Contributions

Conceived and designed the experiments: DON DBC PDM PCT DCB. Performed the experiments: DON DBC PDM PCT DCB. Analyzed the data: DON DBC PDM PCT DCB. Contributed reagents/materials/analysis tools: DON DBC PDM PCT DCB. Wrote the paper: DON DBC PDM PCT DCB.

## References

1. Murray JK, Browne WJ, Roberts MA, Whitmarsh A, Gruffydd-Jones TJ (2010) Number and ownership profiles of cats and dogs in the UK. Veterinary Record 166: 163–168.
2. Asher L, Buckland E, Phylactopoulos CI, Whiting M, Abeyesinghe S, et al. (2011) Estimation of the number and demographics of companion dogs in the UK. BMC Veterinary Research 7: 74.
3. PFMA (2012) The Pet Food Manufacturers' Association 'Statistics'. In: Association TPFM, editor: The Pet Food Manufacturers' Association.
4. Ownby DR, Johnson C, Peterson EL (2002) Exposure to dogs and cats in the first year of life and risk of allergic sensitization at 6 to 7 years of age. Journal of the American Medical Association 288: 963–972.
5. Friedmann E, Son H (2009) The human–companion animal bond: how humans benefit. Veterinary Clinics of North America: Small Animal Practice 39: 293–326.
6. Virués-Ortega J, Buela-Casal G (2006) Psychophysiological effects of human-animal interaction: theoretical issues and long-term interaction effects. Journal of Nervous and Mental Disease 194: 52–57.
7. Walsh F (2009) Human-animal bonds I: the relational significance of companion animals. Family Process 48: 462–480.
8. McGreevy PD, Nicholas FW (1999) Some practical solutions to welfare problems in dog breeding. Animal Welfare 8: 329–341.
9. Rooney NJ (2009) The welfare of pedigree dogs: cause for concern. Journal of Veterinary Behavior: Clinical Applications and Research 4: 180–186.
10. Wayne RK, Leonard JA, Vila C (2006) Genetic analysis of dog domestication. In: Zeder MA, editor. Documenting domestication: new genetic and archaeological paradigms. Berkeley, California: University of California Press. pp. 279–293.
11. Leroy G (2011) Genetic diversity, inbreeding and breeding practices in dogs: results from pedigree analyses. The Veterinary Journal 189: 177–182.
12. McGreevy PD (2007) Breeding for quality of life. Animal Welfare 16: 125–128.
13. Calboli FC, Sampson J, Fretwell N, Balding DJ (2008) Population structure and inbreeding from pedigree analysis of purebred dogs. Genetics 179: 593–601.
14. Lewis TW (2010) Optimisation of breeding strategies to reduce the prevalence of inherited disease in pedigree dogs. Animal Welfare 19: 93–98.
15. Asher L, Diesel G, Summers JF, McGreevy PD, Collins LM (2009) Inherited defects in pedigree dogs. Part 1: disorders related to breed standards. The Veterinary Journal 182: 402–411.
16. Summers JF, Diesel G, Asher L, McGreevy PD, Collins LM (2010) Inherited defects in pedigree dogs. Part 2: Disorders that are not related to breed standards. The Veterinary Journal 183: 39–45.
17. Mellersh CS, Ostrander EA (1997) The canine genome. In: Dodds WJ, James EW, editors. Advances in Veterinary Medicine: Academic Press. pp. 191–216.
18. Starkey MP, Scase TJ, Mellersh CS, Murphy S (2005) Dogs really are man's best friend: canine genomics has applications in veterinary and human medicine! Briefings in Functional Genomics & Proteomics 4: 112–128.
19. BBC (2008) Pedigree Dogs Exposed.
20. Bateson P (2010) Independent inquiry into dog breeding. Cambridge: University of Cambridge.
21. Rooney N, Sargan D (2008) Pedigree dog breeding in the UK: a major welfare concern? Horsham, West Sussex: RSPCA.
22. APGAW (2009) A healthier future for pedigree dogs. London: The Associate Parliamentary Group for Animal Welfare.
23. Collins LM, Asher L, Summers J, McGreevy P (2011) Getting priorities straight: risk assessment and decision-making in the improvement of inherited disorders in pedigree dogs. The Veterinary Journal 189: 147–154.
24. Collins LM, Asher L, Summers JF, Diesel G, McGreevy PD (2010) Welfare epidemiology as a tool to assess the welfare impact of inherited defects on the pedigree dog population. Animal Welfare 19: 67–75.
25. Fleming JM, Creevy KE, Promislow DEL (2011) Mortality in North American dogs from 1984 to 2004: an investigation into age-, size-, and breed-related causes of death. Journal of Veterinary Internal Medicine 25: 187–198.
26. Adams VJ, Evans KM, Sampson J, Wood JLN (2010) Methods and mortality results of a health survey of purebred dogs in the UK. Journal of Small Animal Practice 51: 512–524.
27. Egenvall A, Nødtvedt A, Penell J, Gunnarsson L, Bonnett BN (2009) Insurance data for research in companion animals: benefits and limitations. Acta Veterinaria Scandinavica 51: 42.
28. VetCompass (2013) VetCompass: Health surveillance for UK companion animals. http://wwwrvcacuk/VetCompass. London: RVC Electronic Media Unit.
29. Medivet (2014) Medivet: the veterinary partnership. Medivet Partnership LLP.
30. The VeNom Coding Group (2013) VeNom Veterinary Nomenclature. In: Group TVC, editor. http://wwwvenomcodingorg: VeNom Coding Group.
31. Kearsley-Fleet L, O'Neill DG, Volk HA, Church DB, Brodbelt DC (2013) Prevalence and risk factors for canine epilepsy of unknown origin in the UK. Veterinary Record 172: 338.
32. Epi Info 7 CDC (2012) Centers for Disease Control and Prevention (US): Introducing Epi Info 7. http://wwwncdcgov/epiinfo/7. Atlanta, Georgia: CDC.
33. Willard MD, Tvedten H (2004) Small animal clinical diagnosis by laboratory methods. St. Louis, Miss.: Saunders.
34. Sleator DD, Endre Tarjan R (1983) A data structure for dynamic trees. Journal of Computer and System Sciences 26: 362–391.
35. Irion DN, Schaffer AL, Famula TR, Eggleston ML, Hughes SS, et al. (2003) Analysis of genetic variation in 28 dog breed populations with 100 microsatellite markers. Journal of Heredity 94: 81–87.
36. The Kennel Club (2012) Kennel Club's Breed Information Centre. In: Club TK, editor. http://wwwthe-kennel-cluborguk/services/public/breed/Defaultaspx. London: The Kennel Club.
37. McMillan FD (2001) Rethinking euthanasia: death as an unintentional outcome. Journal of the American Veterinary Medical Association 219: 1204–1206.
38. Aickin M, Gensler H (1996) Adjusting for multiple testing when reporting research results: the Bonferroni vs Holm methods. American Journal of Public Health 86: 726–728.
39. Kirkwood BR, Sterne JAC (2003) Essential Medical Statistics. Oxford: Blackwell Science.
40. Agresti A, Coull BA (1998) Approximate is better than "exact" for interval estimation of binomial proportions. The American Statistician 52: 119–126.
41. Hein HE (1963) Abnormalities and defects in pedigree dogs-II. Hereditary aspects of hip dysplasia. Journal of Small Animal Practice 4: 457–462.
42. Hodgman SFJ (1963) Abnormalities and defects in pedigree dogs-I. An investigation into the existence of abnormalities in pedigree dogs in the British Isles. Journal of Small Animal Practice 4: 447–456.

43. Knight GC (1963) Abnormalities and defects in pedigree dogs–III. Tibio-femoral joint deformity and patella luxation. Journal of Small Animal Practice 4: 463-464.

44. Willis MB (1963) Abnormalities and defects in pedigree dogs—V. Cryptorchidism. Journal of Small Animal Practice 4: 469–474.

45. BVA/KC (2013) Hip Dysplasia Scheme. In: British Veterinary Association/ Kennel Club, editor. London: British Veterinary Association,.

46. BVA/KC (2013) Chiari Malformation/Syringomyelia Scheme (CM/SM Scheme). In: Club BVAK, editor. London: British Veterinary Association.

47. BVA/KC (2013) Elbow Scheme. London: British Veterinary Association.

48. BVA/KC/ISS (2013) Eye Scheme. In: Society BVAKCIS, editor. Loondon: British Veterinary Association,.

49. KC (2013) DNA Screening Schemes and Results. In: The Kennel Club, editor. London: The Kennel Club,.

50. Indrebø A (2007) Animal welfare in modern dog breeding. Acta Veterinaria Scandinavica 50 Supplement S6.

51. Froom P, Froom J (1992) Selection bias in using data from one population to another: common pitfalls in the interpretation of medical literature. Theoretical Medicine 13: 255–259.

52. Bartlett PC, Van Buren JW, Neterer M, Zhou C (2010) Disease surveillance and referral bias in the veterinary medical database. Preventive Veterinary Medicine 94: 264–271.

53. Soll-Johanning H, Hannerz H, Tüchsen F (2004) Referral bias in hospital register studies of geographical and industrial differences in health. Danish Medical Bulletin 51: 207–210.

54. KC (2013) The Kennel Club. London: The Kennel Club,.

55. Platt S, Freeman J, di Stefani A, Wieczorek L, Henley W (2006) Prevalence of unilateral and bilateral deafness in Border Collies and association with phenotype. Journal of Veterinary Internal Medicine 20: 1355–1362.

56. Powers MY, Karbe GT, Gregor TP, McKelvie P, Culp WTN, et al. (2010) Evaluation of the relationship between Orthopedic Foundation for Animals' hip joint scores and PennHIP distraction index values in dogs. Journal of the American Veterinary Medical Association 237: 532–541.

57. Slater MR, Scarlet JM, Donoghue S, Erb HN (1992) The repeatability and validity of a telephone questionnaire on diet and exercise in dogs. Preventive Veterinary Medicine 13: 77–91.

58. Pearce N, Checkoway H, Kriebel D (2007) Bias in occupational epidemiology studies. Occupational and Environmental Medicine 64: 562–568.

59. Gobar GM (1998) Program for surveillance of causes of death of dogs, using the Internet to survey small animal veterinarians. Journal of the American Veterinary Medical Association 213: 251–256.

60. Hudson JI, Pope HG, Glynn RJ (2005) The cross-sectional cohort study: an underutilized design. Epidemiology (Cambridge, Mass) 16: 355–359.

61. Dohoo I, Martin W, Stryhn H (2009) Veterinary Epidemiologic Research. Charlottetown, Canada: VER Inc.

62. Aragon CL, Budsberg SC (2005) Applications of evidence-based medicine: cranial cruciate ligament injury repair in the dog. Veterinary Surgery 34: 93–98.

63. John U, Rumpf H-J, Hapke U (1999) Estimating prevalence of alcohol abuse and dependence in one general hospital: an approach to reduce sample selection bias. Alcohol and Alcoholism 34: 786-794.

64. Chodick G, Freedman MD, Kwok RK, Fears TR, Linet MS, et al. (2007) Agreement between contemporaneously recorded and subsequently recalled time spent outdoors: implications for environmental exposure studies. Annals of Epidemiology 17: 106–111.

65. Edney ATB (1997) An observational study of presentation patterns in companion animal veterinary practices in England. London: University of London. 290 p.

66. Lund EM (1997) Development and evaluation of a model for diagnostic surveillance in companion animal practice. St Paul: University of Minnesota.

67. Glickman L, Glickman N (2012) The National Companion Animal Surveillance System NCASP. Purdue University.

68. Brady S, Norris JM, Kelman M, Ward MP (2012) Canine parvovirus in Australia: the role of socio-economic factors in disease clusters. The Veterinary Journal 193: 522–528.

69. Egenvall A, Bonnett BN, Olson P, Hedhammar Å (1998) Validation of computerized Swedish dog and cat insurance data against veterinary practice records. Preventive Veterinary Medicine 36: 51–65.

70. Lund EM, Armstrong PJ, Kirk CA, Kolar LM, Klausner JS (1999) Health status and population characteristics of dogs and cats examined at private veterinary practices in the United States. Journal of the American Veterinary Medical Association 214: 1336–1341.

71. Rust MK (2005) Advances in the control of Ctenocephalides felis (cat flea) on cats and dogs. Trends in Parasitology 21: 232–236.

72. NOAH (2013) Facts and Figures About the UK Animal Medicines Industry. In: National Office of Animal Health, editor: NOAH,.

73. Royston P, Altman DG, Sauerbrei W (2006) Dichotomizing continuous predictors in multiple regression: a bad idea. Statistics in Medicine 25: 127–141.

74. Mandl KD, Overhage JM, Wagner MM, Lober WB, Sebastiani P, et al. (2004) Implementing syndromic surveillance: a practical guide informed by the early experience. Journal of the American Medical Informatics Association 11: 141–150.

75. Dank G, Segev G, Moshe D, Kent MS (2012) Follow-up study comparing necropsy rates and discrepancies between clinical and pathologic diagnoses at a veterinary teaching hospital: 2009 versus 1989 and 1999. Journal of Small Animal Practice 53: 679–683.

76. Lober WB, Thomas Karras B, Wagner MM, Marc Overhage J, Davidson AJ, et al. (2002) Roundtable on bioterrorism detection: information system–based surveillance. Journal of the American Medical Informatics Association 9: 105–115.

77. Egenvall A, Hedhammar A, Bonnett BN, Olson P (2000) Gender, age and breed pattern of diagnoses for veterinary care in insured dogs in Sweden during 1996. Veterinary Record 146: 551–557.

78. Vilson Å, Bonnett B, Hansson-Hamlin H, Hedhammar Å (2013) Disease patterns in 32,486 insured German Shepherd Dogs in Sweden: 1995–2006. Veterinary Record 173: 116.

79. Bonnett BN, Egenvall A, Hedhammar Å, Olson P (2005) Mortality in over 350,000 insured Swedish dogs from 1995–2000: I. breed-, gender-, age- and cause-specific rates. Acta Veterinaria Scandinavica 46: 105–120.

80. Stone AB, Hautala JA (2008) Meeting Report: Panel on the potential utility and strategies for design and implementation of a National Companion Animal Infectious Disease Surveillance System. Zoonoses and Public Health 55: 378–384.

81. Neff MW, Rine J (2006) A fetching model organism. Cell 124: 229–231.

82. Packer RMA, Hendricks A, Burn CC (2012) Do dog owners perceive the clinical signs related to conformational inherited disorders as 'normal' for the breed? A potential constraint to improving canine welfare. Animal Welfare 21: 81–93.

83. Egenvall A, Bonnett BN, Olson P, Hedhammar Å (2000) Gender, age, breed and distribution of morbidity and mortality in insured dogs in Sweden during 1995 and 1996. Veterinary Record 146: 519–525.

84. Medzhitov R (2010) Inflammation 2010: new adventures of an old flame. Cell 140: 771–776.

85. Mountziaris PM, Spicer PP, Kasper FK, Mikos AG (2011) Harnessing and modulating inflammation in strategies for bone regeneration. Tissue Engineering Part B, Reviews 17: 393–402.

86. Rooney NJ, Sargan DR (2010) Welfare concerns associated with pedigree dog breeding in the UK. Animal Welfare 19: 133–140.

87. Crispin S (2011) Tackling the welfare issues of dog breeding. Veterinary Record 168: 53.

88. Anon (2009) Balancing pedigree dog breed standards and animal welfare - is it possible? Veterinary Record 164: 481–482.

89. Bell J. The clinical truths about pure breeds, mixed breeds, and designer breeds; 2012 Feb 19–23; Las Vegas. 22–23.

90. Page GP, George V, Go RC, Page PZ, Allison DB (2003) "Are we there yet?": Deciding when one has demonstrated specific genetic causation in complex diseases and quantitative traits. The American Journal of Human Genetics 73: 711–719.

91. Marsella R, Girolomoni G (2009) Canine models of atopic dermatitis: a useful tool with untapped potential. The Journal of Investigative Dermatology 129: 2351–2357.

92. Albuquerque C, Morinha F, Requicha J, Martins T, Dias I, et al. (2012) Canine periodontitis: the dog as an important model for periodontal studies. The Veterinary Journal 191: 299–305.

93. Scott DW, Miller WH, Griffin CE, Muller GH (2001) Muller & Kirk's Small Animal Dermatology. Philadelphia: Saunders.

94. Neuber A (2009) Nail diseases in dogs. Companion Animal 14: 56–62.

95. Smith FJD (2003) The molecular genetics of keratin disorders. American Journal of Clinical Dermatology 4: 347–364.

96. Lewis T, Blott S, Woolliams J (2013) Comparative analyses of genetic trends and prospects for selection against hip and elbow dysplasia in 15 UK dog breeds. BMC Genetics 14: 16.

97. German AJ, Hall EJ, Day MJ (2003) Chronic intestinal inflammation and intestinal disease in dogs. Journal of Veterinary Internal Medicine 17: 8–20.

98. Kathrani A, Werling D, Allenspach K (2011) Canine breeds at high risk of developing inflammatory bowel disease in the south-eastern UK. Veterinary Record 169: 635.

99. German AJ (2006) The growing problem of obesity in dogs and cats. The Journal of Nutrition 136: 1940S–1946S.

100. Houlton JE (2008) A survey of gundog lameness and injuries in Great Britain in the shooting seasons 2005/2006 and 2006/2007. Veterinary and comparative Orthopaedics and Traumatology 21: 231–237.

101. Lourenço-Martins AM, Delgado E, Neto I, Peleteiro MC, Morais-Almeida M, et al. (2011) Allergic conjunctivitis and conjunctival provocation tests in atopic dogs. Veterinary Ophthalmology 14: 248–256.

102. Batt RM, Hall EJ (1989) Chronic enteropathies in the dog. Journal of Small Animal Practice 30: 3–12.

103. Pedersen HD, Häggström J (2000) Mitral valve prolapse in the dog: a model of mitral valve prolapse in man. Cardiovascular Research 47: 234–243.

104. Lewis T (2011) Heritability of premature mitral valve disease in Cavalier King Charles Spaniels. The Veterinary Journal 188: 73.

105. Bellumori TP, Famula TR, Bannasch DL, Belanger JM, Oberbauer AM (2013) Prevalence of inherited disorders among mixed-breed and purebred dogs: 27,254 cases (1995–2010). Journal of the American Veterinary Medical Association 242: 1549–1555.

106. Rand JS, Fleeman LM, Farrow HA, Appleton DJ, Lederer R (2004) Canine and feline diabetes mellitus: nature or nurture? The Journal of Nutrition 134: 2072S–2080S.

107. Wood JLN (2002) Heritability and epidemiology of canine hip-dysplasia score and its components in Labrador retrievers in the United Kingdom. Preventive Veterinary Medicine 55: 95–108.

108. Hillier A, Griffin CE (2001) The ACVD task force on canine atopic dermatitis (I): incidence and prevalence. Veterinary Immunology and Immunopathology 81: 147–151.

109. Mellersh C (2012) DNA testing and domestic dogs. Mammalian Genome 23: 109–123.

110. Lewis TW (2010) Genetic evaluation of hip score in UK Labrador Retrievers. PLoS One 5.

111. Wilson B, Nicholas FW, Thomson PC (2011) Selection against canine hip dysplasia: success or failure? The Veterinary Journal 189: 160–168.

112. Gough A, Thomas A (2010) Breed Predispositions to Disease in Dogs and Cats. Chicester, West Sussex: Wiley-Blackwell.

113. Anon. (2013) High profile best of breed winners pass vet checks at Crufts. Veterinary Record 172: 277.

114. Bender R, Lange S (2001) Adjusting for multiple testing - when and how? Journal of Clinical Epidemiology 54: 343–349.

115. Greenland S (2008) Multiple comparisons and association selection in general epidemiology. International Journal of Epidemiology 37: 430–434.

116. Feise R (2002) Do multiple outcome measures require p-value adjustment? BMC Medical Research Methodology 2: 8.

117. CAWC (2006) Breeding and welfare in companion animals: welfare aspects of modifications, through selective breeding or biotechnological methods, to the form, function, or behaviour of companion animals. Sidmouth, Devon: Companion Animal Welfare Council.

# 15

# Linking Bovine Tuberculosis on Cattle Farms to White-Tailed Deer and Environmental Variables Using Bayesian Hierarchical Analysis

**W. David Walter[1]\*, Rick Smith[2], Mike Vanderklok[2], Kurt C. VerCauteren[3]**

**1** U.S. Geological Survey, Pennsylvania Cooperative Fish and Wildlife Research Unit, Pennsylvania State University, University Park, Pennsylvania, United States of America, **2** Animal Industry Division, Michigan Department of Agriculture and Rural Development, Lansing, Michigan, United States of America, **3** United States Department of Agriculture, Animal and Plant Health Inspection Services, Wildlife Services, National Wildlife Research Center, Fort Collins, Colorado, United States of America

## Abstract

Bovine tuberculosis is a bacterial disease caused by *Mycobacterium bovis* in livestock and wildlife with hosts that include Eurasian badgers (*Meles meles*), brushtail possum (*Trichosurus vulpecula*), and white-tailed deer (*Odocoileus virginianus*). Risk-assessment efforts in Michigan have been initiated on farms to minimize interactions of cattle with wildlife hosts but research on *M. bovis* on cattle farms has not investigated the spatial context of disease epidemiology. To incorporate spatially explicit data, initial likelihood of infection probabilities for cattle farms tested for *M. bovis*, prevalence of *M. bovis* in white-tailed deer, deer density, and environmental variables for each farm were modeled in a Bayesian hierarchical framework. We used geo-referenced locations of 762 cattle farms that have been tested for *M. bovis*, white-tailed deer prevalence, and several environmental variables that may lead to long-term survival and viability of *M. bovis* on farms and surrounding habitats (i.e., soil type, habitat type). Bayesian hierarchical analyses identified deer prevalence and proportion of sandy soil within our sampling grid as the most supported model. Analysis of cattle farms tested for *M. bovis* identified that for every 1% increase in sandy soil resulted in an increase in odds of infection by 4%. Our analysis revealed that the influence of prevalence of *M. bovis* in white-tailed deer was still a concern even after considerable efforts to prevent cattle interactions with white-tailed deer through on-farm mitigation and reduction in the deer population. Cattle farms test positive for *M. bovis* annually in our study area suggesting that the potential for an environmental source either on farms or in the surrounding landscape may contributing to new or re-infections with *M. bovis*. Our research provides an initial assessment of potential environmental factors that could be incorporated into additional modeling efforts as more knowledge of deer herd factors and cattle farm prevalence is documented.

**Editor:** Joao Inacio, National Institute for Agriculture and Veterinary Research, IP (INIAV, I.P.), Portugal

**Funding:** Funding for this research was provided by the National Wildlife Research Center of the United States Department of Agriculture, Animal and Plant Health Inspection Service, Wildlife Services. The funders had no role in study design, data collection and analysis, decision to publish, or preparation of the manuscript.

**Competing Interests:** The authors have declared that no competing interests exist.

\* E-mail: wdwalter@psu.edu

## Introduction

Bovine tuberculosis (bTB) is a bacterial disease (*Mycobacterium bovis*) in livestock and wildlife that results in United States Department of Agriculture-mandated depopulation of cattle herds costing farmers millions in lost revenue throughout the world [1,2]. Preliminary efforts by the Michigan Department of Agriculture-Animal Industry Division (MDA) have created protocols that farmers could follow to reduce potential for *M. bovis* infection of cattle in Michigan's Modified Accredited Zone (MAZ) [3]. Basic risk-assessment efforts were needed, however, to address the spatial context of disease epidemiology (i.e., infection probability if a farm is adjacent to a bTB-infected farm) and dynamics of primary reservoirs in the MAZ (i.e., white-tailed deer [*Odocoileus virginianus*]).

The influence of wildlife activity on transmission of *M. bovis* depends on possible hosts and their ability to transmit disease [4–6]. Direct observation of farms in Michigan, USA documented that indirect interactions between cattle and white-tailed deer were dominated by use of pastures and silage storage areas but deer fed from hay racks or silage troughs on only one occasion [7]. Visitation of farm yards and cattle-use areas by sixteen GPS-collared white-tailed deer was documented in Michigan's MAZ and deer were documented using confined feeding areas, water tubs, and pastures [8]. Prevalence of *M. bovis* in deer was as high as 10–12% in some townships but currently can range from 2 to $\geq$5% in some townships due to changes in management regulation for deer and feeding on some cattle farms [3,9,10].

Reoccurrence of *M. bovis* in farms depopulated of cattle in Michigan would suggest an environmental or mammalian host source of re-infection as several farms have become re-infected with *M. bovis* on $\geq$2 separate occasions often spanning 3–7 years between re-infection [3,11]. Under natural shaded conditions on pastures, survival of *M. bovis* in cattle feces was documented to span up to 5 months post-application during winter but only up to 2 months during spring and summer [12]. Effluent plots tested positive for *M. bovis* for up to 29, 13, and 35 days post application for soil, radishes, and lettuce, respectively, in a study in raised garden plots (lined plywood boxes) [13]. Although environmental and anthropogenic variables that influence odds of contracting a disease have been addressed in North America [3,14], only recently has the spatial matrices incorporating proximity to adjacent infected individuals been successfully modeled in disease epidemiology research with advances in software (i.e., WinBUGS; [15–17]). Understanding the spatial dynamics of *M. bovis* will increase our ability to predict future spread or occurrences and variables influencing these occurrences across the MAZ in the northern, lower peninsula of Michigan.

To incorporate spatially explicit data, likelihood of infection probabilities within a geographically designed grid can be determined for cattle herds that tested positive for *M. bovis* and incorporated into a Bayesian hierarchical framework. Although on-farm management practices are believed to influence *M. bovis* transmission, consensus on the most important farm-level factor responsible for transmission is absent and varied across studies in Europe and North America ([11,18,19] but see [3] for a detailed summary). Spatially explicit data on environments that cattle farms occupy is often lacking for researchers attempting to understand the underlying distribution of disease in the landscape and has not been modeled in this system since discovery of *M. bovis* in a free-ranging white-tailed deer in 1975. Our objectives were to model odds of infection with *M. bovis* in cattle farms at the herd level using Bayesian hierarchical analysis by incorporating prevalence of *M. bovis* in the deer population, environmental variables, spatial structure, and unstructured spatial heterogeneity across the MAZ in Michigan. An understanding of conditions that sustain survival of *M. bovis* in the environment would be valuable to our ability to focus surveillance for the disease and predict future spread or occurrences outside of the MAZ in Michigan.

## Materials and Methods

### Study area

We conducted our study in the northern, lower peninsula of Michigan in the MAZ. The 8,062 km$^2$ study area included the entirety of Alcona, Alpena, Montmorency, Oscoda, and Presque Isle counties (Fig. 1). The area encompassed the majority of the cattle farms where *M. bovis* has been found in Michigan. Our study area surrounds Deer Management Unit 452 that has been defined as the bovine tuberculosis core area by the Michigan Department of Natural Resources (MDNR) due to the high prevalence of *M. bovis* in free-ranging deer and the presence of *M. bovis*-positive cattle on farms (Fig. 1; [20,21]). Vegetation categories present in our study area included: *developed* that included roads, development, and barren land; *grass* that included pasture/hay fields and native grasses; *agriculture* that included crops other than forage; *forest* that included upland hardwood stands (*Quercus alba*, *Acer rubrum*, and *A. saccharum*), aspen stands (*Populus tremuloides* and *P. grandidentata*), hardwood/aspen mixed stands, upland conifer stands (*Pinus glauca*, *P. banksiana*, and *P. resinosa*), and hardwood/conifer mixed stands, and swamp that included lowland conifer forests/swamps (*P. glauca*, *P. mariana*, *Thuja occidentalis*, *Abies balsamea*. and *Latrix laricinea*). Elevations in the area ranged from 150–390 m above sea level and the mean annual temperature was 6.6°C, the mean rainfall was 72.5 cm, and there was a mean snowfall of 175 cm [22].

To link the disease status (positive or negative) of each farm in the sample to deer herd and environmental-level predictors, we first overlaid a 5×5 km square grid having a resolution of 25 square kilometers (hereafter referred to as *grid cell*), which is equal to a quarter township in size. We selected quarter townships as the proper resolution given that township would likely be too coarse a

scale and section would be too fine a resolution for model convergence based on previous research with Bayesian hierarchical models [17]. There were a total of 368 grid cells covering the MAZ and we assigned each farm in our study to its appropriate grid cell.

### Observation component

**Cattle farm data.** Our data included 762 cattle farms of known infection status (*observation component*) provided by the Michigan Department of Agriculture and Rural Development (MDA) from mandatory testing of cattle on an annual basis. Based on current knowledge that indirect transmission (i.e., environmental source) of *M. bovis* to cattle may be important, we used replicates for each farm that tested positive on ≥1 occasion over the 11 year span of our study (58 positive, 704 negative) with positive farms coded as 1 and negative farms coded as 0. We included a farm each time it tested positive for *M. bovis* and this was deemed warranted because conditions of that farm or host characteristics in the area were responsible for continued infections of *M. bovis* and replicates would weigh environmental characteristics of farms that tested positive on >1 occasion. Because farms that tested positive for *M. bovis* were depopulated of cattle then re-populated prior to subsequently testing positive, each farm was considered an independent observation for the purposes of our study design. Each farm was tested annually for *M. bovis* but we did not include additional negatives as replicates because that would have likely masked the effects of the positives that we were attempting to model for odds of infection.

We included all cattle farms in this region because we wanted to determine the environmental drivers of disease that were not associated with farm practices and remained unaltered when cattle farms were depopulated or permanently closed (e.g., surrounding habitats, soil composition). Furthermore, we did not include any farm-level covariates (e.g., herd size, feeding practices) in our models because farm mitigation strategies were initiated by the MDA during our study [3], would be difficult to quantify and standardize across the study region, and would only be considered a contamination source (e.g., cattle fed in deer habitat) but would not influence environmental persistence or survival of *M. bovis* in the landscape.

### Process component

**Host-level variables.** The MDNR provided section-level data on deer prevalence for *M. bovis* from 1995 to 2009. We limited our analysis to white-tailed deer prevalence for 2005 to 2009 because deer herd management, ban on baiting deer, and mitigation of on-farm practices indicated that deer prevalence has stabilized within the past 5 years thus, more reflective of current deer prevalence [10,23]. Apparent prevalence of *M. bovis* in deer was determined for each grid cell by dividing the total number of deer testing positive by the total number of deer tested resulting in percent prevalence that was entered into models. Annual deer densities were provided by the MDNR from 2005 to 2009 at the county level for the MAZ based on Sex-Age-Kill reconstruction technique or additional methods if available [24,25]. We averaged deer density over the time period to match deer prevalence (2005–2009) that resulted in a single estimate of deer density per grid cell. Due to the logistical constraints of estimating deer densities at a fine scale, such as to the section-level, we used the only available data to represent deer densities in our study site as deer per square kilometer. We did not select mean deer prevalence or mean deer density for the entire span of sampling of cattle farms because we were interested in modeling the effects of more recent deer

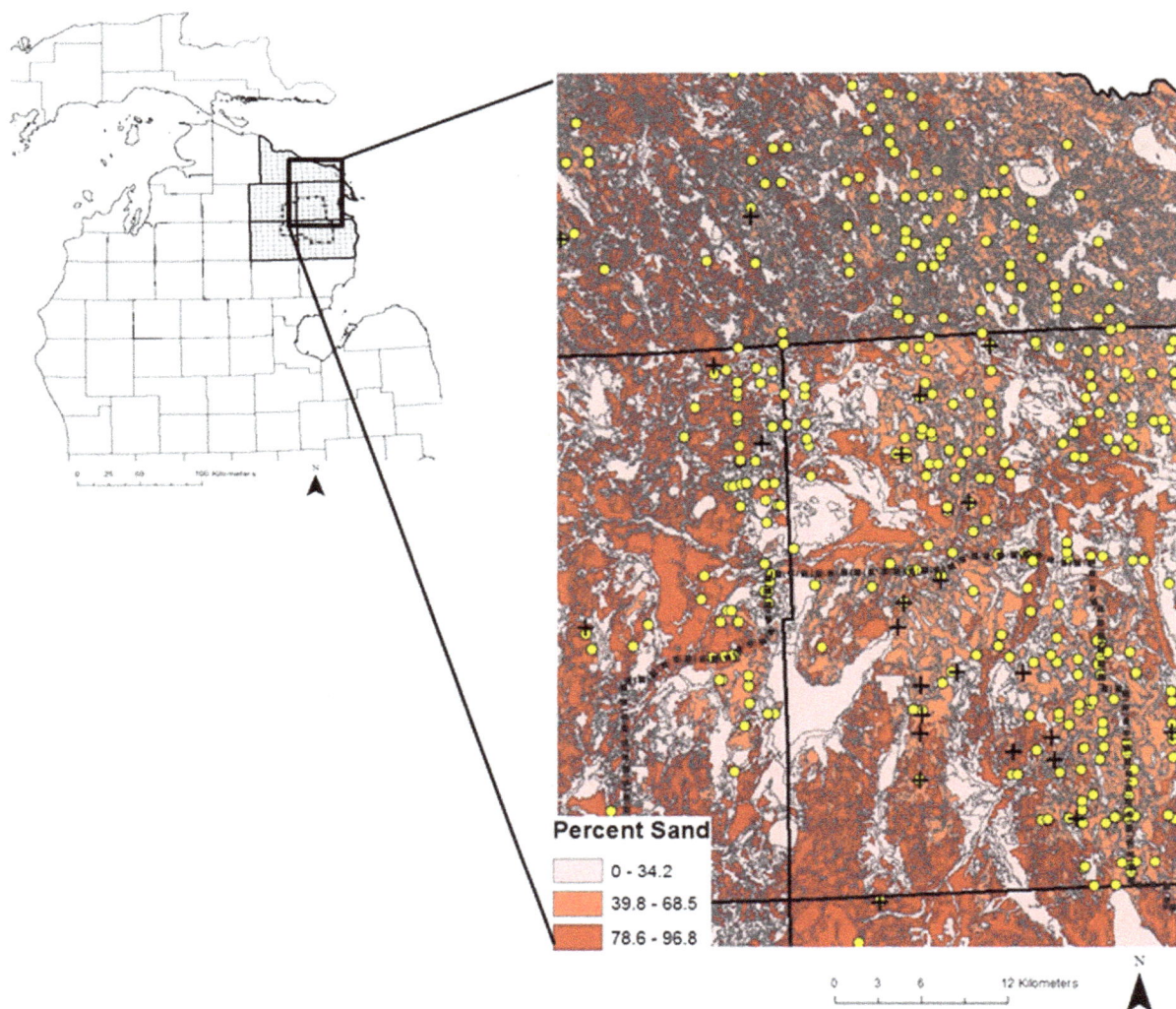

**Figure 1. Sampling grid (25 km² cells) that contained all cattle farms tested for bovine tuberculosis within the Modified Accredited Zone (5 counties in bold) in the upper, lower peninsula of Michigan.** Deer Management Unit 452 (dashed polygon) is considered the bovine tuberculosis core area for surveillance in white-tailed deer (Outset). Cattle farms that tested negative (yellow circles) and positive (black crosses) for *Mycobacterium bovis* used in Bayesian Hierarchical models overlayed on percent sand within a portion of the study area in the upper, lower peninsula of Michigan (Inset).

prevalence that likely would be influenced by initiation of deer and on-farm management practices in 1996.

**Environmental-level variables.** We hypothesized *a priori* that *M. bovis* patterns on farms were structured in part by spatial heterogeneities in features of the landscape, therefore, we identified four environmental-level predictors of infection based on optimal survival characteristics of *M. bovis* identified in the literature [3]. Proportion of sand content in the soil was selected because dry sandy loam soils at the proper pH and moisture promoted bacteria growth [26,27]. Proportion of the landscape ponding frequently and proportion of swamp/wetland were selected because the duration of standing water occurring in non-wetlands (ponding) and soil characteristics of inundated areas (wetlands) were conducive to long-term survival of *M. bovis* [27,28]. Mean soil pH was selected because soil pH from 5.8 to 6.9 was conducive to culture of *M. bovis* at the optimum temperature (37°C) for survival [27,29]. Sand (where "sand" was defined as soil particles with size >2 μm), landscape ponding frequently, and soil

pH was determined using the Advanced Mode of the Soil Data Viewer available through the National Resources Conservation Service of the US Department of Agriculture in ArcMap 9.x (ArcMap; Environmental Systems Research Institute, Redlands, CA, USA). Soil Data Viewer provides interactive mapping software to query the Soil Survey Geographic (SSURGO) database and descriptive characteristics for each soil type. Sand was expressed as the percent sand within a soil type polygon (~2 ha resolution) for each soil map unit [30]. Each grid cell was thus potentially composed of multiple soil type polygons with varying sand contents. Therefore, we calculated the mean percent sand for each 25 km² grid cell using a weighted average based on the area of the various soil type polygons and their associated sand content. Similarly, in the Advanced Mode of the Soil Data Viewer, we identified the proportion of each grid cell that ponded frequently with frequently defined as "ponding occurs, on the average, more than once in 2 years and the chance of ponding is >50% in any year [30]." Similar to sand and ponding frequently, we calculated the mean soil pH for each 25 km$^2$ grid cell using a weighted average based on the area of the various pH polygons and their associated pH value.

We used the National Land Cover Database of 2006 (NLCD) that was created from Landsat 7 imagery to determine the proportion of swamp/wetland across the study site (MRLC 2007). To standardize analyses across the MAZ, we reclassified land cover from the NLCD into 8 categories used in Kaneene et al. [11]: hardwood forest, coniferous forest, mixed forest, open areas and shrubs, wetland/swamp, agricultural use, open water, and other (industrial, residential). We extracted the proportion of wetland/swamp from NLCD within each grid cell with all environmental-level variables, except soil pH, presented as a percentage in a grid cell in modeling efforts. Skewness of data and correlation among covariates was assessed but data transformations and exclusions were not considered necessary prior to entering into models.

## Statistical analysis

We used a Bayesian hierarchical model structure [31,32] with logistic regression models (described below) to examine how recent TB prevalence at the deer herd-level and landscape factors influenced the probability of a farm being infected, while adjusting for the other covariates and spatial structure in the data [33]. To adjust for latent spatial effects we included two types of random effects that captured both the influence of the local neighborhood (i.e., cells sharing a border or vertex with each 25-km$^2$ grid cell; CAR) in determining spatial clustering of *M. bovis*, as well as any spatially independent influences occurring at the 25-km$^2$ spatial resolution of our grid (HET). Our models were constructed hierarchically to accommodate the fact that information from multiple levels (i.e., fixed-effects and spatial random effects) was being used to estimate individual-level infection probabilities. Taking a Bayesian approach, we used Markov Chain Monte Carlo (MCMC) simulation methods available within the program WinBUGS [34] to produce the unnormalized joint posterior density for the parameters of interest across all models examined based on the product of the data likelihood and the prior densities for each parameter. We used this approach to estimate the posterior marginal probability distributions for the parameters governing the influence of the host- and environmental-level, and spatial random effects predictors on the probability of infection. For each model we ran three independent Markov chains with varying initial values for 350,000 iterations and discarded the first 100,000. We thinned the Markov chains by keeping every twentieth iteration for inference. To determine if the three Markov chains used for each model had converged on the same posterior distribution, we used the statistical program R with the package boa [35] and employed several graphical and quantitative diagnostics, including autocorrelation plots, trace plots, and univariate corrected scale reduction factors for each parameter. To assess simultaneous convergence of all parameters for the top models, we calculated the multivariate potential scale reduction factor [32,36,37]. All inferences were based on the mean of each parameter's marginal posterior distribution.

## Likelihood functions

The observation component of the data likelihood specifies each farm's observed *M. bovis* infection status as a Bernoulli random variable with parameter $\varphi_{ij}$:

$$Y_{ij}|\varphi_{ij} \sim \text{Bernoulli}(\varphi_{ij}),$$

where $Y_{ij}$ is the infection status of the $i^{th}$ farm for $i = 1, ..., n$ from the $j^{th}$ grid cell for $j = 1, ..., m$, and $\varphi_{ij}$ represents the probability of infection. Thus, given the probability of infection we assume each farm's infection status is conditionally independent.

The process component of the data likelihood models, via the logit link function, defined as the probability of infection as a function of individual, environmental and spatial covariates as well as random effects that account for spatial variability:

$$\text{logit}(\varphi_{ij}) = \mu + \mathbf{x}'_{ij}\beta + \theta_j + \varphi_j, \tag{1}$$

where $\mu$ defines the baseline *M. bovis* infection probability, $\mathbf{x}'_{ij}$ is the transpose of a $k \times 1$ matrix of covariates for the $i^{th}$ farm from the $j^{th}$ grid cell, $\beta$ is a $k \times 1$ vector of parameter estimates for these covariates, $\theta_j$ is a random effect for the $j^{th}$ grid cell capturing extra-binomial variability over the entire study region at the individual quarter township scale (HET; i.e., 25 km$^2$), and $\phi_j$ is a random effect term for the $j^{th}$ grid cell that models the extra-binomial variability associated with local disease clustering (CAR; i.e., grid cells closer together will have similar infection probabilities due to proximity of cattle farms and pastures).

## Prior distributions

We assumed non-informative $N(0, 100,000)$ prior distributions for each of the $\beta$ parameters, and an improper (flat) prior over the entire real line for $\mu$. For the random effect describing region-wide heterogeneity (HET), we assumed the following:

$$\theta_j \stackrel{iid}{\sim} N(0, \sigma_h^2). \tag{2}$$

To describe the spatial structure, we assumed an intrinsic Gaussian conditional autoregressive prior with a sum to zero constraint [31] for the local clustering random effect (CAR):

$$\varphi_j|\varphi_{j+} \stackrel{iid}{\sim} N\left(\frac{1}{n_{j+}}\sum_{i \bowtie n_{j+}}\varphi_i, \frac{\sigma_c^2}{n_{j+}}\right), \tag{3}$$

where $n_{j+}$ is the number of grid cells that share a border or vertex with the $j^{th}$ grid cell. Thus, the random effect of the $j^{th}$ grid cell is conditional on the values of its $n_{j+}$ (usually = 8) neighboring cells. Adjacency matrices were created with the Adjacency for WinBUGS Tool in ArcMap that provides a matrix relating one areal unit to a collection of neighboring areal units in text files for use in WinBUGS.

Because of the marginal specification for $\sigma_h^2$ and conditional specification for $\sigma_c^2$ of the random effects, we generated prior distributions for the precisions (i.e., $\frac{1}{\sigma_h^2}$ and $\frac{1}{\sigma_c^2}$) using simulations in WinBUGS where we varied the values of the parameters and determined the parameter values that created an expectation of ~0.5 for the *psi* metric [38], where *psi* is as follows:

$$psi = \frac{\sigma_c}{\sigma_c + \sigma_h} \tag{4}$$

These simulations attempted to ensure an equal emphasis on the priors of the standard deviations of the random effects [31]. Based on our simulation results we defined

$$\frac{1}{\sigma_h^2} \sim \text{Gamma}(10.368, 3.22) \text{ and } \frac{1}{\sigma_c^2} \sim \text{Gamma}(1.0, 1.0).$$

## Model Selection

To test our original hypothesis that environmental variables would influence the odds of *M. bovis* infection, our set of candidate models for logistic regression consisted of 12 different structures with strictly additive effects on the logit scale (Table 1). The 12 logistic regression models represented all possible combinations of deer and environmental variables, as well as inherent regional and local spatial structure of the data. Viewing these 12 models as competing hypotheses, we used deviance information criterion (DIC) [15,33,39] to compare the models' respective fits to the data from sampled farms, and then estimated parameters and examined goodness-of-fit and other metrics for the top models. For model comparison we used DIC weights [33], which allow for an intuitive comparison of the evidence in the data for each candidate model. The weights are considered a measure of the strength of evidence in the data for $i^{th}$ model being the "best" model of those within the candidate set, and therefore provide a measure of model selection uncertainty [33,39].

We used parameter estimates from the top model to calculate odds ratios for the effect of variables on *M. bovis* infection odds among farms in that area. Model averaging was not appropriate because DIC, unlike BIC and AIC, is not based on any assumption of a "true" model and is primarily concerned with short-term predictive ability [33]. We treated host-level (deer prevalence, deer density) and environmental-level predictors (percent sand, soil pH,

proportion of wetland/swamp, and area that ponded frequently) as a group of variables, such that they were all entered or removed from the models together (Table 1). To examine the goodness-of-fit of the top model from our candidate set we conducted a numerical posterior predictive check [32]. We examined correlation and trace plots, as well as the estimates of the corrected scale reduction factor for each parameter and multivariate potential scale reduction factors and determined that that the three chains for each model had converged (data not shown). For each dataset, the top models selected via our model selection procedures and their corresponding estimates were similar regardless of prior specification (data not shown; [33]).

## Results

Out of the 762 cattle farms tested on an annual basis, 704 were negative while 37, 9, and 1 tested positive for *M. bovis* on 1, 2, and 3 occasions, respectively. Of our 12 models determined *a priori*, the top two models combined to account for over 95% of the summed weights of all models considered. Models weights of 95% provided strong assurance that some combination of these 2 models and their parameters reflected the underlying infection-generating process far better than other models in the candidate set (Table 1). Parameters in the top model included deer herd factors and local landscape features suggesting that these factors increased the odds of *M. bovis* infection to cattle in the northern, lower peninsula of Michigan (Table 2). As documented since initial diagnosis of a positive white-tailed deer in 1975, deer apparent prevalence ranged from 0.0% to 5.2% and was the most supported variable in the top model (odd ratio = 1.004, 95% CI = 1.001 to 1.007; Table 2). Sand within the vicinity of sampled farms was by far the most supported environmental variable and ranged from 37% to 79% on farms that test positive whereas sand ranged from 17% to 88% for cattle farms that tested negative for *M. bovis* (Fig. 1). The odds of infection for *M. bovis* increased by about 4% for every 1% increase in sand in the area (odd ratio = 1.036, 95% CI = 1.01 to 1.07; Table 2).

Our analyses also identified that an unstructured random effect (HET) dominated over spatial structure (CAR) in influencing the odds of *M.bovis* infection (odd ratio = 3.36, 95% CI = 1.69 to 10.91; Table 2). Inclusion of the unstructured random effect in both our top models would suggest that additional covariates are driving odds of *M. bovis* infection and not spatial occurrence of *M. bovis*-positive farms in our study area.

## Discussion

Our findings support the premise that deer herd-related factors play an important role in sustaining *M. bovis* presence in the northern, lower peninsula of Michigan similar to that found in previous research [11,40]. Because mitigation measures have been implemented to reduce deer access to feeding and cattle use areas [3], we focused our analysis simply on deer density and deer prevalence in the area without reference to farm practices. Farm practices have been the primary focus of most efforts to control *M. bovis* transmission between reservoirs and hosts [11,18,41,42] but are difficult to standardize and document for inclusion in modeling efforts. Bayesian hierarchical models provide the ability to assess spatially the influence of region-wide cattle farm and host-level variables while adjusting for additional covariates [31,43]. The bias that may have been introduced by entering 36% of cattle farms more than once into our models was deemed warranted to achieve our objectives of assessing environmental factors that may lead to continued presence of *M. bovis* on cattle farms. Furthermore, we don't deny that farm-management practices

**Table 1.** Model selection results for the candidate set of models investigating the effect of covariates on the probability of bovine tuberculosis infection from 2005–2010 in Modified Accredited Zone in Michigan, USA using non-informative N (0, 0.00001) prior distributions for the fixed effects parameters and diffuse gamma priors for the random effects with farm-level factors removed.

| Model Terms | Dbar | Dhat | pD | DIC | ΔDIC | Weights |
|---|---|---|---|---|---|---|
| Deer + ------ + HET + Envir | 272.9 | 226.4 | 46.5 | 319.4 | 0.0 | 0.6386 |
| Deer + ------ + HET + ------ | 276.2 | 231.5 | 44.7 | 320.9 | 1.5 | 0.3073 |
| ------ + ------ + HET + Envir | 275.9 | 227.5 | 48.4 | 324.4 | 4.9 | 0.0540 |
| Deer + CAR + ------ + ------ | 289.0 | 235.5 | 53.5 | 342.4 | 23.0 | 0.0000 |
| ------ + CAR + ------ + Envir | 290.5 | 231.7 | 58.8 | 349.3 | 29.8 | 0.0000 |
| Deer + CAR + ------ + Envir | 298.1 | 232.0 | 66.1 | 364.2 | 44.7 | 0.0000 |
| Deer + CAR + HET + ------ | 302.3 | 224.8 | 77.5 | 379.8 | 60.4 | 0.0000 |
| ------ + CAR + HET + Envir | 309.3 | 226.2 | 83.1 | 392.3 | 72.9 | 0.0000 |
| Deer + ------ + ------ + Envir | 387.9 | 380.9 | 7.0 | 394.9 | 75.5 | 0.0000 |
| Deer + ------ + ------ + ------ | 394.2 | 391.2 | 2.9 | 397.1 | 77.6 | 0.0000 |
| ------ + ------ + ------ + Envir | 405.5 | 400.7 | 4.8 | 410.3 | 90.8 | 0.0000 |
| Deer + CAR + HET + Envir | 317.1 | 222.1 | 95.0 | 412.0 | 92.6 | 0.0000 |

"Deer" represents deer herd factors: apparent prevalence of deer and deer density. "Envir" represents the environmental variables: percent sand, percent ponding frequently, percent swamp/wetland, and mean soil pH in each sampled farms quarter township grid cell. "HET" represents the random effect capturing region-wide heterogeneity and "CAR" is the random effect capturing local clustering.

**Table 2.** Mean parameter estimates, standard deviation (SD), Monte Carlo error (MC error), odds ratios (OR), and 95% credible intervals for best-fitting model investigating the effect of covariates on the probability of bovine tuberculosis infection from 2005–2010 in Modified Accredited Zone in Michigan, USA.

| Parameter | Mean | SD | MC error | 2.50% | Median | 97.5% | OR | 95% CI |
|---|---|---|---|---|---|---|---|---|
| Intercept | −3.401 | 2.886 | 0.02 | −9.219 | −3.317 | 2.031 | 0.0333 | 0.00 to 7.622 |
| Deer density | −0.2219 | 0.1454 | 0.00 | −0.515 | 0.219 | 0.056 | 0.8001 | 0.60 to 1.06 |
| Deer prevalence | 0.4147 | 0.1412 | 0.00 | 0.137 | 0.414 | 0.697 | 1.004 | 1.001 to 1.007 |
| Percent wetland | −0.0209 | 0.0262 | 0.00 | −0.074 | −0.020 | 0.029 | 0.9793 | 0.93 to 1.03 |
| Percent sand | 0.0357 | 0.0152 | 0.00 | 0.007 | 0.035 | 0.067 | 1.0363 | 1.01 to 1.07 |
| Soil pH | 0.04212 | 0.3368 | 0.00 | −0.591 | 0.035 | 0.732 | 1.0430 | 0.55 to 2.08 |
| Percent ponding | 0.0240 | 0.035 | 0.00 | −0.043 | 0.023 | 0.095 | 1.0243 | 0.96 to 1.10 |
| HET | 1.213 | 0.4819 | 0.00 | 0.524 | 1.128 | 2.39 | 3.3636 | 1.69 to 10.91 |

"HET" represents the random effect capturing region-wide.

are important in *M. bovis* infection on cattle farms, however, it is very difficult to accurately represent or measure one of these farm practices in a standardized format for hundreds of farms to include in our models. For this reason, we selected objectives that would look at determining new facet in understanding *M. bovis* infection (i.e., environmental variables) as opposed to conducting another study that suggested a different farm practice was responsible for bTB infection in cattle farms as documented in previous research [11,18,41,42].

Although deer densities in the area have been reduced to about 10–15 deer/km$^2$ since 1994 and deer prevalence has remained at just below 2% overall at the DMU 452-level [10], the role of a primary host for *M. bovis* in this region is still influencing transmission of *M. bovis* based on our study. Including mean deer prevalence for the duration of the study (i.e., 1998–2009) in our models would likely have yielded similar results to our current modeling effort but the role of the host would still be supported nonetheless. Due to public pressure about low deer densities and continued occurrence of cattle positive for *M. bovis* on an annual basis, reducing deer densities further is likely not possible. Relatedly, even with our conservative estimate of prevalence of *M. bovis* in deer (i.e., 2005–2009), deer prevalence was in the most supported model even though the odds ratio would likely have been greater if we included 1998–2009.

Our study identified environmental variables that were not possible to assess in previous modeling efforts that can further assist agencies in their attempts to eradicate *M. bovis* in Michigan. Environmental variables have been documented to contribute to presence or viability of infectious agents of disease in several areas in North American and Europe [17,44,45] although environmental sampling has yet to identify *M. bovis* on cattle farms in this region [46,47]. Variables to consider should be based on *a priori* knowledge of the disease agent studied and mechanisms that may hinder or promote survival. Survival of *M. bovis* has been linked to moist, humid environments that maintain the proper soil type and pH [48–50]. Our top model indicated that a combination of landscape variables played an important role in determining infection probability for *M. bovis* on farms which was the impetus for us to select a combination of covariates that were conducive to moist, humid environments with low sunlight exposure on the landscape (e.g., wetlands, ponding frequency, soil types). Percent sand was a significant predictor and increased the odds of *M. bovis* infection by 3.6% for every 1% increase in proportion of sandy soil in the local area (Table 2). Survival of *M. bovis* has been linked to

soil type, temperature and pH [3,29,48] but research in natural settings has limited the advancement of knowledge in this area.

The exact composition of sandy soils or functional role of these soils that make them conducive to the survival of *M. bovis* likely requires further research. Sandy soils are defined as having loose particle sizes (> 2 μm) with structural integrity during desiccation that may promote survival of *M. bovis* when associated with wetlands and areas that routinely have standing water. Moraines that have steep slopes and sandy, well-drained soils dominated by northern hardwood forests were linked to infection of white-tailed with *M. bovis* [51] but are confounded by the fact that they characterize preferred deer habitat in years with heavy oak mast production. Based on prevalence studies on white-tailed deer and our current study of farms positive for *M. bovis*, environmental or landscape-specific characteristics would appear to be a logical focus of future studies and potential assessment of viable *M. bovis* detection in soils or water. Areas that contain these sandy, well-drained soils in northern hardwood forests likely provide moist, humid microclimates conducive to survival of *M. bovis* for extended periods of time and should be considered for focused surveillance for *M. bovis* in deer and cattle as well as the focus of future on-farm mitigation measures.

Since initial detection of *M. bovis* in farms over a decade ago, farms have tested positive on an annual basis. Even after considerable efforts have been implemented to reduce deer densities, limiting or preventing aggregation of deer (e.g., ban on baiting of deer), and limiting deer-cattle interactions through on-farm mitigation measures, Michigan still does not have *M. bovis*-free status. Although modeling efforts are unable to include movements of cattle between farms and its influence on movements and spread of *M. bovis*, repeated positive tests have occurred on numerous farms since the first farm tested positive in 1998 [28]. Repeated positive tests would suggest that potentially an environmental source conducive to survival of the bacteria may be responsible for maintaining *M. bovis* in the region. Mycobacteria have waxy, lipid-rich cell walls that are relatively resistant to biocides used in decontamination procedures thus complicating management of the disease.

Unlike previous work in this region, we were able to assess spatial processes that may be influencing the transmission or presence of *M. bovis* using a Bayesian hierarchical modeling framework [31,43]. We identified that unstructured spatial heterogeneity (HET) was included in the top two models explaining infection of *M. bovis* on farms. If probability of infection was driven by spatial structure or clustering of disease (i.e., contiguous grid cells more alike than 2 arbitrary grid cells) at our site, we would have expected spatial structure (CAR) to be included in our top models but the opposite occurred [43]. Unstructured spatial heterogeneity would suggest that additional covariates that we may not have accounted for in our models were also influencing the disease across our study region. As stated previously, movement of cattle between farms and additional on-farm practices is controlled or mitigated to some extent for some farms but is very difficult to enforce and has been documented to be the cause of contamination of several cattle farms within and outside of the MAZ [21]. Our unstructured spatial heterogeneity could simply be on-farm practices not included in our modeling effort or additional environmental covariates conducive to survival or destruction of *M. bovis* such as slope/aspects conducive to direct exposure to ultraviolet light.

Although host prevalence in DMU 452 and clustering of cattle farms were considered important in *M. bovis* infection in previous research [11,52], our results suggest that less spatially structured components in the landscape are influencing continued occurrence of *M. bovis* in cattle on farms in Michigan. Considering the logistics of managing the host and reservoir through the northern, lower peninsula of Michigan, management efforts could focus on environmental and landscape characteristics that are potentially supporting the continued presence of *M. bovis* in Michigan.

Landscape characteristics that are conducive to survival of *M. bovis* such as habitat inundated with standing water, soil composition, and prime deer habitat should be the focus of future management and research. On-farm mitigations should focus efforts in areas at high risk for continued survival of *M. bovis* prior to mandating complete risk mitigation of farms for an entire area such as DMU 452 (1,479 km$^2$) or the 5 county study area (8,062 km$^2$). Focused surveillance and management of on-farm practices in reservoirs for disease in domestic livestock would provide a logistically feasible approach to combating a disease in an endemic area as well as new areas that the disease has recently been introduced or spread from the endemic area.

## Acknowledgments

We thank the Michigan Department of Natural Resources for deer-related data used in this manuscript. We thank Daniel J. O'Brien, Michigan Department of Natural Resources, for a helpful review of an earlier draft of this manuscript. Any use of trade, firm, or product names is for descriptive purposes only and does not imply endorsement by the U.S. Government.

## Author Contributions

Conceived and designed the experiments: WDW RS MV KCV. Performed the experiments: WDW RS. Analyzed the data: WDW. Wrote the paper: WDW RS MV KCV.

## References

1. de Lisle GW, Bengis RG, Schmitt SM, O'Brien DJ (2002) Tuberculosis in free-ranging wildlife: detection, diagnosis and management. Review Science Technology, OIE 21: 317–334.

2. Kaneene J, Thoen CO (2004) Tuberculosis. Journal of the American Veterinary Medical Association 224: 685–691.

3. Walter WD, Anderson CW, Smith R, Vanderklok M, Averill JJ (2012) On-farm mitigation of transmission of tuberculosis from white-tailed deer to cattle: literature review and recommendations. Veterinary Medicine International 2012: 1–15.

4. Clifton-Hadley RS, Wilesmith JW, Stuart FA (1993) Mycobacterium bovis in the European badger ( Meles meles ): epidemiological findings in tuberculosis badgers from a naturally infected population. Epidemiology and Infection 111: 9–19.

5. Griffin JM, Hahesy T, Lynch K, Salman MD, McCarthy J, et al. (1993) The association of cattle husbandry practices, environmental factors and farmer characteristics with the occurrence of chronic bovine tuberculosis in dairy herds in the Republic of Ireland. Preventive Veterinary Medicine 17: 145–160.

6. Corner LAL (2006) The role of wild animal populations in the epidemiology of tuberculosis in domestic animals: How to assess the risk. Veterinary Microbiology 112: 303–312.

7. Hill JA (2005) Wildlife-cattle interactions in northern Michigan: implications for the transmission of bovine tuberculosis Thesis. Logan: Utah State University. 1–58 p.

8. Berentsen AR, Miller RS, Misiewicz R, Malmberg JL, Dunbar MR (2013) Characteristics of white-tailed deer visits to cattle farms: implications for disease transmission at the wildlife-livestock interface. European Journal of Wildlife Research: In press.

9. O'Brien DJ, Schmitt SM, Fierke JS, Hogle SA, Winterstein SR, et al. (2002) Epidemiology of Mycobacterium bovis in free-ranging white-tailed deer, Michigan, USA, 1995-2000. Preventive Veterinary Medicine 54: 47–63.

10. O'Brien DJ, Schmitt SM, Fitzgerald SD, Berry DE (2011) Management of bovine tuberculosis in Michigan wildlife: Current status and near term prospects. Veterinary Microbiology 151: 179–187.

11. Kaneene JB, Bruning-Fann CS, Granger LM, Miller R, Porter-Spalding BA (2002) Environmental and farm management factors associated with tuberculosis on cattle farms in northeastern Michigan. Journal of the American Veterinary Medical Association 221: 837–842.

12. Williams RS, Hoy WA (1930) The viability of B. tuberculosis (bovinus) on pasture land, in stored faeces and in liquid manure. Journal of Hygeine 30: 413–419.

13. Van Donsel DJ, Larkin EP (1977) Persistence of Mycobacterium bovis BCG in soil and on vegetables spray-irrigated with sewage effluent and sludge. Journal of Food Protection 40: 160–163.

14. Carstensen M, DonCarlos MW (2011) Preventing the establishment of a wildlife disease reservoir: a case study of bovine tuberculosis in wild deer in Minnesota, USA. Veterinary Medicine International 2011: 1–10.

15. Farnsworth ML, Hoeting JA, Hobbs NT, Miller MW (2006) Linking chronic wasting disease to mule deer movement scales: a hierarchical bayesian approach. Ecological Applications 16: 1026–1036.

16. Osnas EE, Heisey DM, Rolley RE, Samuel MD (2009) Spatial and temporal patterns of chronic wasting disease: fine-scale mapping of a wildlife epidemic in Wisconsin. Ecological Applications 19: 1311–1322.

17. Walter WD, Walsh DP, Farnsworth ML, Winkelman DL, Miller MW (2011) Soil clay content underlies prion infection odds. Nature Communications 2: 1–6.

18. Hutchings MR, Harris S (1997) Effects of farm management practices on cattle grazing behaviour and the potential for transmission of bovine tuberculosis from badgers to cattle. The Veterinary Journal 153: 149–162.

19. Mathews F, Lovett L, Rushton S, Macdonald DW (2006) Bovine tuberculosis in cattle: reduced risk on wildlife-friendly farms. Biology Letters 2: 271–274.

20. O'Brien DJ, Schmitt SM, Berry DE, Fitzgerald SD, Vanneste JR, et al. (2004) Estimating the true prevalence of Mycobacterium bovis in hunter-harvested white-tailed deer in Michigan. Journal of Wildlife Diseases 40: 42–52.

21. Okafor CC, Grooms DL, Bruning-Fann CS, Averill JJ, Kaneene JB (2011) Descriptive epidemiology of bovine tuberculosis in Michigan (1975–2010): lessons learned. Veterinary Medicine International 2011.

22. Hughey BD (2003) Are there "hot spots" of bovine tuberculosis in the free-ranging white-tailed deer ( Odocoileus virginianus ) herd of northeastern Michigan? Thesis. East Lansing: Michigan State University. 1–86 p.

23. Okafor CC, Grooms DL, Bruning-Fann CS, Averill JJ, Kaneene JB (2011) Descriptive epidemiology of bovine tuberculosis in Michigan(1975-2010): lessons learned. Veterinary Medicine International 2011: 874924.

24. Eberhardt LL (1960) Estimation of vital characteristics of Michigan deer herds. East Lansing: Department of Conservation.

25. Creed WA, Haberland F, Kohn BE, McCaffery KR (1984) Harvest management: the Wisconsin experience. In: Halls LK, editor. White-tailed deer ecology and management. Harrisburg.

26. Phillips CJC, Foster CRW, Morris PA, Teverson R (2002) Genetic and management factors that influence the susceptibility of cattle to Mycobacterium bovis infection. Animal Health Research Reviews 3: 3–13.

27. Mitscherlich E, Marth EH (1984) Microbial survival in the environment: bacteria and rickettsiae important in human and animal health. Berlin: Springer-Verlag. 1–802 p.

28. Miller R, Kaneene JB (2006) Evaluation of historical factors influencing the occurrence and distribution of *Mycobacterium bovis* infection among wildlife in Michigan. American Journal of Veterinary Research 67: 604–615.

29. Phillips CJC, Foster CRW, Morris PA, Teverson R (2003) The transmission of Mycobacterium bovis infection to cattle. Research in Veterinary Science 74: 1–15.

30. USDA NRCS (2007) Soil Data Viewer 5.2 User Guide. United States Department of Agriculture, Natural Resources Conservation Science.

31. Banerjee S, Carlin BP, Gelfand AE (2004) Hierarchical modeling and analysis for spatial data. New York: Chapman and Hall/CRC. 1–448 p.

32. Gelman A, Carlin JB, Stern HS, Rubin DB (2004) Bayesian data analysis. New York: Chapman and Hall/CRC. 1–696 p.

33. Spiegelhalter DJ, Best NG, Carlin BP, van der Linde A (2002) Bayesian measures of model complexity and fit. Journal of the Royal Statistical SocietySeries B (Statistical Methodology) 64: 583–639.

34. Spiegelhalter D, Thomas A, Best N, Lunn D (2003) WinBUGS Version 1.4 user manual. Cambridge: MRC Biostatistics Unit. 1–60 p.

35. Smith BJ (2007) boa: an R package for MCMC output convergence assessment and posterior inference. Journal of Statistical Software 21: 1–37.

36. Gelman A, Rubin DB (1992) Inference from iterative simulation using multiple sequences. Statistical Science 7: 457–472.

37. Brooks SP, Gelman A (1998) General methods for monitoring convergence of iterative simulations. Journal of Computational and Graphical Statistics 7: 434–455.

38. Eberly LE, Carlin BP (2000) Identifiability and convergence issues for Markov chain Monte Carlo fitting of spatial models. Statistics in Medicine 19: 2279–2294.

39. Burnham KP, Anderson DR (2002) Model selection and multimodel inference: a practical information-theoretic approach. New York: Springer-Verlag. 1–488 p.

40. Miller R, Kaneene JB, Fitzgerald SD, Schmitt SM (2003) Evaluation of the influence of supplemental feeding of white-tailed deer ( Odocoileus virginianus ) on the prevalence of bovine tuberculosis in the Michigan wild deer population. Journal of Wildlife Diseases 39: 84–95.

41. Knust BM, Wolf PC, Wells SJ (2011) Characterization of the risk of deer-cattle interactions in Minnesota by use of an on-farm environmental assessment tool. American Journal of Veterinary Research 72: 924–931.

42. Brook RK (2010) Incorporating farmer observations in efforts to manage bovine tuberculosis using barrier fencing at the wildlife-livestock interface. Preventive Veterinary Medicine 94: 301–305.

43. Besag J, York J, Mollie A (1991) Bayesian image restoration, with two applications in spatial statistics. Annals of the Institute of Statistical Mathematics 43: 1–59.

44. Imrie CE, Korre A, Munoz-Melendez G (2009) Spatial correlation between the prevalence of transmissible spongiform diseases and British soil geochemistry. Environmental Geochemistry and Health 31: 133–145.

45. Fine AE, Bolin CA, Gardiner JC, Kaneene JB (2011) A study of the persistence of Mycobacterium bovis in the environment under natural weather conditions in Michigan, USA. Veterinary Medicine International 2011: 1–12.

46. Witmer G, Fine AE, Gionfriddo J, Pipas M, Shively K, et al. (2010) Epizootiological survey of bovine tuberculosis in northern Michigan. Journal of Wildlife Diseases 46: 368–378.

47. Fine AE, O'Brien DJ, Winterstein SR, Kaneene JB (2011) An effort to isolate Mycobacterium bovis from environmental substrates during investigations of bovine tuberculosis transmission sites (cattle farms and wildlife areas) in Michigan, USA. ISRN Veterinary Science.

48. Duffield BJ, Young DA (1985) Survival of Mycobacterium bovis in defined environmental conditions. Veterinary Microbiology 10: 193–197.

49. Young JS, Gormley E, Wellington EMH (2005) Molecular detection of Mycobacterium bovis and Mycobacterium bovis BCG (Pasteur) in soil. Applied and Environmental Microbiology 71: 1946–1952.

50. Jackson R, de Lisle GW, Morris RS (1995) A study of the environmental survival of Mycobacterium bovis on a farm in New Zealand. New Zealand Veterinary Journal 43: 346–352.

51. Miller R, Kaneene JB, Schmitt SM, Lusch DP, Fitzgerald SD (2007) Spatial analysis of Mycobacterium bovis infection in white-tailed deer ( Odocoileus virginianus ) in Michigan, USA. Preventive Veterinary Medicine 82: 111–122.

52. O'Brien DJ, Schmitt SM, Fitzgerald SD, Berry DE, Hickling GJ (2006) Managing the wildlife reservoir of Mycobacterium bovis: The Michigan, USA, experience. Veterinary Microbiology 112: 313323.

# 16

# Long-Term Health Effects of Neutering Dogs: Comparison of Labrador Retrievers with Golden Retrievers

**Benjamin L. Hart[1]\***, **Lynette A. Hart[2]**, **Abigail P. Thigpen[2]**, **Neil H. Willits[3]**

**1** Department of Anatomy, Physiology and Cell Biology, School of Veterinary Medicine, University of California Davis, Davis, California, United States of America, **2** Department of Population Health and Reproduction, School of Veterinary Medicine, University of California Davis, Davis, California, United States of America, **3** Department of Statistics, University of California Davis, Davis, California, United States of America

## Abstract

Our recent study on the effects of neutering (including spaying) in Golden Retrievers in markedly increasing the incidence of two joint disorders and three cancers prompted this study and a comparison of Golden and Labrador Retrievers. Veterinary hospital records were examined over a 13-year period for the effects of neutering during specified age ranges: before 6 mo., and during 6–11 mo., year 1 or years 2 through 8. The joint disorders examined were hip dysplasia, cranial cruciate ligament tear and elbow dysplasia. The cancers examined were lymphosarcoma, hemangiosarcoma, mast cell tumor, and mammary cancer. The results for the Golden Retriever were similar to the previous study, but there were notable differences between breeds. In Labrador Retrievers, where about 5 percent of gonadally intact males and females had one or more joint disorders, neutering at <6 mo. doubled the incidence of one or more joint disorders in both sexes. In male and female Golden Retrievers, with the same 5 percent rate of joint disorders in intact dogs, neutering at <6 mo. increased the incidence of a joint disorder to 4–5 times that of intact dogs. The incidence of one or more cancers in female Labrador Retrievers increased slightly above the 3 percent level of intact females with neutering. In contrast, in female Golden Retrievers, with the same 3 percent rate of one or more cancers in intact females, neutering at all periods through 8 years of age increased the rate of at least one of the cancers by 3–4 times. In male Golden and Labrador Retrievers neutering had relatively minor effects in increasing the occurrence of cancers. Comparisons of cancers in the two breeds suggest that the occurrence of cancers in female Golden Retrievers is a reflection of particular vulnerability to gonadal hormone removal.

**Editor:** Roger A. Coulombe, Utah State University, United States of America

**Funding:** This work was supported by the Canine Health Foundation (#01488-A) and the Center for Companion Animal Health University of California, Davis (# 2009-54-F/M). The funders had no role in study design, data collection and analysis, decision to publish, or preparation of the manuscript.

**Competing Interests:** The authors have declared that no competing interests exist.

\* Email: blhart@ucdavis.edu

## Introduction

In the last three decades, the practice of spaying female dogs and castrating males (both referred to herein as neutering) has greatly increased. The current estimate is that in the U.S., 83 percent of all dogs are neutered [1] and, increasingly, neutering is being performed prior to 6 mo., as advocated by many veterinarians and animal activists. The impetus for this widespread practice is presumably pet population control, and the belief that mammary gland and prostate cancers are prevented and aggressive male behavior is markedly less likely than in those neutered later. This societal practice in the U.S. continues to contrast with the general attitudes in many European countries, where neutering is commonly avoided and not promoted by animal health authorities [2–4].

In the last decade or so, studies have pointed to some of the adverse effects of neutering in dogs on several long-term health parameters by looking at one disease syndrome in one breed or in pooling data from several breeds. With regard to cancers, a study on osteosarcoma (OSA) in several breeds found a 2-fold increase in neutered dogs relative to intact dogs [5], and in Rottweilers

neutering prior to 1 year of age was associated with an increased occurrence of OSA to 3–4 times that of intact dogs [6].

A study of cardiac hemangiosarcoma (HSA) in spayed females found that the incidence of this cancer was 4 times greater than that of intact females [7] and another on splenic HSA in spayed females found rates 2 times greater than of intact females [8]. A study on lymphosarcoma (lymphoma, LSA) found that neutered females had a higher incidence of the disease than intact females [9]. Cutaneous mast cell tumors (MCT) were studied in several dog breeds revealing an increase in incidence in neutered females to 4 times that of intact females [10]. Another cancer of concern is prostate cancer that, in contrast to humans, is potentiated by the removal of testosterone. One extensive study found that this cancer occurred in neutered males 4 times as frequently as in intact males [11].

The most frequently mentioned advantage of early neutering of female dogs is protection against mammary cancer (MC) [12]. However, a recent meta-analysis of published studies on neutering females and MC found that the evidence linking neutering to a reduced risk of MC is weak [13].

Three very recent studies are particularly relevant in the discussion of neutering and cancers. One was a comprehensive study, from this center, on neutering in 759 Golden Retrievers where males were compared with females and effects of neutering were evaluated in early-neutered (<1 year), late-neutered (>1 year) and intact dogs [14]. Almost 10 percent of early-neutered males were diagnosed with LSA, 3 times more than intact males. There were no cases of MCT in intact females, but in late-neutered females the rate was nearly 6 percent. The incidence of HSA in late-neutered females was also higher than that of intact females. The occurrence of MC was very low and was only seen in a couple of late-neutered females.

A study utilizing the Veterinary Medical Database of over 40,000 dogs found that neutered males and females were more likely to die of cancer than intact dogs, especially of OSA, LSA and MCT [15]. This study included no information on age of neutering. The most recent publication in this area is a study of Vizslas utilizing owner-reported disease occurrence in an online survey, in which the incidence of cancers was reported higher in neutered dogs than in intact dogs [16]. The main cancers related to neutering were LSA, HSA and MCT. The occurrence of MC was very low in females left intact.

With regard to joint disorders, one study of effects of neutering in larger breeds documents a 3-fold increase in excessive tibial plateau angle – a known risk factor for development of cranial cruciate ligament tears or rupture (CCL) [17]. Across several breeds, a study of CCL found that neutered males and females were 2 to 3 times more likely than intact dogs to have this disorder [18]. Neither study examined early versus late neutering with regard to this disorder. The study from this center of neutering in Golden Retrievers (mentioned above with regard to cancers [14]) included examination of joint disorders. Of the early-neutered males, 10 percent were diagnosed with hip dysplasia (HD), double the occurrence of that in intact males. There were no cases of CCL diagnosed in intact males or females, but in early-neutered males and females the occurrences were 5 percent and 8 percent, respectively.

One factor that merits attention with regard to the effects of neutering on joint disorders relates to documented effects of neutering in increasing body weight [19], as reflected in body condition score (BCS). Additional weight on the joints is considered to play a role in the onset of joint disorders [19,20]. While neutering is expected to increase BCS, the issue of concern here is whether neutered dogs with a joint disorder have consistently higher BCSs at the time of diagnosis than do neutered dogs without the joint disorder in the same age range. In the previous analyses on Goldens [14] there was no consistent and major difference in BCS between early neutered dogs with and without a joint disorder. For dogs diagnosed with a joint disorder, some increase in BCS would be expected as a function of less activity due to discomfort from painful joints. Therefore, a modestly higher BCS was predicted for neutered dogs with a joint disorder than in the neutered counterparts without a joint disorder.

The above study on Golden Retrievers [14] raised a major question about breed differences in the effects of neutering, which are relevant for breeders and caregivers of puppies when deciding if, and when, to neuter. A more basic issue concerns insights into the possible pathogenic factors triggering the occurrence of the cancers under consideration. The present study, using the same veterinary hospital database, explored the effects of neutering on joint disorders and cancers in the popular Labrador Retriever to compare with the Golden Retriever, with an addition of several years to the database. The age periods of neutering were refined as

<6 mo., 6–11 mo., 12–23 mo. (1 year), and 2 through 8 years to provide more detailed information on the effects of gonadal hormone removal. The Golden is known for being particularly vulnerable to cancers [21], so we expected some major differences from the Labrador where cancer-related deaths are less frequent than in Goldens [21].

In addition to reporting on the incidence of the individual joint disorders and cancers, a new slant on analyses in the present study combined the incidence of all three joint disorders that have shown evidence of being increased by neutering (HD, CCL, and elbow dysplasia, ED) for one data-point representing the incidence of dogs diagnosed with at least one of the joint disorders, after controlling for multiple diagnoses. This analysis was based on the perspective that for dog owners or breeders, avoidance of any of the debilitating joint disorders would be of prime interest. This analysis was also deemed logical for pathophysiological reasons because a disruption of the growth plate closure by gonadal hormone removal in the joint developmental stage would be expected to apply to all the joint disorders. The study also combined the incidence of dogs diagnosed with at least one of the cancers (LSA, HSA, MCT) for one data point, after controlling for multiple diagnoses, because for dog owners avoidance of any of the cancers would be important. This analysis seemed logical, as there may be a common factor involved in increasing these three particular cancers in neutered dogs because these cancers are repeatedly reported as being increased by neutering in several studies.

## Methods

### Ethics Statement

No animal care and use committee approval was required because, in conformity with campus policy, the only data used were from retrospective veterinary hospital records. Upon approval, faculty from the University of California, Davis (UCD), School of Veterinary Medicine, are allowed use of the record system for research purposes by the Veterinary Medical Teaching Hospital (VMTH). The co-authors of this study were given permission by the VMTH to use their veterinary hospital records for this study.

### Data Collection

The dataset used in this study was obtained from the computerized hospital record system (Veterinary Medical and Administrative Computer System) of the Veterinary Medical Teaching Hospital (VMTH) at UCD. The subjects included were gonadally intact and neutered female and male Labrador Retrievers and Golden Retrievers, from 1 through 8 years of age and admitted to the hospital between January 1, 2000 and December 31, 2012, for 13 years of data. If a disease of interest occurred before 12 months of age or before January 1, 2000, that case was removed for that specific disease analysis, but included in other disease analyses.

Data on patients at 9 years of age or older were not considered. This was deemed an appropriate cut-off point in order to exclude disease information on advanced-aged dogs where the effects of aging would confound interpreting the disease effects related to neutering. Additional inclusion criteria were requirements for information on date of birth, age at neutering (if neutered) and age of diagnosis (or onset of clinical signs) of the joint disorder or cancer. The age at neutering was classified as <6 mo., 6–11 mo., 1 year (12 - <24 mo.), and 2–8 years (2 - <9 years). For all neutered dogs, the neuter status at the time of each visit was reviewed to ensure that neutering occurred prior to onset of the first clinical signs or diagnosis of any disease of interest. If a disease of interest occurred before neutering, the diseased dog was recorded as intact for that specific disease analysis. For the same dog where a different disease occurred after neutering, the dog was recorded as neutered for that disease analysis. Detailed reviews of patient records were performed for evidence of disease occurrence meeting specific diagnostic criteria (see below). Using this screening, only diseases with at least 15 cases in the database were included in the study.

For both breeds, many cases with neutering did not include detailed data on age at neutering. With a very large database for the Labrador, there was a sufficient number of dogs with these data to restrict the analyses to cases for which the age at time of neutering was available from the record system. For the Golden with fewer cases, where additional neutering date information was necessary, telephone calls to the referring veterinarians were made to obtain the neutering dates for case patients born after 2000. Because of the number of neutered dogs where age at neutering was not available from either the record or by phone call, there were proportionately more intact cases in the final data set than would be expected in the population at large.

Golden Retriever cases with complete data for analyses totaled 1,015, with 543 males (315 neutered and 228 intact) and 472 females (306 neutered and 166 intact). Labrador Retriever cases with complete data for analyses totaled 1,500 cases with 808 males (272 neutered and 536 intact) and 692 females (347 neutered and 345 intact). The number of cases analyzed for each disease varied somewhat among diseases because a case could be excluded for one disease analysis, if the diagnosis was made prior to 1 year of age, was unconfirmed, or was outside of study range, but would be included for other diseases if no diagnosis was made or where the diagnoses were confirmed after 1 year of age and within the study range.

Table 1 defines the categories of diagnoses based on information in the record of each case. A patient was considered as having a disease of interest if the diagnosis was made at the VMTH or by a referring veterinarian and later confirmed at the VMTH. Patients diagnosed with HD, ED and/or CCL presented with clinical signs such as difficulty moving, standing up, lameness, and/or joint pain; diagnoses were confirmed with radiographic evidence, orthopedic physical examination and/or surgical confirmation. Diagnoses of the various cancers (LSA, HSA, MCT, MC) were accompanied by clinical signs such as enlarged lymph nodes, lumps on the skin or presence of masses, and confirmed by imaging, appropriate blood cell analyses, chemical panels, histopathology and/or cytology. Pyometra was confirmed by ultrasonic evidence and/or post-surgically after removal of the uterus. When a diagnosis was listed in the record as "suspected" based on clinical signs, but the diagnostic tests were inconclusive, the case was excluded from the analysis for that specific disease, but included for other diseases.

The analyses used in Figures 1 and 2 portray single data-points representing the incidence of dogs diagnosed with at least one joint disorder or at least one cancer, after controlling for multiple diagnoses. The data for incidence of individual joint disorders and cancers are presented in Tables 2 through 5.

Given that body weights are difficult to compare among dogs because of the confounding factor of variations in body height, BCSs were used. The BCS system used by the VMTH is the standard 1–9 range where a score of 5 is the goal [22]. Typically, the clinician assigns the BCS at the time of a patient's visit to the hospital. For this study the BCSs at the time of diagnosis (or clinical signs) of neutered dogs with joint disorders were compared with BCSs of neutered dogs without the disorder at an age that fell

within the range representing 80 percent of the ages of dogs with the disorder at the time of diagnosis. The BCSs were compared between neutered dogs with and without joint disorders for the disorders that were significantly increased in incidence over that of intact dogs and for just the neuter periods where there were such differences. For the few joint disorders associated with neutering at one year or beyond, the BCSs were not included for comparison to maintain uniformity across comparisons. The data are represented as medians to reduce the impact of outliers.

## Statistical Analyses

While the study set out to estimate incidence rates of each disease related to age at neutering, patients were diagnosed at different ages and with differing durations of the disease as well as varying years at risk from the effects of gonadal hormone removal. Cox proportional hazard models (CPH) [23,24] were used to test for group differences with respect to the hazard of a disease while adjusting for the time of neutering and the animal's age at diagnosis. All analyses were run using the SAS software package, version 9.3. Post hoc comparisons among the subgroups were based on least squares means of the hazard within each subgroup. In the Results section the $p$-values were based on these proportional hazard models. For all statistical tests the two-tailed statistical level of significance was set at $p<0.05$.

## Data Availability

In compliance with journal policy the final dataset used for statistical analyses, with the client information removed for confidentiality, is publically available at figshare.com: http://dx.doi.org/10.6084/m9.figshare.1038819.

## Results

With regard to joint disorders and cancers, the incidence rates at various neuter ages were much more pronounced in the Golden Retrievers than in the Labrador Retrievers. Therefore, results will be presented first for the Golden, and then the Labrador, with the two breeds contrasted. For joint disorders, BCSs are reported for those that differed significantly from the intact dogs, only for the neuter periods where the differences occurred. The mean age of diagnosis of joint disorders and cancers for each sex and breed is given to the nearest 0.5 years.

## Golden Retriever Males: Joint Disorders

Figure 1-A presents the incidence of dogs having at least one of the joint disorders. The incidence of at least one joint disorder occurring in intact males was 5 percent. At neuter age <6 mo., at least one of the joint disorders occurred in 27 percent of the males, or five times the incidence of intact males ($p<0.0001$). At neuter age 6–11 mo., this incidence was 14 percent or almost three times that of intact males ($p<0.005$). In the 2–8 year neutering period there was a moderate rise in this measure to double that of intact males ($p = 0.02$).

As shown in Figure 1-A and in Table 2, the main joint disorder related to neutering in males was HD, which was significantly higher than that of intact males for the <6 mo. and 6–11 mo. neuter periods ($p<0.001$; $p<0.05$, respectively). The mean age of diagnosis of HD in males was 4 years. The other important joint disorder was CCL, which was never diagnosed in intact males, and was significantly higher than intact males in the <6 mo. and 6–11 mo. neuter periods ($p<0.001$; $p = 0.004$, respectively). The mean age of diagnosis of this joint disorder in males was 5 years. In this breed the occurrence of ED was relatively minor compared with the other joint disorders and not significantly above that of

**Table 1.** Categories used in determining diagnosis for joint disorders and cancers of interest in Golden Retrievers and Labrador Retrievers (1–8 years old) admitted to the Veterinary Medical Hospital, University of California, Davis, from 2000–2012.

| Classification | Definition |
| --- | --- |
| No disease | No evidence of a joint disorder or cancer of interest in the medical records |
| VMTH | Diagnosed at the VMTH |
| Referring Veterinarian/VMTH | Diagnosed by referring veterinarian and confirmed at the VMTH through treatment or further testing |
| Referring Veterinarian | Diagnosed by referring veterinarian but no confirming diagnostic tests done at the VMTH. Unconfirmed cases were excluded from analysis for the specific joint disorder or cancer |
| Invalid (suspected) | Diagnosis was suspected based on clinical signs, but diagnostic tests were inconclusive or not done. Unconfirmed cases were excluded from analysis for the suspected joint disorder or cancer |
| Invalid (confirmed) | Diagnosed prior to January 2000 or before 1 year of age. Invalid cases were excluded from analysis for the specific joint disorder or cancer. |

intact males for any neuter period. When it did occur, mean age of diagnosis of ED was 2.5 years.

The median BCS of neutered males with HD was 6.0, and the median BCS of neutered males without HD was 5.5. In intact males with and without HD the median BCS was 5. For neutered males with CCL, the median BCS was 5.5 and for neutered males without CCL, 6.0. In intact males without CCL the median BCS was 5.0.

## Golden Retriever Males: Cancers

Figure 2-A presents the incidence in dogs having at least one of the cancers followed. The level in the intact males was 11 percent. At neuter ages <6 mo. and 6–11 mo. the occurrence of one or more cancers was 15–17 percent, but not significantly different than intact males. However, as Table 3 reveals, the main cancer elevated by neutering in males, LSA, reached 11.5 percent at the 6–11 mo. period, significantly higher than the 4 percent level of intact males ($p = 0.007$). The mean age of diagnosis of LSA in males was 5.5 years.

## Golden Retriever Females: Joint Disorders

Figure 1-A portrays the incidence of dogs having at least one of the joint disorders at different neuter periods. The incidence of at least one joint disorder occurring in intact females was 5 percent, virtually the same as males. At neuter age <6 mo. at least one of the joint disorders occurred in 20 percent of dogs, four times that of the intact females ($p < 0.001$). At the 6–11 mo. neuter age, 13 percent had at least one joint disorder, which was over twice that of intact females, but did not reach significance.

As shown in Table 2, the main joint disorders related to neutering females at the <6 mo. period were HD and CCL, occurring at 10–11 percent. The occurrence of HD did not reach significance compared with intact females (4 percent), but CCL, which was not seen in any of the intact females, was significantly higher at the <6 mo., 6–11 mo. and 2–8 year neuter periods ($p < 0.001$ to $p = 0.03$). The mean age of diagnosis of CCL in females was 5.5 years. As with males, the occurrence of ED in neutered females was not significant over that of intact females. The mean age of diagnosis of ED in females, when it did occur, was 1.5 years.

The median BCS of neutered females with CCL was 6.0 and the median BCS of the neutered females without CCL was 5.5. In intact females without CCL the median BCS was 5.0.

## Golden Retriever Females: Cancers

Figure 2-A presents the incidence of females having at least one of the cancers where the incidence of cancers in intact females was

just 3 percent. The increase in cancers over all the neuter periods ranged from 8 to 14 percent. Combining all of the neuter periods beyond 6 mo. (to have a larger data set for analyses), the elevated incidence level across all these neuter periods was significantly higher than that of intact females ($p = 0.049$). The results reveal that neutering through 8 years of age increases the risk of acquiring at least one of the cancers to a level 3–4 times that of leaving the female dog intact.

Examination of Table 3 shows that the main cancer resulting from neutering females at <6 mo. and 6–11 mo. was LSA where at 6–11 mo. the increased risk over that of intact females reached significance ($p = 0.014$). The mean age of diagnosis of LSA in females was 5.5 years. The main cancer that was increased at the 2–8 year period of neutering was MCT ($p = 0.013$). The occurrence of HSA, although increased by neutering beyond 1 year, did not reach significance over intact females. The mean age of diagnosis of both MCT and HSA in females was 6.5 years.

The occurrence of MC was not seen in any of the intact females. This cancer was seen only in dogs neutered in the 2–8 year period where the incidence was 3.5 percent. The occurrence of pyometra in intact females was 1.8 percent, which was diagnosed at the mean age of 6 years.

## Labrador Retriever Males: Joint Disorders

Figure 1-B illustrates the incidence of males having at least one of the joint disorders. The only neuter period where this measure was significantly increased above the 5 percent level of intact males, was at <6 mo., where this measure was 12.5 percent ($p = 0.014$). Examining the joint disorders individually (Table 4), HD was not increased by neutering at any time. However, at the <6 mo. neuter period, both CCL and ED were significantly increased over that of intact males ($p = 0.02$; 0.02). For ED, there was a moderate increased risk with the 2–8 year neuter period to about 2 percent compared with the low 0.57 percent incidence in intact males ($p = 0.006$). The mean age of diagnosis of ED in males was 3 years, considerably less than that for CCL, which was 4.5 years.

The median BCS of neutered males with CCL was 6.0 and the median BCS of the neutered males without CCL was 5.0. In intact males with CCL the median BCS was 6.0 and for intact males without CCL the median BCS was 5. The median BCS of neutered males with ED was 6.5 and the median BCS of the neutered males without ED was 5.0. In intact males with and without ED the BCS was 5.0.

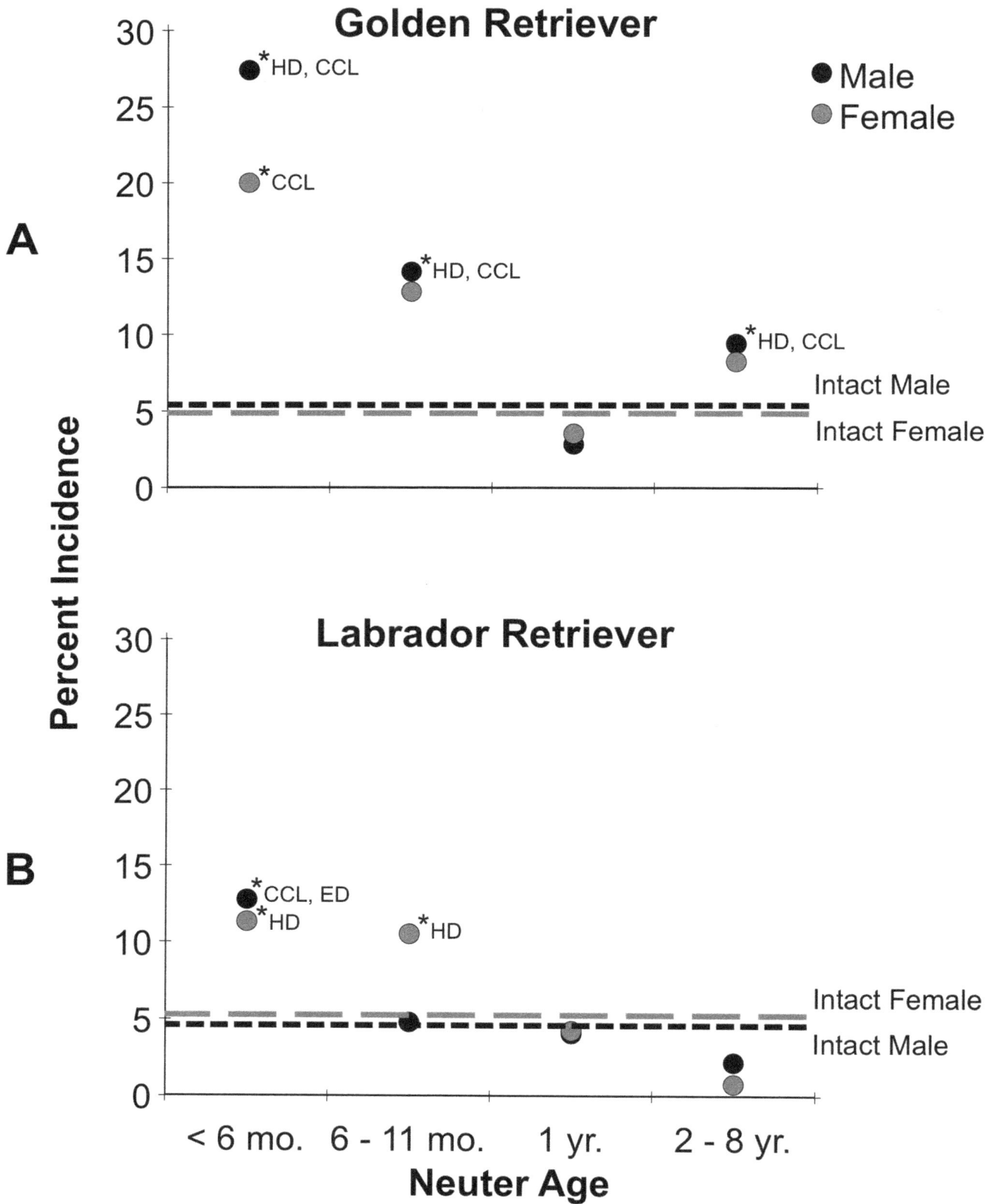

**Figure 1. Incidence of the occurrence of at least one joint disorder in male and female Golden Retrievers (top) and Labrador Retrievers (bottom), as a function of age at neutering.** The occurrences in intact males and females for the same measure are shown by the horizontal lines. The asterisks indicate significance from the intact level, and the abbreviations reveal the joint disorders contributing to the dots when significant.

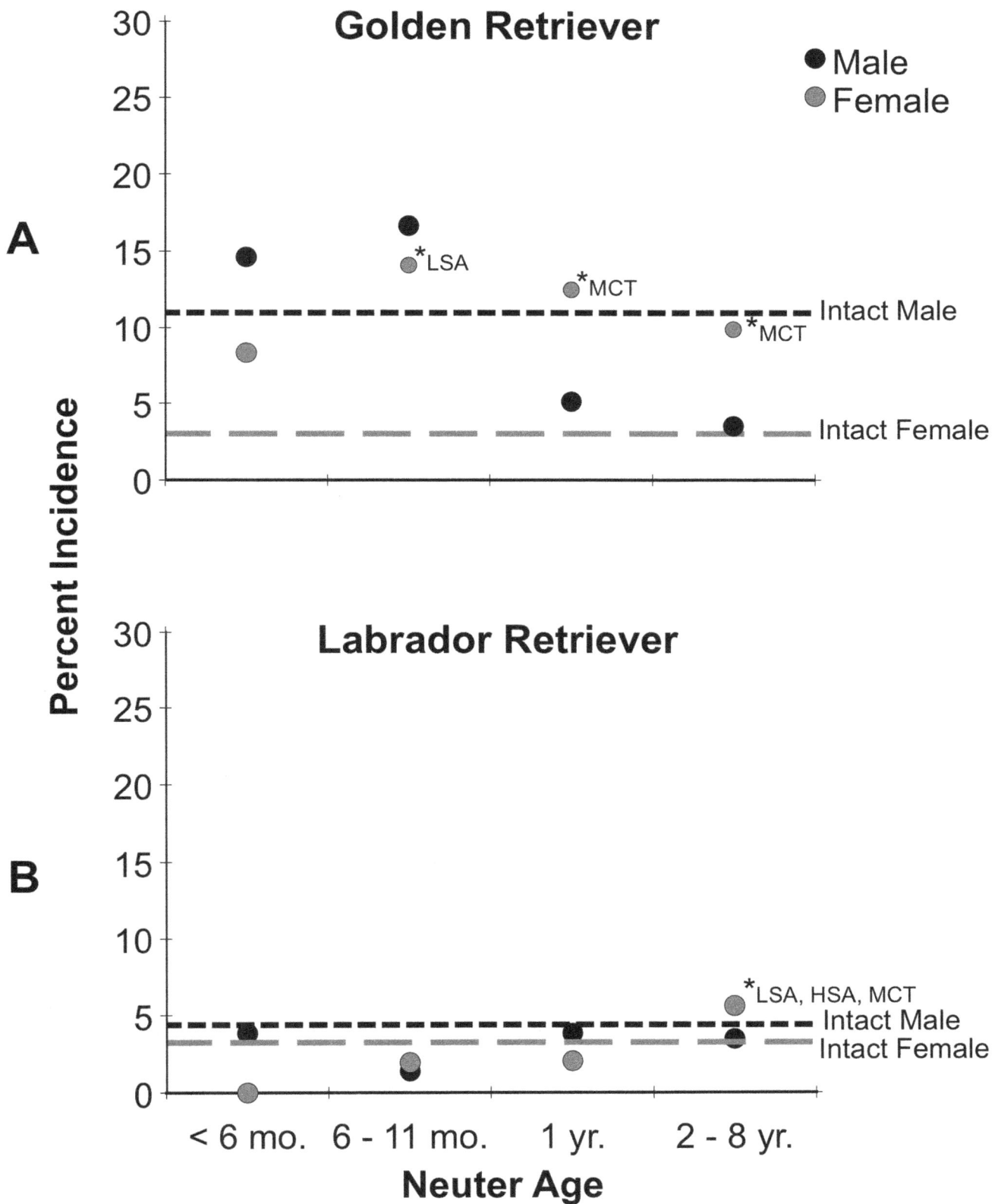

**Figure 2. Incidence of the occurrence of at least one cancer in male and female Golden Retrievers (top) and Labrador Retrievers (bottom), as a function of age at neutering.** The occurrences in intact males and females for the same measures are shown by the horizontal lines. The asterisks indicate significance from the intact level, and the abbreviations reveal the cancers contributing to the dots when significant.

**Table 2.** Golden Retriever males and females, joint disorders.

| | HD | CCL | ED |
|---|---|---|---|
| Male <6 months | **11/75 (14.67)** | **8/89 (8.99)** | 5/84 (5.95) |
| Male 6–11 months | **9/113 (7.96)** | **4/123 (3.25)** | 4/116 (3.45) |
| Male 1 year | 1/38 (2.63) | 0/41 (0) | 0/38 (0) |
| Male 2–8 years | **4/55 (7.27)** | **2/59 (3.39)** | 0/59 (0) |
| Male Intact | 9/221 (4.07) | 0/226 (0) | 5/222 (2.25) |
| Female <6 months | 9/92 (9.78) | **11/101 (10.89)** | 0/97 (0) |
| Female 6–11 months | 4/79 (5.06) | **4/81 (4.94)** | 3/81 (3.7) |
| Female 1 year | 0/30 (0) | 0/32 (0) | 1/30 (3.33) |
| Female 2–8 years | 4/86 (4.65) | **3/89 (3.37)** | 0/88 (0) |
| Female Intact | 6/163 (3.68) | 0/165 (0) | 2/164 (1.22) |

For ages 1 through 8 years, for each neuter period, the joint disorders are: hip dysplasia (HD), cranial cruciate ligament tear or rupture (CCL), and elbow dysplasia (ED). Shown are number of cases over number in the pool, with percentages given in parentheses. When bolded the incidence is significantly above that of intact dogs.

## Labrador Retriever Males: Cancers

The underlying rate of intact males having at least one of the cancers was 4.6 percent. Neutering at any age period had virtually no effect on this measure of cancer occurrence above the level of intact males (Figure 2-B and Table 5).

## Labrador Retriever Females: Joint Disorders

As portrayed in Figure 1-B, at neuter periods <6 mo. and 6–11 mo. the risk of dogs having at least one of the joint disorders increased to about double the 5 percent level of intact females ($p = 0.044$; 0.043). In contrast to male Labradors, the females seemed to be vulnerable to the effects of early neutering on HD but not on ED. The neutering effects on HD were evident through 1 year, where the incidence was 4–5 percent compared to 1.5 percent in intact females (Table 4) ($p = 0.02$–0.046). The mean age of diagnosis of HD was 3.5 years, and for ED, 2.5 years. As in male Labradors, CCL in females was increased by early neutering, but in this sex, not significantly so. The mean age of diagnosis of CCL in females was 5.5 years.

The median BCS of neutered females with HD was 5.5, and the median BCS of neutered females without HD was 5.5. In intact females with HD the median BCS was 7 and for those without HD the median BCS was 5.0.

## Labrador Retriever Females: Cancers

As seen in Figure 2-B, the underlying rate of intact females having at least one cancer of those tracked was 3.2 percent, close to that of males. In contrast to female Goldens, the only increase in the incidence of dogs having at least one cancer, was with the 2–8 year neuter period where the incidence was modestly increased to 5.6 percent ($p = 0.03$), a reflection of the increased occurrence of LSA and MCT (Table 5). The mean age of diagnosis of these two cancers in females was 5.5 and 6.5 years, respectively.

With regard to MC, only 1.4 percent of the intact females were diagnosed with MC. With the 2–8 year neuter period MC was diagnosed in 2 percent of females. Pyometra was diagnosed in just less than 4 percent of intact females. The mean age of diagnosis of pyometra was 5.5 years.

## Discussion

Both the Golden Retriever and Labrador Retriever are very popular breeds that have found wide acceptance as family pets and

**Table 3.** Golden Retriever males and females, cancers.

| | LSA | MCT | HSA |
|---|---|---|---|
| Male <6 months | 6/89 (6.74) | 3/90 (3.33) | 5/90 (5.56) |
| Male 6–11 months | **14/122 (11.48)** | 4/124 (3.23) | 2/122 (1.64) |
| Male 1 year | 0/41 (0) | 1/40 (2.5) | 1/39 (2.56) |
| Male 2–8 years | 0/58 (0) | 2/60 (3.33) | 0/59 (0) |
| Male Intact | 9/226 (3.98) | 8/225 (3.56) | 8/220 (3.64) |
| Female <6 months | 4/98 (4.08) | **3/102 (2.94)** | 1/102 (0.98) |
| Female 6–11 months | **9/82 (10.98)** | 1/81 (1.23) | 1/79 (1.27) |
| Female 1 year | 2/32 (6.25) | **1/32 (3.13)** | 1/32 (3.13) |
| Female 2–8 years | 1/84 (1.19) | **5/88 (5.68)** | 2/84 (2.38) |
| Female Intact | 3/166 (1.81) | 0/165 (0) | 2/165 (1.21) |

For ages 1 through 8 years, for each neuter period, the cancers are: lymphosarcoma (LSA), mast cell tumor (MCT), and hemangiosarcoma (HSA). Shown are number of cases over number in the pool, with percentages given in parentheses. When bolded the incidence is significantly above that of intact dogs.

**Table 4.** Labrador Retriever males and females, joint disorders.

|  | HD | CCL | ED |
|---|---|---|---|
| Male <6 months | 0/48 (0) | **4/53 (7.55)** | **2/48 (4.17)** |
| Male 6–11 months | 1/68 (1.47) | 2/72 (2.78) | 0/67 (0) |
| Male 1 year | 1/50 (2.00) | 1/52 (1.92) | 0/49 (0) |
| Male 2–8 years | 0/92 (0) | 0/93 (0) | **2/93 (2.15)** |
| Male Intact | 9/528 (1.7) | 12/531 (2.26) | 3/525 (0.57) |
| Female <6 months | **3/56 (5.36)** | 3/59 (5.08) | 1/57 (1.75) |
| Female 6–11 months | **5/99 (5.05)** | 5/101 (4.95) | 0/103 (0) |
| Female 1 year | **2/47 (4.26)** | 0/50 (0) | 0/50 (0) |
| Female 2–8 years | 0/131 (0) | 1/128 (0.78) | 0/132 (0) |
| Female Intact | 6/345 (1.74) | 8/343 (2.33) | 4/343 (1.17) |

For ages 1 through 8 years, for each neuter period, the joint disorders are: hip dysplasia (HD), cranial cruciate ligament tear or rupture (CCL), and elbow dysplasia (ED). Shown are number of cases over number in the pool, with percentages given in parentheses. When bolded the incidence is significantly above that of intact dogs.

as service dogs for those with disabilities. The two breeds are similar in body size, conformation and in behavioral characteristics [25], and they share a similar developmental background as upland game retrievers. Using the same database and methodology, the two breeds were contrasted with regard to the effects of neutering on three joint disorders (HD, CCL, ED) and three cancers (LSA, HSA, MCT). In addition to reporting the occurrence of the three joint disorders and the three cancers, an analysis of cases with at least one of the joint disorders, or at least one of the cancers, was plotted graphically (Figures 1 and 2). The findings on the Golden Retriever closely resemble the picture presented in the earlier study drawn from this same database with a somewhat smaller data set [14].

The present study reveals that the breeds respond very differently to the effects of neutering on joint disorders and certain devastating cancers. With regard to the occurrence of one or more joint disorders, in Golden Retrievers, neutering at <6 mo. resulted in an incidence of 27 percent in males and 20 percent in females, 4–5 times the 5 percent level for intact males and females. In male and female Labrador Retrievers, with the same underlying occurrence of joint disorders in intact dogs, neutering at <6 mo. resulted in an incidence of 11–12 percent for one or more joint

disorders, roughly double that of intact males and females. Thus, for both breeds, neutering at the standard <6 mo. period markedly and significantly increased the occurrence of joint disorders, although the increase was worse in the Golden than the Labrador. A difference in the specific joints affected was that in male Goldens HD and CCL were mostly increased, but in male Labradors CCL and ED were increased. The effects of neutering in the first year of a dog's life, especially in larger breeds, undoubtedly reflects the vulnerability of joints to delayed closure of long-bone growth plates from gonadal hormone removal [26,27]. Differences in the two breeds studied here could be due to differences in sensitivities of the growth plates to gonadal hormone removal.

The BCSs in neutered dogs with the different joint disorders were compared with neutered dogs without the joint disorders. Although dogs with the disorders were expected to have a modestly higher BCS as a function of reduced activity from painful joints, the issue of concern was if those with a joint disorder had a consistently and markedly higher BCS than comparable neutered dogs without a joint disorder. The BCS comparisons revealed variable differences, in the range of 0.5 to 1.0 (except for ED in male Labradors where the difference was 1.5). The general picture

**Table 5.** Labrador Retriever males and females, cancers.

|  | LSA | MCT | HSA |
|---|---|---|---|
| Male <6 months | 0/52 (0) | 2/53 (3.77) | 0/53 (0) |
| Male 6–11 months | 0/72 (0) | 0/73 (0) | 1/73 (1.37) |
| Male 1 year | 1/52 (1.92) | 0/51 (0) | 1/51 (1.96) |
| Male 2–8 years | 0/93 (0) | 2/89 (2.25) | 1/93 (1.08) |
| Male Intact | 4/530 (0.75) | 12/533 (2.25) | 7/531 (1.32) |
| Female <6 months | 0/59 (0) | 0/60 (0) | 0/60 (0) |
| Female 6–11 months | 0/104 (0) | 2/103 (1.94) | 0/104 (0) |
| Female 1 year | 0/49 (0) | 1/50 (2) | 0/50 (0) |
| Female 2–8 years | 2/131 (1.53) | 5/126 (3.97) | 0/133 (0) |
| Female Intact | 4/342 (1.17) | 6/344 (1.74) | 1/345 (0.29) |

For ages 1 through 8 years, for each neuter period, the cancers are: lymphosarcoma (LSA), mast cell tumor (MCT), and hemangiosarcoma (HSA). Shown are number of cases over number in the pool, with percentages given in parentheses. When bolded the incidence is significantly above that of intact dogs.

of BCSs of neutered dogs with joint disorders being usually, but not always, a bit higher than the BCSs of neutered dogs without joint disorders, is consistent with the perspective that the increase in joint disorders in neutered dogs is primarily due to the effect of gonadal hormonal removal on bone growth plates and not to greater weight on the joints.

Data on the effects of neutering on the occurrence of cancers in the two breeds also reveal important breed differences. In both breeds the occurrence of one more cancers in intact dogs ranged from 3 to 5 percent, except for Golden Retriever males where the level in intact dogs was 11 percent. In Golden Retriever females neutering females at any neuter period beyond 6 months elevated the risk of one or more cancers to 3 to 4 times the level of intact females (Figure 2). In male Golden Retrievers neutering appeared to have little effect in the occurrence of one or more of the three cancers. An exception was LSA that was increased significantly at the <6 mo. period. In both male and female Labrador Retrievers, neutering at any period appeared to have little effect in increasing cancers.

The striking effect of neutering in female Golden Retrievers compared to male and female Labradors, and male Golden Retrievers, suggests that for this gender and breed the presence of gonadal hormones has a protective effect against cancers over most years of the dog's life. This may reflect a particular sensitivity of receptor sites of some potentially metastatic cancer cells to gonadal hormone removal and/or prolonged levels of the gonadotropin hormone, follicle stimulating hormone [28]. Gonadotropin receptors have been identified in some extragonadal tissues. For example, in the dog these receptor sites have been found in the skin [29] and urinary tract [30]. Treatment of one or more of these cancers by a receptor-site blocking agent may be worth exploring. The relatively high occurrence of one or more of

these cancers in intact male Goldens, coupled with the relative absence of an effect of neutering, except with regard to LSA, points to a relatively high underlying rate of cancer occurrence in this gender and breed that is not affected by gonadal hormone removal.

The findings presented here are clinically relevant in two realms. For dog owners of the popular Golden Retrievers and Labrador Retrievers, the study points to the importance of acquiring information needed to decide if, and when, to neuter. Aside from avoiding increased risks of joint disorders and cancers, there is an indication that age-related cognitive decline could be accelerated by neutering [31]. This is particularly relevant for service dogs where active cognition is important for the expected tasks.

The findings of this study also have important implications for investigators looking for canine models for research on various forms of cancer [32,33]. For some cancers of interest, not only may breeds vary in predisposition but also the possibility of interactions between gender, gonadal hormone influences, and timing of gonadal hormone alteration should be taken into account in selecting the model and in investigating causal factors to be explored.

## Acknowledgments

Special thanks are extended to Marty Bryant, Cristina Bustamante, Valerie Caceres, Madeline Courville, Siobhan Aamoth and Roger Pender.

## Author Contributions

Conceived and designed the experiments: BLH LAH. Performed the experiments: APT BLH LAH. Analyzed the data: NHW APT BLH LAH. Wrote the paper: BLH LAH APT. Edited manuscript: NHW.

## References

1. Trevejo R, Yang M, Lund EM (2011) Epidemiology of surgical castration of dogs and cats in the United States. J Am Vet Med Assoc 238: 898–904.
2. Sallander M, Hedhammer A, Rundgren M, Lindberg JE (2001) Demographic data of population of insured Swedish dogs measured in a questionnaire study. Acta Vet Scand 42: 71–80.
3. Kubinyi E, Turcsan B, Miklosi A (2009) Dog and owner demographic characteristics and dog personality trait associations. Behav Processes 81: 392–401.
4. Diesel G, Brodbelt D, Laurence C (2010) Survey of veterinary practice policies and opinions on neutering dogs. Vet Rec 166: 455–458.
5. Ru G, Terracini B, Glickman LT (1998) Host related risk factors for canine osteosarcoma. Vet J 156:31–39.
6. Cooley DM, Beranek BC, Schlittler DL, Glickman MW, Glickman LT, et al. (2002) Endogenous gonadal hormone exposure and bone sarcoma risk. Cancer Epidemiol Biomarkers Prevent 11: 1434–1440.
7. Ware WA, Hopper DL (1999) Cardiac tumors in dogs: 1982–1995. J Vet Intern Med 13: 95–103.
8. Prymak C, McKee LJ, Goldschmidt MH, Glickman LT (1988) Epidemiologic, clinical, pathologic, and prognostic characteristics of splenic hemangiosarcoma and splenic hematoma in dogs: 217 cases (1985). J Am Vet Med Assoc 193: 706–712.
9. Villamil JA, Henry CJ, Hahn AW, Bryan JN, Tyler JW, et al. (2009) Hormonal and sex impact on the epidemiology of canine lymphoma. J Cancer Epidemiol 2009: 1–7. doi:10.1155/2009/591753
10. White CR, Hohenhaus AE, Kelsey J, Procter-Grey E (2011) Cutaneous MCTs: Associations with spay/neuter status, breed, body size, and phylogenetic cluster. J Am Anim Hosp Assoc 47: 210–216.
11. Teske E, Naan EC, van Dijk E, Van Garderen E, Schalken JA (2002) Canine prostate carcinoma: epidemiological evidence of an increased risk in castrated dogs. Mol Cell Endocrinol 197: 251–255.
12. Root Kustritz MV (2007) Determining the optimal age for gonadectomy of dogs and cats. J Am Vet Med Assoc 231: 1665–1675.
13. Beauvais W, Cardwell JM, Brodbelt DC (2012) The effect of neutering on the risk of mammary tumours in dogs – a systematic review. J Small Anim Pract 53: 314–322.
14. Torres de la Riva G, Hart BL, Farver TB, Oberbauer AM, McV Messam LL, et al. (2013) Neutering Dogs: Effects on Joint Disorders and Cancers in Golden Retrievers. PLOS ONE 2013; 8(2): e55937. doi:10.1371/journal.pone.0055937

15. Hoffman JM, Creevy KE, Promislow DEL (2013) Reproductive capability is associated with lifespan and cause of death in companion dogs. PLOS ONE 2013; 8(4): e6 1082. doi: 10.1371/journal.pone.0061082
16. Zink MC, Farhoody P, Elser SE, Ruffini LD, Gibbons TA, et al. (2014) Evaluation of the risk and age of onset of cancer and behavioral disorders in gonadectomized Vizslas. J Am Vet Med Assoc 244: 309–319.
17. Duerr FM, Duncan CG, Savicky RS, Park RD, Egger EL, et al. (2007) Risk factors for excessive tibial plateau angle in large-breed dogs with cranial cruciate disease. J Am Vet Med Assoc 231: 1688–1691.
18. Witsberger TH, Villamil JA, Schultz LG, Hahn AW, Cook JL (2008) Prevalence of, and risk factors for, hip dysplasia and cranial cruciate ligament deficiency in dogs. J Am Vet Med Assoc 232: 1818–1824.
19. Dobson JM (2013) Breed-predispositions to cancer in pedigree dogs. Vet Sci 2013: 1–23.
20. Kasström H (1975) Nutrition, weight gain and development of hip dysplasia. An experimental investigation in growing dogs with special reference to the effect of feeding intensity. Acta Radiologica 344: 135–179, Supplementum.
21. Duval JM, Budsberg SC, Flo GL, Sammarco Jl (1999) Breed, sex, and body weight as risk factors for rupture of the cranial cruciate ligament in young dogs. J Am Vet Med Assoc 215: 811–814.
22. Baldwin K, Bartges J, Buffington T, Freeman LM, Grabow M, et al. (2010) AAHA nutritional assessment guidelines for dogs and cats. J Am Anim Hosp Assoc 46: 285–296.
23. Cox DR (1972) Regression models and life tables (with discussion). Journal of the Royal Statistical Society, series B, 34: 187–220.
24. Rothman KJ, Greenland S (1998) Modern Epidemiology. Philadelphia: Lippincott Williams & Wilkins.
25. Hart BL, Hart LA (1988) The Perfect Puppy. How to Choose Your Dog by Its Behavior. New York: W.H. Freeman and Co.
26. Salmeri KR, Bloomberg MS, Scruggs SL, Shille V (1991) Gonadectomy in immature dogs: Effects on skeletal, physical, and behavioral development. J Am Vet Med Assoc 198: 1193–1203.
27. Grumbach M (2000) Estrogen, bone growth and sex: a sea of change in conventional wisdom. J Ped Endocrinol Metab 13: 1439–1455.
28. Concannon PW (1993) Biology of gonadotrophin secretion in adult and prepubertal female dogs. J Reprod Fert Supp 47: 3–27.
29. Reichler IM, Welle M, Eckrich C, Sattler U, Barth A, et al. (2008) Spaying-induced coat changes: the role of gonadotropins, GnRH and GnRH treatment on the hair cycle of female dogs. Vet Dermatol 19: 77–87.

30. Fields MJ, Shemesh M (2004) Extragonadal luteinizing hormone receptors in the reproductive tract of domestic animals. Biol Reprod 71: 1412–1418.
31. Hart BL (2001) Effects of gonadectomy on subsequent development of age-related cognitive impairment in dogs. J Am Vet Med Assoc 219: 51–56.
32. Vail DM, MacEwen EG (2002) Spontaneously occurring tumors of companion animals as models for human cancer. Cancer Invest 18: 781–792.
33. Khanna C, Lindblad-Toh K, Vail D, London C, Bergman P, et al. (2006) The dog as a cancer model. Nat Biotechnol 24: 1065–1066.

# 17

# Prevalence of Bovine Tuberculosis and Risk Factor Assessment in Cattle in Rural Livestock Areas of Govuro District in the Southeast of Mozambique

Ivânia Moiane[1,2,3◊], Adelina Machado[3◊], Nuno Santos[1,2], André Nhambir[3], Osvaldo Inlamea[3], Jan Hattendorf[5], Gunilla Källenius[4], Jakob Zinsstag[5], Margarida Correia-Neves[1,2]*

1 Life and Health Sciences Research Institute (ICVS), School of Health Sciences, University of Minho, Braga, Portugal, 2 ICVS/3B's, PT Government Associate Laboratory, Braga/Guimarães, Portugal, 3 Paraclinic Department, Veterinary Faculty, Eduardo Mondlane University, Maputo, Mozambique, 4 Department of Clinical Science and Education, Södersjukhuset, Karolinska Institutet, Stockholm, Sweden, 5 Swiss Tropical and Public Health Institute, Basel, Switzerland

## Abstract

*Background:* Bovine tuberculosis (bTB), caused by *Mycobacterium bovis,* is an infectious disease of cattle that also affects other domestic animals, free-ranging and farmed wildlife, and also humans. In Mozambique, scattered surveys have reported a wide variation of bTB prevalence rates in cattle from different regions. Due to direct economic repercussions on livestock and indirect consequences for human health and wildlife, knowing the prevalence rates of the disease is essential to define an effective control strategy.

*Methodology/Principal findings:* A cross-sectional study was conducted in Govuro district to determine bTB prevalence in cattle and identify associated risk factors. A representative sample of the cattle population was defined, stratified by livestock areas (n = 14). A total of 1136 cattle from 289 farmers were tested using the single comparative intradermal tuberculin test. The overall apparent prevalence was estimated at 39.6% (95% CI 36.8–42.5) using a diagnostic threshold cut-off according to the World Organization for Animal Health. bTB reactors were found in 13 livestock areas, with prevalence rates ranging from 8.1 to 65.8%. Age was the main risk factor; animals older than 4 years were more likely to be positive reactors (OR = 3.2, 95% CI: 2.2–4.7). *Landim* local breed showed a lower prevalence than crossbred animals (*Landim* × *Brahman*) (OR = 0.6, 95% CI: 0.4–0.8).

*Conclusions/Significance:* The findings reveal an urgent need for intervention with effective, area-based, control measures in order to reduce bTB prevalence and prevent its spread to the human population. In addition to the high prevalence, population habits in Govuro, particularly the consumption of raw milk, clearly may potentiate the transmission to humans. Thus, further studies on human tuberculosis and the molecular characterization of the predominant strain lineages that cause bTB in cattle and humans are urgently required to evaluate the impact on human health in the region.

**Editor:** Pere-Joan Cardona, Fundació Institut d'Investigació en Ciències de la Salut Germans Trias i Pujol, Universitat Autònoma de Barcelona, CIBERES, Spain

**Funding:** The research leading to these results has received funding from the European Union's Seventh Framework Program (FP7/2007–2013) under grant agreement n° 221948, ICONZ (Integrated Control of Neglected Zoonoses). The contents of this publication are the sole responsibility of the authors and do not necessarily reflect the views of the European Commission. The funders had no role in study design, data collection and analysis, decision to publish, or preparation of the manuscript.

**Competing Interests:** The authors have declared that no competing interests exist.

* E-mail: mcorreianeves@ecsaude.uminho.pt

◊ These authors contributed equally to this work.

## Introduction

Bovine tuberculosis (bTB) is an infectious disease of cattle caused by *Mycobacterium bovis,* a member of the *Mycobacterium tuberculosis* complex. This chronic disease also affects a wide range of other domestic and wildlife animals and may also cause disease in humans [1].

Worldwide, bTB is considered one of the seven most neglected endemic zoonoses, presenting a complex epidemiological pattern and with the highest prevalence rates in cattle found in African countries, part of Asia and of the Americas [2]. In affected countries, the disease has an important socio-economic and public health-related impact, and represents also a serious constraint in the trade of animals and their products [3]. In developed countries, bTB was regarded as one of the major diseases of domestic animals until the 1920s [4], when preventive and control measures based on tuberculin skin test and subsequent slaughter of positive reactors and sanitary surveillance in slaughterhouses, began to be systemically applied [5]. After implementation of the control programs, bTB in cattle populations was greatly reduced or even eradicated [3]. Nevertheless, wildlife species are still considered a significant source of infection and responsible for the failure of the complete eradication of livestock bTB in some developed countries [6]. Unfortunately, a vaccination strategy for animals is not available and present bTB control strategies are expensive and difficult to implement. Consequently, in developing countries, where bTB remains of economic and public health importance [7], these strategies are often not in use or not applied systematically [1,8]. In addition, it is estimated that in Africa 90% of the milk is consumed raw or fermented, increasing the risk of bTB transmission to humans [9].

In order to develop an effective national program for bTB surveillance and control in developing countries, accurate data on bTB prevalence is needed [10]. In Mozambique, data on bTB epidemiology is still scarce and mostly unpublished. However, bTB is estimated to be one of the most important causes of economic losses in cattle production, due to rejection of carcasses at the slaughterhouse and limitations on trade, both intra-community and between districts [11]. Surveillance and control programs based on the tuberculin skin test in cattle at the farm and subsequent slaughter of positive reactors are not applied system-atically and do not cover the small holder sector due to the costs with replacement of slaughtered animals [11]. Additionally, there are no effective measures for preventing the transmission of zoonotic diseases and a "bridge" between control programs of bTB and human tuberculosis has not been implemented.

In Mozambique's Govuro district, a great proportion of the population holds livestock animals (especially cattle and goats). According to the findings of positive skin test reactors, associated with lesions compatible with bTB found at slaughterhouses, the Provincial Livestock Services (SPP) considered Govuro positive for bTB [11] but accurate information on the bTB prevalence and its role in human tuberculosis is missing. Control measures are nowadays only based on compulsory test for bTB in cattle to be transferred for breeding or rearing purposes. While slaughter for local consumption is uncommon (only in traditional ceremonies), animals are frequently sold to be consumed in the south of the country. In Govuro there is extensive consumption of untreated milk, direct contact between people and livestock, together with malnutrition and a high prevalence rate of HIV infection, all of which constitute risk factors for this zoonosis. Also still unknown (but crucial to minimize disease propagation) are the main risk factors contributing to the spread of the disease between animals.

Previous studies conducted in Govuro in 2008, using the single intradermal tuberculin test (SITT) in the caudal fold and in the middle neck region of cattle, found prevalence values of 61.94% (n = 268) [11]. This represents the highest recorded prevalence in

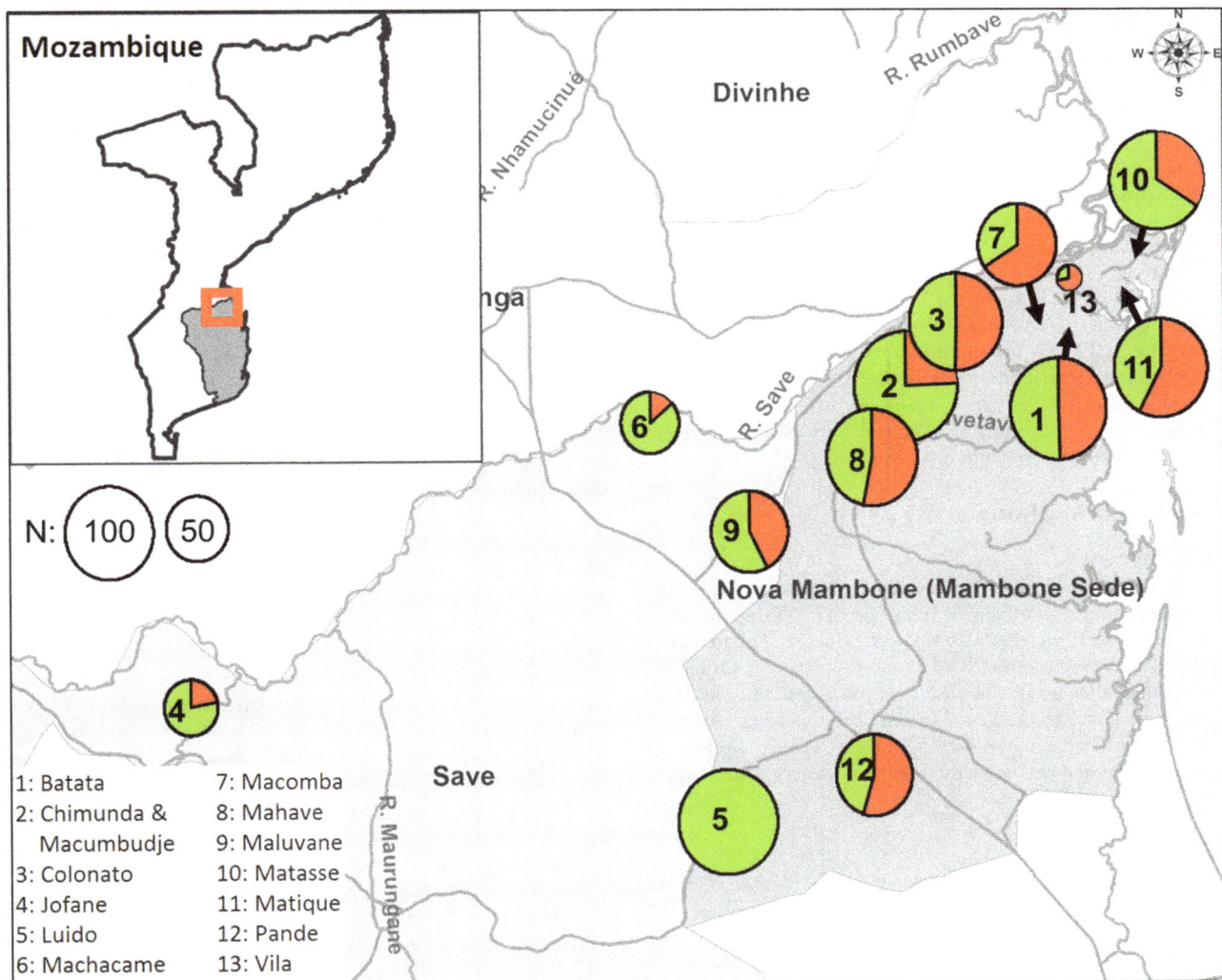

Figure 1. Location of the study district Govuro and spatial distribution of positive reactor cattle. The circle size is proportional to the number of animals tested in each location, and red area denotes the proportion of positive animals.

**Table 1.** Basic characteristics of the sample.

| Characteristics | Classes | n | % |
|---|---|---|---|
| Gender | Female | 773 | 68.0 |
| | Male | 362 | 31.9 |
| | Not recorded | 1 | 0.1 |
| Age | 0–1 yr (calf) | 38 | 3.3 |
| | 1–4 yrs (steer) | 245 | 21.6 |
| | >4 yrs (bull, cow, ox) | 852 | 75.0 |
| | Not recorded | 1 | 0.1 |
| Breed | Landim | 468 | 41.2 |
| | Crossbred (Landim × Brahman) | 534 | 47.0 |
| | Bonsmara | 88 | 7.7 |
| | Other | 11 | 1.0 |
| | Not recorded | 35 | 3.1 |
| Body condition score | Good | 705 | 62.1 |
| | Reasonable | 337 | 29.7 |
| | Poor | 86 | 7.6 |
| | Very poor | 2 | 0.2 |
| | Not recorded | 6 | 0.5 |

cattle in the country, however only two livestock areas of the district were analyzed. In order to determine the prevalence rate of bTB in Govuro we conducted a cross-sectional survey covering a representative sample of the cattle population of all livestock areas within the district. The single comparative intradermal tuberculin test (SCITT) was used since its specificity is higher than the one from the SITT [12]. While the SITT is the standard diagnostic test used in the Mozambican Bovine Tuberculosis Control Program, the SCITT is the confirmatory test and can also be used as screening test in herds with a history of cross-reactivity. We also assessed intrinsic determinants of disease associated with SCITT positivity in the study area in order to define strategies suitable to bTB control in cattle in Govuro.

## Materials and Methods

### Ethics Statement

The purpose of this study was explained to the cattle owners and an informed consent was obtained. While the SITT is the standard diagnostic test used in the Mozambican Bovine Tuberculosis Control Program we used the SCITT due to its higher specificity and to the fact that using this more complete test the data for SITT was also obtained. The Mozambican National Animal Health authority (*Direcção Nacional de Serviços Veterinários*) approved the present study and provided the ethical clearance (Nota 162/MINAG/DNSV/900/2013).

### Study Area

A cross-sectional study was carried out in the Govuro district (Figure 1) located in the northern part of Inhambane province, south-eastern Mozambique. The region is bordered on the north by the Machanga district of the Sofala province (across the Save River), on the east by the Indian Ocean, on the south by Inhassoro district and on the west by the Mabote district. The district covers an area of 3,960 km$^2$ with an estimated population of 35,500 inhabitants. The climate is tropical dry in the interior and humid close to the coast with an average temperature of 25.5°C (18–33°C). The rainy and dry seasons generally occur around October to March and April to September, respectively [13]. Govuro comprises 2 administrative posts (Nova Mambone and Save), 5 localities, 14 livestock areas and 45 villages containing an estimated number of 773 farmers and 8,760 cattle heads.

### Animals and Production Systems Tested for Bovine TB

The animals included in this study were from the small holder sector or from the commercial sector. In the small holder sector most animals were longhorn *Landim* cattle (local breed, mixed *Bos indicus* and *Bos taurus*) and crossbreeds (*Landim × Brahman*) and with herds typically comprised of both these cattle breeds. Cattle were kept traditionally in a free-range grazing system using communal grazing grounds (without supplementation) and watering points such as small puddles (formed throughout the grazing area during the rainy season) or the Save River (during the dry season) [11]. Animals received little veterinary assistance, mostly restricted to vaccination. Animals from the commercial sector were mostly of *Simmental* (*Bos taurus*), *Brahman* (*Bos indicus*) and *Bonsmara* (mixed *Bos indicus* and *Bos taurus*) breeds. They were reared under semi-intensive farming with limited grazing areas (maintained in fences separated from cattle of the small holder sector) and with established water sources. Veterinary assistance and supplementation were provided. Whilst in the commercial sector the livestock production was mainly market-oriented, in the small holder farming animals were frequently used to till the ground and to transport material and people. Livestock trading in the small holder sector is restricted to special occasions, essentially when there is scarcity in agriculture production; in case of diseases and medical assistance is needed; to raise money for children's school fees or other essential livelihood assets for the family such as food items, soap and clothes.

**Table 2.** Apparent prevalence of bTB in Govuro per livestock area.

| Livestock area | Animals tested | | Bovine PPD SCITT reactors | | | Bovine PPD SITT reactors | | | Avian PPD SITT reactors | | |
|---|---|---|---|---|---|---|---|---|---|---|---|
| | Total | Read | n | % | 95% CI | n | % | 95% CI | n | % | 95% CI |
| Batata | 133 | 117 | 58 | 49.6 | 40.7–58.5 | 78 | 66.7 | 57.7–74.6 | 17 | 14.5 | 9.3–22.0 |
| Macomba | 101 | 79 | 52 | 65.8 | 54.9–75.3 | 60 | 75.9 | 65.5–84.0 | 7 | 8.9 | 4.4–17.2 |
| Colonato | 173 | 111 | 56 | 50.5 | 42.3–59.6 | 70 | 63.1 | 53.8–71.5 | 12 | 10.8 | 6.3–18.0 |
| Jofane | 37 | 37 | 8 | 21.6 | 11.4–37.2 | 11 | 29.7 | 17.5–45.8 | 1 | 2.7 | 0.5–13.8 |
| Maluvane | 84 | 76 | 32 | 42.1 | 31.7–53.3 | 39 | 51.3 | 40.3–62.2 | 4 | 5.3 | 2.1–12.8 |
| Matasse | 123 | 115 | 39 | 33.9 | 25.9–43.0 | 53 | 46.1 | 37.2–55.2 | 16 | 13.9 | 8.6–21.4 |
| Chimunda | 75 | 62 | 27 | 43.5 | 31.9–56.0 | 37 | 59.7 | 47.2–71.0 | 16 | 25.8 | 16.6–37.9 |
| Mahave | 150 | 105 | 56 | 53.3 | 43.8–62.6 | 74 | 70.5 | 61.2–78.4 | 15 | 14.3 | 8.9–22.2 |
| Matique | 142 | 111 | 64 | 57.7 | 48.4–66.4 | 83 | 74.8 | 66.0–82.0 | 22 | 19.8 | 13.5–28.2 |
| Pande | 95 | 74 | 41 | 55.4 | 44.1–66.2 | 46 | 62.2 | 50.8–72.4 | 8 | 10.8 | 5.6–19.9 |
| Luido | 130 | 125 | 0 | 0.0 | 0.0–3.0 | 1 | 0.8 | 0.1–4.4 | 8 | 6.4 | 3.3–12.1 |
| Vila | 43 | 7 | 5 | 71.4 | 35.9–91.8 | 5 | 71.4 | 35.9–91.8 | 0 | 0.0 | 0.0–35.4 |
| Machacame | 45 | 43 | 6 | 14.0 | 6.6–27.3 | 9 | 20.9 | 11.4–35.2 | 3 | 7.0 | 2.4–18.6 |
| Mucumbudje | 90 | 74 | 6 | 8.1 | 3.8–16.6 | 20 | 27.0 | 18.2–38.1 | 8 | 10.8 | 5.6–19.9 |
| Total | 1421 | 1136 | 450 | 39.6 | 36.8–42.5 | 586 | 51.6 | 48.7–54.5 | 137 | 12.1 | 10.3–14.1 |

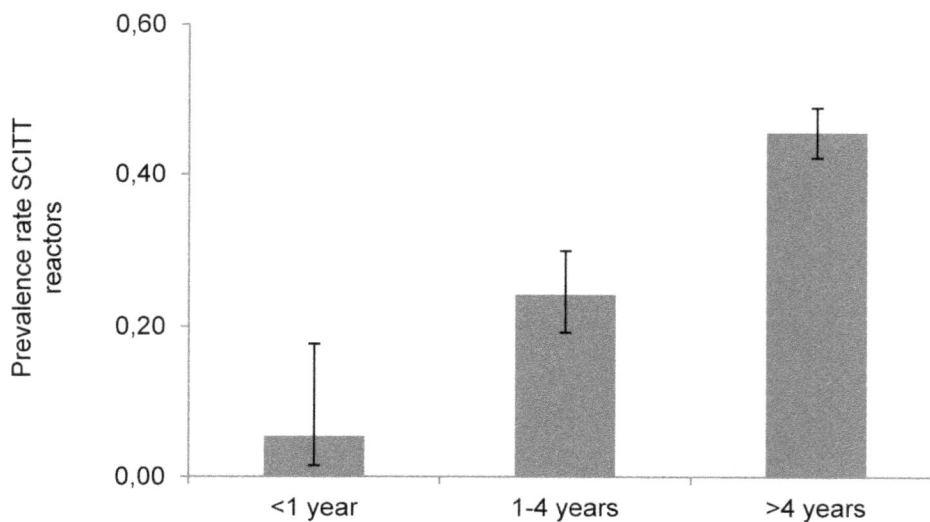

**Figure 2. Prevalence rates among SICTT reactors (95% confidence intervals) by age classes.**

## Sample Size Calculation and Study Animals

To obtain a sample size representative of the Govuro district cattle population, the number of animals to be tested was calculated with Epicalc 2000 (Brixton Books v.1 2), using an expected prevalence of 10% and precision measured as one-half length of the 95% confidence interval of 5%. Sample sizes were calculated for each livestock area and corrected for finite population sizes. The epidemiological unit of this study was the livestock area, which corresponds to the cattle from several owners belonging to the same village. Even belonging to distinct owners, animals have regular direct contact between them and share natural pasture areas and watering sites (grazing groups) or even cowsheds. All cattle of the district (estimated as n = 8,763) was included in the sampling frame. The required sample sizes for the livestock areas ranged from 45 to 139 animals and resulted in a total sample size of n = 1,443 (Details are provided in Appendix S1).

All cattle owners from each livestock area were contacted to participate. The vast majority of the owners brought their animals to pre-defined locations. For the owners that could not bring the animals to the testing place we went to their home place. As a result more than 6,000 cattle participated, out of an estimated population of 8,760. Animals were selected randomly by systematic sampling according to the sample size previously determined and the number of cattle present on the day of the test. They were moved through a cattle chute and every $k^{th}$ animal was selected for sampling, being k the number of animals presented for testing in that livestock area divided by the intended sample size for that same livestock area. At the time of SCITT testing, each animal was identified by a numbered ear tag and individual animal data on age, gender, breed, body condition score (BCS) and owner were registered. Information regarding the age of the animals was provided by the farmers and the breed was determined according to the phenotypic characteristics. The body condition was scored using the guidelines established by Nicholson and Butterworth [14]; all study animals were categorized in four groups: very poor (1), poor (2 to 3), reasonable (4 to 6) and good (score, 7 to 9).

## Single Comparative Intradermal Tuberculin Test

The purpose of the study was explained to the owners with the assistance of local veterinary services (SDAE), community leaders, the local prosecutor and trusted intermediaries. SCITT was performed by intradermal injections of both avian and bovine purified protein derivates (PPD) in the middle neck region (usually on the right side) according to the method described by the World Organization for Animal Health standards [2]. Briefly, two sites of about 2 cm$^2$ diameter, approximately 12 to 15 cm apart, were shaved and the skin thickness was measured using a manual caliper. Aliquots of 0.1 ml containing 20,000 IU/ml of bovine PPD (Bovituber PPD, Synbiotics Europe, Lyon, France) and 0.1 ml with 25,000 IU/ml of avian PPD (Avituber PPD, Synbiotics Europe, Lyon, France) were injected using two different syringes into the dermis in the corresponding shaved area. Palpation of a small grain-like thickening at each site of injection was done to confirm the correct intradermal injection. Three days after injection, the tested animals were brought back for reading. The relative change in skin appearance was classified as swelling or induration followed by measurement of skin thickness at both injection sites. Skin thickness measurements on testing and reading day were performed by the same person to avoid errors related to individual variations in technical procedure.

The SCITT results were analyzed and interpreted according to the recommendations of the World Organization for Animal Health standards [2]. The reaction was considered positive if the increase in skin thickness at the bovine PPD site of injection ($B_{72}$-$B_0$) was at least 4 mm greater than the reaction at the avian PPD injection site ($A_{72}$-$A_0$). The livestock area was considered positive for bTB if at least one positive reactor was found.

Additionally we determined the SITT results by analyzing the same dataset taking into consideration only the bovine PPD data, using the same cutoff. Also, to assess the prevalence of reactors to other sensitising organisms such as *Mycobacterium avium*, the skin reactions at the injection site of the avian PPD alone were analyzed; animals that reacted to the avian PPD with an increase in skin thickness equal or superior to 4 mm were considered reactors to *M. avium*. Geographical coordinates were registered at the central point of each livestock area by a hand held global positioning system.

**Table 3.** Risk factors associated with positive reaction to SCITT.

| Risk factor | Category | Positive/total | Positive (%) | Univariate analysis | | Multivariate analysis | | |
|---|---|---|---|---|---|---|---|---|
| | | | | OR | 95% CI | OR | 95% CI | p |
| Age | ≤4 yrs | 62/283 | 22 | reference | | reference | | |
| | >4 yrs | 388/854 | 45 | 2.9 | 2.0–4.1 | 3.2 | 2.2–4.7 | <0.001 |
| Gender | Female | 259/773 | 38 | reference | | reference | | |
| | Male | 155/362 | 43 | 1.1 | 0.8–1.4 | 1.2 | 0.9–1.6 | 0.300 |
| Breed | Landim × Brahman | 265/534 | 50 | reference | | reference | | |
| | Landim | 167/468 | 36 | 0.7 | 0.5–0.9 | 0.6 | 0.4–0.8 | 0.002 |
| | Bonsmara[a] | 0/88 | 0 | nd | | nd | | |
| Body condition score | Good | 250/705 | 35 | reference | | reference | | |
| | Reasonable | 153/337 | 45 | 1.0 | 0.8–1.4 | 1.0 | 0.7–1.4 | 0.820 |
| | Poor and Very poor | 44/88 | 50 | 1.4 | 0.8–2.3 | 1.3 | 0.7–2.1 | 0.410 |

[a]Excluded from the multivariate model to avoid quasi separation.

## Data Analysis

All data at individual animal level were entered into a Microsoft Access database. Data analysis was performed in R statistical software (v2.15.1). Prevalence, odds ratios (OR) and their 95% confidence intervals were adjusted for correlation within livestock areas using generalized linear mixed models with binary outcome and livestock area as random effect.

## Results

### Sample Characteristics

Over the study period a total of 1,419 cattle were injected with PPDs and measurements were obtained from 1,136 animals (80%) belonging to 289 farmers. Table 1 shows the main characteristics of the sample tested. One hundred and twenty five (11%) animals came from the commercial sector (all from the Luido area) and 1,011 (89%) from the small holder sector. About two third of the cattle were female. The age distribution was as follows: 3% of the animals between 0 to 1 years old (calf - "<1 year"); 22% between 1 to 4 years old (steer - "1–4 years"); and 75% were older than 4 years (bull, cow and ox - ">4 years"). Almost half (49%) of the animals were of crossbreeds (*Landim × Brahman*), 43% *Landim* and 8% *Bonsmara*. *Simmental*, *Brahman* and *Limousine* were tested only in one herd from the commercial sector in Luido representing 1% of the sample. Sixty-two percent of all animals tested were classified as having good BCS, 30% reasonable BCS, and a small proportion presented poor (8%) and very poor (0.2%) BCS. Characteristic measures were not recorded for a few animals (Table 1).

### Cattle bTB Prevalence in Govuro

The results of the SCITT are presented in Table 2 as prevalence per livestock area. The overall apparent prevalence of SCITT positive reactors was 39.6% (95% CI: 36.8–42.5). Except in Vila, where most of the PPD-inoculated animals failed the reading day, representative samples were obtained for each of the other 13 livestock areas. Among them, only in Luido, where the animals were all from the commercial sector, no SCITT positive reactors were detected (Table 2). In addition, data shows that bTB prevalence rates vary remarkably between livestock areas (ranging from undetectable up to 65.8%).

SCITT results showed that 137 (12%; 95% CI: 10.3–14.1) out of 1,136 cattle tested were positive reactors to avian PPD (Table 2). Among the 137 cattle with a positive reaction to avian PPD, 49 (36%; 95% CI: 28.2–44.1) had an overall SCITT test also positive but 24 (18%; 95% CI: 12.1–24.8) showed a stronger response to avian PPD than to bovine PPD.

### Risk Factors Associated with Positive Reaction to SCITT

Univariate and multivariate analysis showed that age and breed represented intrinsic risk factors associated with positive reaction to SCITT (Table 3). Animals older than 4 years were more likely to be infected compared to young animals (45.4% *vs* 21.9%; OR = 3.2, 95% CI 2.2–4.7) (Table 3), and this difference was statistically significant even when considering the age classes "<1 year", "1–4 years" and ">4 years" ($\chi^2 = 55.56$; d.f. = 2, P<0.001) (Figure 2). Male animals tended to show higher prevalence rates for bTB (42.7% *vs* 37.2% in females), but there was no statistically significant difference in reactivity to the SCITT test between gender ($\chi^2 = 2.20$; d.f. = 1; P>0.05).

The rates of SCITT bTB reactors were higher in crossbreeds (*Landim × Brahman*) when compared to local *Landim* breed. Out of 468 of the *Landim* breed animals tested, 167 were found to be positive for the disease (35.7%; 95% CI 31.5–40.1) whereas 265 out of 534 (49.6%; 95% CI 45.4–53.9) in the crossbred (*Landim* × *Brahman*) cattle were positive reactors (Table 3). These data revealed a statistically significant association between the type of breeds and bTB prevalence, where the *Landim* breed seemed to be at lower risk for infection (OR = 0.6; 95% CI 0.4–0.8). All animals of the breed *Bonsmara* belonged to two private farmers from the livestock area Luido, where no positive reactors were found (0/88).

## Discussion

Our results show that bTB is highly prevalent in Govuro district, with an overall prevalence rate of 39.6%. The sample size in each livestock area was slightly lower than targeted and the observed prevalence was closer to 50%, consequently, the precision associated with the prevalence estimates for the single livestock areas was lower than planned in the sample size calculation. However, the overall prevalence and risk factors were associated with high precision and narrow interval estimates. The SCITT has a less than perfect sensitivity, with a range of 52.0–95.5%, dependent on local factors [12]. Adjusting for the relatively low sensitivity of the SCITT, we estimated that the true prevalence in Govuro district is likely to be substantially higher than the apparent prevalence. The Rogan-Gladen estimator yielded a true prevalence of 65%, assuming a test specificity of 0.96 and sensitivity of 0.59, recalculated from data on Chadian cattle [15].

A high prevalence of bTB was observed in almost all livestock areas where small scale farming was practiced, in sharp contrast with what was observed in the commercial sector (only present in Luido), where no SCITT positive animals were detected. While in the commercial sector animals are normally tested for bTB and kept in quarantine before being introduced, trading of animals among breeders in the small holder sector is frequently performed without previous information about bTB status of the animals. In addition, the two tested farms in Luido were established in 2008, only four years before sampling. Interestingly, in the two livestock areas with the lowest bTB prevalence in the small holder sector (Mucumbudje and Machacame), livestock was just recently introduced (years 2007–2008). Our data show that age of the animals was an important intrinsic risk factor, most probably associated with increased exposure to *M. bovis* with lifetime. The type of management system applied in the small holder sector in Govuro, with sharing of water points and grazing areas, and close contact between animals from the same or different herds, promotes the spread of respiratory diseases such as bTB [4,16,17]. Additionally, during vaccination campaigns or external deworming, the animals from different farmers or herds use the same dip tanks. In contrast, animals from the commercial sector are kept inside fences and reared on a rotational grazing system with no contact with cattle from the small holder sector.

A study carried out in 2008 in the same region reported a bTB prevalence rate of 61.9% (95% CI: 55.8–67.8) [11]. Together with the present study, these data suggests that bTB is stable at an extremely high prevalence in the region. In the previous study the covered sample was limited to two livestock areas (Colonato and Vila), whereas in the present study all livestock areas were included. In addition, this study by Macucule et al. [11] made use of the single intradermal tuberculin test (SITT) while in the present study we made use of the SCITT. When our data were analyzed taking in consideration only the bovine PPD result, which corresponds to the SITT, the prevalence rates obtained (63.6%, 95% CI: 0.55–0.72) were similar to what was reported from these two livestock areas in 2008.

The choice of the SCITT instead of the SITT has been shown to be of relevance to differentiate between animals infected with *M. bovis* and those responding to bovine PPD possibly as a result of exposure to other mycobacteria. In fact, in our study the overall prevalence of bTB, taking into consideration only the bovine PPD results, was 51.6% (95% CI: 48.7–54.5), clearly higher than the one determined using the SCITT. This higher rate of positive SITT reactors can be attributed to sensitization with cross-reactive antigens among mycobacterial species and related genera [2].

According to the definitions of positivity, the animals that reacted equally to both PPDs (avian and bovine) were classified as negative reactors to SCITT [2]. Reactivity to the avian PPD may indicate infection or simply exposure to species of the *M. avium* complex or other environmental mycobacteria. This reactivity, however, may indicate a mixed reaction to both agents and hence the classification of bTB negative might also lead to some false negatives. The equal reactivity in both sites of injections (avian and bovine PPD) could be related with a generalized sensitization in which the immune response is not specific to a particular mycobacteria species.

In our study we found 137 (12%) animals that reacted positively to the avian PPD, a finding that has also been previously described. In a cross-sectional study done in Uganda, Inangolet et al. [18] attributed the high number of avian reactors in cattle with the existence of large poultry population in the studied areas, where chicken production in a free-ranging system is common. Fecal contamination of the watering sources was indicated as the main route of transmission of *M. avium* to cattle. In our study area, poultry production is a common activity, nevertheless the system where cattle are kept in corrals (mainly during the night), away from residences, do not promote direct and frequent contact between these two species. The reactivity in the avian PPD in Govuro could be associated with the high population density of cattle egret (*Bubulcus ibis*) in the district. This species is usually found along grazing cattle (removing ticks and flies from the animals). In fact, the presence of *M. avium* subsp. *avium* was already found in fecal samples of cattle egret [19] which could constitute a source of spread to the cattle.

The causative agent of avian tuberculosis, *M. avium* subsp. *avium*, was the predominant MAC isolated from tuberculous lesion in cattle [20]. The role of small ruminants (goats and sheep) as vector of *M. avium* subsp. *avium* and *Mycobacterium avium* subsp. *paratuberculosis* has also been identified [3]. In Govuro, the predominant production system is the communal/pastoral system, where the small ruminants graze together with cattle. Sharing of pastures and watering points could represent a potential source of infection of *M. avium* to cattle. However, according to Okuni et al. [21], paratuberculosis in cattle was not reported in Mozambique. Further studies are necessary to clarify the source of the avian PPD reactions found in cattle in Govuro.

In accordance with findings from numerous cross-sectional studies conducted in both developed and developing countries [e.g. 18,22–25], our results show that age was the main individual risk factor. Some authors suggest that it could be related to increased duration of exposure with age, with older cattle being more likely to have been exposed than the younger [24,26]. Out of 38 calves tested only 2 (5.26%) had a positive result on SCITT. The low number of positive cases in young animals may be associated with the predominance of gamma delta ($\gamma\delta$) T cells in calves that have been shown to play a relevant role in antimycobacterial immunity [27]. The positive calves (although in low number) could be due to congenital transmission in utero [28]. In addition, ingestion of contaminated colostrum has already been reported as another route of bTB transmission [29], as well as pseudo-vertical transmission (close contact between cow and its calf) [30].

The analysis of our bTB reactors according to gender showed that, although the reactivity among males was slightly higher (43% *versus* 38%) the difference was not statistically significant. Male cattle were identified as being the group at highest risk in other studies due to their particular longevity in the herd, given their use as draught oxen, facilitating maintenance of the infection in the herds [22]. Higher reactivity of females than males was previously reported in dairy cows [18,25] and associated with their maintenance in the same herd for several years [5]. In Govuro, however, male cattle tend to be maintained for longer periods in the herds since they are commonly used for plowing the land and pull carts for transportation of people and goods.

Most of the cattle included in the present study were crossbreed (*Landim* × *Brahman*) and *Landim* local breed and bTB prevalence rates were found to be significantly higher in this later breed. The cattle recorded as *Simmental* and *Bonsmara* breed, from the two commercial sector farms in Luido, were too few to allow a relevant comparison of susceptibility. Several studies [31,32] have shown a variation in susceptibility to bTB among cattle breeds, with European breeds (*Bos taurus*) being less resistant compared to Zebu cattle (*Bos indicus*). Although crossbred cattle in Ethiopia (local *Bos indicus* breed Arsi × Holstein *Bos taurus* breed) has been suggested to exhibit intermediate levels of susceptibility [31], our data does not support this observation, as animals with more Zebu background (*Landim* × *Brahman*) showed higher bTB prevalence than *Landim* cattle. It should be mentioned that differences in bTB prevalence between breeds - as observed in several studies - can be influenced by different husbandry conditions; however, genetic variations among cattle breeds are also likely to have an influence on susceptibility to infection with *M. bovis*. The genetic variations among cattle breeds have an influence on susceptibility to infection with *M. bovis*. In diverse breeds of British cattle, the genomic regions INRA111 and BMS2753 were strongly associated with bTB infection status [33]. Two others loci have also been linked to susceptibility in Holstein cattle, namely, a variant in the TLR1 gene [34] and BTA 22 [35].

Several studies reported a correlation between body condition and bTB [e.g. 10,36]. In our study animals in reasonable and poor or very poor body condition showed more positive skin test results than animals in good body condition, however this difference did not reach statistical significance. Following recommendations by Humblet *et al.* [5], this parameter should be analyzed carefully, since while a poor BCS might be a cause of disease, it is also extremely influenced by the seasonal climatic changes (rain or dry season) and the consequently more or less availability of pasturage and/or prevalence of intestinal parasites (in the small scale small holder farming of Govuro deworming for internal parasites is

uncommon). It was reported previously [10,36] that animals in very poor body condition could be non-responsive to the SCITT due to anergy caused by immune-suppression. Our results do not support this finding. In addition, in cross-sectional studies, the status of the animal before becoming infected is not known, and thereby it is impossible to distinguish if the poor body condition was a risk factor or if it is a consequence of advanced stage of bTB.

This is the first systematic study on bTB prevalence encompassing a representative sampling of all livestock areas of a particular district in Mozambique. The data clearly show that bTB is a serious problem in Govuro district with extremely high prevalence rates being maintained for several years. Our results strengthen the notion that if strong measures were undertaken, as was the case among the commercial sector, the disease might be controlled. It is of relevance to stress that drinking raw milk is a common habit in Mozambique, especially for young children that take in charge the livestock grazing. In addition, due to their stature, children that graze animals may be extremely exposed to *M. bovis* airborne transmission from infected animals. Taking all this into account and the fact that studies on human tuberculosis have not been systematically performed in Govuro (neither for *M. tuberculosis* nor *M. bovis*) our results reinforce the need not just to undertake bTB control measures in the region but also the urgency to investigate the prevalence of tuberculosis in humans, especially in children in Govuro.

## Acknowledgments

Disclaimer: The contents of this publication are the sole responsibility of the authors and do not necessarily reflect the views of the European Commission.

The authors thank Yolanda Vaz for critical analysis of the data, Nadine Santos for her careful reading of the manuscript, and important advice and the Provincial Livestock Services of Inhambane Province, District Services of Economic Activities of Govuro district and the field staff for their valuable help and support during fieldwork.

## Author Contributions

Conceived and designed the experiments: IM AM JH GK JZ MCN. Performed the experiments: IM AM AN OI MCN. Analyzed the data: IM AM NS JH GK MCN. Contributed reagents/materials/analysis tools: AM JH GK MCN. Wrote the paper: IM AM NS JH GK MCN.

## References

1. Etter E, Donado P, Jori F, Caron A, Goutard F, et al. (2006) Risk analysis and bovine tuberculosis, a re-emerging zoonosis. Ann N Y Acad Sci 1018: 61–73.

2. OIE (2009) Manual of diagnostic tests and vaccines for terrestrial animals. World Animal Health Organization. Paris, France. Version adopted by the World Assembly of Delegates of the OIE in May 2009. Available: http://www.oie.int/eng/normes/mmanual/A_summry.htm. Accessed 2013 Jul 12.

3. Biet F, Boschiroli ML, Thorel MF, Guilloteau LA (2005) Zoonotic aspects of *Mycobacterium bovis* and *Mycobacterium avium-intracellulare* complex (MAC). Vet Res 36: 411–436.

4. Cosivi O, Grange JM, Daborn CJ, Raviglione MC, Fujikura T, et al. (1998) Zoonotic tuberculosis due to *Mycobacterium bovis* in developing countries. Emerg Infect Dis 4(1): 59–70.

5. Humblet MF, Gilbert M, Govaerts M, Fauville-Dufaux M, Walravens K, et al. (2009) New assessment of bovine tuberculosis risk factors in Belgium based on nationwide molecular epidemiology. J Clinic Microb 48(8): 2802–2808.

6. Schiller I, Oesch B, Vordermeier M, Palmer M, Harris B, et al. (2010) Bovine tuberculosis: a review of current and emerging diagnostic techniques in view of their relevance for disease control and eradication. Transb Emerg Dis 57(4): 205–220.

7. Awah-Ndukum J, Kudi AC, Bah GS, Bradley G, Tebug SF, et al. (2012) Bovine tuberculosis in cattle in the highlands of Cameroon: seroprevalence estimates and rates of tuberculin skin test reactors at modified cut-offs. Vet Med Int 2012, article ID 798502, doi:10.1155/2012/798502.

8. Ayele WY, Neill SD, Zinsstag J, Weiss MG, Pavlik I (2004) Bovine tuberculosis: an old disease but a new threat to Africa. Int J Tub Lung Dis 8: 924–937.

9. Ibrahim S, Cadmus SIB, Umoh JU, Ajogi I, Farouk UM, et al. (2012) Tuberculosis in humans and cattle in Jigawa state, Nigeria: risk factors analysis. Vet Med Int 2012, article ID 865924, doi:10.1155/2012/865924.

10. Tschopp R, Schelling E, Hattendorf J, Aseffa A, Zinsstag J (2009) Risk factors of bovine tuberculosis in cattle in rural livestock production systems of Ethiopia. Prev Vet Med 89(3–4): 205–211.

11. Macucule BA (2008) Study of the prevalence of bovine tuberculosis in Govuro District, Inhambane Province, Mozambique. MSc Thesis – University of Pretoria, South Africa. 66 p.

12. de la Rua-Domenech R, Goodchild AT, Vordermeier HM, Hewinson RG, Christiansen KH, et al. (2006) Ante mortem diagnosis of tuberculosis in cattle: a review of the tuberculin tests, γ-interferon assay and other ancillary diagnostic techniques. Res Vet Sci 81: 190–210.

13. Ministério da Administração Estatal (2005) Perfil do Distrito de Govuro – Província de Inhambane. Available: http://www.govnet.gov.mz/, 39 p. Accessed 2013 Jul 12.

14. Nicholson MJ, Butterworth MH (1986) A guide to condition scoring in Zebu cattle. Addis Abeba, Ethiopia: International Livestock Centre for Africa. 29 p. Available: http://ftpmirror.your.org/pub/misc/cd3wd/1005/_ag_zebu_cattle_condition_score_ilcaenlp118060.pdf. Accessed 2013 Jul 12.

15. Müller B, Vounatsou P, Ngandolo BNR, Diguimbaye-Djaïbe C, Schiller I, et al. (2009) Bayesian receiver operating characteristic estimation of multiple tests for diagnosis of bovine tuberculosis in Chadian cattle. PLoS ONE 4(12): e8215, doi:10.1371/journal.pone.0008215.

16. Ameni G, Vordermeier M, Firdessa R, Aseffa A, Hewinson G, et al. (2011) Mycobacterium tuberculosis infection in grazing cattle in central Ethiopia. Vet J 188(3–4): 359–361.

17. Boukary AR, Thys E, Abatih E, Gamatié D, Ango I, et al. (2011) Bovine tuberculosis prevalence survey on cattle in the rural livestock system of Torodi (Niger). PLoS ONE 6(9): e24629, doi:10.1371/journal.pone.0024629.

18. Inangolet FO, Demelash B, Oloya J, Opuda-Asibo J, Skjerve E (2008) A cross-sectional study of bovine tuberculosis in the transhumant and agro-pastoral cattle herds in the border areas of Katakwi and Moroto districts, Uganda. Trop Anim Healt Prod 40: 501–508.

19. Dvorska L, Matlova L, Ayele WY, Fischer OA, Amemori T, et al. (2007) Avian tuberculosis in naturally infected captive water birds of the Ardeideae and Threskiornithidae families studied by serotyping, IS901 RFLP typing, and virulence for poultry. Vet Microb 119(2–4): 366–374.

20. Pavlik I, Matlova L, Dvorska L, Shitaye JE, Parmova I (2005) Mycobacterial infections in cattle and pigs caused by Mycobacterium avium complex members and atypical mycobacteria in the Czech Republic during 2000–2004. Vet Med Cz 50: 281–290.

21. Okuni JB, Dovas CI, Loikopoulos P, Bouzalas IG, Kateete DP, et al. (2012) Isolation of Mycobacterium avium subspecies paratuberculosis from Ugandan cattle and strain differentiation using optimized DNA typing. BMC Vet Res 8: 99, doi:10.1186/1746-6148-8-99.

22. Kazwala RR, Daborn CJ, Sharp JM, Kambarage DM, Jiwa SFH, et al. (2001) Isolation of Mycobacterium bovis from human cases of cervical adenitis in Tanzania: a cause for concern? Int J Tub Lung Dis 5(1): 87–91.

23. Ameni G, Aseffa A, Engers H, Young D, Hewinson G, et al. (2006) Cattle husbandry in Ethiopia is a predominant factor for affecting the pathology of bovine tuberculosis and gamma interferon responses to mycobacterial antigens. Clin Vac Imm 13: 1030–1036.

24. Cleaveland S, Shaw DJ, Mfinanga SG, Shirima G, Kazwala RR, et al. (2007) Mycobacterium bovis in rural Tanzania: risk factors for infection in human and cattle populations. Tuberc 87(1): 30–43.

25. Dinka H, Duressa A (2011) Prevalence of bovine tuberculosis in Arsi zone of Oromia, Ethiopia. Afric J Agr Res 6(16): 3853–3858.

26. Cook AJ, Tuchili LM, Buve A, Foster SD, Godfrey-Fausett P, et al. (1996) Human and bovine tuberculosis in the Monze District of Zambia–a cross-sectional study. Brit Vet J 152(1): 37–46.

27. Kennedy HE, Welsh MD, Bryson DG, Cassidy JP, Forster FI, et al. (2001) Modulation of immune responses to Mycobacterium bovis in cattle depleted of WC1+ γδ T cells. Inf Imm 70(3): 1488–1500.

28. Ozyigit MO, Senturk S, Akkoc A (2007) Suspected congenital generalized tuberculosis in a newborn calf. Vet Rec 160(9): 307–308.

29. Zanini MS, Moreira E, Lopes MT, Mota P, Salas CE (1998) Detection of Mycobacterium bovis in milk by polymerase chain reaction. J Vet Med B 45: 473–479.

30. Phillips CJ, Foster CR, Morris PA, Teverson R (2003) The transmission of Mycobacterium bovis infection to cattle. Res Vet Sci 74(1): 1–15.

31. Vordemeier M, Ameni G, Berg S, Bishop R, Robertson B, et al. (2012) The influence of cattle breed on susceptibility to bovine tuberculosis in Ethiopia. Comp Imm Microb Inf Dis 35: 227–232.

32. Ameni G, Aseffa A, Engers H, Young D, Gordon S, et al. (2007) High prevalence and increased severity of pathology of bovine tuberculosis in Holsteins compared to zebu breeds under field cattle husbandry in Central Ethiopia. Clin Vac Imm 14(10): 1356–1361.

33. Driscoll EE, Hoffman JI, Green LE, Medley GF, Amos W (2011) A preliminary study of genetic factors that influence susceptibility to bovine tuberculosis in the British cattle Herd. PLoS ONE 6(4): e18806, doi:10.1371/journal.pone.0018806.

34. Sun L, Song Y, Riaz H, Yang H, Hua G, et al. (2012) Polymorphisms in toll-like receptor 1 and 9 genes and their association with tuberculosis susceptibility in Chinese Holstein cattle. Vet Imm Immunopat 147(3–4): 195–201.

35. Finlay EK, Berry DP, Wickham B, Gormley EP, Bradley DG (2012) A genome wide association scan of bovine tuberculosis susceptibility in Holstein-Friesian dairy cattle. PLoS ONE 7(2): e30545, doi:10.1371/journal.pone.0030545.

36. Nega M, Mazengia H, Mekonen G (2012) Prevalence and zoonotic implications of bovine tuberculosis in Northwest Ethiopia. Int J Med Sci 2(9): 188–192.

# 18

# Subcutaneous Immunization with Inactivated Bacterial Components and Purified Protein of *Escherichia coli, Fusobacterium necrophorum* and *Trueperella pyogenes* Prevents Puerperal Metritis in Holstein Dairy Cows

Vinícius Silva Machado, Marcela Luccas de Souza Bicalho, Enoch Brandão de Souza Meira Junior, Rodolfo Rossi, Bruno Leonardo Ribeiro, Svetlana Lima, Thiago Santos, Arieli Kussler, Carla Foditsch, Erika Korzune Ganda, Georgios Oikonomou, Soon Hon Cheong, Robert Owen Gilbert, Rodrigo Carvalho Bicalho*

Department of Population Medicine & Diagnostic Sciences, College of Veterinary Medicine, Cornell University, Ithaca, New York, United States of America

## Abstract

In this study we evaluate the efficacy of five vaccine formulations containing different combinations of proteins (FimH; leukotoxin, LKT; and pyolysin, PLO) and/or inactivated whole cells (*Escherichia coli, Fusobacterium necrophorum,* and *Trueperella pyogenes*) in preventing postpartum uterine diseases. Inactivated whole cells were produced using two genetically distinct strains of each bacterial species (*E. coli, F. necrophorum,* and *T. pyogenes*). FimH and PLO subunits were produced using recombinant protein expression, and LKT was recovered from culturing a wild *F. necrophorum* strain. Three subcutaneous vaccines were formulated: Vaccine 1 was composed of inactivated bacterial whole cells and proteins; Vaccine 2 was composed of proteins only; and Vaccine 3 was composed of inactivated bacterial whole cells only. Two intravaginal vaccines were formulated: Vaccine 4 was composed of inactivated bacterial whole cells and proteins; and Vaccine 5 was composed of PLO and LKT. To evaluate vaccine efficacy, a randomized clinical trial was conducted at a commercial dairy farm; 371 spring heifers were allocated randomly into one of six different treatments groups: control, Vaccine 1, Vaccine 2, Vaccine 3, Vaccine 4 and Vaccine 5. Late pregnant heifers assigned to one of the vaccine groups were each vaccinated twice: at 230 and 260 days of pregnancy. When vaccines were evaluated grouped as subcutaneous and intravaginal, the subcutaneous ones were found to significantly reduce the incidence of puerperal metritis. Additionally, subcutaneous vaccination significantly reduced rectal temperature at $6\pm1$ days in milk. Reproduction was improved for cows that received subcutaneous vaccines. In general, vaccination induced a significant increase in serum IgG titers against all antigens, with subcutaneous vaccination again being more effective. In conclusion, subcutaneous vaccination with inactivated bacterial components and/or protein subunits of *E. coli, F. necrophorum* and *T. pyogenes* can prevent puerperal metritis during the first lactation of dairy cows, leading to improved reproduction.

**Editor:** Daniela Flavia Hozbor, Universidad Nacional de La Plata, Argentina

**Funding:** This study was funded by a grant from Merck Animal Health. The funders had no role in study design, data collection and analysis, decision to publish, or preparation of the manuscript.

**Competing Interests:** Rodrigo Carvalho Bicalho, Robert Owen Gilbert, Marcela Luccas de Souza Bicalho, and Vinicius Silva Machado have a pending patent entitled "Vaccine for the prevention of uterine diseases" (Application number 61/731,333) on the vaccine technology described in this manuscript. This study was funded by Merck Animal Health. There are no further patents, products in development or marketed products to declare.

* E-mail: rcb28@cornell.edu

## Introduction

Postpartum uterine diseases of dairy cows compromise animal welfare and may result in early removal from the herd or impaired reproductive performance. Puerperal metritis is defined by an abnormally enlarged uterus and a fetid, watery, red-brown uterine discharge associated with signs of systemic illness (decreased milk yield, dullness, or other signs of toxemia) and temperature >39.5°C within 21 d after parturition. Endometritis refers to inflammation of the uterus without systemic illness, happening later than 21 d postpartum [1]. In North America, metritis affects 10% to 20% of cows [2], whereas the incidence of endometritis is approximately 28%, ranging from 5.3% to 52.6% [3,4]. Puerperal metritis is commonly treated with antibiotics like penicillin or third-generation cephalosporins. However, antibiotic resistance worldwide is recognized already as a top public health challenge facing the 21st century, and thus there is growing concern regarding the potential impact of extensive use of antibiotics in food animals, including later-generation cephalosporins [5,6]. Overton and Fetrow (2008) reported the cost of each case of metritis to be approximately US$329–386, due to antibiotic treatment and the detrimental effects of metritis on reproductive performance, milk production, and survivability [7].

An efficacious vaccine against uterine diseases will have a significant positive impact on the dairy industry, limiting the use of antibiotics, and decreasing economic losses due to these disorders. Owing to the multifactorial nature of puerperal metritis and endometritis, a vaccine should likely be multivalent, including antigens from the most important etiological agents of uterine infections.

*Escherichia coli, Trueperella pyogenes* and *Fusobacterium necrophorum* are the primary bacterial causes of uterine diseases [8–10]. In the first days postpartum, *E. coli* is the predominant bacteria in the infected uterus, and is highly associated with uterine inflammation and impaired reproductive performance [11–13]. This early uterine contamination with *E. coli* leads to subsequent infection by *F. necrophorum* and *T. pyogenes* at 7 and >25 days postpartum, respectively [12,14], which are associated with both metritis [9,11,12] and endometritis [15,16].

Recently, two studies reported that FimH, an *E. coli* type 1 pilus adhesive protein that plays a critical role in adhesion to mannosides [17] and colonization of epithelial surfaces [18], is an important virulence factor that enables intrauterine *E. coli* to colonize the endometrium and initiate the uterine infection process [10,19]. *E. coli* strains expressing type 1 pili containing FimH are the most important cause of urinary tract infection (**UTI**) in humans [20]. Immunization against FimH prevented *E. coli* colonization of the bladder mucosa in mice [21]. Additionally, the prevalence of liver abscesses, caused by *F. necrophorum* and *T. pyogenes* [22], was reduced successfully with a single dose of a vaccine containing inactivated *F. necrophorum* leukotoxin (**LKT**) and *T. pyogenes* pyolysin (**PLO**) [23]. Therefore, pre-partum immunization of cows with FimH, LKT and PLO may also reduce potentially the incidence of uterine diseases in dairy cattle.

Both intravaginal and systemic immunization against FimH, LKT, PLO, and relevant isolates of *E. coli*, *F. necrophorum* and *T. pyogenes* appear to be interesting strategies to successfully prevent bovine uterine diseases. Intravaginal immunization with a whole-cell vaccine has been shown to be very promising in the prevention of human urinary tract infection (UTI) [24,25], increasing total vaginal and urinary IgG and IgA [24], and decreasing the risk of UTI in women [25]. On the other hand, results from other studies suggest that a systemic antibody response has a key role in local immunological protection in the bovine reproductive tract [26,27], because most of the bovine intrauterine immunoglobulin is serum-derived [26], and opsonic activity of cervicovaginal mucus from cows immunized systemically was higher than from cows immunized intravaginally [27].

Our hypothesis was that pre-partum immunization against relevant antigens for postpartum uterine diseases would prevent the occurrence of puerperal metritis and endometritis. For this purpose, we formulated 5 different vaccines (3 subcutaneous and 2 intravaginal) containing different combinations of proteins (FimH, LKT, PLO) and/or inactivated whole cells (*E. coli*, *F. necrophorum* and *T. pyogenes*). We report here that subcutaneous immunization effectively reduced the incidence of puerperal metritis, leading to enhanced reproductive performance.

## Materials and Methods

### Ethics statement

The field trial was conducted in a commercial dairy farm located near Ithaca, NY. This farm was selected because of its long working relationship with the Ambulatory and Production Medicine Clinic at Cornell University, and the trial was authorized by the farm owner, who was aware of all procedures. The research protocol was reviewed and approved by the Institutional Animal Care and Use Committee of Cornell University (Protocol number: 2011-0111).

### Inactivated bacterial components

*E. coli* strains 4612-2 and 12714-2 were selected because they possess virulence factors found to be associated with the occurrence of metritis (Bicalho et al., 2010). Each strain possess FimH and at least one of astA, cdt, kpsII, ibeA, and hly, which are virulence factors common to extraintestinal and enteroaggregative *E. coli*. Strains were grown aerobically on Luria-Bertani (LB) broth (Sigma-Aldrich) at 37°C. They were inoculated with 1% of an overnight culture and grown in 800 ml of medium, with agitation (150 rpm). For strain 12714-2, cells were harvested at 4 h, with an $OD_{600}$ of 0.432 and $1.0 \times 10^9$ CFU/ml; for strain 4612-2, cells were harvested at 3.5 h, $OD_{600}$ of 0.473 and $1.2 \times 10^9$ CFU/ml. The cultures were inactivated with 0.1% formalin for 12 h, and the cells were concentrated 4-fold (final volume of 200 ml), so 0.25 ml of each strain would be present in the final vaccine formulation, with approximately $10^9$ CFU per dose.

*Trueperella pyogenes* strains 10481-8 and 6375-1 were isolated from the uterine lumen of dairy cows. Strains were grown on VersaTREK REDOX 1 (Trek Diagnostic Systems, OH) in 7% $CO_2$ at 37°C. Cells were harvested at 48 h, with $1.3 \times 10^8$ and $0.5 \times 10^8$ CFU/ml for strains 10481-8 and 6375-1, respectively. The cultures were inactivated with 0.1% formalin for 12 h, and 1 ml of each strain was added to the final vaccine formulation, with approximately $10^8$ CFU per dose.

*Fusobacterium necrophorum* strains 5663 and 513 were isolated from the uterine lumen of dairy cows. Strains were grown on VersaTREK REDOX 2 (Trek Diagnostic Systems, OH) anaerobically at 37°C. All cultures were inactivated with 0.1% formalin for 12 h before the cells were concentrated. Cells were harvested at 12 h, with $1.6 \times 10^{12}$ and $1.8 \times 10^{12}$ CFU/ml for strains 513 and 5663, respectively. The cultures were inactivated with 0.1% formalin for 12 h, and 0.01 ml of each strain was added to the final vaccine formulation, with approximately $10^{10}$ CFU per dose.

### Recombinant protein expression and purification

To generate the expression plasmids encoding PLO, The *PLO* gene, lacking the coding region for the predicted signal sequence, was amplified from *T. pyogenes* ATCC49698 genomic DNA by PCR with a 5′ primer containing an *Xho*I site (5′-ACAG-CATCCTCGAGTGCCGGATTGGGAAAC-3′) and a 3′ primer containing an *Eco*RI site (5′-TGGAATTCCCTAGGATTTGA-CATTGT-3′) [28]. The 1.5-kb amplicon was digested with *Xho*I-*Eco*RI and cloned into *Xho*I-*Eco*RI-digested pTrcHisB (Invitrogen, NY).

The portion of the *FimH* gene encoding the signal peptide and the first 156 amino acids (the mannose-binding lectin domain, LD, [29]) of the mature protein was amplified from plasmid pET-22b(+)-F3-LD [30], provided by Dr. Evgeni Sokurenko, University of Washington, WA. The 5′ primer used contained a *Bam*HI site (5′-CGCGGATCCATGAAACGTGTTATTACCCTG-3′) and the 3′ primer contained a *Hin*dIII site (5′-CCCAAGCTTC-TAGTGATGGTGATGGTGATGGCCGCCAGTAGGCAC-CAC-3′) and a six-histidine tag following the authentic sequence of the protein. The amplicon, approximately 0.6 kb, was digested with *Bam*HI-*Hin*dIII and cloned into *Bam*HI-*Hin*dIII-digested pTrcHisA (Invitrogen).

Bacteria were harvested after 5 hours of induction and cells were disrupted by two passages through a French pressure cell (Amicon) at 20,000 psi (138 Mpa), and the insoluble material was removed by centrifugation at 12,000×g for 30 min. His-tagged recombinant proteins were purified using TALON metal affinity resin (Clontech, CA) according to the manufacturer's instructions. Isolated pure protein fraction was concentrated using a fiber concentration/desalting system using a filter with a molecular weight exclusion of 10 kDa (Amicon ultra 100K, Millipore, MA) and subjected to SDS-PAGE (15%) using the Mini-PROTEAN Tetra Cell electrophoresis system (Bio-Rad, CA), following standard protocols. Protein concentration was determined by the Bradford method [31].

A total of 30 liters of culture was grown to produce a total of 321.24 mg of His-PLO. The final volume of His-PLO was 41 ml and the final concentration was 7.83 mg/ml. A total of 92 liters of culture was grown to produce 216.34 mg of $FimH_{1-156}$-His. The final volume of $FimH_{1-156}$-His was 172.5 ml and the concentration was 1.25 mg/ml.

**Culture concentrated supernatant and affinity purification of Leukotoxin.** *F. necrophorum* strain 6586 was grown in VersaTREK REDOX 2 for 12 h anaerobically at 37°C. The culture supernatant was concentrated at 4°C in a hollow fiber concentration/desalting system using a filter with a molecular weight exclusion of 100 kDa (Amicon ultra 100K, Millipore, MA). Affinity purification of LKT was performed to evaluate the concentration of LKT in the *F. necrophorum* 6586 culture concentrated supernatant, as described in [32]. Briefly, purified mAb F7B10 (3.5 mg) was coupled to 5 ml of Affi-Gel 10 affinity support (Bio-Rad, CA) and packed in a 1×20 cm column. The *F. necrophorum* 6586 culture concentrated supernatant was applied to the column, and non-binding materials were removed by passing 15 mL of 0.5 M NaCl in PBS through the column. Purified LKT was eluted with 0.2 M glycine-HCl (pH 3.0), immediately neutralized with NaOH, and washed and concentrated using an Amicon ultra 10K. Purity of the toxin was determined by SDS-PAGE.

A total of 10 L of *F. necrophorum* 6586 was grown to produce 220 mL of concentrated supernatant containing 0.186 mg/ml of LKT. The presence and concentration of LKT in the concentrated supernatant was determined by affinity purification.

## Vaccine formulation

Five different vaccine formulations were made: three subcutaneous vaccines (Vaccines 1–3) and two intravaginal vaccines (Vaccine 4–5). Vaccine 1 was composed of inactivated bacterial whole cells (*E. coli*, *T. pyogenes* and *F. necrophorum*) and proteins (FimH, PLO and LKT); Vaccine 2 was composed only of proteins (FimH, PLO and LKT); and Vaccine 3 was composed only of inactivated bacterial whole cells (*E. coli*, *T. pyogenes* and *F. necrophorum*). Vaccine 4 was composed of inactivated bacterial whole cells (*E. coli*, *T. pyogenes* and *F. necrophorum*) and proteins (FimH, PLO and LKT), and Vaccine 5 was composed only of proteins (PLO and LKT). The adjuvant for the subcutaneous vaccines was aluminum hydroxide (Rehydragel HPA, General Chemical, NJ). The adjuvant volume used in the subcutaneous vaccines was 25% of the final vaccine volume. Aluminum hydroxide was added to each component separately, and it was gently stirred overnight. The adjuvant for the intravaginal vaccines was 20 μg/dose of Cholera toxin (List Biological Laboratories, Inc., CA).

All vaccine components were tested for sterility before the final vaccine was assembled and bottled. Sterility was evaluated by culturing 100 μl of vaccine component aerobically in LB broth, aerobically in 7% $CO_2$ on VersaTREK REDOX 1 and anaerobically on VersaTREK REDOX 2 at 37°C for 48 h. Components were considered contaminated if there was bacterial growth in any of the three culture media by the end of the incubation period.

Assessment of endotoxin levels was performed using the LAL Endpoint Assay (Hycult Biotech, The Netherlands) following the manufacturer's instructions. All vaccine formulations had endotoxin levels below $10^5$ EU/ml.

## Farm and management

Holstein pregnant heifers were enrolled from May 24, 2012 to August 16, 2012; the follow-up period continued until April 30, 2013. The farm milked 3,300 Holstein cows 3 times daily in a double 52-stall parallel milking parlor. All animals were subjected to the same immunization protocol prior and during the study period. At three months of age, all animals we immunized with Vista 5 SQ (Merck Animal Health, NJ), Covexin (Merck Animal Health, NJ), and Piliguard Pinkeye Triview (Merck Animal Health, NJ). They received a booster of each vaccine 2 weeks later. At 11 months, they received another dose of Vista 5 SQ. Furthermore, at 200 days of pregnancy, they were immunized with Triangle 9 (Boehringer Ingelheim Vetmedica, Inc., MO), and Covexin. At 250 and 264 they were immunized with J-Vac (Merial, GA), and Scourguard (Zoetis, NJ). Finally, at 35 DIM, they were immunized with Vista 5 SQ and J-Vac, and at the first pregnancy diagnosis date, they received another dose of J-Vac.

The heifers were housed in freestall barns with concrete stalls covered with mattresses and bedded with manure solids. All cows were offered a total mixed ration (TMR) consisting of approximately 55% forage (corn silage, haylage, and wheat straw) and 45% concentrate (corn meal, soybean meal, canola, cottonseed, and citrus pulp) on a dry matter basis of the diet. The diet was formulated to meet or exceed the NRC nutrient requirements for lactating Holstein cows weighing 650 kg and producing 45 kg of 3.5% fat corrected milk. The chemical composition of pre-fresh and fresh diets is presented in table S1. The reproductive management utilized a combination of Presynch [33], Ovsynch [34], Resynch [35], and detection of estrus, with 25% to 30% of cows bred via timed artificial insemination and the remainder bred after detection of estrus solely by activity monitors (ALPRO; DeLaval, Kansas City, MO).

## Treatment groups and Case definition

Prior to commencement of the study, statistical power and sample size calculations were performed. Based on the farm's average metritis incidence among primiparous cows, we assumed that the puerperal metritis incidence in the control group would be close to 30%. Considering a statistical power of 0.8, a *P*-value of 0.05, and that vaccination would decrease the puerperal metritis incidence to 10%, a sample size of 100 and 50 cows for control and treatment group, respectively, was considered sufficient.

Late pregnant heifers were enrolled on a weekly basis; inclusion criteria for enrollment were: 230±3 days of pregnancy, 629 to 734 days of age and body condition score (BCS) greater than 2.5. Heifers that were visually lame were not included in the study. A total randomized field trial study design was used; heifers were randomly allocated into one of six different treatment groups using the random number function of Excel (Microsoft, Redmond, MA). A total of 371 pregnant heifers were enrolled in the study; 105, 54, 53, 53, 53, and 53 heifers were randomly allocated to the control, Vaccine 1, Vaccine 2, Vaccine 3, Vaccine 4 and Vaccine 5 groups, respectively. Heifers assigned to the vaccine groups received two doses of vaccine: at 230±3 days of pregnancy and 260±3 days of pregnancy. Heifers assigned to the control group did not receive a placebo.

Information regarding ease of calving was gathered by farm workers, and a 5-point scale was used: EASE 1 was defined as calvings that occurred easily without assistance; EASE 2 was defined as unassisted, but more difficult than EASE 1, calvings; EASE 3 was defined as calvings requiring easy assistance from a person; EASE 4 was defined as vaginally delivered calvings requiring the calf position to be corrected or hard traction to be applied to deliver the calf; and EASE 5 was defined as calvings requiring fetotomy or caesarian section. Dystocia was defined as calving with EASE greater than 2.

Body condition scores were determined for all study cows at $230 \pm 3$ days of gestation, $260 \pm 3$ days of gestation, $2 \pm 1$ days in milk (DIM), $6 \pm 1$ DIM and at $35 \pm 3$ DIM by a single investigator blinded to treatment group using a five-point scale with a quarter-point system as described by [36]. To obtain serum samples, blood was collected from a coccygeal vein/artery using a Vacutainer tube without anticoagulant and a 20 gauge$\times$2.54 cm Vacutainer needle (Becton, Dickinson and Company, Franklin Lakes, NJ). All blood samples were transported to the laboratory on ice and spun in a centrifuge at $2,000 \times g$ for 15 min at $4°C$; serum was harvested and frozen at $-80°C$. Serum samples were collected at $230 \pm 3$ days of gestation, $260 \pm 3$ days of gestation, $1 \pm 2$ DIM, $6 \pm 1$ DIM and $35 \pm 3$ DIM. Rectal temperature was measured at $6 \pm 1$ DIM using a digital thermometer (GLA M750, GLA Agriculture Electronics, CA) equipped with an angle probe (11.5 cm, 42°).

Cervical swabs were collected at $2 \pm 1$ DIM and $6 \pm 1$ DIM; cows were restrained and the perineum area was cleansed and disinfected with 70% ethanol solution. The swab was manipulated inside the cervix and exposed to uterine secretion. The swabs were kept inside a sterile vial at $4°C$ until processed in the laboratory. Swabs collected at $2 \pm 1$ DIM were cultured aerobically on Chromagar (Difco) at $37°C$ and *E. coli* colonies were distinguished by a blue color; swabs collected at $6 \pm 1$ DIM were cultured anaerobically on LKV agar (Anaerobe Systems) and *F. necrophorum* colonies were distinguished by morphology.

Retained placenta, puerperal metritis, ketosis, and clinical mastitis were diagnosed and treated by trained farm personnel who followed a specific diagnostic protocol designed by veterinarians from the Ambulatory and Production Medicine Clinic, Cornell University. Farm personnel were blinded to the treatments.

After parturition, cows were kept in the same pen until around 20 DIM. This pen was monitored by farm employees, and cows were submitted to a complete physical exam if they were showing signs of dullness and depression; cows with fetid, watery, red-brown uterine discharge accompanied with fever were diagnosed with puerperal metritis and treated by farm employees. Retained placenta was defined as a condition where cows failed to release their fetal membranes within 24 h of calving [37]. Puerperal metritis diagnosis by the research team was performed at $6 \pm 1$ DIM. Puerperal metritis was defined as the presence of fetid, watery, red-brown uterine discharge and rectal temperature greater than $39.5°C$ [1]. Information regarding puerperal metritis diagnosis was not exchanged between farm personnel and the research team. Data regarding health traits and reproduction were extracted from the farm's DairyComp 305 database (Valley Agricultural Software, Tulare, CA).

Clinical endometritis diagnosis was evaluated at $35 \pm 3$ DIM by visual inspection of a uterine lavage sample for the presence of purulent secretion as described [38]. To obtain uterine lavage samples, the cows were restrained, the perineum area was cleansed and disinfected with 70% ethanol, and a plastic infusion pipette was introduced into the cranial vagina and manipulated through the cervix into the uterus. A total of 20 ml of sterile saline solution was infused into the uterus and agitated gently, and a sample of the fluid was aspirated. The volume of recovered fluid ranged from 5 to 15 ml. All samples were visually scored by one investigator, who assessed the presence of a purulent or mucopurulent secretion in the uterine lavage sample. The score ranged from 0 to 2, with 0 indicating absence of a purulent or mucopurulent secretion, 1 indicating a bloody but not purulent sample, and 2 indicating the presence of pus in the lavage sample. Cows with a score of 2 were considered as diagnosed with clinical endometritis. Samples were kept on ice until they were cultured on Mueller–Hinton agar plates (BBL$^{TM}$) supplemented with 5% defibrinated sheep blood for 48 h aerobically in 5% $CO_2$ at $38°C$. Typical *T. pyogenes* colonies were distinguished by colony morphology, post-incubation hemolysis, and characteristic appearance on Gram's stain.

## Enzyme-linked immunosorbant assays (ELISAs)

Portions of the antigens produced for preparation of vaccines were used in ELISAs. *E. coli* strains were pooled together as a single antigen. The same was done for *F. necrophorum* and *T. pyogenes* strains.

The selected ELISA protocols were as follows. ELISA microtiter plates (Greiner Bio-One, Germany) were coated with either 0.295 µg/ml of FimH$_{1-156}$-His, 0.036 µg/ml of His-PLO, 0.186 µg/ml of LKT, $10^7$ cells/ml of *E. coli*, $10^{10}$ cells/ml of *F. necrophorum*, and $10^7$ cells/ml of *T. pyogenes* for anti-FimH, anti-LKT, anti-PLO, anti-*E. coli*, anti-*F. necrophorum*, and anti-*T. pyogenes* IgG assays, respectively. Serum samples were diluted in proportions of 1:1000, 1:5000, 1:5000, 1:150, 1:500, and 1:150 for anti-FimH, anti-LKT, anti-PLO, anti-*E. coli*, anti-*F. necrophorum*, and anti-*T. pyogenes* IgG assays, respectively. The optimal antigen and antibody concentrations were determined by performing the quantitative ELISA protocol with varying concentrations.

## Statistical analyses

Descriptive statistics analysis was undertaken in SAS using the FREQ procedure (SAS Institute INC., Cary, NC). To assess the effect of vaccination on the odds of RDPMET, FDPMET, endometritis, *E. coli*, *F. necrophorum*, and *T. pyogenes* culture outcomes, logistic regression models were fitted in SAS using the Logistic procedure. Contrasts were performed to compare the effect of subcutaneous vaccines composed by proteins (Vaccine 1 and Vaccine 2), and inactivated whole cells (Vaccine 1 and Vaccine 3) versus control. The effect of subcutaneous and intravaginal vaccines on reproduction was analyzed by Cox's proportional hazard using the proportional hazard regression procedure in SAS. To illustrate the effect of vaccination on reproduction, Kaplan-Meier survival analysis was performed using Medcalc version 10.4.0.0 (Mariakerke, Belgium). To assess the effect of vaccination on rectal temperature at $6 \pm 1$ DIM, mixed general linear models were fitted to the data using JMP PRO9. To assess the effect of vaccination on ELISA detecting serum IgG against vaccine antigens, mixed general linear models were fitted to the data using JMP PRO9. For all models described above, independent variables and their respective interactions were kept when $P<0.10$ in an attempt to reduce the type II error risk while maintaining a stringent type I error risk of 5%. The variable *treatment* was forced into all statistical models even in the absence of statistical significance. Age in days at enrollment, BCS at enrollment, and dystocia were offered to all models.

## Results

### Descriptive statistics

Descriptive statistics regarding average age at enrollment (days), average BCS at enrollment and at $6 \pm 1$ days postpartum, average gestation length at enrollment, and total number of animals enrolled are presented in Table 1. Only pregnant heifers were

**Table 1.** Descriptive statistics of treatment groups.

|  | Control | Vaccine 1 | Vaccine 2 | Vaccine 3 | Vaccine 4 | Vaccine 5 |
|---|---|---|---|---|---|---|
| Average age (days) at enrollment (± SE) | 664 (3.72) | 655 (5.2) | 665 (5.24) | 669 (5.24) | 666 (5.24) | 668 (5.24) |
| Average body condition score at enrollment (± SE) | 3.71 (0.03) | 3.76 (0.05) | 3.74 (0.05) | 3.65 (0.05) | 3.72 (0.05) | 3.66 (0.05) |
| Average body condition score at 6±1 (± SE) | 3.5 (0.02) | 3.49 (0.03) | 3.52 (0.03) | 3.49 (0.03) | 3.44 (0.03) | 3.50 (0.03) |
| Average days of gestation at enrollment (± SE) | 230 (0.21) | 230 (0.29) | 230 (0.29) | 230 (0.29) | 230 (0.29) | 230 (0.29) |
| Total enrolled animals (%) | 105 (28.3) | 54 (14.5) | 53 (14.3) | 53 (14.3) | 53 (14.3) | 53 (14.3) |

enrolled in this study, allowing us to have as little variation between animals as possible.

## Effect of vaccination on incidence of researcher diagnosed puerperal metritis (RDPMET), farm diagnosed puerperal metritis (FDPMET), and rectal temperature at 6±1 DIM

The effect of vaccination on the incidence of RDPMET is presented in Table 2. When evaluated separately, there was no difference between incidence of RDPMET between treatment groups ($P$-value = 0.153). However, when vaccines were evaluated grouped as either subcutaneous or intravaginal vaccines, the subcutaneous vaccines were associated with a significant reduction in the incidence of RDPMET ($P$-value = 0.018). Additionally, contrasts showed a significant reduction on the incidence of RDPMET for cows subcutaneously immunized with inactivated whole cells (Vaccine 1 & 3, $P$-value = 0.035).

The effect of vaccination on incidence of FDPMET is present in Table 3. When the vaccines were evaluated separately, the incidence of FDPMET tended to be different among the treatments ($P$-value = 0.056). When compared to control, Vaccine 1 reduced the incidence of FDPMET ($P$-value = 0.019). Additionally, when the vaccines were evaluated grouped as subcutaneous or intravaginal vaccines, the subcutaneous vaccines were associated with a significantly lower odds of FDPMET ($P$-value = 0.034). Furthermore, contrasts showed a significant reduction on the incidence of RDPMET for cows subcutaneously immunized with proteins (Vaccine 1 & 2, $P$-value = 0.010), and inactivated whole cells (Vaccine 1 & 3, $P$-value = 0.026).

The effect of vaccination on rectal temperature at 6±1 DIM is presented in Figure 1. Rectal temperature was not statistically different among the treatment groups when the vaccines were evaluated separately ($P$-value = 0.14); rectal temperature was 38.96°C (SEM = 0.05), 38.79°C (SEM = 0.07), 38.75°C (SEM = 0.07), 38.83°C (SEM = 0.07), 38.90°C (SEM = 0.07), and

**Table 2.** Effects of different vaccine formulations on incidence of researcher diagnosed puerperal metritis.

| Model and variables | Puerperal metritis incidence (%) | Coefficients (SE) | Odds ratio (95% CI) | Individual $P$-value | Overall $P$-value |
|---|---|---|---|---|---|
| **Model 1** |  |  |  |  |  |
| Control | 12.1 | Ref. | baseline |  |  |
| Vaccine 1 | 6.2 | −0.14 (0.56) | 0.44 (0.11–1.67) | 0.226 |  |
| Vaccine 2 | 4.1 | −0.73 (0.65) | 0.24 (0.05–1.17) | 0.078 |  |
| Vaccine 3 | 2.0 | −1.32 (0.87) | 0.13 (0.02–1.08) | 0.060 | 0.153 |
| Vaccine 4 | 13.5 | 0.68 (0.43) | 0.99 (0.35–2.78) | 0.989 |  |
| Vaccine 5 | 14.0 | 0.80 (0.43) | 1.12 (0.40–3.12) | 0.832 |  |
| Intercept |  | −2.15 (0.27) |  |  |  |
| **Model 2** |  |  |  |  |  |
| Control | 12.1 | Ref. | baseline |  |  |
| Subcutaneous | 4.1 | −0.90 (0.32) | 0.27 (0.09–0.75) | 0.013 | 0.018 |
| Intravaginal | 13.7 | 0.47 (0.26) | 1.05 (0.45–2.46) | 0.905 |  |
| Intercept |  | −1.88 (0.22) |  |  |  |
| **Contrasts** |  |  |  |  |  |
| Control | 12.1 | Ref. | baseline |  |  |
| Vaccine 1 & 2 | 5.1 | −1.12 (0.57) | 0.32 (0.10–1.01) | 0.051 |  |
| Vaccine 1 & 3 | 4.1 | −1.42 (0.67) | 0.24 (0.06–0.91) | 0.035 |  |

Vaccines were evaluated separately in Model 1, and grouped in Model 2. Age in days, dystocia, and body condition score at enrollment were offered to both models.

**Table 3.** Effects of different vaccine formulations on incidence of farm diagnosed puerperal metritis.

| Model and variables | Puerperal metritis incidence (%) | Coefficients (SE) | Odds ratio (95% CI) | Individual P-value | Overall P-value |
|---|---|---|---|---|---|
| **Model 1** | | | | | |
| Control | 27.6 | Ref. | baseline | | |
| Vaccine 1 | 11.1 | −0.73 (0.38) | 0.31 (0.12–0.82) | 0.019 | |
| Vaccine 2 | 17.0 | −0.29 (0.33) | 0.49 (0.21–1.14) | 0.100 | |
| Vaccine 3 | 20.7 | −0.01 (0.31)- | 0.65 (0.29–1.45) | 0.297 | 0.056 |
| Vaccine 4 | 34.0 | 0.67 (0.28) | 1.27 (0.62–2.62) | 0.504 | |
| Vaccine 5 | 19.2 | −0.08 (0.32) | 0.60 (0.27–1.37) | 0.226 | |
| Intercept | | −1.06 (0.18) | | | |
| **Model 2** | | | | | |
| Control | 27.6 | Ref. | baseline | | |
| Subcutaneous | 16.2 | −0.46 (0.18) | 0.48 (0.26–0.88) | 0.018 | 0.034 |
| Intravaginal | 26.7 | 0.18 (0.18) | 0.91 (0.49–1.68) | 0.766 | |
| Intercept | | −0.91 (0.17) | | | |
| **Contrasts** | | | | | |
| Control | 27.6 | Ref. | baseline | | |
| Vaccine 1 & 2 | 14.0 | −0.93 (0.36) | 0.39 (0.19–0.80) | 0.010 | |
| Vaccine 1 & 3 | 15.9 | −0.35 (0.35) | 0.45 (0.22–0.91) | 0.026 | |

Vaccines were evaluated separately in Model 1, and grouped in Model 2. Age in days, dystocia, and body condition score at enrollment were offered to both models.

38.87°C (SEM = 0.07) for control, Vaccine 1, Vaccine 2, Vaccine 3, Vaccine 4, and Vaccine 5 cows, respectively. However, rectal temperature was statistically different between the treatment groups when the vaccines were evaluated grouped as control, subcutaneous vaccines or intravaginal vaccines (P-value = 0.018); rectal temperature was 38.96°C (SEM = 0.05), 38.78°C (SEM = 0.04), and 38.89°C (SEM = 0.05) for control, subcutaneous vaccinated, and intravaginally vaccinated cows, respectively. Subcutaneous vaccination was associated with a significant reduction in rectal temperature at 6 ± 1 DIM.

## Effect of vaccination on incidence of endometritis and uterine secretion culture outcomes

Vaccines were not effective in preventing endometritis, when evaluated separately or when grouped as subcutaneous and intravaginal vaccines (P-value = 0.99). Endometritis incidence was 8.6%, 7.9%, 12.1%, 7.5%, 9.1%, and 9.8% for control, vaccine 1, vaccine 2, vaccine 3, vaccine 4, and vaccine 5, respectively. The incidence of endometritis was 9.0% and 9.5% for subcutaneous and intravaginal vaccines, respectively. Additionally, there was no significant effect of vaccination on the likelihood of intrauterine bacterial contamination (Table 4).

## Effect of vaccination on reproduction

Cows that received subcutaneous vaccination were 1.36 times more likely to conceive when compared to control cows (P-value = 0.04, Figure 2). However, for cows that received intravaginal vaccines, the likelihood of conceiving was not statistically different from control cows (Hazard ratio = 1.12, P-value = 0.46). Age in days at enrollment and BCS at enrollment were retained in the model for this analysis (P-value = 0.02 and 0.01, respectively).

## Serological responses to vaccination

The effect of vaccination on ELISA-detected serum IgG against several antigens is presented in Figure 3. Vaccine 1 and 2 increased serum IgG titers against *E. coli*, while cows from all other treatment groups did not respond to this antigen. Additionally, cows vaccinated with vaccines 1, 2, and 4 had increased IgG levels against to FimH. However, it seems that the animals naturally responded to LKT and *F. necrophorum*, because all animals have elevated IgG titers against these antigens after parturition. Cows vaccinated with vaccine 1 and 3 had increased IgG levels against *T. pyogenes*, while vaccine 1 and 2 had increased IgG titers against PLO.

## Discussion

We evaluated here the effects of 5 different vaccine formulations (3 subcutaneous vaccines and 2 intravaginal vaccines) containing different combinations of proteins (FimH, LKT, PLO) and inactivated whole cells (*E. coli*, *F. necrophorum* and *T. pyogenes*) on the uterine health of dairy cows. We demonstrated that subcutaneous vaccination significantly decreased the incidence of puerperal metritis, whereas intravaginal vaccination was not effective.

Puerperal metritis is characterized by inflammation of the entire thickness of the uterine walls, and is associated with signs of systemic illness such as dullness, decreased milk yield and fever [1]. The signs of puerperal metritis (presence of fetid, watery, red-brown uterine discharge and rectal temperature greater than 39.5°C) used for the diagnosis of metritis in this study is widely used by researchers and veterinarians. In a recent study, it was reported that there is a considerable inconsistency between observers to classify animals as healthy or metritic based on the assessment of vaginal discharge odor [39], suggesting that the classification of disease based on the signs used is prone to errors. However, we expect that errors occurred equally among all

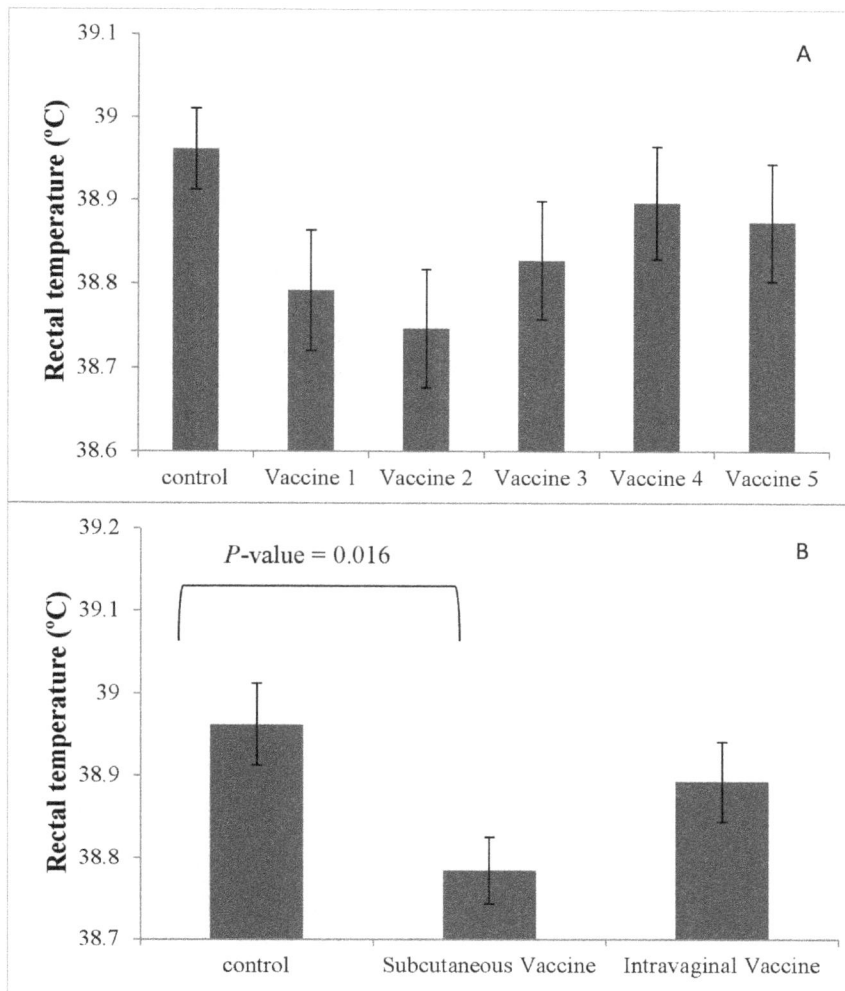

**Figure 1. Effect of vaccination on rectal temperature at 6±1 DIM.** Vaccines were evaluated separately (A, $P$-value = 0.14), and grouped (B, $P$-value = 0.018). Standard errors of the means are represented by the error bars.

treatment groups. When diagnosed by our research group, puerperal metritis incidence was 12.1% and when diagnosed by farm workers it was 27.6%. This discrepancy can be attributed to the period during which the cows were monitored; whereas farm workers monitored the cows daily during their first 20 days after parturition, the research team examined the cows only at 6±1 days after calving. Cows were examined at this time point because metritis peaks in the first 7 days after calving [40]. However, it is important to highlight that, in general, the effect of vaccination on puerperal metritis was consistent between the research group's and the farm workers' diagnoses; subcutaneous vaccination significantly lowered the incidence of puerperal metritis, whereas intravaginal vaccine was not effective in preventing the disease.

*E. coli* and *F. necrophorum* are gram-negative bacteria, characterized by the presence of lipopolysaccharide (**LPS**) in their outer membrane, and are known etiological agents of puerperal metritis; LPS is known to cause increased body temperature in cattle [41]. Although vaccination did not significantly decrease the percentage of cows that were positive for intrauterine *E. coli* and *F. necrophorum*, subcutaneously vaccinated cows did have a lower rectal temperature at 6±1 DIM. The differences of the rectal temperature between treatment groups was small; however, control cows had

higher rectal temperature, suggesting that more cows in the control group were found with fever. This suggests that, even in the presence of bacteria in the uterus, immunized cows were less likely to develop systemic signs caused by LPS released from *E. coli* and *F. necrophorum*. It is known that reducing the bacterial load of *E. coli* decreases the severity of the disease [1]; therefore, we can also speculate that immunization decreased the pathogen-load inside the uterus. However, further investigation is needed to address questions regarding the mechanisms of action of the vaccine.

The relationship between poor immune status around calving and uterine diseases is already well established [42–46]. Recruitment of polymorphonuclear cells (**PMNs**) to the endometrial surface and the uterine lumen is critical for the immune defense of the uterus [13]. A vaccine against uterine diseases would have great potential for enhancing the immune status around parturition, by inducing production of pathogen-specific immunoglobulins in bovine endometrial secretions, which would act by lysing bacteria, by serving as opsonins to enhance phagocytosis, and by stimulating the complement pathways [47].

Although it was found that subcutaneous immunization effectively prevented puerperal metritis, we did not observe the

**Table 4.** Effects of different vaccine formulations on incidence of intrauterine *Escherichia coli* at 2±1 DIM, *Fusobacterium necrophorum* at 6±1 DIM and *Trueperella pyogenes* at 35±3 DIM.

| Model and variables | Cows positive for intrauterine culture (%) | Coefficients (SE) | Odds ratio (95% CI) | P-value |
|---|---|---|---|---|
| **Model 1** | *E. coli* | | | |
| Control | 55.0 | Ref. | baseline | |
| Vaccine 1 | 47.1 | −0.01 (0.26) | 0.73 (0.37–1.45) | |
| Vaccine 2 | 46.1 | −0.09 (0.25) | 0.67 (0.34–1.34) | |
| Vaccine 3 | 40.4 | −0.36 (0.26) | 0.52 (0.26–1.03) | 0.57 |
| Vaccine 4 | 50.9 | 0.10 (0.25) | 0.82 (0.42–1.61) | |
| Vaccine 5 | 50.0 | 0.05 (0.26) | 0.78 (0.39–1.55) | |
| Intercept | | 1.91 (1.14) | | |
| **Model 2** | *E. coli* | | | |
| Control | 55.0 | Ref. | baseline | |
| Subcutaneous | 44.5 | −0.23 (0.14) | 0.63 (0.38–1.06) | 0.21 |
| Intravaginal | 50.5 | −0.01 (0.46) | 0.80 (0.46–1.40) | |
| Intercept | | 1.89 (1.13) | | |
| **Model 3** | *F. necrophorum* | | | |
| Control | 49.0 | Ref. | baseline | |
| Vaccine 1 | 36.0 | −0.39 (0.26) | 0.59 (0.29–1.18) | |
| Vaccine 2 | 48.0 | 0.11 (0.26) | 0.96 (0.49–1.90) | |
| Vaccine 3 | 48.0 | 0.11 (0.26) | 0.96 (0.49–1.90) | 0.76 |
| Vaccine 4 | 47.2 | 0.07 (0.25) | 0.93 (0.48–1.81) | |
| Vaccine 5 | 44.0 | −0.05 (0.26) | 0.82 (0.41–1.62) | |
| Intercept | | −0.19 (0.11) | | |
| **Model 4** | *F. necrophorum* | | | |
| Control | 49.0 | Ref. | baseline | |
| Subcutaneous | 44.0 | −0.09 (0.14) | 0.82 (0.49–1.36) | 0.74 |
| Intravaginal | 45.6 | −0.02 (0.16) | 0.87 (0.50–1.52) | |
| Intercept | | −0.15 (0.11) | | |
| **Model 5** | *T. pyogenes* | | | |
| Control | 14.5 | Ref. | baseline | |
| Vaccine 1 | 5.3 | −0.80 (0.63) | 0.30 (0.06–1.46) | |
| Vaccine 2 | 21.2 | 0.77 (0.42) | 1.44 (0.48–4.32) | |
| Vaccine 3 | 12.5 | 0.05 (0.46) | 0.70 (0.21–2.30) | 0.37 |
| Vaccine 4 | 12.1 | 0.06 (0.50) | 0.70 (0.20–2.52) | |
| Vaccine 5 | 7.3 | −0.49 (0.54) | 0.41 (0.10–1.61) | |
| Intercept | | −16.55 (5.48) | | |
| **Model 6** | *T. pyogenes* | | | |
| Control | 14.5 | Ref. | baseline | |
| Subcutaneous | 12.6 | 0.01 (0.26) | 0.74 (0.30–1.82) | 0.50 |
| Intravaginal | 9.5 | −0.32 (0.31) | 0.53 (0.19–1.53) | |
| Intercept | | −16.66 (5.48) | | |

Vaccines were evaluated separately in Model 1, Model 3 and Model 5; and grouped in Model 2, Model 4 and Model 6. Age in days, dystocia, and body condition score at enrollment were offered to both models.

same effect on endometritis. Metritis and endometritis appear to be linked uterine diseases; however, metritis is not necessary for the development of endometritis [13,48]. This finding suggests that immunization against the targeted, while important to prevent puerperal metritis, was not effective to decrease the incidence of endometritis. Further investigation is needed to evaluate if addition of others antigens to these vaccines would contribute to prevention of endometritis. A potential candidate would be the

fimbriae subunit FimA; the gene FimA is highly prevalent in *T. pyogenes* isolated from the uterus of dairy cows [49], and it was associated with development of metritis [12,49] and endometritis [12].

Mucosal immune responses can be effectively induced by the administration of vaccines onto mucosal surfaces, whereas subcutaneous and intramuscular vaccines typically fail to induce mucosal immunity, and are less effective in preventing infection of

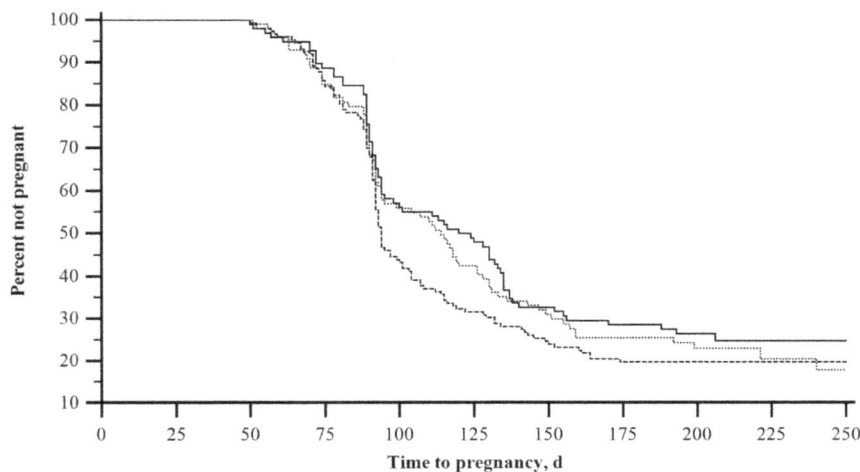

**Figure 2. Effect of subcutaneous and intravaginal vaccines on reproduction.** The median calving-to-conception interval for subcutaneously vaccinated cows (inner interrupted line), intravaginally vaccinated cows (middle interrupted line), and control cows (solid line) was 94, 114, and 120 respectively. (*P*-value = 0.04).

mucosal surfaces [50]. Promising results regarding prevention of human UTI by intravaginal immunization with a whole-cell vaccine have already been reported [24,25]. However, it is not known how local synthesis of specific antibodies by uterine antibody-secreting cells contributes to uterine immunity [47]. In the present study, intravaginal immunization was not effective in preventing uterine diseases, suggesting that mucosal immunization of the vagina, considering dose and composition used, does not affect the immunological status of the uterus. Nevertheless, it is important to highlight that the uterus is an immune tolerant environment during pregnancy [51], and this might have prevented the uterus to develop an immune response to the intravaginal vaccines. Further investigation is needed to evaluate if intravaginal vaccination administered prior to pregnancy would elicit a uterine immune response capable of prevent uterine diseases, and conclude if local synthesis of specific antibodies by the uterine mucosa is important for the prevention of puerperal metritis and endometritis in heifers.

In general, subcutaneous vaccination increased the serum levels of IgG against *E. coli*, FimH, *F. necrophorum*, LKT, *T. pyogenes*, and PLO. This suggests that there is a significant contribution of circulating specific IgG to the postpartum uterine immunity, a conclusion supported by previous studies. After intramuscular immunization with *Histophilus somni*, most of the IgG in uterine secretions of cattle at estrus were derived from serum [26]. Additionally, it has been reported that systemic immunization with *Campylobacter fetus* increased the IgG activity in the bovine reproductive tract. It is possible that IgG proteins work as opsonins in the bovine genital tract [27], hence contributing to phagocyte-dependent clearance of infection of the uterus.

It has already been documented that prevention of other diseases such as liver abscess and UTI are caused by some of the agents present as antigens within the vaccines tested in this study. It has been reported that a single injection of a bivalent *T. pyogenes* – *F. necrophorum* bacterin-toxoid reduced the prevalence of liver abscess when given to cattle entering a feedlot; reductions of 48.4% and 37.5% in the prevalence of liver abscess in the two trials reported [23]. It is known that *F. necrophorum* LKT is highly toxic to bovine PMNs [52], inducing apoptosis-mediated killing of them [53]; this toxicity is dose-dependent [54]. It is possible that immunizing the cows against LKT might have reduced the

detrimental effect of this toxin on intrauterine PMNs, improving the ability of the innate immune system to eliminate bacterial infections from the uterus through phagocytosis. Recruited PMNs are key players in the immune defense of the uterus; reduced migration of PMNs 2 weeks before calving is associated with retained placenta [46], and lower phagocytic activity and oxidative burst capacity of PMNs are associated with occurrence of metritis and endometritis [43,45].

Furthermore, it has been reported that systemic vaccination with FimH protects mice and cynomolgus monkeys from UTI [21,55]. Mice that were immunized with FimH vaccines and challenged with an uropathogenic *E. coli* isolate exhibited a 100- to 1000-fold reduction in the number of organisms recovered from their bladders as compared to controls [21]. Additionally, cynomolgus monkeys immunized with FimH and further infected with a type 1-piliated *E. coli* isolate were protected against bladder infection, while control monkeys were affected with cystitis [55]. Although we did not observe a significant reduction in intrauterine presence of *E. coli* (the percentage of positive cows for *E. coli* culture was numerically lower for systemically vaccinated cows). Furthermore, based on our serological findings, systemic FimH immunization was an important factor for prevention of puerperal metritis.

This study evaluated the effect of multivalent vaccines; therefore, it is not possible to relate the effectiveness of the vaccines to any particular antigen. Published literature reported the multifactorial etiology of uterine diseases; therefore, we designed multivalent vaccines, aiming to successfully immunize cows against the most relevant known pathogens associated with uterine infections. Although our serological findings suggest that most of the antigens were partially important for the effectiveness of the subcutaneous vaccines, we do not know if certain antigens were potentially more important. Further research is needed to elucidate how important each antigen is for the effectiveness of the vaccines, and perhaps simplify the vaccine formulations.

In conclusion, the incidence of puerperal metritis was significantly decreased with prepartum subcutaneous vaccination with vaccines containing different combinations of proteins (FimH, LKT, PLO) and inactivated whole cells (*E. coli*, *F. necrophorum* and *T. pyogenes*). In contrast, intravaginal vaccination was not effective in decreasing the incidence of puerperal metritis. We can therefore

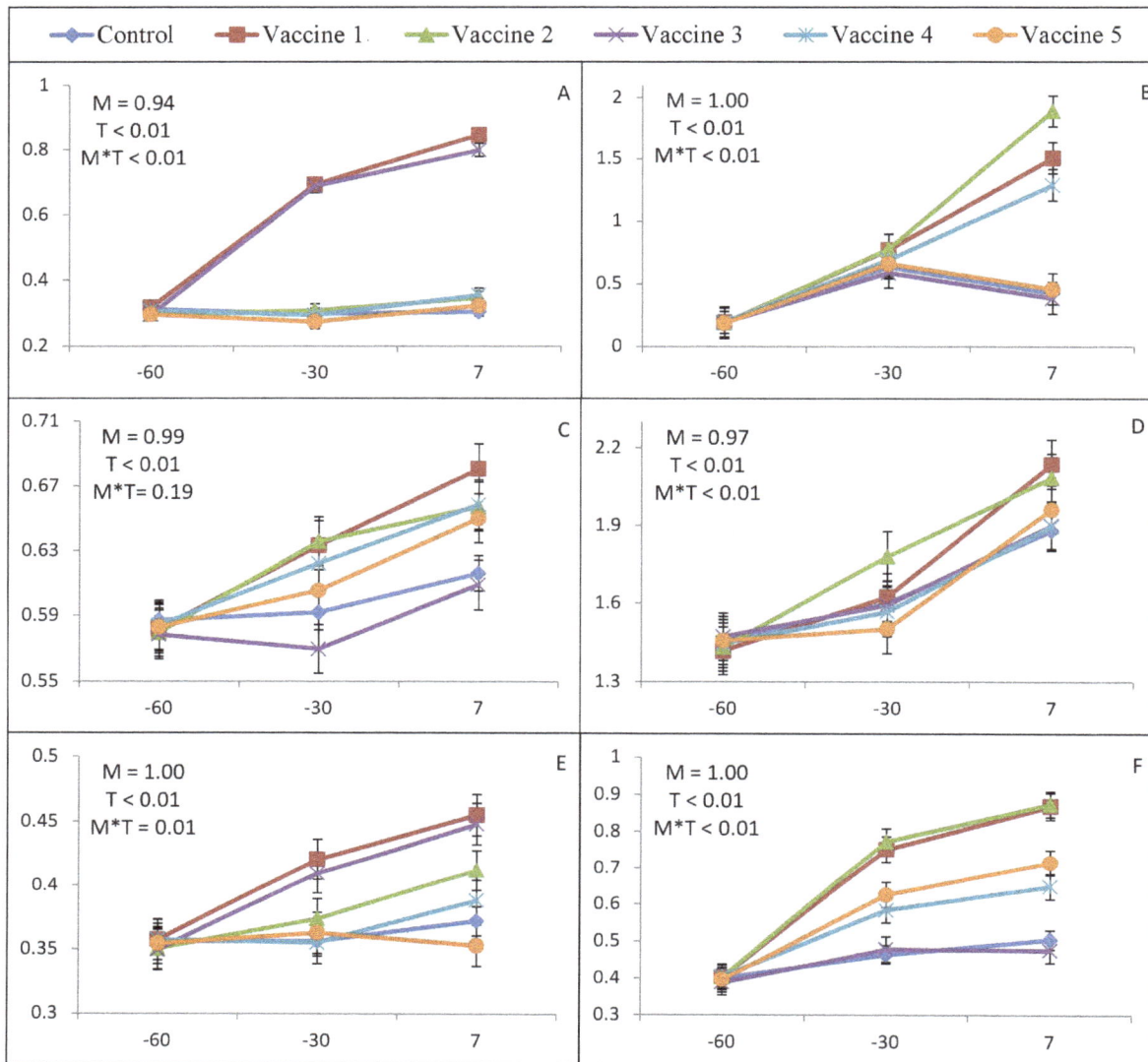

**Figure 3. Effect of vaccination on ELISA-detected serum IgG against** *E. coli* **(A), FimH (B),** *F. necrophorum* **(C), LKT (D),** *T. pyogenes* **(E), and PLO (F). X-axis represents days relative to calving, while Y-axis represents $OD_{650}$ of ELISA-detected serum IgG against several antigens.** Standard errors of the means are represented by the error bars.

suggest that commercial production of a vaccine against metritis may be feasible. Such a vaccine could become an integral part of a preventive strategy against metritis, leading to reduced incidence of the disease, reduced use of antibiotics and therefore alleviating both animal distress and the overall negative economic impact of metritis on the dairy industry.

## Supporting Information

**Table S1    Chemical composition (mineral and vitamins) of pre-fresh and lactating cows diets.** Pre-fresh diets were

fed from 3 week prepartum through parturition and fresh diets were fed from parturition through week 35 postpartum.

## Author Contributions

Conceived and designed the experiments: RCB VSM ROG SHC. Performed the experiments: VSM MLdSB EBdSM RR BLR SL TS AK CF EKG. Analyzed the data: RCB VSM. Contributed reagents/materials/analysis tools: RCB. Wrote the paper: VSM RCB GO.

## References

1. Sheldon IM, Lewis GS, LeBlanc S, Gilbert RO (2006) Defining postpartum uterine disease in cattle. Theriogenology 65: 1516–1530.
2. LeBlanc SJ, Osawa T, Dubuc J (2011) Reproductive tract defense and disease in postpartum dairy cows. Theriogenology 76: 1610–1618.
3. Cheong SH, Nydam DV, Galvao KN, Crosier BM, Ricci A, et al. (2012) Use of reagent test strips for diagnosis of endometritis in dairy cows. Theriogenology 77: 858–864.
4. Dubuc J, Duffield TF, Leslie KE, Walton JS, LeBlanc SJ (2010) Definitions and diagnosis of postpartum endometritis in dairy cows. J Dairy Sci 93: 5225–5233.

5. Aust V, Knappstein K, Kunz HJ, Kaspar H, Wallmann J, et al. (2012) Feeding untreated and pasteurized waste milk and bulk milk to calves: Effects on calf performance, health status and antibiotic resistance of faecal bacteria. J Anim Physiol Anim Nutr (doi: 10.1111/jpn.12019).

6. Dolejska M, Jurcickova Z, Literak I, Pokludova L, Bures J, et al. (2011) IncN plasmids carrying bla CTX-M-1 in escherichia coli isolates on a dairy farm. Vet Microbiol 149: 513–516.

7. Overton M, Fetrow J (2008) Economics of postpartum uterine health. Proc Dairy Cattle Reproduction Council: 39–44.

8. Miller AN, Williams EJ, Sibley K, Herath S, Lane EA, et al. (2007) The effects of arcanobacterium pyogenes on endometrial function in vitro, and on uterine and ovarian function in vivo. Theriogenology 68: 972–980.

9. Santos TM, Gilbert RO, Bicalho RC (2011) Metagenomic analysis of the uterine bacterial microbiota in healthy and metritic postpartum dairy cows. J Dairy Sci 94: 291–302.

10. Bicalho RC, Machado VS, Bicalho ML, Gilbert RO, Teixeira AG, et al. (2010) Molecular and epidemiological characterization of bovine intrauterine escherichia coli. J Dairy Sci 93: 5818–5830.

11. Machado VS, Bicalho ML, Pereira RV, Caixeta LS, Bittar JH, et al. (2012) The effect of intrauterine administration of mannose or bacteriophage on uterine health and fertility of dairy cows with special focus on escherichia coli and arcanobacterium pyogenes. J Dairy Sci 95: 3100–3109.

12. Bicalho ML, Machado VS, Oikonomou G, Gilbert RO, Bicalho RC (2012) Association between virulence factors of escherichia coli, fusobacterium necrophorum, and arcanobacterium pyogenes and uterine diseases of dairy cows. Vet Microbiol 157: 125–131.

13. Bondurant RH (1999) Inflammation in the bovine female reproductive tract. J Anim Sci 77 Suppl 2: 101–110.

14. Dohmen MJ, Joop K, Sturk A, Bols PE, Lohuis JA (2000) Relationship between intra-uterine bacterial contamination, endotoxin levels and the development of endometritis in postpartum cows with dystocia or retained placenta. Theriogenology 54: 1019–1032.

15. Machado VS, Oikonomou G, Bicalho ML, Knauer WA, Gilbert R, et al. (2012) Investigation of postpartum dairy cows' uterine microbial diversity using metagenomic pyrosequencing of the 16S rRNA gene. Vet Microbiol 159: 460–469.

16. Williams EJ, Fischer DP, Pfeiffer DU, England GC, Noakes DE, et al. (2005) Clinical evaluation of postpartum vaginal mucus reflects uterine bacterial infection and the immune response in cattle. Theriogenology 63: 102–117.

17. Krogfelt KA, Bergmans H, Klemm P (1990) Direct evidence that the FimH protein is the mannose-specific adhesin of escherichia coli type 1 fimbriae. Infect Immun 58: 1995–1998.

18. Mooi FR, de Graaf FK (1985) Molecular biology of fimbriae of enterotoxigenic escherichia coli. Curr Top Microbiol Immunol 118: 119–138.

19. Sheldon IM, Rycroft AN, Dogan B, Craven M, Bromfield JJ, et al. (2010) Specific strains of escherichia coli are pathogenic for the endometrium of cattle and cause pelvic inflammatory disease in cattle and mice. PLoS One 5: e9192.

20. Kaper JB, Nataro JP, Mobley HL (2004) Pathogenic escherichia coli. Nat Rev Microbiol 2: 123–140.

21. Langermann S, Palaszynski S, Barnhart M, Auguste G, Pinkner JS, et al. (1997) Prevention of mucosal escherichia coli infection by FimH-adhesin-based systemic vaccination. Science 276: 607–611.

22. Nagaraja TG, Lechtenberg KF (2007) Liver abscesses in feedlot cattle. Vet Clin North Am Food Anim Pract 23: 351–369.

23. Jones G, Jayappa H, Hunsaker B, Sweeny D, Rapp-Gabrielson V, et al. (2004) Efficacy of an Arcanobacterium pyogenes-Fusobacterium necrophorum Baterin-toxoid as an aid in the prevention of liver abscesses in feedlot cattle. Bovine Pract 38: 36–44.

24. Uehling DT, Hopkins WJ, Dahmer LA, Balish E. (1994) Phase I clinical trial of vaginal mucosal immunization for recurrent urinary tract infection. J Urol 152: 2308–2311.

25. Uehling DT, Hopkins WJ, Elkahwaji JE, Schmidt DM, Leverson GE (2003) Phase 2 clinical trial of a vaginal mucosal vaccine for urinary tract infections. J Urol 170: 867–869.

26. Butt BM, Besser TE, Senger PL, Widders PR (1993) Specific antibody to haemophilus somnus in the bovine uterus following intramuscular immunization. Infect Immun 61: 2558–2562.

27. Corbeil LB, Schurig GD, Duncan JR, Corbeil RR, Winter AJ (1974) Immunoglobulin classes and biological functions of campylobacter (vibrio) fetus antibodies in serum and cervicovaginal mucus. Infect Immun 10: 422–429.

28. Billington SJ, Jost BH, Cuevas WA, Bright KR, Songer JG (1997) The arcanobacterium (actinomyces) pyogenes hemolysin, pyolysin, is a novel member of the thiol-activated cytolysin family. J Bacteriol 179: 6100–6106.

29. Choudhury D, Thompson A, Stojanoff V, Langermann S, Pinkner J, et al. (1999) X-ray structure of the FimC-FimH chaperone-adhesin complex from uropathogenic escherichia coli. Science 285: 1061–1066.

30. Aprikian P, Tchesnokova V, Kidd B, Yakovenko O, Yarov-Yarovoy V, et al. (2007) Interdomain interaction in the FimH adhesin of escherichia coli regulates the affinity to mannose. J Biol Chem 282: 23437–23446.

31. Bradford MM (1976) A rapid and sensitive method for the quantitation of microgram quantities of protein utilizing the principle of protein-dye binding. Anal Biochem 72: 248–254.

32. Tan ZL, Nagaraja TG, Chengappa MM, Staats JJ (1994) Purification and quantification of fusobacterium necrophorum leukotoxin by using monoclonal antibodies. J Vet Microbiol 42: 121–133.

33. Moreira F, Orlandi C, Risco CA, Mattos R, Lopes F, et al. (2001) Effects of presynchronization and bovine somatotropin on pregnancy rates to a timed artificial insemination protocol in lactating dairy cows. J Dairy Sci 84: 1646–1659.

34. Pursley JR, Mee MO, Wiltbank MC (1995) Synchronization of ovulation in dairy cows using PGF2alpha and GnRH. Theriogenology 44: 915–923.

35. Fricke PM, Caraviello DZ, Weigel KA, Welle ML (2003) Fertility of dairy cows after resynchronization of ovulation at three intervals following first timed insemination. J Dairy Sci 86: 3941–3950.

36. Edmonson AJ, Lean IJ, Weaver LD, Farver T, Webster G (1989) A body condition scoring chart for holstein dairy cows. J Dairy Sci 72: 68–78.

37. Kelton DF, Lissemore KD, Martin RE (1998) Recommendations for recording and calculating the incidence of selected clinical diseases of dairy cattle. J Dairy Sci 81: 2502–2509.

38. Machado VS, Knauer WA, Bicalho ML, Oikonomou G, Gilbert RO, et al. (2012) A novel diagnostic technique to determine uterine health of holstein cows at 35 days postpartum. J Dairy Sci 95: 1349–1357.

39. Sannmann I, Burfeind O, Suthar V, Bos A, Bruins M, et al. (2013) Technical note: Evaluation of odor from vaginal discharge of cows in the first 10 days after calving by olfactory cognition and an electronic device. J Dairy Sci 96: 5773–5779.

40. LeBlanc SJ (2008) Postpartum uterine disease and dairy herd reproductive performance: A review. Vet J 176: 102–114.

41. Bannerman DD, Paape MJ, Hare WR, Sohn EJ (2003) Increased levels of LPS-binding protein in bovine blood and milk following bacterial lipopolysaccharide challenge. J Dairy Sci 86: 3128–3137.

42. Hammon DS, Evjen IM, Dhiman TR, Goff JP, Walters JL (2006) Neutrophil function and energy status in holstein cows with uterine health disorders. Vet Immunol Immunopathol 113: 21–29.

43. Cai TQ, Weston PG, Lund LA, Brodie B, McKenna DJ, et al. (1994) Association between neutrophil functions and periparturient disorders in cows. Am J Vet Res 55: 934–943.

44. Galvao KN, Flaminio MJ, Brittin SB, Sper R, Fraga M, et al. (2010) Association between uterine disease and indicators of neutrophil and systemic energy status in lactating holstein cows. J Dairy Sci 93: 2926–2937.

45. Kim IH, Na KJ, Yang MP (2005) Immune responses during the peripartum period in dairy cows with postpartum endometritis. J Reprod Dev 51: 757–764.

46. Kimura K, Goff JP, Kehrli ME Jr, Reinhardt TA (2002) Decreased neutrophil function as a cause of retained placenta in dairy cattle. J Dairy Sci 85: 544–550.

47. Singh J, Murray RD, Mshelia G, Woldehiwet Z (2008) The immune status of the bovine uterus during the peripartum period. Vet J 175: 301–309.

48. Dubuc J, Duffield TF, Leslie KE, Walton JS, LeBlanc SJ (2010) Risk factors for postpartum uterine diseases in dairy cows. J Dairy Sci 93: 5764–5771.

49. Santos TM, Caixeta LS, Machado VS, Rauf AK, Gilbert RO, et al. (2010) Antimicrobial resistance and presence of virulence factor genes in arcanobacterium pyogenes isolated from the uterus of postpartum dairy cows. Vet Microbiol 145: 84–89.

50. Neutra MR, Kozlowski PA (2006) Mucosal vaccines: The promise and the challenge. Nat Rev Immunol 6: 148–158.

51. Oliveira LJ, Barreto RS, Perecin F, Mansouri-Attia N, Pereira FT, et al. (2012) Modulation of maternal immune system during pregnancy in the cow. Reprod Domest Anim 47 Suppl 4: 384–393.

52. Tan ZL, Nagaraja TG, Chengappa MM, Smith JS (1994) Biological and biochemical characterization of fusobacterium necrophorum leukotoxin. Am J Vet Res 55: 515–521.

53. Narayanan S, Stewart GC, Chengappa MM, Willard L, Shuman W, et al. (2002) Fusobacterium necrophorum leukotoxin induces activation and apoptosis of bovine leukocytes. Infect Immun 70: 4609–4620.

54. Tan ZL, Nagaraja TG, Chengappa MM (1992) Factors affecting the leukotoxin activity of fusobacterium necrophorum. Vet Microbiol 32: 15–28.

55. Langermann S, Mollby R, Burlein JE, Palaszynski SR, Auguste CG, et al. (2000) Vaccination with FimH adhesin protects cynomolgus monkeys from colonization and infection by uropathogenic escherichia coli. J Infect Dis 181: 774–778.

# 19

# The Impact of Movements and Animal Density on Continental Scale Cattle Disease Outbreaks in the United States

Michael G. Buhnerkempe[1][*][¤], Michael J. Tildesley[2], Tom Lindström[3], Daniel A. Grear[1], Katie Portacci[4], Ryan S. Miller[4], Jason E. Lombard[4], Marleen Werkman[2], Matt J. Keeling[2], Uno Wennergren[3], Colleen T. Webb[1]

1 Department of Biology, Colorado State University, Fort Collins, Colorado, United States of America, 2 Center for Complexity Science, Mathematics Institute, University of Warwick, Coventry, United Kingdom, 3 Department of Physics, Chemistry, and Biology, Linköping University, Linköping, Sweden, 4 United States Department of Agriculture, Animal and Plant Health Inspection Service, Centers for Epidemiology and Animal Health, Fort Collins, Colorado, United States of America

## Abstract

Globalization has increased the potential for the introduction and spread of novel pathogens over large spatial scales necessitating continental-scale disease models to guide emergency preparedness. Livestock disease spread models, such as those for the 2001 foot-and-mouth disease (FMD) epidemic in the United Kingdom, represent some of the best case studies of large-scale disease spread. However, generalization of these models to explore disease outcomes in other systems, such as the United States's cattle industry, has been hampered by differences in system size and complexity and the absence of suitable livestock movement data. Here, a unique database of US cattle shipments allows estimation of synthetic movement networks that inform a near-continental scale disease model of a potential FMD-like (i.e., rapidly spreading) epidemic in US cattle. The largest epidemics may affect over one-third of the US and 120,000 cattle premises, but cattle movement restrictions from infected counties, as opposed to national movement moratoriums, are found to effectively contain outbreaks. Slow detection or weak compliance may necessitate more severe state-level bans for similar control. Such results highlight the role of large-scale disease models in emergency preparedness, particularly for systems lacking comprehensive movement and outbreak data, and the need to rapidly implement multi-scale contingency plans during a potential US outbreak.

Editor: Alessandro Vespignani, Northeastern University, United States of America

Funding: Funding provided by the Research and Policy for Infectious Disease Dynamics (RAPIDD) Program, Science and Technology Directorate, US Department of Homeland Security, and Fogarty International Center, National Institutes of Health; Foreign Animal Disease Modeling Program, Science and Technology Directorate, US Department of Homeland Security (Grant ST-108-000017); and USDA Cooperative Agreements 11-9208-0269-CA 11-1 and 09-9208-0235-CA. Data included in this analysis were provided by the US Department of Agriculture, Animal and Plant Health Inspection Service, Veterinary Services. However, the views and conclusions contained in this document are those of the authors and should not be interpreted as necessarily representing the official policies, either expressed or implied, of USDA-APHIS-Veterinary Services or the US Department of Homeland Security. The authors also acknowledge the National Institute for Mathematical and Biological Synthesis for supporting the Modeling Bovine Tuberculosis working group, where the initial ideas for using ICVI data were developed. The funders had no role in study design, data collection and analysis, decision to publish, or preparation of the manuscript.

Competing Interests: The authors have declared that no competing interests exist.

* E-mail: michael.buhnerkempe@gmail.com

¤ Current address: Department of Ecology and Evolutionary Biology, University of California Los Angeles, Los Angeles, California, United States of America; Fogarty International Center, National Institutes of Health, Bethesda, Maryland, United States of America

## Introduction

Outbreaks of rapidly spreading infections in populations of livestock around the world can have far reaching economic impacts. Direct costs of the 1997 FMD epidemic in Taiwan were estimated at $387.6 million, while the total cost was determined to be closer to $1.6 billion [1]. Similarly, the 2001 epidemic in the UK was estimated to have cost £3.1 billion to agriculture with similar, associated losses to tourism [2]. With a cattle population that is nearly an order of magnitude larger than that in the UK, the potential impacts of a rapidly spreading disease like FMD on the US economy are staggering. Mechanistic models of the spread of an FMD-like disease in the US can help to mitigate these potential costs by providing robust explorations of the effects of

scale and regionalization on potential surveillance and control measures. In particular, retrospective models of the 2001 UK outbreak provide insights on the influence of premises and animal densities on spatial dynamics of transmission [3–8] and the utility of detailed animal movement information in prediction of long-range disease spread [9–14].

Long-distance transmission is of particular concern when studying outbreaks at a larger spatial scale, and although mechanisms (e.g., tagging of certain animals) exist in the US to support animal tracing during an outbreak, these data are not readily available. Most publicly available information on livestock distribution in the US is aggregated at the county level owing to confidentiality concerns [15], and even the best source of national animal movement data (i.e., Interstate Certificates of Veterinary

Inspection; ICVIs) is incomplete owing to reporting requirements designed to ensure compliance with state and federal animal health import requirements as opposed to comprehensive movement tracking (see Materials and Methods). Previous characterizations of US cattle movements were therefore based on coarse summary data describing the volume of cattle moving between a subset of states [16], and existing models of disease spread in the US cattle industry lack an explicit, data driven movement network encompassing the entire industry [17–19]. In all, US livestock disease models face three inherent challenges not encountered in previous livestock disease models: 1) incomplete cattle movement information to characterize long-distance spread; 2) spatially aggregated premises location data prohibiting models of distance-based premises-to-premises spread; and 3) lack of outbreak data to parameterize epidemiological rates. We address the first challenge using a unique sample of ICVI records that, when incorporated into a spatially explicit movement kernel parameterized through Bayesian inference, allows us to create the first comprehensive cattle movement network model for the US. To address challenge two, a novel county-level metapopulation model is used to capture disease spread and assess control strategies. The parsimony of this model allows for extensive sensitivity analyses of epidemiological parameters to explore the impacts of challenge three (see Section E in Text S1) and also allows for the potential to fit the model during the early stages of a US outbreak.

## Materials and Methods

### ICVI Data

When livestock cross state lines, they are usually required to be accompanied by an Interstate Certificate of Veterinary Inspection (ICVI). A notable exception to this ICVI import requirement is cattle going directly to slaughter, although these movements are less important for transmission dynamics. ICVIs are official documents issued by a veterinarian accredited by USDA Animal and Plant Health Inspection Service-Veterinary Services who certifies animal health during an inspection prior to shipment. Additional copies of the ICVI are sent for approval and storage to the state veterinarian's office in both the state where the shipment originated and the state of destination. Because ICVIs are issued by individual states, forms differ from state to state. However, all ICVIs list the origin and destination address for the livestock shipment providing a useful source of data on interstate cattle movements. In addition, ICVIs contain varying quality information on the following: shipment date, purpose (e.g., feeding, breeding, show/exhibition), production type (i.e., beef or dairy), breed, sex, and age [20].

To facilitate sampling, we requested that state veterinarians' offices sample 2009 export ICVIs (see Section A in Text S1). ICVIs were sampled systematically by taking every 10th cattle record. In most cases states either sent the 10% sample or sent all of their 2009 export ICVIs, which were subsequently sampled using the same design (see Section A in Text S1 for exceptions). Our ICVI sample contains 19234 non-slaughter movement records from 49 states and 2433 counties with New Jersey being the only state that did not provide data.

### ICVI Network

Network models consist of a set of nodes representing the individual units of study and a set of edges that describe interactions between nodes. In our case, nodes are defined as either counties or states in the US, and edges indicate that nodes are connected by a shipment of cattle. Edges in the model are directed (i.e., shipments have a defined start and end point) and

weighted by the total number of shipments that move between nodes. Movement between nodes can now be described by paths, or any sequence of steps that can be taken to get from one node to another. We calculated several statistics that capture the overall structure of the US cattle movement network, including the diameter (i.e., the longest, shortest path length between any two nodes using unweighted edges) and the giant strongly connected component (i.e., GSCC, the largest set of nodes for which all pairs are reachable by a path in either direction). We also calculated a node's in-degree (i.e., the total number of imports to a node) and out-degree (i.e., the total number of exports from a node). We calculated the network statistics using the igraph package [21] for R statistical software [22].

### Bayesian Networks

Due to the partial observation of the cattle movement network, some method of estimating the total number of movements between counties is required to simulate disease spread on this network. Contact heterogeneities induced by spatial clustering as well as industry structure are known to have important consequences for disease spread dynamics [23] and hence need to addressed in this estimation. We therefore used a spatially explicit kernel method based on Bayesian inference that makes three different assumptions about the cattle movement in the US system: 1) the probability of movement between counties decreases with distance; 2) the probability of movement is dependent on the number of premises in a county; and 3) cattle industry infrastructure and production are highly variable between states influencing the number of shipments sent and received [24]. The model, parameter estimation and validation are comprehensively described in Lindström et al. [24], or see Section C in Text S1 for a brief description).

### Disease Model

A novel, stochastic metapopulation disease model [25,26] was developed that operates at the county scale and incorporates both local density-dependent spread and movement-based spread (see Table 1) along with culling of identified infected premises (IP). The disease simulations are based on a conceptualization where the premises is the basic unit of infection (see Section D in Text S1 for a complete description); that is, all animals within a premises become rapidly infected such that the entire premises can be classified as Susceptible, Exposed, Infectious or Removed. Premises-to-premises transmission occurs by two routes. First, local, non-movement contacts can result in aerosol, fence-line contact, or fomite transmission that are captured by a density- and distance-dependent spread process that is spatially localized within a county and between adjacent counties (see Table 1 and Figure S1). Second, long range movement transmission due to the shipping of animals between premises can occur between any two counties in the US (Table 1). However, while we consider transmission at the individual premises scale, data are only available at the county scale. This county-based aggregation leads to a stochastic metapopulation model whereby the population is divided geographically into a number of discrete patches, which we define as US counties [27–29].

Within each county, the population is considered to be well-mixed, consistent with the metapopulation formulation. However, in keeping with our conceptualization of the processes, local contacts are implicitly spatial and therefore depend on local density. We use the total number of cattle premises in each county from the 2007 Census of Agriculture conducted by the USDA National Agricultural Statistics Service (NASS) data as the base population in each county [15] and work with the number of

**Table 1.** Disease transmission routes in the model.

| | Movement spread[*] | Non-movement spread | |
| --- | --- | --- | --- |
| | | **Within-county** | **Local cross-border** |
| **Cause** | Animal Shipments | Aerosol, fence-line contact, or fomite transmission | Aerosol, fence-line contact, or fomite transmission |
| **Spatial Scale** | All counties in the US | Premises within an infected county | All neighboring counties |
| **Assumptions** | 1) Premises density-dependent; 2) Spatially explicit[†]; 3) Differs by state and production type | 1) Premises density-dependent; 2) Premises size dependent | 1) Premises density-dependent[‡]; 2) Premises size dependent[‡]; 3) Spatially implicit[§] |
| **Informed by or data from** | 1) ICVI records; 2) Number of premises by county and production type[¶]; 3) State cattle inflows [38] | 1) 2001 UK FMD outbreak [39]; 2) US premises density and size distributions[¶] | 1) 2001 UK FMD outbreak [39]; 2) US premises density and size distributions[¶]; 3) Shared county border length |
| **Parameter Uncertainty** | Estimated through Bayesian inference and incorporated in the simulations via multiple realizations of shipment networks. | Broad parameter ranges explored in a sensitivity analysis[‖]. | Broad parameter ranges explored in a sensitivity analysis[‖]. |

[*]See Section C in Text S1 and Lindström et al. [24].
[†]Based on county centroids.
[‡]In both the focal and neighboring counties.
[§]Based on randomly distributed premises in the focal and neighboring counties.
[¶]See Section B in Text S1 and NASS census data [15].
[‖]See Section E in Text S1.

premises of each epidemiological classification in each county (Susceptible, Exposed, Infectious, or Removed). At the start of the simulation all premises are assumed to be susceptible. These become infected through estimates of localized within- or between-county transmission, or movement-based transmission and move into the exposed class. Unless stated otherwise, we assume disease parameters for a rapidly spreading FMD-like disease. The mean exposed (latent) period is 5 days after which the premises becomes infectious and actively transmits (see Table 2). The mean delay from a premises becoming infectious and that premises being removed is 7 days (see Table 2), in line with previous work for time

to depopulation in the 2001 UK epidemic [3,6]. A thorough sensitivity analysis of transmission parameters was also performed (see Section E in Text S1 and Table 2).

When studying the effect of movement restrictions, we assumed that any movement ban was 100% effective, in that all movements to and from the movement ban area would stop once introduced, and that a movement ban was introduced on the same day that the first infectious premises in a region was removed (i.e. a 7 day delay from a premises becoming infectious). We also explored the effect of movement ban effectiveness of stopping 100%, 90%, 75% and 50% of movements, coupled with a time delay to implementation

**Table 2.** Disease simulation model parameters.

| Type | Parameter | Value | Range | Description |
| --- | --- | --- | --- | --- |
| Transmission | $\beta$ | 0.0003508[*] | $[2\times10^{-5}, 4\times10^{-2}]$ | Transmission rate between cattle on different premises |
| | $\alpha$ | 4.6[†] | [2.1, 6] | Shape of the local, non-movement spatial kernel |
| | $\theta$ | 1.6[‡] | [1,6] | Scale of the local, non-movement spatial kernel |
| | $p$ | 0.414[†] | [0, 1] | Non-linear scaling of the effect of premises size (i.e., number of cattle) on susceptibility to infection |
| | $q$ | 0.424[†] | [0, 1] | Non-linear scaling of the effect of premises size (i.e., number of cattle) on transmission of infection |
| Control | $\varepsilon$ | 100%[†] | [50%,100%] | Percentage of movements to/from an area that are stopped by a movement ban |
| | $\lambda$ | 7[§] | 7, 14, 21 | The delay between a premises becoming infected and subsequently being identified and removed, which triggers movement bans |
| Other | $\sigma$ | 5[§] | NA[¶] | The latent period; amount of time between a premises being exposed to infection and becoming infectious |

[*]Units in Premises (days)$^{-1}$.
[†]Unit-less parameter.
[‡]Units in kilometers.
[§]Units in days.
[¶]Sensitivity analysis was not performed on this parameter.

of the movement ban from the first premises becoming infectious of 7 days, 14 days and 21 days.

For all of the analyses described in this paper, 100 epidemics were seeded in each of the 3109 counties in turn to allow for an investigation of the impact of the precise location of the source of the outbreak upon the spread of disease. For each epidemic, we measured the epidemic extent (i.e., number of counties infected) and the epidemic size (i.e., number of farms infected). Across all simulations, we also measured each county's infection risk (i.e., the proportion of epidemics a county is affected by when seeding infection in each of the 3109 counties). Each of the 100 simulations in a given county utilized a different realization (as sampled from the posterior predictive distribution of movements) of the Bayesian movement kernel described above. The model was programmed in FORTRAN.

## Results and Discussion

### Cattle Movement Networks

Movement patterns are dominated by movements to and from the Central Plains states (Figure 1). These states boast the majority of US feeder cattle, reflecting the large percentage of sampled ICVIs filed for feeding purposes (44.8%), although breeding (16.8%) and show/exhibition/rodeo (7.2%) movements are also common. Shipments were generally small with 81.7% containing fewer than 100 head of cattle and 38.2% containing fewer than 10, which, in general, matches the prevalence of US premises with fewer than 100 head of cattle (90.4% of beef premises [30]; 76.7% of dairy premises [31]). These general trends in the sampled ICVIs are consistent with a large central feeding system that amasses

cattle from numerous relatively small holdings [30-32]. Although this database is the first of its kind, we note that we are limited to a single year of data, and multiple factors can change with time to affect cattle movement patterns (e.g., drought, fuel prices, and feed prices). However, we are encouraged that, in addition to the similarities to trends in the U.S. cattle industry noted above, large scale patterns (i.e., state-to-state cattle flows) are similar between summary ICVI data from 2000–2001 [16] and our sampled ICVI data (Figure 1). Thus, despite the potential for yearly variation, our sampled ICVI data are at least good qualitative indicators of the major cattle movement patterns that appear robust to such variation.

To characterize these patterns and consider spatial heterogeneity in shipments, we aggregated ICVI data at both the state and county scales to create movement networks, with the number of shipments determining the weight of directed edges between nodes. At the state scale, the cattle network consists almost entirely of one giant strongly connected component (GSCC), with the only exception being New Jersey due to its lack of export data (Figure 2A). This GSCC results in a network with a relatively small linear size (i.e., a diameter of 3), potentially allowing cattle, and hence infection, to move between states in a small number of steps. Several geographically central states show higher import and export activity in the cattle movement network (Figures 3A and 4A). At the county scale, the GSCC contains 1551 of the 2433

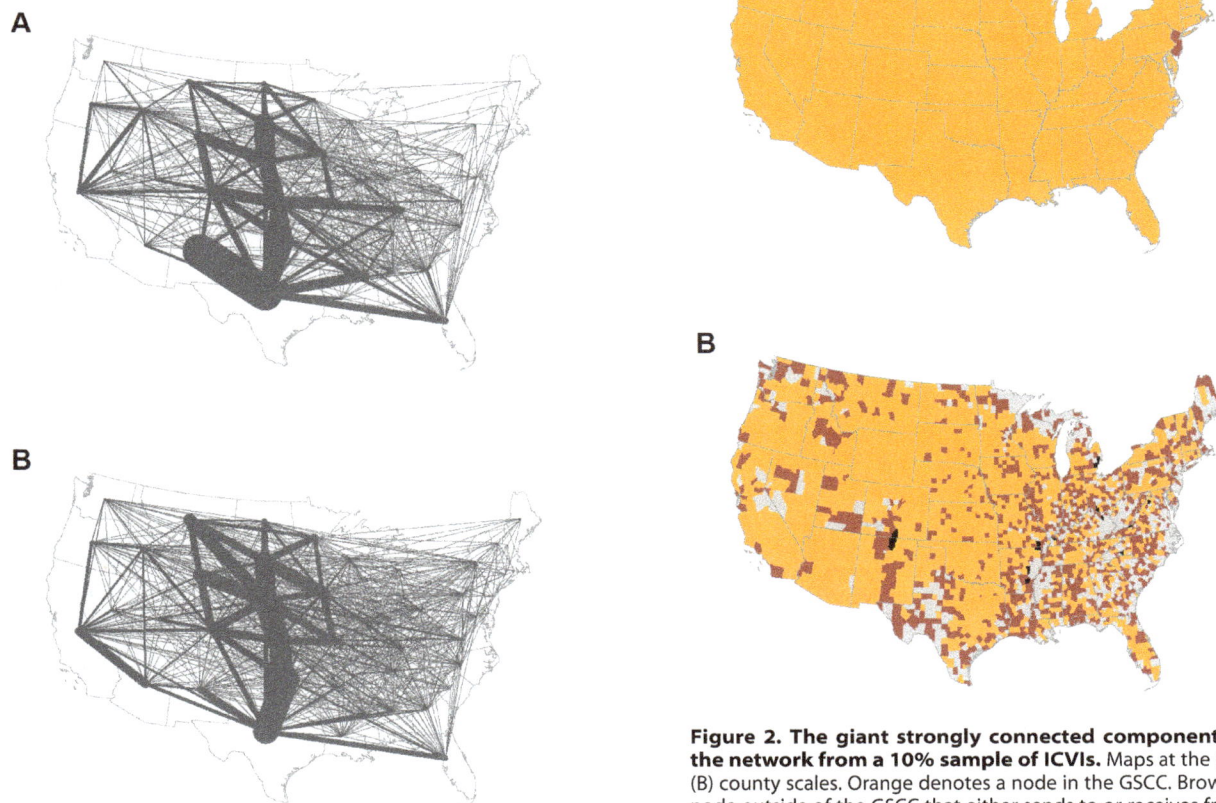

**A**

**B**

**Figure 1. State-to-state cattle flows.** Given for the (A) ERS ICVI summary data [16] and (B) 10% sample of paper ICVIs.

**A**

**B**

**Figure 2. The giant strongly connected component (GSCC) of the network from a 10% sample of ICVIs.** Maps at the (A) state and (B) county scales. Orange denotes a node in the GSCC. Brown denotes a node outside of the GSCC that either sends to or receives from nodes in the GSCC but not both, and black indicates nodes that are isolated from the GSCC. Gray indicates no data. New Jersey is outside the state level GSCC because it was the only state not to supply ICVI data.

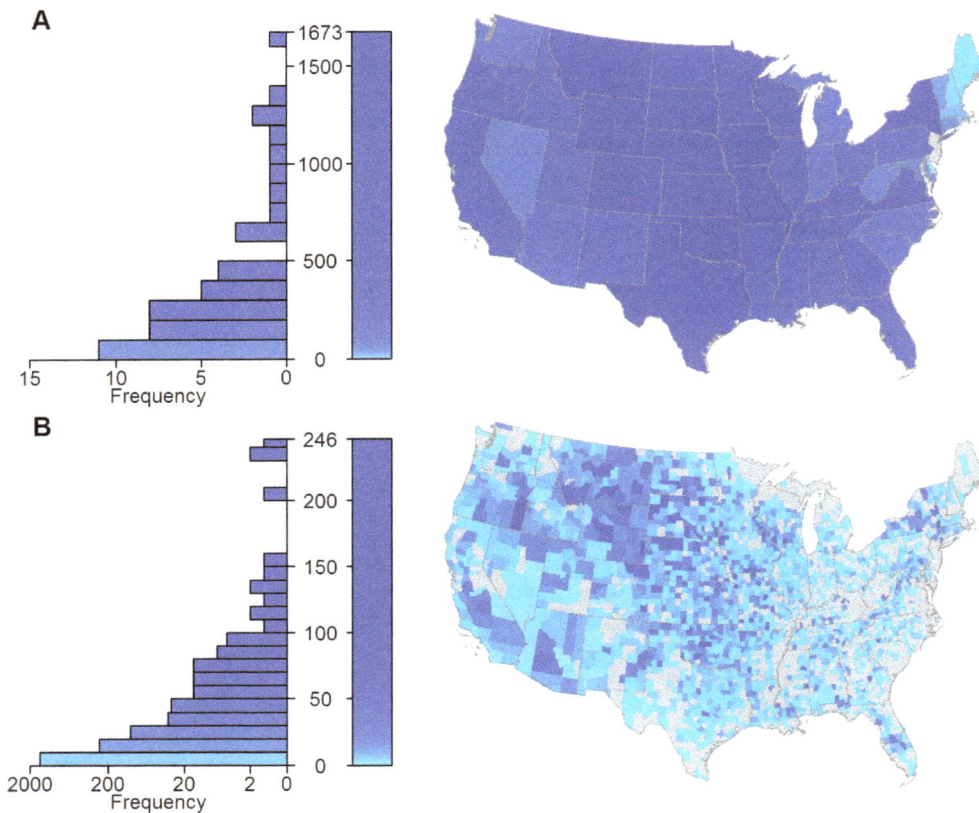

**Figure 3. Out-degree distributions of the cattle movement network from a 10% sample of ICVIs.** The network is aggregated into (A) state and (B) county nodes. The left-hand graphs show the frequency distribution of node out-degrees, while the maps show the value for that area. A logarithmic color scale is used to differentiate high (dark blue) from low (light blue) out-degree. Counties with no sampled out-shipments are indicated in gray.

counties in the network, with other counties being either isolated or only connected in one direction (i.e., by imports or exports but not both) to the GSCC (Figure 2B); in addition, there is a substantial increase in the network distance between nodes (i.e., a diameter of 12). At the county level, import and export activity centers are shifted spatially and exist both within and outside of their state-level counterparts (Figures 3B and 4B). As such, the state scale network aggregates over heterogeneities that are potentially important for disease spread and targeted disease surveillance and control [32].

Owing to the resolution of the available data and the heterogeneities present, we suggest that epidemics are more effectively studied at the county scale. Our ICVI data are a sample of interstate movements, but the data contained numerous short-distance interstate movements. We therefore extrapolate this data to inform the full pattern of movements using a heterogeneous spatial kernel and Bayesian inference methods to generate complete movement networks, including within-state movements [24]. Rather than simulating disease with past movement patterns to determine the spread of infection [10–12,33], we use replicated Bayesian estimates of complete movement networks [24] (i.e., scaling up to all cattle shipments including within-state movements) to explore uncertainty in movement patterns (see Sections C and D in Text S1).

## Metapopulation Disease Model

Our model shows that epidemic behavior is strongly dependent on the site of introduction although results are highly stochastic. The largest generated epidemics (i.e., upper $97.5^{th}$ percentile) are capable of reaching 40% of US counties (the epidemic extent; Figure 5A) and infecting over 120,000 premises (the epidemic size; Figure S2A). When analyzing epidemics, we focus on the upper $97.5^{th}$ percentile for outbreaks because epidemic extent and size are bimodal: most outbreaks affect 1 or 2 counties (Figure S3A) and less than 10 farms (Figure S2B), but emergency preparedness must address the potential for sustained nationwide epidemics, such as those that arise from the Central Plains and Ohio River Valley in our simulations (Figures 5A and S2A). These regions also experience the greatest risk of infection following introduction elsewhere pointing to potential surveillance and vaccine targets (Figure 5B).

With large epidemics spawned from diverse regions of the US, insight for control and surveillance can be gained through an understanding of the heterogeneity in disease spread processes that create the mosaic of outbreak sizes. Because the outputs of our disease simulations were a product of a mixture of local and global processes, simple correlational analyses between a county's disease outputs and its movements (measured here by the mean out-degree of a county over the 100 predicted networks used in the disease simulations) are confounded by the effect of local spread processes (measured by premises density). To circumvent this

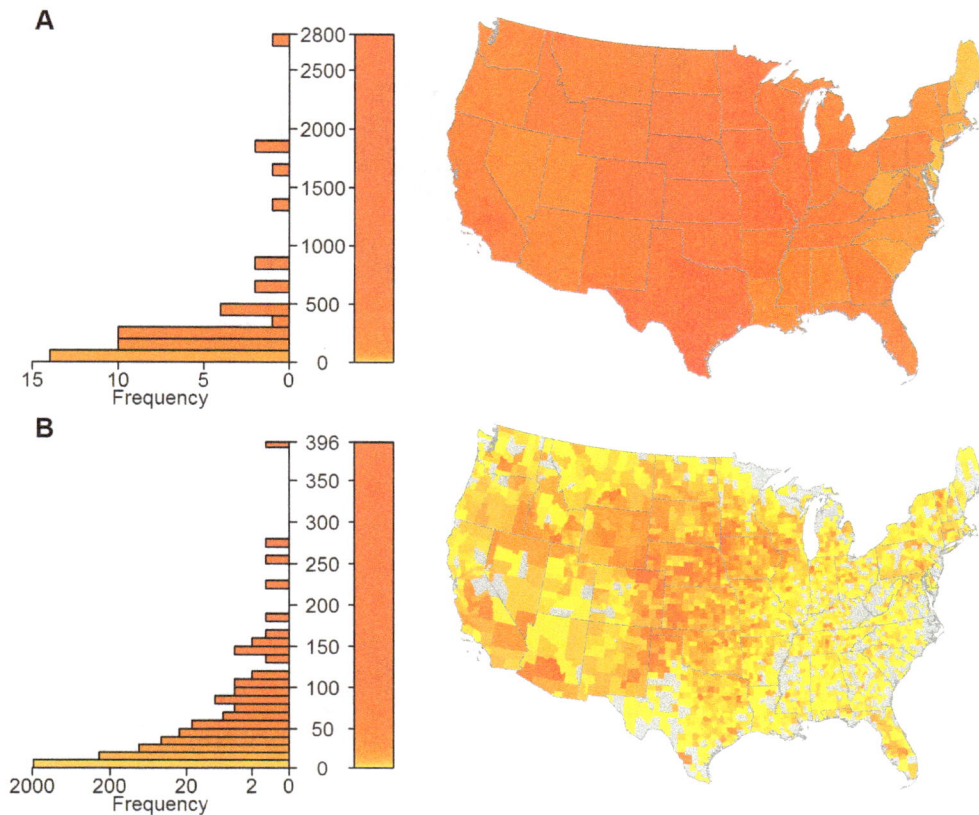

**Figure 4. In-degree distributions of the cattle movement network from a 10% sample of ICVIs.** The network is aggregated into (A) state and (B) county nodes. The left-hand graphs show the frequency distribution of node in-degrees, whilst the maps show the value for that area. A logarithmic color scale is used to differentiate high (red) from low (yellow) in-degree. Counties with no sampled in-shipments are indicated in gray.

problem, we used a principal component analysis on the counties' out-degrees and premises densities to remove any correlations between the two processes. When we consider the largest epidemic extents (i.e., the counties that generate the largest 20% of uncontrolled epidemic extents denoted by the colored dots in Figure 6A), we see no discernible pattern in the relationship between epidemic extent and these principal components. Spatially, however, we find that counties where movement was relatively more important are found within the clusters of counties that generate large outbreaks (i.e., green to blue regions in Figure 6B). These movement centers are in turn juxtaposed with regions where density is relatively more important (i.e., the orange to red regions in Figure 6B). Thus, local spread processes, here modeled with density-dependence, can result in slow, diffusive spread capable of sustaining itself without long-distance movement but potentially triggering epidemic spread when it reaches a nearby movement hub. Disease spread in the Ohio River Valley appears to be driven almost exclusively due to the impacts of local spread as measured by the effect of cattle density (Figure 6B) requiring potentially different approaches to disease control.

## Controlling Disease Spread with Movement Bans

When infection is detected, cattle shipments from the infected area are likely to be banned to prevent further spread. We focus on movement bans from any county (or state) with known infection. With rapid detection, county-level bans substantially reduce epidemic extent, size and infection risk (Figures 5C-D, S2C-D, and S3C-D) while state bans have little additional benefit (Figures

5E-F, S2E-F, and S3E-F). The sufficiency of county restrictions results from the fragmented distribution of movement centers (Figures 3B and 6B). Local spread away from movement centers is relatively slow in many areas, such that rapid IP removal alone is adequate to prevent the majority of spread across county borders. This means that when infection can be controlled locally, bans beyond the county scale have little additional impact. However, this result will ultimately be modified by the relative influence of local processes on disease spread. Increased density-dependence will decrease the effectiveness of local bans by promoting local, cross-border spread. Thus, the performance of control strategies must be considered in the context of the mechanisms underlying disease spread.

For the results above, we assumed the delay from a farm becoming infectious to its removal was 7 days (i.e., the infectious period), at which point a 100% effective movement ban was also introduced (i.e., all movements to/from and within the targeted area are prevented). Although this assumption is based on observed detection for the UK [3,6], it may be optimistic in the US where the scale of the industry may hamper detection and control. Longer delays before IP culling and movement bans increase the epidemic extent dramatically for some source counties (Figures 7 and S4), as these delays allow both a greater degree of local spread and a greater risk of moving infected cattle. Consequently, for a delay of 21 days, a county ban cannot readily contain infection, and a state ban results in marked reductions in epidemic extent (Figure 7). Less effective movement bans (i.e., where a proportion of shipments still occur) result in an increase in

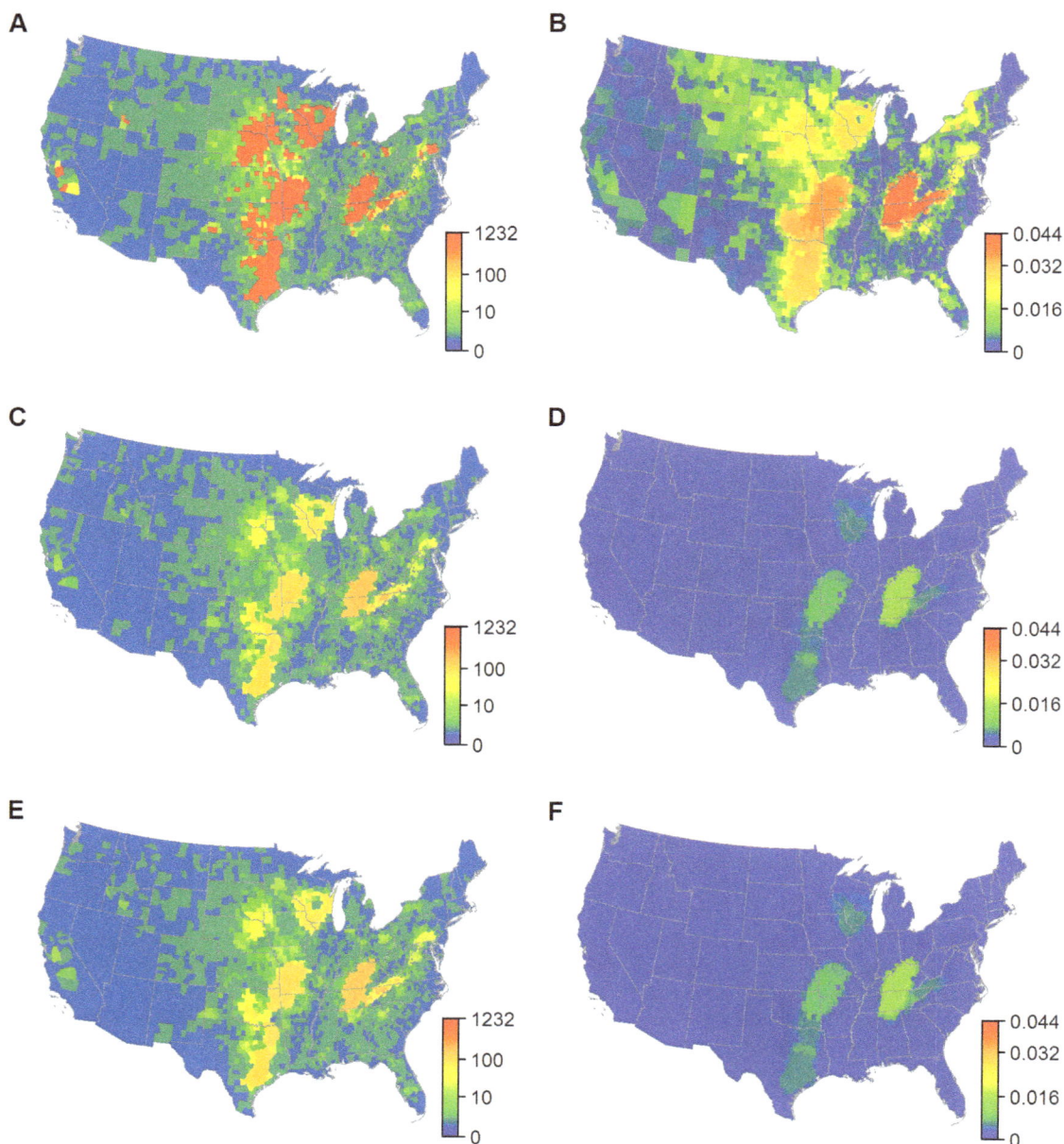

**Figure 5. Epidemic extent and infection risk with unrestricted, county and, state movement bans.** Upper tail of the distribution (based on the 97.5th percentile of 100 simulations) for epidemic extent and infection risk when infections are introduced to each of the 3109 counties of the continental US. (A & B) assume standard movements while (C & D) assume a county-level movement ban and (E & F) assume a state-level movement ban. (A, C, & E) the epidemic extent (the number of counties infected) for an infection seeded in each county. (B, D, & F) the infection risk (the proportion of all simulated outbreaks that infect a county).

the mean epidemic extents due to counties that produce epidemics that ultimately affect over 1000 additional counties, a scale rarely observed under a completely effective ban (Figure S4). As the effectiveness decreases from 100% to 50%, even more differentiation between the state and county bans is observed (Figure 7). We therefore conclude that IP removal and movement control must be introduced rapidly and with reasonable effectiveness for county level control to be sufficient. Any significant delays in detection favor the use of a state ban with an emphasis on ban effectiveness.

## Conclusions

Generalizing kernel-based disease models in UK cattle [3–8] to larger cattle systems, such as the United States, has been difficult with insufficient spatial resolution and alignment among often-times incomplete data sets to capture inherently complex contact networks. By integrating novel movement data, network scaling advances, and metapopulation disease models that absorb location uncertainties with a flexible kernel-based spread model to explore disease impacts, we illustrate the potential to explore disease spread and control in large, complex, and relatively data-poor systems like the US cattle industry. Our modeling framework

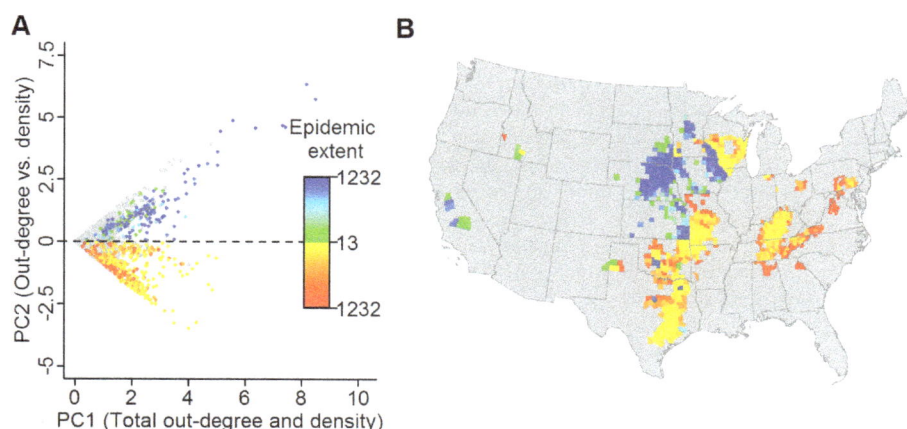

**Figure 6. Relative importance of movement vs. local spread determined through a Principal component analysis.** (A) Plot of PC1 (0.7071*Out−degree+0.7071*Premises density) vs. PC2 (0.7071*Out−degree+0.7071*Premises density) for each county. Colored dots represent counties in the upper 20% of simulated epidemic extents with the counties where movement is relatively more important (i.e., PC2 > 0) ranging from green to blue and the counties where density is relatively more important (i.e., PC2 < 0) ranging from yellow to red based on epidemic extent. (B) Map depicting the spatial distribution of the counties within the upper 20% of epidemic extents.

advances previous models of cattle disease spread in the US [17–19] by using the sampled ICVI data to estimate complete contact networks for the entire country, which is a noted gap in applying previous FMD models, even to regional spatial scales [34,35]. In addition, parametric distance distributions have been used to describe local transmission processes among individual premises in previous US simulation models spanning county [18] and national scales [17]. Notably, our model represents a trade-off in scale: the coarse data and modeling resolution (relative to individual premises modeling) does not require information on the spatial locations of all cattle premises in the US. Rather, in this study, county-level demographic information is sufficient to characterize disease spread and inform policy at epidemiologically and policy relevant spatial scales.

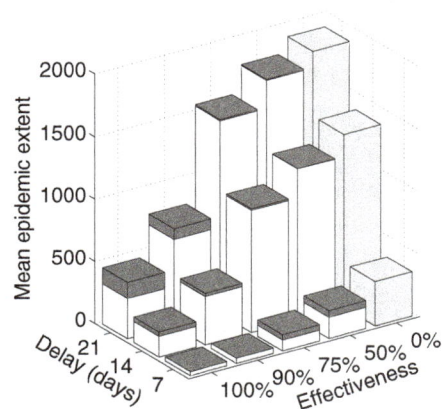

**Figure 7. Sensitivity analysis for disease control parameters.** Sensitivity of epidemic extent (i.e., number of counties infected) to changes in the delay to implementation and effectiveness of movement bans (i.e., proportion of movements from an area that are stopped). Bars give the mean extent for epidemics begun in the 5% of counties that generate the largest uncontrolled epidemics (as depicted in Figure 5A). The white bars represent a state-level ban while the dark gray bars show the additional epidemic extent if only a county-level ban were introduced. The light gray bars show the no movement ban case.

Yet without a previous significant epidemic, disease models in the US need to be largely informed by outbreak data from countries with cattle industries of different size and structure. Therefore, when faced with an outbreak in the US, rapid estimation of epidemiological parameters is crucial to assess appropriate control measures. Indeed, model sensitivity analyses (see Section E in Text S1) show that levels of infection are strongly parameter dependent (Figure S5A), supporting the need for quick parameterization of models during an outbreak. In contrast to previous U.S. simulation models [17,19], the relatively parsimonious model structure used in this study facilitates such estimation due to the small number of parameters to be estimated. However, despite the sensitivity of model outputs to specific parameter values, the relative pattern of county-level heterogeneities is robust against parameter variation (Figure S5B). Thus, despite considerable uncertainty in parameter values, spatial patterning in disease impacts is qualitatively, although not necessarily quantitatively, consistent.

However, parameter variation is not the only potential source of uncertainty to be addressed in models of disease spread in the US cattle industry. Recent work has found that daily fluctuations in cattle movement patterns can be an important feature of European network models affecting node centrality and transmission potential in both time and space [36,37]. Unfortunately, daily networks resulting from our ICVI data are sparse owing to current data constraints. Thus, care must be taken to identify a temporal resolution (e.g., seasonal) that captures actual trends in movement, as opposed to sampling artifacts, in future modeling efforts. In addition, logistical constraints necessarily limited our data collection to cattle ICVIs. However, spread of some livestock diseases (e.g., FMD) may impact species outside of cattle. Future data collection efforts in the US should focus on the potential interaction between livestock industries and in particular, the interaction between long-distance movements and inter-specific local spread.

Despite these potential limitations, our model provides the first truly nationwide assessment of the potential mechanisms, spatial patterns, and impacts of an FMD-like disease outbreak in US cattle. Given the difference in spatial scale between the US and the more well-studied European systems, it is valuable to identify such risk areas for targeted planning and control as we have done here.

In particular, the near-continental scale of our model makes state-scale interventions more similar to national-scale interventions in European contexts. We found that more local movement controls, contrary to national or state-scale moratoriums, are often sufficient to control the largest epidemics, although the scale of intervention critically depends on the speed and effectiveness of control. Local movement controls enhance business continuity, a finding with wide appeal for food security, animal welfare, and economic issues not only in the US but also internationally where these local movement controls have not been thoroughly explored. Thus, this modeling framework provides a crucial tool for assessing the efficiency of disease mitigation control measures not only in the US cattle industry, but in numerous data-poor systems where disease spread over large regions is a concern. Future models must continue to explore a wide variety of potential strategies and epidemiological scenarios.

## Supporting Information

**Figure S1 Graphical representation of the spatial variables found in $\Omega_C$ and $\Omega_{C,C1}$ (see Section D in Text S1).**

**Figure S2 Upper tail of and median epidemic size with unrestricted, county, and state movement bans.** Epidemic size (the number of premises infected) when infections are seeded in each of the 3109 counties of mainland USA. (A, C, E) show the upper tail of the distribution (based on the 97.5th percentile of 100 simulations seeded in a county), while (B, D, F) show the median epidemic size (based on the median of 100 simulations seeded in a county) under (A, B) standard movements, (C, D) a county-level movement ban, and (E, F) a state-level movement ban.

**Figure S3 Median epidemic extent and infection risk under unrestricted, county, and state movement bans.** Median epidemic extents and infection risks (based on the medians of 100 simulations) when infections are seeded in each of the 3109 counties of mainland USA. (A, C, E) show the median epidemic extents (the number of counties infected), while (B, D, F) show the median infection risks under (A, B) no movement ban, (C, D) a county-level movement ban, and (E, F) a state-level movement ban. The bimodality in epidemic behavior is apparent when comparing epidemic extents here to the much larger epidemics seen in Figure 5.

## References

1. Yang PC, Chu RM, Chung WB, Sung HT (1999) Epidemiological characteristics and financial costs of the 1997 foot-and-mouth disease epidemic in Taiwan. Vet Rec 145: 731–734.
2. Thompson D, Muriel P, Russell D, Osborne P, Bromley A, et al. (2002) Economic costs of the foot and mouth disease outbreak in the United Kingdom in 2001. Rev Sci Tech 21: 675–687.
3. Keeling MJ, Woolhouse MEJ, Shaw DJ, Matthews L, Chase-Topping M, et al. (2001) Dynamics of the 2001 UK foot and mouth epidemic: stochastic dispersal in a heterogeneous landscape. Science 294: 813–817.
4. Ferguson NM, Donnelly CA, Anderson RM (2001) The foot-and-mouth epidemic in Great Britain: pattern of spread and impact of interventions. Science 292: 1155–1160.
5. Keeling MJ, Woolhouse MEJ, May RM, Davies G, Grenfell BT (2003) Modelling vaccination strategies against foot-and-mouth disease. Nature 421: 136–142.
6. Tildesley MJ, Savill NJ, Shaw DJ, Deardon R, Brooks SP, et al. (2006) Optimal reactive vaccination strategies for a foot-and-mouth outbreak in the UK. Nature 440: 83–86.
7. Chis Ster I, Ferguson NM (2007) Transmission parameters of the 2001 foot and mouth epidemic in Great Britain. PLoS ONE 2: e502. doi:10.1371/journal.pone.0000502

**Figure S4 Sensitivity of epidemic extent to delay to implementation and effectiveness of a movement ban.** The frequency distributions of epidemic extent for a 7-day (top panel), 14-day (middle panel), and 21-day (bottom panel) delay to the implementation of a county (blue bars) or state (green/yellow bars) movement ban. Ban effectiveness decreases from 100% (county ban – dark blue; state ban – dark green) to 75% (county ban – blue; state ban – light green), and 50% (county ban – light blue; state ban – yellow) of movements stopped. The results for the no movement ban case are shown in red.

**Figure S5 Sensitivity analysis for disease transmission parameters.** Sensitivity analysis results are from the binomial mixed-model describing the mean number of counties infected in the US. (A) Effect sizes for the fixed effects, including main effects of the parameters and all pair-wise interactions, of the transmission parameters. All fixed effects were significantly different from zero ($p < 0.05$), although the main effects had the largest magnitude effect sizes. (B) Variability in the random, county effects on the transmission parameters. Dashed lines indicate zero values.

**Text S1 Supplementary methods.** Contains sections with descriptions of (A) Interstate Certificate of Veterinary Inspection (ICVI) collection and entry; (B) Premises density and size data; (C) Bayesian kernel model for complete network estimation; (D) Metapopulation disease model; and (E) Sensitivity analysis of disease transmission parameters.

## Acknowledgments

We would like to thank the State Veterinarian's Offices that helped obtain the ICVI data.

## Author Contributions

Conceived and designed the experiments: MGB MJT TL DAG KP RSM JEL UW CTW. Performed the experiments: MGB MJT TL DAG KP RSM MW CTW. Analyzed the data: MGB MJT DAG MW. Contributed reagents/materials/analysis tools: MGB MJT TL DAG KP RSM MJK UW CTW. Wrote the paper: MGB MJT TL DAG KP RSM JEL MW MJK UW CTW. Collected ICVI data: MGB DAG KP RSM CTW. Performed network analysis on ICVI data: MGB DAG. Performed Bayesian estimation of complete networks: TL UW. Developed the metapopulation disease model: MGB MJT DAG MJK UW CTW. Ran disease simulations and analysis: MGB MJT DAG MW.

8. Chis Ster I, Singh BK, Ferguson NM (2009) Epidemiological inference for partially observed epidemics: the example of the 2001 foot and mouth epidemic in Great Britain. Epidemics 1: 21–34.
9. Green DM, Kiss IZ, Kao RR (2006) Modelling the initial spread of foot-and-mouth disease through animal movements. Proc Biol Sci 273: 2729–2735.
10. Kao RR, Danon L, Green DM, Kiss IZ (2006) Demographic structure and pathogen dynamics on the network of livestock movements in Great Britain. Proc Biol Sci 273: 1999–2007.
11. Kiss IZ, Green DM, Kao RR (2006) The network of sheep movements within Great Britain: network properties and their implications for infectious disease spread. J R Soc Interface 3: 669–677.
12. Ortiz-Pelaez A, Pfeiffer DU, Soares-Magalhães RJ, Guitian FJ (2006) Use of social network analysis to characterize the pattern of animal movements in the initial phases of the 2001 foot and mouth disease (FMD) epidemic in the UK. Prev Vet Med 76: 40–55.
13. Kao RR, Green DM, Johnson J, Kiss IZ (2007) Disease dynamics over very different time-scales: foot-and-mouth disease and scrapie on the network of livestock movements in the UK. J R Soc Interface 4: 907–916.
14. Robinson SE, Everett MG, Christley RM (2007) Recent network evolution increases the potential for large epidemics in the British cattle population. J R Soc Interface 4: 669–674.

15. National Agricultural Statistics Service, US Department of Agriculture (2007) Census of Agriculture. Available: http://www.nass.usda.gov/census.

16. Shields DA, Mathews KH (2003) Interstate livestock movements. USDA ERS Outlook Report LDP-M-108-01. Available: http://www.ers.usda.gov/media/312234/ldpm10801_1_.pdf.

17. Harvey N, Reeves A, Schoenbaum MA, Zagmutt-Vergara FJ, Dubé C, et al. (2007) The North American Animal Disease Spread Model: a simulation model to assist decision making in evaluating animal disease incursions. Prev Vet Med 82: 176–197.

18. Bates TW, Thurmond MC, Carpenter TE (2003) Description of an epidemic simulation model for use in evaluating strategies to control an outbreak of foot-and-mouth disease. Am J Vet Res 64: 195–204.

19. Speck DE (2008) Overview of the Multiscale Epidemiologic/Economic Simulation and Analysis (MESA) decision support system. US Department of Energy Report LLNL-TR-404724. Available: https://e-reports-ext.llnl.gov/pdf/360630.pdf.

20. Portacci K, Miller RS, Riggs PD, Buhnerkempe MG, Abrahamsen LM (2013) Assessment of paper Interstate Certificates of Veterinary Inspection to support disease tracing in cattle. J Am Vet Med Assoc 234: 555–560.

21. Csardi G, Nepusz T (2006) The igraph software package for complex network research. InterJournal Complex Systems 1695.

22. R Development Core Team (2012) R: a language and environment for statistical computing. Vienna, Austria: R Foundation for Statistical Computing.

23. Lindström T, Lewerin SS, Wennergren U (2012) Influence on disease spread dynamics of herd characteristics in a structured livestock industry. J R Soc Interface 9: 1287–1294.

24. Lindström T, Grear DA, Buhnerkempe M, Webb CT, Miller RS, et al. (2013) A Bayesian approach for modeling cattle movements in the United States: scaling up a partially observed network. PLoS ONE 8: e53432. doi: 10.1371/journal.pone.0053432

25. Sattenspiel L, Dietz KA (1995) structured epidemic model incorporating geographic mobility among regions. Math Biosci 128: 71–91.

26. Hanski I, Gaggiotti OE, editors (2004) Ecology, Genetics and Evolution of Metapopulations. Burlington, MA: Elsevier Academic Press. 696 p.

27. Smith DL, Lucey B, Waller LA, Childs JE, Real LA (2002) Predicting the spatial dynamics of rabies epidemics on heterogeneous landscapes. Proc Natl Acad Sci USA 99: 3668–3672.

28. Ovaskainen O, Hanski I (2001) Spatially structured metapopulation models: global and local assessment of metapopulation capacity. Theor Popul Biol 60: 281–302.

29. Ovaskainen O (2002) The effective size of a metapopulation living in a heterogeneous patch network. Am Nat 160: 612–628.

30. US Department of Agriculture (2011) Small-scale U.S. Cow-calf Operations. Report 596.0411, USDA–APHIS–VS, CEAH, Fort Collins, CO.

31. US Department of Agriculture (2008) Dairy 2007, Part II: Changes in the U.S. Dairy Cattle Industry, 1991-2007. Report N481.0308, USDA–APHIS–VS, CEAH, Fort Collins, CO.

32. Buhnerkempe MG, Grear DA, Portacci K, Miller RS, Lombard JE, et al. (2013) A national-scale picture of U.S. cattle movements obtained from Interstate Certificate of Veterinary Inspection data. Prev Vet Med 112: 318–329.

33. Vernon MC, Keeling MJ (2012) Impact of regulatory perturbations to disease spread through cattle movements in Great Britain. Prev Vet Med 105: 110–117.

34. National Research Council (2010) Evaluation of a Site-Specific Risk Assessment for the Department of Homeland Security's Planned National Bio- and Agro-Defense Facility in Manhattan, Kansas. Washington, DC: National Academies Press.

35. National Research Council (2012) Evaluation of the Updated Site-Specific Risk Assessment for the National Bio- and Agro-Defense Facility in Manhattan, Kansas. Washington, DC: National Academies Press.

36. Bajardi P, Barrat A, Natale F, Savini L, Colizza V (2011) Dynamical patterns of cattle trade movements. PLoS ONE 6: e19869. doi:10.1371/journal.pone.0019869

37. Bajardi P, Barrat A, Savini L, Colizza V (2012) Optimizing surveillance for livestock disease spreading through animal movements. J R Soc Interface 9: 2814–2825.

38. National Agricultural Statistics Service, US Department of Agriculture (2012) Quick stats Washington, DC. Available: http://quickstats.nass.usda.gov/.

39. Tildesley MJ, Deardon R, Savill NJ, Bessell PR, Brooks SP, et al. (2008) Accuracy of models for the 2001 foot-and-mouth epidemic. Proc Biol Sci 275: 1459–1468.

# 20

# Evaluation of Monoclonal Antibody-Based Sandwich Direct ELISA (MSD-ELISA) for Antigen Detection of Foot-and-Mouth Disease Virus Using Clinical Samples

**Kazuki Morioka, Katsuhiko Fukai, Kenichi Sakamoto, Kazuo Yoshida, Toru Kanno\***

Exotic Disease Research Station, National Institute of Animal Health, National Agriculture and Food Research Organization, Josuihoncho Kodaira, Tokyo, Japan

## Abstract

A monoclonal antibody-based sandwich direct ELISA (MSD-ELISA) method was previously developed for foot-and-mouth disease (FMD) viral antigen detection. Here we evaluated the sensitivity and specificity of two FMD viral antigen detection MSD-ELISAs and compared them with conventional indirect sandwich (IS)-ELISA. The MSD-ELISAs were able to detect the antigen in saliva samples of experimentally-infected pigs for a longer term compared to the IS-ELISA. We also used 178 RT-PCR-positive field samples from cattle and pigs affected by the 2010 type-O FMD outbreak in Japan, and we found that the sensitivities of both MSD-ELISAs were about 7 times higher than that of the IS-ELISA against each sample (P<0.01). In terms of the FMD-positive farm detection rate, the sensitivities of the MSD-ELISAs were about 6 times higher than that of the IS-ELISA against each farm (P<0.01). Although it is necessary to conduct further validation study using the other virus strains, MSD-ELISAs could be appropriate as a method to replace IS-ELISA for FMD antigen detection.

**Editor:** Herman Tse, The University of Hong Kong, Hong Kong

**Funding:** This study was supported by Grants-in-Aid for Scientific Research from the Foot-and-Mouth Disease Control Project of the Ministry of Agriculture, Forestry and Fisheries of Japan. URL http://www.s.affrc.go.jp/docs/pdf/2008_project_2_1.pdf. The funders had no role in study design, data collection and analysis, decision to publish, or preparation of the manuscript.

**Competing Interests:** The authors have declared that no competing interests exist.

\* E-mail: kannot@affrc.go.jp

## Introduction

Foot-and-mouth disease (FMD) is caused by the FMD virus (FMDV), a member of the family *Picornaviridae*, genus *Aphthovirus*. FMD is highly contagious and has the economic effect of limiting international trade in livestock and livestock products [1]. FMDV can cause blistering, vesicles and ulcers in the epithelia of the mouth, snout, feet and teat. FMDV consists of seven immunologically distinct serotypes: O, A, C, Asia1, South African Territories (SAT) 1, SAT2 and SAT3. There are some genetically and geographically distinct evolutionary lineages (topotypes) which differ by at least 15% in their VP1 sequences within various serotypes. For example, FMDV type O can be divided into eight topotypes [2]. Antigenic diversity often influences immunoassays for FMDV diagnosis and/or vaccine selection [3,4]. The FMDV antigenic diagnostic methods mentioned in the World Organization for Animal Health's Office International des Epizooties (OIE) manual [5] are virus isolation, immunological methods—i.e., indirect sandwich–enzyme-linked immunosorbent assays (IS-ELISAs) and the complement fixation test—and nucleic acid detection methods such as reverse transcription-polymerase chain reaction (RT-PCR) and real-time RT-PCR. However, the IS-ELISA is able to do serotyping FMDV, but it does not have sufficient sensitivity [6–8].

In an extensive outbreak, it is difficult to collect vesicular fluid and/or vesicular epithelial samples from every suspect farm. In fact, in the 2010 FMD outbreak in Japan, most of the diagnostic samples were oral or nasal swabs, and initial diagnosis was conducted only by RT-PCR for the reason of sensitivity of IS-

ELISA which is appropriate for vesicular fluid and/or vesicular epithelial samples. Thus, an antigen-detection ELISA which has high sensitivity enough to detect a viral antigen in samples of saliva and/or nasal discharge must be valuable for the case like 2010 outbreak in Japan.

In our previous study [7], monoclonal antibody (MAb)-based sandwich direct ELISAs (MSD-ELISAs) were developed for multiserotypes (MS) and single serotypes (SS) for FMDV types O, A and Asia1. The MSD-ELISAs were able to detect the different FMDV strains except for MSD-ELISA/SS/Asia1, which showed a weak cross-reaction to type O antigens. In clinical samples, MSD-ELISA/MS and SS/O were able to detect specific FMDV antigens from the saliva and plasma of pigs inoculated with O/TAW/97 (Cathay topotype) [7], and the detection limits of these assays were about 100 to 1000 PFU, as determined by real-time RT-PCR results.

In this study, we evaluated the sensitivity and specificity of the MSD-ELISA reported and compared it with the currently used IS-ELISA, using both experimental samples of other topotypes of serotype O and serotypes A and Asia1 and field samples from the 2010 outbreak of serotype O FMD in Japan.

## Materials and Methods

### Cells and viruses

The virus strains FMDV O/JPN/2000 (ME-SA topotype) [9,10], O1 BFS 1860 (EURO-SA topotype), A15 TAI 1/60 (ASIA topotype), and Asia1 Shamir ISR were used for animal experiments. Each of these viruses was propagated in the cell lines IBRS-2 [11] and/or BHK-21, which were maintained in Eagle's minimum essential medium containing 5% fetal bovine serum, 0.3 mg/mL of L-glutamine and 1.125 mg/mL of $NaHCO_3$, and used as inoculum.

## Ethics statement

Animal experiments carried out in this study were approved by the ethics committee of National Institute of Animal Health, Japan (approval #787, 08–122, 09–029). Field samples used in this study were submitted from Miyazaki prefecture for diagnosis of FMD occurred in 2010 in Japan. These oral and nasal swabs and vesicular epithelial tissues were collected by veterinarians in accordance with the guidelines of Act on Domestic Animal Infectious Diseases Control.

## Laboratory clinical samples

Animal experiments were conducted in a biosafety level 3ag-approved biocontainment facility at our institute. For each virus strains, six or two two-month old pigs were inoculated intradermally with $10^7$ $TCID_{50}$ at the right and front heel bulbs. Saliva samples were collected by cotton swab until 6 days when the clinical signs were definitely observed, and undiluted saliva samples were used for the detection of FMD viral antigens in each assay.

## Field samples

In addition to the samples from animal experiments, a total of 178 RT-PCR-positive samples (135 oral swab samples, 7 nasal samples, 24 oral and nasal swabs soaked in about 10-times volumes of PBS (about 2 ml) and 12 samples of 10% emulsion of homogenized epithelial tissues) collected from cattle and pigs from 78 farms that were affected by the 2010 type O FMD outbreak in Japan caused by O/JPN/2010 (SEA topotype) [12] were used for the comparative studies.

Field samples were submitted from Miyazaki prefecture for diagnosis of FMD occurred in 2010 in Japan. These samples were collected by veterinarians in accordance with the guidelines of Act on Domestic Animal Infectious Diseases Control in which the veterinarian should collect samples such as epithelium or swabs from a lesion and soaked them in 2 ml of PBS.

## Monoclonal antibody-based sandwich direct eLISA for foot-and-mouth disease virus antigen detection

In MSD-ELISAs: the MSD-ELISA for multiserotypes (MS) and the MSD-ELISA for single serotypes (SS) for each serotype (O, A, Asia1), MAb 1H5 (which was produced against O/JPN/2000), which reacts with all seven serotypes of FMDV is used as an antigen-capture-antibody. For the detection of each antigen, the MAbs 1H5, 70C4 (which was produced against O/JPN/2000), 16C6 (which was produced against A15 TAI 1/60), and 12C7 (which was produced against Asia1 Shamir ISR) were used as horseradish-peroxidase (HRPO)-labeled-MAbs for MS, SS for O, A and Asia1, respectively. To improve the specificity of SS for Asia1, MAb 12C7 was used in this study instead of MAb 7C2, which showed slight cross-reaction with the type O strains in previous study. In addition, for the detection of all seven FMDV serotypes in MS, MAb was changed from 71F2 (which was produced against O/JPN/2000) to 1H5. The protocol of the MSD-ELISAs is described in detail in our previous report [7].

## Foot-and-mouth Disease Virus Antigen Detection Indirect Sandwich ELISA

The IS-ELISA by the World Reference Laboratory of FMD was conducted in accord with the OIE manual [5]. The reagents of IS-ELISA (rabbit anti-sera and guinea pig anti-sera) in a lot which we used for this study are as follows: type O (O Taiwan 98 (Cathay topotype)), type A (A 4164 (Asia topotype)), and type Asia1 (Asia1 CAM 9/80).

## Statistics

For analyzing the statistical significance of the differences in virus detection rates between the MSD-ELISAs and IS-ELISA, the Pearson's chi-square test was used.

## RT-PCR

For the RT-PCR for detection of FMDV nucleic acid, the SuperScript III One-Step RT-PCR System with Platinum Taq DNA Polymerase (Invitrogen, Carlsbad, CA) and primers for the 3D region were used [9].

## Real-time RT-PCR

A TaqMan probe and primers for 3D region of FMDV were designed according to the OIE manual [5]. The sequences were as follows: forward primer 5'- ACT GGG TTT TAC AAA CCT GTG A -3', reverse primer 5'- GCG AGT CCT GCC ACG GA - 3', TaqMan probe 5'-FAM- TCC TTT GCA CGC CGT GGG AC -TAMRA-3'. The program was 48°C for 30 min, 95°C for 10 min, and 40 cycles of 60°C for 15 seconds and 95°C for 1 min. Serial 10-fold dilutions of each FMD virus containing $10^6$ plaque forming unit (PFU)/0.1 ml were used as the positive samples to construct the standard curve.

## Results

### Laboratory clinical samples

Table 1 shows the FMDV antigen detection by the MSD-ELISAs and the IS-ELISA obtained using FMDV (O/JPN/2000, O1 BFS 1860, A15 TAI 1/60 and Asia1 Shamir ISR)-inoculated pig saliva samples. On average, about 0.3 ml of saliva samples were recovered from experimental cotton swabs. In these viruses, O/JPN/2000, A15 TAI 1/60 and Asia1 Shamir ISR are homologous to MAbs used for the MSA-ELISA/SS and heterologous to rabbit and guinea-pig immune sera use in IS-ELISAs. However, O1 BFS 1860 is heterologous antigen for both of the MSD-ELISAs and IS-ELISA. The MSD-ELISAs (especially the MSD-ELISA/SSs) were able to detect each FMDV serotype antigen with high sensitivity and specificity compared to the IS-ELISA. Among the inoculated viruses, the FMDV O/JPN/2000 strain was a low pathogenic virus that showed lower levels of clinical signs compared to the other inoculated FMDV strains (data not shown), and the virus excretion levels of the O/JPN/2000 strain were also lower than those of the other strains (Table 1). Therefore, the IS-ELISA did not show positive results against most of the samples of O/JPN/2000-virus-inoculated pigs. Regarding pigs inoculated with the other FMDV strain (O1 BFS 1860, A15 TAI 1/60 and Asia1 Shamir ISR), the MSD-ELISAs were able to detect FMDV antigens for a longer term compared to the IS-ELISA. The two MSD-ELISAs could detect FMDV antigen at about the same time when the obvious vesicular appeared except for the inoculation site and some samples of inoculated pigs with O1 BFS 1860 and A15 TAI 1/60 showed positive before the vesicular forming. It was generally able to detect about 2 to 3 days after vesicular forming and becoming

**Table 1.** Comparison of the results of FMDV antigen detection methods using saliva of FMDV-inoculated pigs.

| Inoculated virus | Pig no. | Methods* | Days post-inoculation | | | | | | |
|---|---|---|---|---|---|---|---|---|---|
| | | | 0 | 1 | 2 | 3 | 4 | 5 | 6 |
| O/JPN/2000 | 1 | MS | -† | - | - | + | ‖+ | - | - |
| | | SS | - | - | - | ‡‡ | + | + | - |
| | | IS | - | - | - | - | - | - | - |
| | | rPCR | ‡ | - | + | ‡‡ | ‡‡ | ‡‡ | + |
| | 2 | MS | - | - | - | - | - | + | - |
| | | SS | - | - | - | - | - | ‡‡ | - |
| | | IS | - | - | - | - | - | - | - |
| | | rPCR | - | - | - | + | ‡‡ | ‡‡ | + |
| | 3 | MS | - | - | + | + | ‡‡ | - | - |
| | | SS | - | - | - | ‡‡ | + | - | - |
| | | IS | - | - | - | - | - | - | - |
| | | rPCR | - | - | ‡‡ | ‡‡ | ‡‡ | + | + |
| | 4 | MS | - | - | + | + | + | - | - |
| | | SS | - | - | + | ‡‡ | + | - | - |
| | | IS | - | - | - | - | - | - | - |
| | | rPCR | - | - | ‡‡ | ‡‡ | ‡‡ | + | + |
| | 5 | MS | - | - | - | + | - | - | - |
| | | SS | - | - | + | + | - | - | - |
| | | IS | - | - | - | - | - | - | - |
| | | rPCR | - | - | + | ‡‡ | ‡‡ | + | + |
| | 6 | MS | - | - | + | + | - | - | - |
| | | SS | - | - | ‡‡ | + | - | - | - |
| | | IS | - | - | + | - | - | + | - |
| | | rPCR | - | - | + | ‡‡ | ‡‡ | + | - |
| O1 BFS1860 | 1 | MS | - | + | ‡‡ | + | + | - | - |
| | | SS | - | ‡‡ | ‡‡ | ‡‡ | + | + | - |
| | | IS | - | - | - | - | - | + | - |
| | | rPCR | - | ‡‡ | - | ‡‡ | ‡‡ | + | - |
| | 2 | MS | - | - | + | + | - | - | - |
| | | SS | - | + | ‡‡ | ‡‡ | - | - | - |
| | | IS | - | - | - | - | - | - | - |
| | | rPCR | - | ‡‡ | ‡‡ | ‡‡ | + | + | - |
| | 3 | MS | - | - | + | ˢ | | | |
| | | SS | - | - | ‡‡ | | | | |

| Inoculated virus | Pig no. | Methods* | Days post-inoculation | | | | | | |
|---|---|---|---|---|---|---|---|---|---|
| | | | 0 | 1 | 2 | 3 | 4 | 5 | 6 |
| A15 TAI 1/60 | 1 | MS | - | + | + | + | - | - | - |
| | | SS | - | ‡‡ | ‡‡ | ‡‡ | + | + | + |
| | | IS | - | + | + | - | + | + | - |
| | | rPCR | - | ‡‡ | ‡‡ | ‡‡ | + | + | + |
| | 2 | MS | - | - | ‡‡ | + | + | + | - |
| | | SS | - | - | ‡‡ | ‡‡ | ‡‡ | + | + |
| | | IS | - | - | ‡‡ | - | - | - | - |
| | | rPCR | - | + | ‡‡ | ‡‡ | ‡‡ | + | + |
| | 3 | MS | - | - | + | + | ‡‡ | + | - |
| | | SS | - | - | + | ‡‡ | ‡‡ | + | - |
| | | IS | - | - | - | + | - | - | - |
| | | rPCR | - | + | ‡‡ | ‡‡ | ‡‡ | + | + |
| | 4 | MS | - | - | + | + | + | - | - |
| | | SS | - | - | + | ‡‡ | + | - | - |
| | | IS | - | - | - | - | - | - | - |
| | | rPCR | - | + | ‡‡ | ‡‡ | ‡‡ | + | + |
| | 5 | MS | - | + | ‡‡ | + | + | + | - |
| | | SS | - | ‡‡ | ‡‡ | ‡‡ | + | - | - |
| | | IS | - | - | + | + | - | - | - |
| | | rPCR | - | ‡‡ | ‡‡ | ‡‡ | ‡‡ | + | + |
| | 6 | MS | - | + | + | + | + | - | - |
| | | SS | - | ‡‡ | ‡‡ | ‡‡ | + | + | - |
| | | IS | - | - | + | - | - | - | - |
| | | rPCR | - | ‡‡ | ‡‡ | ‡‡ | ‡‡ | + | + |
| Asia1 Shamir | 1 | MS | - | - | + | + | + | - | - |
| | | SS | - | - | + | + | + | - | - |
| | | IS | - | - | - | - | - | - | - |
| | | rPCR | - | - | - | + | ‡‡ | + | - |
| | 2 | MS | - | - | - | + | ‡‡ | + | + |
| | | SS | - | - | - | - | - | - | - |
| | | IS | - | - | - | - | - | - | - |
| | | rPCR | - | + | ‡‡ | ‡‡ | ‡‡ | + | + |

**Table 1.** Cont.

| Inoculated virus | Pig no. | Methods* | 0 | 1 | 2 | 3 | 4 | 5 | 6 |
|---|---|---|---|---|---|---|---|---|---|
| | | IS | - | - | - | | | | - |
| | | rPCR | - | + | ++ | | | | |
| | 4 | MS | - | + | § | | | | |
| | | SS | - | +++ | § | | | | |
| | | IS | - | - | | | | | |
| | | rPCR | - | ++ | | | | | |
| | 5 | MS | - | - | ++ | +++ | - | - | - |
| | | SS | - | + | +++ | +++ | + | - | - |
| | | IS | - | + | + | + | - | + | - |
| | | rPCR | - | +++ | ++ | ++ | + | + | - |
| | 6 | MS | - | - | ++ | ++ | § | | |
| | | SS | - | + | +++ | +++ | | | |
| | | IS | - | - | + | - | | | |
| | | rPCR | - | ++ | ++ | | | | |

*MS: MSD-ELISA for multi-serotypes; SS: MSD-ELISA for single serotypes (O, A, Asia1); IS: Indirect sandwich-ELISA for each serotype (O, A, Asia1); rPCR: real-time RT-PCR.

†The OD results (average sample OD-average buffer OD) of the MS, SS and IS ELISAs were as +++, >1.0; ++, 0.5–1.0; +, 0.1–0.5; and −, <0.1.

‡The results-related plaque-forming unit of rPCR were as +++, >$10^4$; ++, $10^2$–$10^3$; +, $10^0$–$10^2$; and −, <$10^0$.

§The pigs inoculated with virus were euthanized.

||Squares mean the day the obvious vesicular appeared except for the inoculated site.

**Table 2.** Sensitivities of the MSD-ELISAs and the IS-ELISA against the FMDV-positive field samples by RT-PCR.

| Subject* | | MSD-ELISA | | IS-ELISA |
|---|---|---|---|---|
| | | MS | SS (type O) | type O |
| Sample | | | | |
| | oral swab | 56.30%[†] (76/135)[‡] | 62.50% (85/135) | 7.40% (10/133[§]) |
| | nasal swab | 42.86% (3/7) | 57.14% (4/7) | 0% (0/7) |
| | oral/nasal swab | 62.50% (15/24) | 70.83% (17/24) | 4.17% (1/24) |
| | epithelial tissue | 66.67% (8/12) | 66.67% (8/12) | 33.33% (4/12) |
| | Total | 57.30% (102/178) | 64.04% (114/178) | 8.52% (15/176) |
| Farm | | | | |
| | | 84.62% (66/78)[||] | 87.18% (68/78) | 14.10% (11/78) |

*A total of 178 RT-PCR-positive samples (135 oral swab samples, 7 nasal samples, 24 oral and nasal swab samples, 12 samples of 10% emulsion of homogenized epithelial tissue) collected in the 2010 type O FMD outbreak in Japan from 78 farms were used.
[†]In both the MSD-ELISAs and the IS-ELISA, OD results (= sample OD − average negative OD) of 0.1 or more were judged as positive.
[‡]Fractions in parentheses show ELISA-positive samples or farms/RT-PCR-positive samples or farms.
[§]The amounts of two samples were insufficient for the test.
[||]The sensitivities against farm units were calculated using the sensitivities against samples.

undetectable with decrease in virus shedding. In all samples, the peak of amounts of detected virus genome (Ct values) and virus antigens (OD values) were almost coincided. The correlation coefficient of the OD values of each ELISA and Ct values are as follows: the MSD-ELISA/MS ($r = 0.529$, $p = 0.021$), the MSD-ELISA/SS ($r = 0.622$, $p = 0.004$) and the IS-ELISA ($r = 0.31$, $p = 0.240$).

### Field samples

In addition to these samples from animal experiments, we used 178 RT-PCR-positive field samples (135 oral swab samples, 7 nasal samples, 24 oral and nasal swabs soaked in about 10-times volumes of PBS (about 2 ml) and 12 samples of 10% emulsion of homogenized epithelial tissues) from cattle and pigs affected by the 2010 type-O FMD outbreak in Japan to compare the sensitivity of the MSD-ELISAs (MS and SS/O) and IS-ELISA. In the results, the positive sample detection rate of the IS-ELISA was 8.52%, while on the other hand, those of the MSD-ELISA/MS and MSD-ELISA/SS/O were 57.30% and 64.04%, respectively (Table 2). It means that the sensitivities of both MSD-ELISAs were about 7 times higher than that of the IS-ELISA against each sample (P<0.01). However the detection rates of IS-ELISA against oral and/or nasal swabs were low, it seems to depend on the amount of antigen of each sample.

Based on the sample detection results, we calculated the FMD-positive farm detection rate. In the FMD diagnosis for the FMD free country, if the ELISA showed positive on at least one sample from FMD-suspected farm, it should be regarded as FMD-positive and conduct on immediately stamping-out for control and eradication of the disease. In terms of farm units, the IS-ELISA detected 14.1% of positive farms, and the MSD-ELISA/MS and MSD-ELISA/SS/O detected 84.62% and 87.18% of positive farms, respectively (Table 2). It means that the sensitivities of the MSD-ELISAs were about 6 times higher than that of the IS-ELISA against each farm (P<0.01).

### Discussion

Here we found that the sensitivity of the two MSD-ELISAs against oral and nasal swabs were higher than that of the conventional IS-ELISA. Since RT-PCR is one of the most sensitive diagnostic methods, it was generally used as the primary diagnosis tool for FMD diagnosis in the FMD free countries. However, RT-PCR cannot distinguish serotypes and is at risk for developing contamination. In addition to these reasons, the laboratory diagnosis should be performed by several methods especially for the disease causing severe economic loss for the country, such as FMD. Therefore, an MSD-ELISA could be appropriate as a method to replace IS-ELISA, and it can perform an early serotyping of FMDV using saliva and oral or nasal swabs in which the amount of virus might be low, not to mention epithelial suspensions, vesicular fluids or cell culture supernatants. In this study, we used undiluted saliva samples from inoculated pigs. However, undiluted saliva samples from inoculated cattle generally produced a false negative result, and it could be solved by two times dilution with PBS plus 0.05% Tween 20 (data not shown). Therefore, we considered that there is some inhibition factor against ELISA (antigen–antibody reaction) in saliva of cattle. As for the antigenic matching between viruses and detector antibodies of each ELISA, O/JPN/2010 belongs to SEA topotype, therefore both MSD-ELISA (70C4 originated from O/JPN/2000 (ME-SA topotype)) and IS-ELISA (antisera for Cathay topotype) were heterologous to O/JPN/2010 strain. As a result, we suppose the influence of the antigenic matching between viruses and detector antibodies is not important matter to compare the results of MSD-ELISAs and IS-ELISA in this study.

The MSD-ELISAs could detect FMDV antigen about 2 to 3 days after vesicular forming. Although it was the data from animal experiments, the detectable period would shorter than those of RT-PCR/real-time RT-PCR, also in the field. It is vital for the detection of FMDV antigen by these methods including IS-ELISA that diagnostic samples should be collected from early-stage of disease.

The advantage of using MAbs is to be able to select highly efficient MAbs for high specificity and sensitivity, and uniform affinity to the antigen leads to minimum disparity between the lots compared to polyclonal anti-sera. However, a MAb recognize a single epitope, thus it should be evaluated broad intra- and inter-type reactivity of the MAbs to cover the antigenic variability of FMD viruses. In regard to this point, we have carried out making the panel of our MAbs against recent pandemic FMDV strains in preparation for antigenic varieties (data not shown). Therefore it will be possible to change or combine antigen detection MAbs according to epidemic FMDV strains as needed. To be a lager diagnostic use of the MSD-ELISAs, further validation study should be conducted using field samples of the other virus strains, which are epidemic in especially Asian countries.

## References

1. Alexandersen S, Zhang Z, Donaldson AI, Garland AJ (2003) The pathogenesis and diagnosis of foot-and-mouth disease. J. Comp. Pathol. 129: 1–36.
2. Samuel AR, Knowles NJ (2001) Foot-and-mouth disease type O viruses exhibit genetically and geographically distinct evolutionary lineages (topotypes). J. Gen. Virol. 82: 609–621.
3. Mumford JA (2007) Vaccines and viral antigenic diversity. Rev. Sci. Tech. Off. Int. Epiz. 26: 69–90.
4. Paton DJ, Valarcher J-F, Bergmann I, Matlho OG, Zakharov VM, et al. (2005) Selection of foot and mouth disease vaccine strains – a review. Rev. Sci. Tech. Off. Int. Epiz. 24: 981–993.
5. World Organization for Animal Health. (2012) Chapter 2. 1. 5. Foot and mouth disease. In: Manual of diagnostic tests and vaccines for terrestrial animals 2012. OIE, Paris, France, Available: http://www.oie.int/fileadmin/Home/eng/Health_standards/tahm/2.01.05_FMD.pdf.
6. Mohapatra JK., Subramaniam S, Tosh C, Hemadri D, A Sanyal, et al. (2007) Genotype differentiating RT-PCR and sandwich ELISA: handy tools in epidemiological investigation of foot and mouth disease. J. Virol. Methods 143: 117–121.
7. Morioka K, Fukai K, Yoshida K, Yamazoe R, Onozato H, et al. (2009) Foot-and-mouth disease virus antigen detection enzyme-linked immunosorbent assay using multiserotype-reactive monoclonal antibodies. J. Clin. Microbiol. 47: 3663–3668.
8. Reid SM, Forsyth MA, Hutchings GH, Ferris NP (1998) Comparison of reverse transcription polymerase chain reaction, enzyme linked immunosorbent assay and virus isolation for the routine diagnosis of foot-and-mouth disease. J. Virol. Methods 70: 213–217.
9. Sakamoto K, Kanno T, Yamakawa M, Yoshida K, Yamazoe R, et al. (2000) Isolation of foot-and-mouth disease virus from Japanese black cattle in Miyazaki Prefecture, Japan, 2000. J. Vet. Med. Sci. 64: 91–94.
10. Morioka K, Fukai K, Ohashi S, Sakamoto K, Tsuda T, et al. (2007) Comparison of the characters of the plaque-purified viruses from foot-and-mouth disease virus O/JPN/2000. J. Vet. Med. Sci. 70: 653–658.
11. Chapman WG, Ramshaw IA (1971) Growth of the IB-RS-2 pig kidney cell line in suspension culture and its susceptibility to foot-and-mouth disease virus. Appl. Environ. Microbiol. 22: 1–5.
12. Fukai K, Morioka K, Yoshida K (2011) An experimental infection in pigs using a foot-and-mouth disease virus isolated from the 2010 epidemic in Japan. J. Vet. Med. Sci. 73: 1207–1210.

## Author Contributions

Conceived and designed the experiments: KM KY. Performed the experiments: KM KF KY. Analyzed the data: KM. Contributed reagents/materials/analysis tools: KM KF KY TK. Wrote the paper: KM KF KS KY TK.

# PERMISSIONS

All chapters in this book were first published in PLOS ONE, by The Public Library of Science; hereby published with permission under the Creative Commons Attribution License or equivalent. Every chapter published in this book has been scrutinized by our experts. Their significance has been extensively debated. The topics covered herein carry significant findings which will fuel the growth of the discipline. They may even be implemented as practical applications or may be referred to as a beginning point for another development.

The contributors of this book come from diverse backgrounds, making this book a truly international effort. This book will bring forth new frontiers with its revolutionizing research information and detailed analysis of the nascent developments around the world.

We would like to thank all the contributing authors for lending their expertise to make the book truly unique. They have played a crucial role in the development of this book. Without their invaluable contributions this book wouldn't have been possible. They have made vital efforts to compile up to date information on the varied aspects of this subject to make this book a valuable addition to the collection of many professionals and students.

This book was conceptualized with the vision of imparting up-to-date information and advanced data in this field. To ensure the same, a matchless editorial board was set up. Every individual on the board went through rigorous rounds of assessment to prove their worth. After which they invested a large part of their time researching and compiling the most relevant data for our readers.

The editorial board has been involved in producing this book since its inception. They have spent rigorous hours researching and exploring the diverse topics which have resulted in the successful publishing of this book. They have passed on their knowledge of decades through this book. To expedite this challenging task, the publisher supported the team at every step. A small team of assistant editors was also appointed to further simplify the editing procedure and attain best results for the readers.

Apart from the editorial board, the designing team has also invested a significant amount of their time in understanding the subject and creating the most relevant covers. They scrutinized every image to scout for the most suitable representation of the subject and create an appropriate cover for the book.

The publishing team has been an ardent support to the editorial, designing and production team. Their endless efforts to recruit the best for this project, has resulted in the accomplishment of this book. They are a veteran in the field of academics and their pool of knowledge is as vast as their experience in printing. Their expertise and guidance has proved useful at every step. Their uncompromising quality standards have made this book an exceptional effort. Their encouragement from time to time has been an inspiration for everyone.

The publisher and the editorial board hope that this book will prove to be a valuable piece of knowledge for researchers, students, practitioners and scholars across the globe.

# LIST OF CONTRIBUTORS

**Krister Blodörn, Sara Hägglund and John Pringle**
Swedish University of Agricultural Sciences, Host Pathogen Interaction Group, Department of Clinical Sciences, Uppsala, Sweden

**Jenna Fix, Catherine Dubuquoy, Jean-François Eléouët and Sabine Riffault**
INRA, Unité de Virologie et Immunologie Moléculaires, Jouy-en-Josas, France

**Boby Makabi-Panzu, Michelle Thom and Geraldine Taylor**
The Pirbright Institute, Pirbright, Surrey, United Kingdom

**Per Karlsson**
National Veterinary Institute, Department of Virology, Immunology, and Parasitology, Uppsala, Sweden

**Jean François Valarcher**
Swedish University of Agricultural Sciences, Host Pathogen Interaction Group, Department of Clinical Sciences, Uppsala, Sweden
National Veterinary Institute, Department of Virology, Immunology, and Parasitology, Uppsala, Sweden

**Jean-Louis Roque**
Clinique Veterinaire des Mazets, Riom es Montagnes, France

**Erika Karlstam**
National Veterinary Institute, Department of Pathology and Wildlife Diseases, Uppsala, Sweden

**Ross S. Davidson and Michael R. Hutchings**
1 Disease Systems Team, SRUC, Edinburgh, United Kingdom

**Jamie C. Prentice**
Disease Systems Team, SRUC, Edinburgh, United Kingdom
Biomathematics and Statistics Scotland, Edinburgh, United Kingdom
Environment Department, University of York, York, United Kingdom

**Glenn Marion**
Biomathematics and Statistics Scotland, Edinburgh, United Kingdom

**Piran C. L. White**
Environment Department, University of York, York, United Kingdom

**Gregorio Mentaberre, Ignasi Marco, Nora Navarro-González, Roser Velarde and Santiago Lavín**
Servei d9Ecopatologia de Fauna Salvatge (SEFaS), Departament de Medicina i Cirurgia Animal, Facultat de Veterina`ria, Universitat Auto`noma de Barcelona, Bellaterra, Barcelona, Spain

**Emmanuel Serrano**
Servei d9Ecopatologia de Fauna Salvatge (SEFaS), Departament de Medicina i Cirurgia Animal, Facultat de Veterinária, Universitat Autònoma de Barcelona, Bellaterra, Barcelona, Spain
Estadística i Investigació Operativa, Departament de Matemàtica. Universitat de Lleida, Lleida, Spain

**Beatriz Romero, Lucía de Juan, Ana Mateos and Lucas Domínguez**
VISAVET Health Surveillance Centre. Universidad Complutense, Madrid, Spain
Departamento de Sanidad Animal. Facultad de Veterinaria, Universidad Complutense, Madrid, Spain

**Xavier Olivé -Boix**
Reserva Nacional de Cac¸a dels Ports de Tortosa i Beseit, Roquetes, Tarragona, Spain

**Tariq Halasa and Anette Boklund**
Section of Epidemiology, the National Veterinary Institutes, Technical University of Denmark, Copenhagen, Denmark

**Christopher S. Jennelle, Viviane Henaux and Bala Thiagarajan**
Department of Forest and Wildlife Ecology, University of Wisconsin, Madison, Wisconsin, United States of America

**Gideon Wasserberg**
Biology Department, University of North Carolina, Greensboro, North Carolina, United States of America

**Robert E. Rolley**
Wisconsin Department of Natural Resources, Madison, Wisconsin, United States of America

**Michael D. Samuel**
U.S. Geological Survey, Wisconsin Cooperative Wildlife Research Unit, University of Wisconsin, Madison, Wisconsin, United States of America

**Amber N. Barnes**
College of Public Health and Health Professions, University of Florida, Gainesville, Florida, United States of America

**Ali M. Messenger and Gregory C. Gray**
College of Public Health and Health Professions, University of Florida, Gainesville, Florida, United States of America
Emerging Pathogens Institute, University of Florida,Gainesville, Florida, United States of America

**Calvin Sindato**
National Institute for Medical Research, Tabora, Tanzania
Department of Veterinary Medicine and Public Health, Sokoine University of Agriculture, Morogoro, Tanzania,
Southern Africa Centre for Infectious Disease Surveillance, Morogoro, Tanzania

**Esron D. Karimuribo**
Department of Veterinary Medicine and Public Health, Sokoine University of Agriculture, Morogoro, Tanzania
Southern Africa Centre for Infectious Disease Surveillance, Morogoro, Tanzania

**Dirk U. Pfeiffer**
Royal Veterinary College, London, United Kingdom

**Leonard E. G. Mboera**
National Institute for Medical Research, Dar es Salaam, Tanzania

**Fredrick Kivaria**
Food and Agriculture Organization of the United Nations, Dar es Salaam, Tanzania

**George Dautu**
Department of Disease Control, University of Zambia, Lusaka, Zambia

**Bett Bernard**
International Livestock Research Institute, Nairobi, Kenya

**Janusz T. Paweska**
Center for Emerging and Zoonotic Diseases, National Institute for Communicable
Diseases, of the National Health Laboratory Service, Sandringham, South Africa
School of Pathology, Faculty of Health Sciences, University of the Witwatersrand, Johannesburg, South Africa

**Marcello Ceccarelli and Luca Galluzzi**
Department of Biomolecular Sciences, University of Urbino "Carlo Bo", Fano (PU), Italy

**Antonella Migliazzo**
Istituto Zooprofilattico Sperimentale della Sicilia, Palermo (PA), Italy

**Mauro Magnani**
Department of Biomolecular Sciences, University of Urbino "Carlo Bo", Urbino (PU), Italy

**Dennis M. Heisey, Robin E. Russell and Daniel P. Walsh**
United States Geological Survey, National Wildlife Health Center, Madison, Wisconsin, United States of America

**Christopher S. Jennelle**
Department of Forest and Wildlife Ecology, University of Wisconsin, Madison, Wisconsin, United States of America

**M. D. Salman**
Animal Population Health Institute, College of Veterinary Medicine and Biomedical Sciences, Colorado State University, Fort Collins, Colorado, United States of America

**Kurt C. VerCauteren**
United States Department of Agriculture, Animal Plant and Health Inspection Service, Wildlife Services, National Wildlife Research Center, Fort Collins, Colorado, United States of America

**Christine K. Ellis**
Animal Population Health Institute, College of Veterinary Medicine and Biomedical Sciences, Colorado State University, Fort Collins, Colorado, United States of America,
United States Department of Agriculture, Animal Plant and Health Inspection Service, Wildlife Services, National Wildlife Research Center, Fort Collins, Colorado, United States of America

**Randal S. Stahl**
United States Department of Agriculture, Animal Plant and Health Inspection Service, Wildlife Services, National Wildlife Research Center, Fort Collins, Colorado, United States of America

**Matthew McCollum, Pauline Nol and Jack C. Rhyan**
United States Department of Agriculture, Animal Plant and Health Inspection Service, Veterinary Services, Wildlife Livestock Disease Investigations Team, Fort Collins, Colorado, United States of America

**W. Ray Waters and Mitchell V. Palmer**
United States Department of Agriculture, Agricultural Research Service, National Animal Disease Center, Ames, Iowa, United States of America

**Joshua B. Smith, Jonathan A. Jenks and Troy W. Grovenburg**
Department of Natural Resource Management, South Dakota State University, Brookings, South Dakota, United States of America

**Robert W. Klaver**
Iowa Cooperative Fish and Wildlife Research Unit and Department of Natural Resource Ecology and Management, Iowa State University, Ames, Iowa, United States of America

**Martin Jeffrey, Stuart Martin and Lorenzo González**
Animal Health and Veterinary Laboratories Agency (AHVLA-Lasswade), Pentlands Science Park, Bush Loan, Penicuik, Midlothian, Scotland, United Kingdom

**Francesca Chianini, Samantha Eaton and Mark P. Dagleish**
Moredun Research Institute, Pentlands Science Park, Bush Loan, Penicuik, Midlothian, Scotland, United Kingdom

**Kate D. Halsby, Amanda L. Walsh and Dilys Morgan**
Gastrointestinal, Emerging and Zoonotic Infections Department, Public Health England, London, United Kingdom

**Colin Campbell**
Centre for the Epidemiological Study of Sexually Transmitted Infections and AIDS of Catalonia (CEEISCAT) – ICO, Hospital Universitari Germans Trias i Pujol, Badalona, Spain

**Kirsty Hewitt**
Gastrointestinal, Emerging and Zoonotic Infections Department, Public Health England, London, United Kingdom
London/KSS Specialty School of Public Health, London Deanery, London, United Kingdom

**Dan G. O9Neill and Dave C. Brodbelt**
Veterinary Epidemiology, Economics and Public Health, Royal Veterinary College, London, United Kingdom

**David B. Church**
Small Animal Medicine and Surgery Group, Royal Veterinary College, London, United Kingdom

**Paul D. McGreevy and Peter C. Thomson**
Faculty of Veterinary Science, University of Sydney, Sydney, New South Wales, Australia

**W. David Walter**
U.S. Geological Survey, Pennsylvania Cooperative Fish and Wildlife Research Unit, Pennsylvania State University, University Park, Pennsylvania, United States of America

**Rick Smith and Mike Vanderklok**
Animal Industry Division, Michigan Department of Agriculture and Rural Development, Lansing, Michigan, United States of America

**Kurt C. VerCauteren**
United States Department of Agriculture, Animal and Plant Health Inspection Services, Wildlife Services, National Wildlife Research Center, Fort Collins, Colorado, United States of America

**Benjamin L. Hart**
Department of Anatomy, Physiology and Cell Biology, School of Veterinary Medicine, University of California Davis, Davis, California, United States of America,

**Lynette A. Hart and Abigail P. Thigpen**
Department of Population Health and Reproduction, School of Veterinary Medicine, University of California Davis, Davis, California, United States of America

**Neil H. Willits**
Department of Statistics, University of California Davis, Davis, California, United States of America

**Nuno Santos and Margarida Correia-Neves**
Life and Health Sciences Research Institute (ICVS), School of Health Sciences, University of Minho, Braga, Portugal
ICVS/3B's, PT Government Associate Laboratory, Braga/Guimarães, Portugal

**Ivânia Moiane**
Life and Health Sciences Research Institute (ICVS), School of Health Sciences, University of Minho, Braga, Portugal
ICVS/3B's, PT Government Associate Laboratory, Braga/Guimarães, Portugal
Paraclinic Department, Veterinary Faculty, Eduardo Mondlane University, Maputo, Mozambique

**André Nhambir, Adelina Machado and Osvaldo Inlamea**
Paraclinic Department, Veterinary Faculty, Eduardo Mondlane University, Maputo, Mozambique

**Gunilla Källenius**
Department of Clinical Science and Education, Södersjukhuset, Karolinska Institutet, Stockholm, Sweden

**Jakob Zinsstag and Jan Hattendorf**
Swiss Tropical and Public Health Institute, Basel, Switzerland

**Vinícius Silva Machado, Marcela Luccas de Souza Bicalho, Enoch Brandão de Souza Meira Junior, Rodolfo Rossi, Bruno Leonardo Ribeiro, Svetlana Lima, Thiago Santos, Arieli Kussler, Carla Foditsch, Erika Korzune Ganda, Georgios Oikonomou, Soon Hon Cheong, Robert Owen Gilbert and Rodrigo Carvalho Bicalho**
Department of Population Medicine & Diagnostic Sciences, College of Veterinary Medicine, Cornell University, Ithaca, New York, United States of America

**Colleen T. Webb, Michael G. Buhnerkempe and Daniel A. Grear**
Department of Biology, Colorado State University, Fort Collins, Colorado, United States of America

**Michael J. Tildesley, Marleen Werkman and Matt J. Keeling**
Center for Complexity Science, Mathematics Institute, University of Warwick, Coventry, United Kingdom

**Tom Lindström and Uno Wennergren**
Department of Physics, Chemistry, and Biology, Linköping University, Linköping, Sweden

**Katie Portacci, Ryan S. Miller and Jason E. Lombard**
United States Department of Agriculture, Animal and Plant Health Inspection Service, Centers for Epidemiology and Animal Health, Fort Collins, Colorado, United States of America

**Kazuki Morioka, Katsuhiko Fukai, Kenichi Sakamoto, Kazuo Yoshida and Toru Kanno**
Exotic Disease Research Station, National Institute of Animal Health, National Agriculture and Food Research Organization, Josuihoncho Kodaira, Tokyo, Japan

# Index

# Vegetable Crops: Quality Evaluation and Management